CELL AND TISSUE TRANSPLANTATION INTO THE ADULT BRAIN

TIMOTHY O.T. TS'O, M.D., PH.D.
P.O. BOX 147
LIBERTYVILLE, IL 60048

ANNALS OF THE NEW YORK ACADEMY OF SCIENCES
Volume 495

CELL AND TISSUE TRANSPLANTATION INTO THE ADULT BRAIN

Edited by Efrain C. Azmitia and Anders Björklund

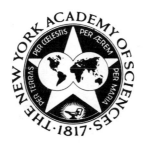

The New York Academy of Sciences
New York, New York
1987

Cover: *A photograph of an adult dorsal raphe neuron co-transplanted with fetal hippocampus into adult hippocampus (paperback volume only). The serotonergic neuron and fetal hippocampus were allowed to grow in the adult host for 1 month.*
See the paper by E. C. Azmitia (pp. 362-377), which includes a black-and-white version of this photograph, for more details.

Library of Congress Cataloging-in-Publication Data

Cell and tissue transplantation into the adult brain.

(Annals of the New York Academy of Sciences, ISSN 0077-8923; v. 495)
Based on a conference held in New York, N.Y. on Apr. 2-4, 1986 by the New York Academy of Sciences.
Includes bibliographies and index.
1. Fetal nerve tissue—Transplantation—Immunological aspects—Congresses. 2. Surgery, Experimental—Congresses. 3. Parkinsonism—Surgery—Congresses. 4. Alzheimer's disease—Surgery—Congresses. I. Azmitia, Efrain C. II. Björklund, Anders, 1945-   . III. New York Academy of Sciences. IV. Series. [DNLM: 1. Brain—surgery—congresses. 2. Nerve Tissue—transplantation—congresses. W1 AN626YL v.495/WL 368 C393 1986]
Q11.N5 vol. 495   500 s   87-15408
[RD594]   [616.8'3306]
ISBN 0-89766-385-3
ISBN 0-89766-386-1 (pbk.)

PCP
Printed in the United States of America
ISBN 0-89766-385-3 (cloth)
ISBN 0-89766-386-1 (paper)
ISSN 0077-8923

ANNALS OF THE NEW YORK ACADEMY OF SCIENCES

Volume 495
June 30, 1987

CELL AND TISSUE TRANSPLANTATION INTO THE ADULT BRAIN[a]

Editors and Conference Organizers
EFRAIN C. AZMITIA and ANDERS BJÖRKLUND

CONTENTS

---

[a] This volume is the result of a conference entitled Cell and Tissue Transplantation into the Adult Brain, which was held in New York, New York on April 2-4, 1986 by the New York Academy of Sciences.

Theme II. Models of Aging, Dementia, and Neurodegenerative Diseases
Part IV. Grafting in Rodent Models of Aging and Dementia

Financial assistance was received from:

- Hoechst-Roussel Pharmaceutical
- Lilly Research Laboratories/A Division of Eli Lilly and Company
- Miles Laboratories
- National Institute of Aging/NIH
- National Institute of Mental Health/NIH
- U.S. Army Medical Research and Development Command
- U.S. Office of Naval Research/Department of Navy Grant N00014-86-G-0077

Preface

The first attempts to graft central nervous system tissue into the adult central nervous system were made by Thompson at New York University nearly a century ago; however, the tremendous potential of this elegant procedure only began to be realized about a decade ago. In 1986, when the papers constituting this volume were presented, a single surgical team was experimenting with transplanting tissue into patients with Parkinson's disease; today, however, clinical trials with adrenal medullary grafts have been performed in parkinsonian patients in at least four countries (China, Mexico, Sweden, and the United States), and significant positive results have been reported by the Mexican team.

The acceptance by the international medical community of cell and tissue transplantation into human patients reflects the advances made in basic research on experimental animals over the last several years. Cell and tissue transplantation has made available a procedure for mixing cells from different locations, species, and ages in the intact brain of mammals. For instance, endocrine adrenal medullary cells can be removed and transplanted into the caudate of human parkinsonian patients. Human fetal oligodendroglial cells can be placed into the brains of mutant mice lacking these myelin-producing cells. Finally, monoaminergic neurons from a fetal brainstem can be transplanted into target sites within the brains of aged rodents. In some cases, the new cells appear to be able to migrate into the host brain, and the donor cells can send out neuronal axons and dendrites into the host. There is now considerable evidence that the rich mixture of growth factors, hormones, neuropeptides, chemical transmitters, and metabolic substances secreted by the donor tissue can modify or influence host brain function.

This volume provides detailed reports on the work currently in progress in the laboratories of many of the leading neuroscientists engaged in brain transplantation. Many important studies are not represented, however, because of our focus on the adult mammalian brain, or, more particularly, the ability of adult tissue to support the survival and maturation of fetal or developing neurons, and important research dealing with neuroendocrine regulation, spinal cord experiments, and other subjects relevant to the general field of the adult mammalian brain could not be included because of our desire to focus on two key areas: cellular and molecular mechanisms and models of aging, dementia, and neurodegenerative diseases.

In the first area, the role of astroglial cells (nonneuronal cells) in the integration of donor and host neurons was stressed by a variety of workers using different experimental designs. These included immunocytochemistry, tissue culture, radioautography, electron microscopy, horseradish peroxidase injections, and prior trauma to the brain. The glial cells were reported to possess both beneficial and detrimental properties, and approaches to activate these two responses separately were presented. Another aspect emphasized in the first area was the ability of the host tissue to support the survival and maturation of the transplanted donor cells. Specific growth factors, the concentrations of which were increased after damage to the host target areas, increased the number of surviving neurons and enhanced the growth of these neurons into the host brain. The papers in this first area provide timely procedures for enhancing the integration of host and donor cells. The efforts of the basic scientists involved in these aspects served to provide a foundation for the subsequent reports on the more clinically oriented research.

In the second area, a variety of rodent systems demonstrated that transplanted cells can reverse at least some types of functional deficits, and the importance of multidisciplinary approaches was stressed. The final part of this area covered recent studies in applying the technology developed in rodents to primates (monkeys and humans). Several presentations dealt with the advantages of using 1-methyl-4-phenyl-1,2,3,6-tetrahydropyridine to produce a model of Parkinson's disease. The presentation of clinical research performed in Sweden since 1982 sparked extensive questioning concerning the future of cell and tissue transplantation in human parkinsonian patients. The many important questions raised in the Final Discussion concerning cell and tissue transplantation into human patients will be highly relevant when the use of grafting techniques in clinical trials becomes more widespread.

A special word of thanks should be given to those who served as session chairmen at the conference. As distinguished neuroscientists not directly involved in the field of brain transplantation, they provided, as we had hoped, some fresh insights to the proceedings; furthermore, they proved to be remarkably efficient at maintaining a smooth flow of information, summarizing the talks in their sessions, and in structuring the discussions. The discussions they led may influence the direction of research in brain transplantation. In addition, sincere appreciation should be extended to our many financial sponsors, especially those that were the main source of our funding: the National Institute of Mental Health and the National Institute of Aging. Finally, we would like to thank the staff of the New York Academy of Sciences for their guidance, support, patience, and time in making the meeting in New York and this volume a reality.

EFRAIN C. AZMITIA
ANDERS BJÖRKLUND

Growth and Connectivity of Axotomized Retinal Neurons in Adult Rats with Optic Nerves Substituted by PNS Grafts Linking the Eye and the Midbrain[a]

A. J. AGUAYO, M. VIDAL-SANZ,
M. P. VILLEGAS-PÉREZ, AND G. M. BRAY

Neurosciences Unit
Montreal General Hospital and McGill University
Montreal, Quebec H3G 1A4, Canada

During development, nerve cells elongate processes that reach specific targets and connect with other neurons or with effector and receptor organs.[1] After injury in adult animals, certain types of neurons can replicate some or all of these developmental events. Indeed, in all vertebrates, including adult mammals, an extensive regrowth follows the severing of axons in the peripheral nervous system (PNS), and, in fish and amphibia, certain injured central nervous system (CNS) neurons can regain their anatomical and functional connections. After interruption of the optic nerve in the goldfish, for example, vision is restored as axotomized retinal ganglion cells regenerate and synapse appropriately with nerve cells in the optic tectum.[2] Conversely, the cutting of the optic nerve in mammals is followed by abortive axonal growth and retrograde degeneration of many retinal neurons.[3-5] Largely as a result of their failure to regrow, retinal and other injured neurons in the adult mammalian brain and spinal cord remain permanently disconnected from their natural fields of innervation. Paradoxically, this well-documented failure of axons to regenerate within the CNS of adult mammals appears to coexist with a preserved ability of many central neurons to sustain lengthy fiber regrowth. The regenerative capacity of mature central neurons has been tested experimentally by transplanting long segments of peripheral nerve into different regions of the CNS where they act as "bridges" between widely separated regions of the neuraxis. Under these experimental circumstances, the injured neurons appear to establish critical interactions with nonneuronal components of the PNS and successfully regrow axons several centimeters long. These findings suggest that fiber elongation in the mature CNS is either prevented by local inhibitory influences or requires additional cellular and extracellular components that stimulate axonal growth. Although analogous elements in the CNS of developing vertebrates and in certain regions of the brain and spinal cord of anamniotes (amphibia and fish) appear to promote or

[a]Research grants were provided by the Medical Research Council, the Multiple Sclerosis Society of Canada, and the Muscular Dystrophy Association of Canada. M. Vidal-Sanz and M. P. Villegas-Pérez were supported by the Spanish Ministry of Education and Science.

1

permit nerve fiber extension, the maturation of the mammalian CNS is accompanied by changes in the extraneuronal milieu that restrict the elongation of regenerating axons.

Some of the features that characterize the growth of CNS axons into PNS grafts have been investigated in adult rats with the help of electrophysiological techniques and new anatomical tracing methods.[6] Little is known, however, of either the ability of these regenerated central axons to make terminal connections or the molecular mechanisms that regulate the diverse responses of neurons whose axons are injured within the CNS and PNS environments.[7-13]

The retina contains a functionally and anatomically well-characterized group of CNS neurons that are experimentally convenient for further investigations of the regenerative potentials that are realized by nerve graft placement. Because of the wide separation that normally exists between the eye and the contralateral superior colliculus, which is the natural target of most ganglion cells in the rat, the reconnection of neurons in these two regions of the visual system requires, first, the promotion and guidance of axonal elongation and, second, an ability of the regenerated terminals to reform terminal synapses.

The experiments reviewed here were recently carried out to investigate the regenerative capacities of axotomized ganglion cells in adult rats and to explore the role of neuron-substrate and neuron-neuron interactions on the regrowth and connectivity of these nerve cells of the mammalian CNS.[14]

METHODS

So and Aguayo[15] demonstrated that axotomized ganglion cells from a sector of the adult rat retina regenerate into segments of autologous sciatic nerve inserted through the sclera into the retina. To obtain grafts that contain axons from larger numbers of retinal ganglion cells, Vidal-Sanz et al.[14,16] have developed a technique whereby the entire optic nerve is replaced by a peripheral nerve graft that can be used as a bridge between the eye and the dorsal mesencephalon (FIG. 1). With this method, the optic nerve in each experimental animal, an adult Sprague-Dawley rat, was transected a few millimeters from the eye; care was taken to avoid the retinal blood supply. One end of a 2-4-cm-long autologous peroneal nerve segment was then apposed to the retinal stump of the transected optic nerve and attached to the sclera with fine sutures. The remainder of the PNS graft was placed under the scalp with its caudal tip tied with a silk suture and temporarily left over the opposite occipital bone (FIG. 1a).

Two to 3 months later, the blind-ended tips of such grafts were exposed and transected in 19 experimental animals. Retrogradely transported labels were then applied to permit the identification of the retinal cells whose axons had elongated through the grafts. In the studies reviewed here, the tracer horseradish peroxidase (HRP) (Sigma VI, 30%) was applied for 1 hr to the cut end of the graft, and, 2 days later, the animals were perfused with fixative solution (4% formaldehyde in 0.1 M phosphate buffer). Normal and grafted retinas were processed, reacted by a modified Hanker-Yates method,[17] and examined as flattened whole-mounts to determine the number, size, and distribution of HRP-labeled neurons.

A second group of experimental animals was used to investigate the fate of the regenerated retinal axons that reach their targets in the dorsal midbrain through the

PNS bridges. For this purpose, in 18 rats prepared as in the first group, the transected caudal end of the graft was eventually divided into several small fascicles and inserted into the contralateral superior colliculus (FIG. 1b) with the help of a micropipette. One to 2 months later, HRP was injected into the grafted eyes of these animals (FIG. 1c) to label the endings of the regenerated axons by orthograde transport.[18] Two days later, these animals were perfused with fixative solution (2.5% glutaraldehyde and 1% formaldehyde in 0.1 M phosphate buffer). To visualize the anterogradely transported HRP reaction product and to stabilize it for electron microscopy, serial 50-μ-thick sections of the midbrain were cut with a vibrating microtome and reacted first with tetramethylbenzidine (TMB) and then with diaminobenzidine (DAB).[19] Wet mounts of the reacted sections were surveyed by light microscopy and selected for further light microscopic study after thionin staining or for electron microscopy after osmication and flat-embedding in epoxy resin.

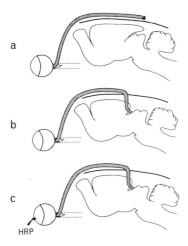

a

b

c

HRP

FIGURE 1. Diagrams of peripheral nerve segments grafted to the optic nerves in adult rats. (**a**) The optic nerve was transected near the eye and replaced by a segment of autologous peroneal nerve (hatched region). The end of the graft was left for 2-3 months beneath the scalp over the posterior skull on the opposite side. To visualize the cell bodies of the retinal neurons that had grown along the graft, HRP was applied to the reexposed end of the graft. Two days later, the retina (stippled region) was reacted for histochemical demonstration of HRP reaction product. (**b**) In another group of animals, the distal end of the graft was inserted into the dorsal midbrain 2-3 months after the grafting. (**c**) To identify the terminals of the axons that had reentered the midbrain, HRP was injected into the grafted eye, and sections of the midbrain reacted to demonstrate the orthogradely transported label.

CHARACTERISTICS OF RETINAL GANGLION CELLS WITH REGENERATED AXONS

Numbers of Retinal Neurons

In the previous experiments[15] in which peripheral nerve grafts were inserted into the retinas of adult rats, it was determined that only axotomized retinal ganglion cells regrew their axons into the grafts. In the present studies in which all ganglion cells were cut by transecting the optic nerve at the time of grafting, the regrowth of axons into the PNS segment was proven by the retrograde labeling of retinal neurons after the extracranial application of HRP to the caudal tip of the graft 3.0-3.5 cm away from the eye. In this group of 19 animals, the numbers of ganglion cells labeled ranged from 949 to 12 385 (mean: 3500) (FIG. 2a). No labeled neurons were identified in the control (unoperated) retinas of these animals. Because there are approximately 110 000 ganglion cells[20] in the intact retinas of adult rats, more than 10% of the normal retinal ganglion cell population was proven to have regenerated axons about 3 cm long. Because some regenerated axons may not have reached the tip of the graft at the time of HRP application, and some of those that did may have not incorporated the label, it is reasonable to assume that an even larger proportion of retinal ganglion cells had regenerated axons into the graft. Furthermore, because many ganglion cells degenerate after cutting the optic nerve in these experimental animals, the incidence of axonal regrowth from the surviving neurons has been estimated to be considerably higher than that suggested by the above figures (unpublished observations).

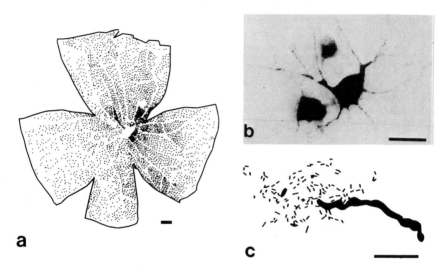

FIGURE 2. (a) Schematic representation of the location of 3323 neurons (dots) in the retina of an animal grafted and processed for retrograde labeling of HRP as depicted in FIGURE 1a (bar: 500 μ). (b) Photograph of three HRP-labeled neurons in a retinal whole-mount such as that illustrated in FIGURE 2a (bar: 20 μ). (c) Camera lucida reconstruction of the HRP-labeled terminal arborization at the end of a nerve graft in the dorsal midbrain. The other end of the graft was attached to the retinal stump of the transected optic nerve, as illustrated in FIGURE 1a (bar: 20 μ).

Size of Retinal Neurons

Retinal ganglion cells have different functional characteristics that correlate with the size of their cell bodies and with the pattern of their dendritic arborizations.[21] Although HRP labeling does not permit consistent visualization of the dendrites (FIG. 2b), we did compare the perikaryial areas of populations of neurons retrogradely labeled in grafted retinas with the areas of retinal ganglion cells in the retina of an intact rat 48 hr after the application of HRP to the transected retinal stump of the optic nerve. The areas of 680 HRP-labeled neuronal cell bodies, measured in one retina, ranged from 60 to 614 μ² (normal range: 52 to 483 μ²; $N = 653$). These data indicate that retinal ganglion cells of different sizes, and presumably different functional properties, had grown into the grafts.

TERMINATION OF REGENERATING AXONS

The animals with bridges linking the retina and the dorsal mesencephalon were examined for anterograde axonal labeling after HRP injection into the eye. Once the grafts were located in the dorsal midbrain of these animals, the branches of these grafts were followed by light and electron microscopy to establish the course and termination of the regenerating retinal axons that reached the colliculus. An injury tract delineated by hemosiderin-containing macrophages usually extended beyond the tip of the graft, presumably the result of the micropipette-aided grafting procedure.[22] The HRP-labeled axon profiles were usually observed near these tracts and in the proximity of blood vessels. The presence of profiles containing HRP reaction product suggested that they were the endings of axons whose cell bodies had incorporated the tracer injected into the PNS-grafted eyes. Several types of labeled profiles were observed within the dorsal midbrain. One type of labeled profile typically extended radially from the injury tracts but only for distances of less than 1 mm. Along this short course away from the substrate formed by the graft and the injury tract, these HRP-labeled profiles were associated with blood vessels and with CNS structures that included astrocytic and oligodendroglial processes; no peripheral nerve components such as Schwann cells, basal laminas, or fibroblasts appeared to have accompanied these labeled structures into the targeted regions of the dorsal midbrain beyond the anatomical tip of the graft. These labeled axons contained prominent collections of neurofilaments and mitochondria and resembled the terminal bulbs seen after transection of the optic nerve in goldfish[23] or rats.[4] Many of the radial profiles that extended from the ends of the grafts actually terminated as short arborizations (FIG. 2c). By electron microscopy, small, heavily labeled profiles in the vicinity of the arborizations were often seen apposed to dendrites. Synaptic vesicles and occasional postsynaptic specializations were identified in some of the less heavily labeled profiles. Because the HRP-injected eye and the contralateral midbrain can only be linked by nerve fibers that had extended through the PNS bridge, the HRP-labeled profiles found in the region of the superior colliculus are presumed to be the terminals of ganglion cell axons reentering the CNS after regenerating about 3 cm along the graft but less than 1 mm within the superior colliculus. Although these observations suggest that, along their short course into the CNS, the regenerating axons of retinal ganglion cells can make synaptic connections with central neurons located within the restricted region they penetrate, we do not know if the synapses observed are appropriate or sustained. Furthermore, although we have recently demonstrated electrophysiologically that some axotomized ganglion cells that regenerate and extend fibers along PNS grafts retain or regain their normal functional responses to light,[24] it remains to be proven that this activity can be relayed transsynaptically to collicular or other neurons.

The magnitude of the regenerative response of the ganglion cells is underscored by the observation that the lengths of the regrown axons within these grafts are nearly twice those of the normal retinal projections to the midbrain (about 2.0 cm in the intact rat). We interpret the extensive growth of retinal axons along the PNS bridge and their limited axonal elongation into the CNS as further evidence of the decisive influence of the two different nonneuronal environments on fiber growth.[6,25]

Another remarkable characteristic of the regenerating retinal axons is the development of multiple small branches once they penetrate the CNS. This phenomenon was also observed when axons regenerating from fetal mesencephalic neurons were directed along peripheral nerve grafts into the striatum of adult rats.[26,27] It would therefore appear that although the peripheral nerve milieu is more conducive to axonal elongation, the CNS environment promotes or permits axonal branching.

CONCLUDING REMARKS

The wide gap that separated the retina from its targets of innervation in the dorsal midbrain was bridged with a long PNS graft following the transection of one optic nerve in adult rats. The approach used for these studies has not only permitted an evaluation of the neuronal capacities and substrate conditions that stimulate or inhibit axonal extension but has also provided some new insights into renewed synaptic connectivity.

In the vertebrate visual system, complex conditions are thought to influence the regeneration of severed retinotectal axons in anamniotes,[2] the regrowth of retinotectal projections into the injured superior colliculus of immature rodents,[28] and the short-range growth of transplanted fetal rat retinal cells into the host tectum.[29] Our present findings suggest that it may also be possible to investigate renewed retinocollicular interactions in adult mammals to determine if some of the developmental conditions that promote the orderly synaptic arrangement of the normal retinal projections can be recapitulated by axon terminals from indigenous retinal neurons regenerating into the brain.

ACKNOWLEDGMENTS

The authors thank M. David, J. Laganière, S. Shinn, J. Trecarten, and W. Wilcox for their expert technical assistance.

REFERENCES

1. PURVES, D. & J. W. LITCHMAN. 1984. Principles of Neural Development. Sinauer. Sunderland, MA.
2. GRAFSTEIN, B. 1986. Regeneration in ganglion cells. *In* The Retina. R. Adler & D. Farber, Eds.: 275-335. Academic Press. Orlando, FL.
3. GRAFSTEIN, B. & N. A. INGOGLIA. 1982. Intracranial transection of the optic nerve in adult mice: Preliminary observations. Exp. Neurol. **76:** 318-330.
4. RICHARDSON, P. M., V. M. K. ISSA & S. SHEMIE. 1982. Regeneration and retrograde degeneration of axons in the rat optic nerve. J. Neurocytol. **11:** 949-966.
5. MISANTONE, L. J., M. GERSHENBAUM & M. MURRAY. 1984. Viability of retinal ganglion cells after optic nerve crush in adult rats. J. Neurocytol. **13:** 449-465.
6. AGUAYO, A. J. 1985. Axonal regeneration from injured neurons in the adult mammalian central nervous system. *In* Synaptic Plasticity. C. W. Cotman, Ed.: 457-484. Guilford Press. New York, NY.
7. SCHWAB, M. & H. THOENEN. 1985. Dissociated neurons regenerate into sciatic but not optic nerve explants in culture irrespective of neurotrophic factors. J. Neurosci. **5:** 2415-2423.
8. SKENE, J. H. P. & E. M. SHOOTER. 1983. Denervated sheath cells secrete a new protein after nerve injury. Proc. Natl. Acad. Sci. USA **80:** 4169-4173.

9. SCHWARTZ, M., M. BELKIN, A. HAREL, A. SOLOMON, V. LAVIE, M. HADANI, I. RACHAILOVICH & C. STEIN-IZSAK. 1985. Regenerating fish optic nerves and regeneration-like responses in injured optic nerves of adult rabbits. Science 228: 600-603.
10. MATTHEW, W. D. & P. H. PATTERSON. 1983. The production of a monoclonal antibody that blocks the action of a neurite outgrowth promoting factor. Cold Spring Harbor Symp. Quant. Biol. 48: 625-631.
11. RICHARDSON, P. M. & R. J. RIOPELLE. 1984. Uptake of nerve growth factor along peripheral and spinal axons of primary sensory neurons. J. Neurosci. 4: 1683-1689.
12. LANDER, A. D., D. K. FUJII & L. F. REICHARDT. 1985. Laminin is associated with the "neurite outgrowth-promoting factors" found in conditioned media. Proc. Natl. Acad. Sci. USA 82: 2183-2187.
13. LIESI, P. 1985. Laminin-immunoreactive glia distinguish regenerative adult CNS systems from nonregenerative ones. EMBO J. 4(10): 2505-2511.
14. VIDAL-SANZ, M., G. M. BRAY, M. P. VILLEGAS-PÉREZ, S. THANOS & A. J. AGUAYO. 1987. Axonal regeneration and synapse formation in the superior colliculus by retinal ganglion cells in the adult rat. J. Neurosci. In press.
15. SO, K.-F. & A. J. AGUAYO. 1985. Lengthy regrowth of cut axons from ganglion cells after peripheral nerve transplantation into the retina of adult rats. Brain Res. 328: 349-354.
16. VIDAL-SANZ, M., M. VILLEGAS-PÉREZ, P. COCHARD & A. J. AGUAYO. 1985. Axonal regeneration from the rat retina after total replacement of the optic nerve by a PNS graft. Soc. Neurosci. Abstr. 11: 254.
17. HANKER, J. S., P. E. YATES, C. B. METZ & A. RUSTIONI. 1977. A new specific, sensitive and non-carcinogenic reagent for the demonstration of horseradish peroxidase. Histochem. J. 9: 789-792.
18. MESULAM, M.-M. & E. J. MUFSON. 1980. The rapid anterograde transport of horseradish peroxidase. Neuroscience 5: 1277-1286.
19. RYE, D. B., C. B. SAPER & B. H. WAINER. 1984. Stabilization of the tetramethylbenzidine (TMB) reaction product: Application for retrograde and anterograde tracing, and combination with immunohistochemistry. J. Histochem. Cytochem. 32: 1145-1154.
20. PERRY, V. H. 1981. Evidence for an amacrine cell system in the ganglion cell layer of the rat retina. Neuroscience 6: 931-944.
21. FUKUDA, Y. 1977. A three-group classification of rat retinal ganglion cells: Histological and physiological studies. Brain Res. 119: 327-344.
22. BENFEY, M., U. BUENGER, M. VIDAL-SANZ, G. M. BRAY & A. J. AGUAYO. 1985. Axonal regeneration from GABA-ergic neurons in the adult thalamus. J. Neurocytol. 14: 279-296.
23. LANNERS, H. N. & B. GRAFSTEIN. 1980. Early stages of axonal regeneration in the goldfish optic tract: An electron microscopic study. J. Neurocytol. 9: 733-751.
24. DAVID, S. & A. J. AGUAYO. 1981. Axonal elongation into peripheral nervous system "bridges" after central nervous system injury in adult rats. Science 214: 931-933.
25. AGUAYO, A. J., A. BJÖRKLUND, U. STENEVI & T. CARLSTED. 1984. Fetal mesencephalic neurons survive and extend long axons across peripheral nervous system grafts inserted into the adult rat striatum. Neurosci. Lett. 45: 53-58.
26. GAGE, F. H., U. STENEVI, T. CARLSTEDT, G. FOSTER, A. BJÖRKLUND & A. J. AGUAYO. 1985. Anatomical and functional consequences of grafting mesencephalic neurons into a peripheral nerve "bridge" connected to the denervated striatum. Exp. Brain Res. 60: 584-589.
27. KEIRSTEAD, S. A., M. VIDAL-SANZ, M. RASMINSKY, A. J. AGUAYO, M. LEVESQUE & K.-F. SO. 1985. Responses to light of retinal neurons regenerating axons into peripheral nerve grafts in the rat. Brain Res. 359: 402-406.
28. SCHNEIDER, G. E., S. JHAVERI, M. A. EDWARDS & K.-F. SO. 1985. Regeneration, rerouting and redistribution of axons after early lesions: Changes with age and functional impact. *In* Recent Achievements in Restorative Neurology: Upper Motor Neuron Functions and Dysfunctions. J. C. Eccles & M. R. Dimitrijevic, Eds.: 291-310. Karger. Basel.
29. McLOON, S. C. & R. D. LUND. 1983. Development of fetal retina, tectum and cortex transplanted to the superior colliculus of adult rats. J. Comp. Neurol. 217: 376-389.

DISCUSSION OF THE PAPER

C. SOTELO (*INSERM U106, CMC Foch, Suresnes*): This is a beautiful demonstration of what we hoped for years would eventually happen to CNS fibers growing along sciatic nerve grafts. If I understood correctly, you injected HRP within the posterior chamber of the eye. You showed terminals in the superior colliculus, and you used DAB to visualize peroxidase activity. I'm very surprised that you have a physiological uptake of HRP and physiological transport of HRP to the terminals since HRP must be in membrane-bound organelles and not diffusable within the axoblasts.

AGUAYO: For these experiments we used the technique of Lemann *et al.* (*Brain Res. Bull.* **14:** 227-282, 1985) to visualize the HRP product. With this method, the HRP-TMB reaction product appears as crystals that are then stabilized by DAB.

SOTELO: Do you have any idea about the possibility of identifying these retinal terminals? In normal animals, the retinal terminals have mitochondria and other characteristics that allow them to be recognized. The two terminals you showed were very difficult to compare to the morphology of normal retinal axons.

AGUAYO: One of the difficulties that we have had is that many terminals or many profiles were heavily labeled. This makes it difficult for us to identify the structures that we really want to see, which are the synaptic vesicles and the postsynaptic differentiated profiles. We have not yet been able to make a careful study of the structures that are present in these terminals.

P. PASIK (*Mount Sinai School of Medicine, New York, NY*): Are the fibers leaving the retina into the graft myelinated?

AGUAYO: It is difficult to answer this question because within the peripheral nerve graft there are many "contaminants," that is, axons of peripheral rather than central origin. These are fibers that come from nerves in the meninges and nearby muscles that are interrupted at the time of the surgical procedure. We know that many of the fibers within the grafts are myelinated, but we cannot prove that the fibers from the retina are themselves myelinated. However, in the electrophysiologic studies, one can use criteria that help to answer this question. We believe that conduction velocities of up to 9 meters per second in fibers within the graft which respond to retinal stimulation by light (Keirstead *et al., Brain Res.* **359:** 402-406, 1985) must reflect the presence of at least a thin myelin sheath along fibers regenerating from axotomized retinal ganglion cells.

On the other hand, we do have evidence that some of these axons (all of which in intact animals are myelinated in the optic nerve by oligodendroglial cells) that course along these grafts behave electrophysiologically and appear by electron microscopy as C fibers, that is, as unmyelinated fibers surrounded only by Schwann cell processes. This change in the type of ensheathment from myelinated to unmyelinated may have resulted from peculiar interactions between the central axons and their new ensheathing cells or from the normal interplay of axon caliber and myelin formation where small axons such as those that arise from the retina would not be myelinated by Schwann cells.

QUESTIONER: Do the axons terminate also on the large cells in the intermediate layer of the superior colliculus, or do they terminate only on the neurons of the superficial layers?

AGUAYO: The objective of these studies was to determine that synaptic connectivity may be the end result of growth. At this moment, studies are being conducted of what type of synapse is made, of how sustained these synapses are, and of how appropriate these synapses are in terms of the regions of the superior colliculus. The only thing that I am reporting is that connectivity appears to be in some cases the end result of growth.

R. F. VALENTINI (*Brown University, Providence, RI*): I was wondering if you had quantified the amount of labeling in your anterograde versus your retrograde HRP staining?

AGUAYO: No, we have not done that.

Onset and Duration of Astrocytic Response to Cells Transplanted into the Adult Mammalian Brain[a]

PATRICIA M. WHITAKER-AZMITIA,[b] ANTONIO
RAMIREZ,[c] LEO NOREIKA,[b] PATRICK J. GANNON,[d]
AND EFRAIN C. AZMITIA[c]

[b]Department of Psychiatry
State University of New York at Stony Brook
Stony Brook, New York 11794

[c]Department of Biology
New York University
New York, New York 10003

[d]Department of Otolaryngology
Mount Sinai School of Medicine
New York, New York 10029

INTRODUCTION

Traumatic insult to central nervous system (CNS) tissue results in an astrocytic response that may limit recovery of the affected area.[1-4] Such an insult is incurred during the transplantation of tissue into the mammalian brain. Thus it is important to understand the properties and the extent of the astroglial response in order to better predict the survival and subsequent functional state of the transplanted tissue.

Initial observations of the gliotic response indicated that the astrocytes were inhibitory or detrimental to the integration of transplanted tissue or to the regeneration and recovery of damaged tissue.[5-8] For example, the astrocytes are well known for their ability to remove cellular debris through phagocytosis.[9,10] Furthermore, astrocytes have been reported to form a barrier around wound areas resulting in the formation of a scar. Such scar tissue within the CNS may then become the site of a functional disability such as observed in epilepsy.[11,12]

More recently, however, the properties of astroglial cells have been viewed in a more positive light. Many neuronal growth factors, including nerve growth factor (NGF), are produced by astroglial cells.[13-17] Moreover, these cells can produce the extracellular matrix components, such as laminin, over which neurons grow during development. Astrocytes also maintain homeostasis in the mature brain[18] and have a

[a]This work was supported by Grant BNS 86-07425 (to P. M. Whitaker-Azmitia) and Grant BNS 79-06474 (to E. C. Azmitia) from the National Science Foundation and by a grant from the Dreyfus Foundation (to P. M. Whitaker-Azmitia).

10

role in the uptake[19-21] and metabolism of neurotransmitters.[22] It has recently become apparent that neurons communicate with astrocytes by means of neurotransmitter-specific receptors on the membranes of the astrocytes.[23-26] These receptors are responsible for glycogenolysis[27] and the release of inhibitory factors such as taurine[28-30] in addition to playing a major role in development, including the production of growth factors.[31]

In order to study the astroglial response to transplanted CNS tissue, we have used an antibody raised against the glial-specific protein glial fibrillary acidic protein (GFAP) to immunocytochemically stain these cells following transplantation of tissue. As a source of CNS transplant tissue, we have used the raphe regions from 14-day-old fetal rat brain or primary cultures of brainstem astroglial cells. The response has been studied from 6 hr to 6 months after transplantation. In addition, we have attempted to determine the source of the glial response by three measures: 1) Proliferation, by using the antimitotic, cytosine arabinoside, for 1 week after transplantation; 2) Migration, by the use of serial lesions; and 3) Differentiation, by pretreating with phenytoin (diphenylhydantoin; Dilantin).

METHODS

Tissue Source

Fetal Tissue

Pregnant Sprague-Dawley rats (15-17 days gestation) were etherized, and the fetuses were transferred into sterile Hanks' balanced salt solution (HBSS) containing 1% glucose. The fetuses were decapitated, their brains removed, and a raphe strip dissected from between the mesencephalic and pontine flexures. The dissected tissue pieces were minced and dissociated in EDTA with gentle repipetting. The neurons were centrifuged at 800 g for 10 min and resuspended at a concentration of 10^6 cells/ 3 µl.

Primary Astroglial Cultures

Newborn rat pups were decapitated, and the brains were removed into sterile HBSS. Brainstem regions, freed of meninges, were minced and dissociated with EDTA using gentle repipetting. The cells were centrifuged at 800 g for 10 min and resuspended in complete medium (minimum essential medium with 10% horse serum and 5% fetal calf serum). The cells were plated into 35-mm Falcon culture dishes at a concentration of one brain per plate. One day after plating, the cultures were shaken to remove nonadhering cells, and the medium was changed. After 1 week, the cultures were scraped and centrifuged at 800 g for 10 min. The resulting pellet was resuspended at a final concentration of 10^6 cells/3 µl.

Inhibiting Treatments

Cytosine arabinoside was injected intraperitoneally for 1 week after transplantation (75 mg/kg, twice daily). Phenytoin animals were injected intraperitoneally with 100 mg/kg phenytoin 30 min before transplantation.

For serial lesions, a glass pipette was introduced into the hippocampus 2 weeks before transplantation, either into the ipsi- or contralateral side.

Transplantation

Adult male Sprague-Dawley rats (150 g) were anesthetized with chloral hydrate/ketamine. Cell suspensions (3 μl) were injected into either the hippocampus (4.5 mm anterior to the lambda; 1.5 mm lateral and 3.7 mm vertical from the skull) or the midbrain (1.0 mm anterior to the lambda; 4.5 mm lateral and 7.5 mm vertical from the skull) using a glass pipette and at a rate of 0.2 μl/min.

Immunocytochemistry

Animals were killed 6 hr, 1 week, 1 month, and 6 months after transplantation. Two hundred milliliters of 4% paraformaldehyde in a 0.1 M phosphate buffer (pH 7.2) was transcardially perfused over 20 min. The brains were fixed overnight and sliced on an oscillating tissue slicer (from Frederick Haer).

The slices were incubated overnight at room temperature with primary antibodies against GFAP (1:1000) (from Dakopatts) or serotonin (1:2000) (a gift from Dr. J. Lauder). The slices were processed using the indirect method described by Sternberger. Both the secondary (sheep antirabbit) and peroxidase-antiperoxidase antibodies were used at a dilution of 1:100 (both from Dakopatts). The final substrate was diaminobenzidine (DAB) (from Sigma).

Morphometric Analysis

Representative serotonin-immunoreactive cells were traced onto paper using a drawing tube. After the paper was enlarged, the surface area of the cells was determined using mass analysis.

RESULTS

Transplantation of Fetal Tissue

Six Hours

The astroglial cells surrounding the transplant region and the needle tract were more intensely stained for GFAP than cells in adjacent regions. There was as yet no sign of a concentration of immunoreactive cells around the wound area.

Twenty-four Hours

Beginning at this time, a graduation of GFAP-immunoreactive cells became evident. The number of intensely stained cells was greatest in the areas immediately adjacent to the transplant region.

One Week

GFAP-immunoreactive cells were now clearly visible and were concentrated around the transplant region (FIG. 1). The cells, however, did not form a complete border. There were almost no immunoreactive cells within the transplant region itself.

Serotonin-immunoreactive cells were clearly visible and were evenly distributed throughout the transplant region. Very few processes passed into the host tissue, and the cell bodies remained within the injection area.

One Month

The GFAP-positive cells formed a thick and almost continuous border around the transplant region (FIG. 2). Very few weakly staining cells were visible within the transplant.

Serotonin-immunoreactive cells were now larger and had positioned themselves along the astroglial border. Very few cell bodies were seen to have left the transplant. The cells had highly branched dendrites and numerous varicosities in the axons.

Similar staining profiles were seen in the hippocampus and in the midbrain.

Six Months

The astroglial border was as intense as observed at 1 month (FIG. 3). Cells within the transplant were now more visibly stained for GFAP. In a few cases, no evidence of a transplant was observed, with only a glial "scar" remaining.

The serotonin-immunoreactive cells were fewer in number and were found almost exclusively along the border formed by the astroglial cells.

Transplantation of Primary Astrocytes

The intensity of GFAP staining in host tissue in response to trauma was less in the astroglial transplants than in serum-free medium injections alone. Little evidence of the formation of an astroglial border by the host tissue was evident at any time following the transplantation of astrocytes.

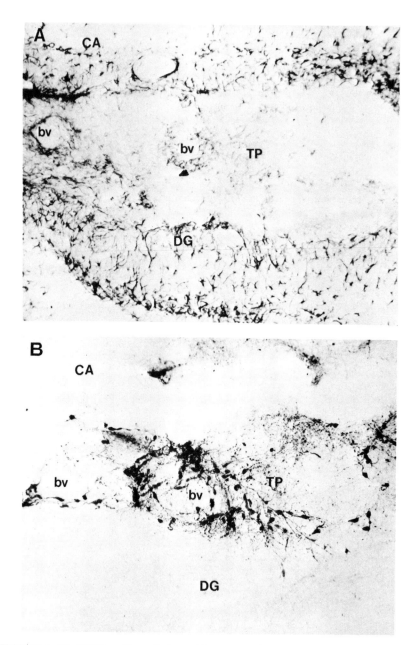

FIGURE 1. (A) GFAP-positive cells in rat hippocampus 1 week after transplantation of fetal raphe cells. The cells have become reactive but do not form a complete border. There are no cells visible within the transplant. (B) Serotonin-positive cells in a section adjacent to that in **A.** Immunoreactive cells are spread throughout the transplant region. CA: cornus ammonus; DG: dentate gyrus; TP: transplant; bv: blood vessel.

Inhibiting Treatments

Antimitotics

Cytosine arabinoside did not have any effect on the onset or intensity of the astroglial response.

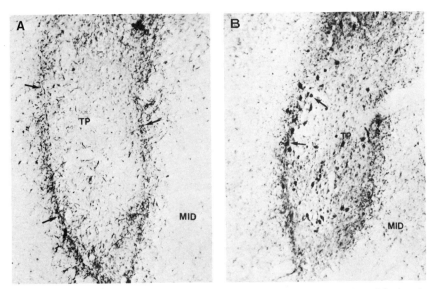

FIGURE 2. (A) GFAP-positive cells in midbrain 1 month after transplantation of fetal raphe cells. The cells have migrated to form a visible border around the transplant. Some cells are visible within the transplant. **(B)** Serotonin-positive cells in a section adjacent to that in **A**. The cells have migrated to the periphery of the transplant, but do not migrate into the host tissue. MID: midbrain; TP: transplant.

Phenytoin

The administration of diphenylhydantoin before transplantation appeared to significantly decrease the astrocytic response, that is, the intensified staining, at 24 hr. This effect was not so pronounced at 1 week.

Serial Lesions

At 1 week after transplantation, the glial response in ipsilaterally lesioned animals was markedly attenuated (FIG. 4). There was little indication of an astroglial border;

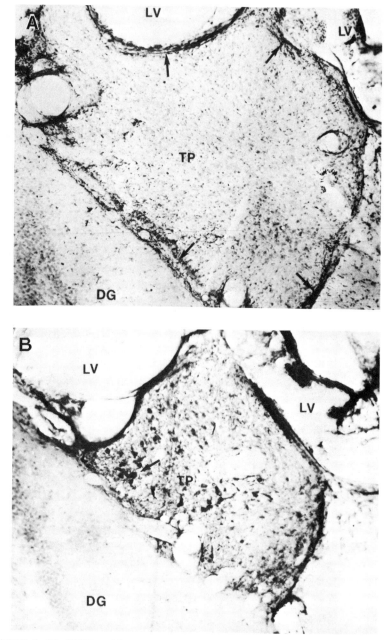

FIGURE 3. (A) GFAP-positive cells adjacent to the rat hippocampus 6 months after the transplantation of fetal raphe cells. The cells form a complete border around the transplant. (B) Serotonin-positive cells in a section adjacent to that in A. The number of remaining immunoreactive cells is less. DG: dendate gyrus; TP: transplant; LV: lateral ventricle.

furthermore, intensely staining astroglial cells were observed within the transplant region. These results were still observable at 1 month. In animals that had received a contralateral lesion, GFAP-positive cells were also evident within the transplant region at 1 week and 1 month after transplantation. The astroglial border from the host tissue was also not as intense as in control animals, but the diminution was not as great as that seen in ipsilaterally lesioned animals (FIG. 5).

Morphometric Analysis

The serotonin-immunoreactive cells appeared to increase in size up to 20 days after transplantation, when their growth was arrested. These results are given in TABLE 1.

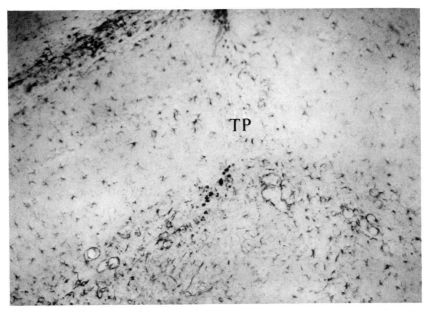

FIGURE 4. GFAP-positive cells in the hippocampus 1 week after the transplantation of fetal raphe cells and 3 weeks after ipsilateral lesioning. There is little evidence of cell concentration around the transplant. Positive cells are visible within the transplant. Compare to FIGURE 1A.

DISCUSSION

The astroglial response to transplanted cells that we are reporting appears to occur in two stages. First, the cells in the area surrounding the transplant become more intensely stained for GFAP, suggesting a differentiation of these cells into reactive astrocytes. This is evident as early as 6 hr after transplantation. Interestingly, this

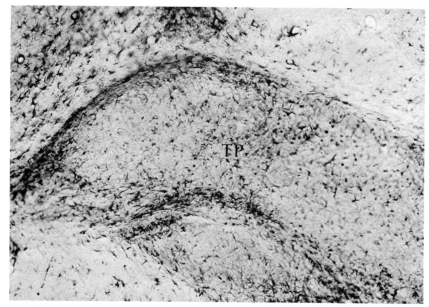

FIGURE 5. GFAP-positive cells 1 week after the transplantation of fetal raphe cells and 3 weeks after contralateral lesioning. A border is evident, and positive cells are visible within the transplant. Compare to FIGURES 1A & 4.

observation is paralleled in tissue culture, where astrocytes become more intensely stained as early as 6 hr after the withdrawal of serum[32] or the addition of cAMP.[18,19] Second, the astroglial cells in the host tissue form a border around the transplant. This border is evident, though sparse, at 24 hr and is complete by 1 month. The resulting concentration of glial cells (sometimes referred to as a "glial scar") is still evident at 6 months after transplantation.

Our work with transplantation of astroglial cultures suggests that the glial response is primarily induced by neurons.

The serotonin-immunoreactive cells within the transplant initially appear to do well: they form branched dendrites and varicose axons. They begin to migrate toward the periphery of the transplant, apparently in an attempt to integrate with the host tissue. In fact, some processes and a few cell bodies do pass into the surrounding tissue, but many more remain behind. The morphometric analysis of these cells gives

TABLE 1. Area of Serotonin-immunoreactive Cells in the Midsections of 14-day-old Fetal Raphe Transplants into the Hippocampus

Days after Transplantation	Area ± SEM (μ^2)
5	200 ± 16
13	213 ± 11
20	356 ± 67
26	318 ± 19

a similar profile. In the initial stages, the surface areas of the cell bodies increase dramatically, but by 26 days, the growth appears to have stopped. It is interesting to speculate that this two-stage pattern in the growth of the transplanted cells is related to the two-stage astroglial response. This would imply that the initial reactive changes of the astrocytes is beneficial to the transplanted neurons, but by 1 month, when the formation of the glial border around the transplant is complete, the influence of the cells becomes detrimental.

Our results with the various "gliosis-inhibiting" measures suggest two sources of the response, which may result in the two-stage pattern we have seen.

The lack of effect of pretreatment with cytosine arabinoside is unusual considering that such a pretreatment is known to be beneficial in reducing gliosis in optic nerves[33] and cortex.[34] This suggests that although proliferation may be a source of the glial response in some brain regions, it is not in the hippocampus. However, the two remaining sources of gliosis—differentiation (into "reactive" astrocytes) and migration—both appear to contribute.

In our studies, lesioning of the brain induced a migration of astrocytes such that subsequent transplantation did not induce further movement and formation of a glial scar. Futhermore, the host astrocytes showed better penetration into the transplant region. Together, these observations suggest a better integration of transplanted tissue into previously lesioned brain that may partially explain the reports of enhanced graft survival under similar conditions.[35,36]

Our use of phenytoin was based on several of its known *in vivo* effects. First, phenytoin protects against posttraumatic brain ischemia.[37-39] Second, phenytoin inhibits the rise in cAMP that normally accompanies brain injury.[40-42] We speculated that these two *in vivo* situations may be modeled in tissue culture by the withdrawal of serum and the addition of dibutyryl cAMP, respectively. If in tissue culture models these measures lead to reactive astroglial formation, it is possible that inhibiting edema and/or cAMP formation *in vivo* (with phenytoin) would also inhibit formation of reactive astrocytes. This, in fact, is what we have observed. It is possible, however, that this pretreatment is detrimental to transplant survival. We have hypothesized that the initial reactive changes are beneficial, in that the astroglial cells may produce growth factors. It is interesting to note that neurons developing in culture[43] or *in vivo*[44,45] in the presence of phenytoin do not survive or mature as well as untreated neurons.

In conclusion, our work has shown that the astroglial response to tissue transplanted into the hippocampus is from two sources that may have distinct time courses and roles. The initial response (beginning at 6 hr) is due to the transformation of astrocytes to a reactive state and may be beneficial. The second response, which is complete at 1 month, is due to the migration of astrocytes from surrounding regions. This results in the formation of a glial border and may limit subsequent integration of the transplant.

REFERENCES

1. CAVANAUGH, J. B. 1970. The proliferation of astrocytes around a needle wound in the rat brain. J. Anat. **106:** 471-487.
2. LATOV, N., G. NILAVER, E. A. ZIMMERMAN, W. G. JOHNSON, A.-J. SILVERMAN, R. DEFENDINI & L. COTE. 1979. Fibrillary astrocytes proliferate in response to brain injury. Dev. Biol. **72:** 381-384.

3. PRIVAT, A., J. VALAT & J. FULCRAND. 1981. Proliferation of neuroglial cells in the degenerating optic nerve of young rats. J. Neuropathol. Exp. Neurol. **40:** 46-60.
4. AZMITIA, E. C. & P. M. WHITAKER. 1983. Formation of a glial scar following microinjection of fetal neurons into the hippocampus or midbrain of the adult rat: An immunocytochemical study. Neurosci. Lett. **38:** 145-150.
5. RAMON Y CAJAL, S. 1928. Degeneration and Regeneration of the Nervous System. Vol. 1. Hafner. New York, NY.
6. CLEMENTE, C. C. Regeneration in the vertebrate central nervous system. Int. Rev. Neurobiol. **6:** 257-301.
7. LASEK, R. J., I. G. MCQUARRIE & J. R. WUJEK. 1981. The central nervous system regeneration problem: Neuron and environment. *In* Posttraumatic Peripheral Nerve Regeneration: Experimental Basis and Clinical Implications. A. Gorio, H. Mallesi & S. Meingrino, Eds.: 59-70. Raven Press. New York, NY.
8. WINDLE, W. F. 1956. Regeneration of axons in the vertebrate central nervous system. Physiol. Rev. **36:** 427-440.
9. SOREIDE, A. J. 1981. Variation in the perineuronal glial changes after different types of nerve lesions: Light and electron microscopic investigations on the facial nucleus of the rat. Neuropathol. Appl. Neurobiol. **7:** 195-204.
10. TORVIK, A. 1972. Phagocytosis of nerve cells during retrograde degeneration. J. Neuropathol. Exp. Neurol. **31:** 132-146.
11. BROTCHI, J. 1979. Activated astrocytes and epileptogenic focus. Acta Neurol. Belg. **79:** 137-304.
12. POLLEN, D. A. & M. C. TRACHTENBERG. 1970. Neuroglia: Gliosis and focal epilepsy. Science **167:** 1252-1253.
13. BURNHAM, P. A., C. RAIBORN & S. VARON. 1972. Replacement of nerve growth factor by ganglionic nonneuronal cells for the survival *in vitro* of dissociated ganglionic neurons. Proc. Natl. Acad. Sci. USA **69:** 3556-3560.
14. VARON, S., C. W. RAIBORN, JR. & S. NORR. 1974. Association of antibody to nerve growth factor with ganglionic nonneurons (glia) and consequent interference with their neuron-supportive action. Exp. Cell Res. **88:** 247-256.
15. PEREZ-POLO, J. R., K. HALL, K. LIVINGSTON & K. WESTHIND. Steroid induction of nerve growth factor synthesis in cell culture. Life Sci. **1:** 1535-1544.
16. BARDE, Y. A., R. M. LINDSAY, D. MONARD & H. THOENEN. 1978. New factor released by cultured glioma cells supporting survival and growth of sensory neurons. Nature (London) **274:** 818.
17. LINDSAY, R. M. 1979. Adult rat brain astrocytes support survival of both NGF-dependent and NGF-insensitive neurons. Nature (London) **282:** 80-82.
18. HERTZ, L. 1978. An intense potassium uptake into astrocytes, its further enhancement by high concentrations of potassium, and its possible involvement in potassium homeostasis at the cellular level. Brain Res. **145:** 202-208.
19. HERTZ, L. 1978. Kinetics of adenosine uptake into astrocytes. J. Neurochem. **31:** 55-62.
20. HENN, F. A. & A. HAMBERGER. 1971. Glial cell function: Uptake of transmitter substances. Proc. Natl. Acad. Sci. USA **69:** 2686-2690.
21. WHITAKER, P. M., C. K. VINT & R. MORIN. 1983. [^{3}H]Imipramine labels sites on brain astroglial cells not related to serotonin uptake. J. Neurochem. **41(5):** 1319-1323.
22. HANSSON, E. 1984. Enzyme activities of monoamine oxidase, cathecol-O-methyltransferase and α-aminobutryric acid transaminase in primary astroglial cultures and adult rat brain from different brain regions. Neurochem. Res. **9(1):** 45-57.
23. HERTZ, L. & S. MUKERJI. 1980. Diazepam receptors on mouse astrocytes in primary cultures: Displacement by pharmacologically active concentrations of benzodiazepines or barbiturates. Can. J. Physiol. Pharmacol. **58:** 217-220.
24. HOSLI, L., E. HOSLI, U. SCHNEIDER & W. WIGET. 1984. Evidence for the existence of histamine H_1- and H_2-receptors on astrocytes of cultured rat central nervous system. Neurosci. Lett. **48:** 287-291.
25. MCCARTHY, K. D. & J. DEVELLIS. 1979. The regulation of adenosine 3',5'-cyclic monophosphate accumulation in glia by α-adrenergic agonists. Life Sci. **24:** 639-650.
26. WHITAKER-AZMITIA, P. M. & E. C. AZMITIA. 1986. [^{3}H]5-Hydroxytryptamine binding

to brain astroglial cells: Differences between intact and homogenized preparations and mature and immature cultures. J. Neurochem. **46**(4): 1186-1189.

27. OPLER, L. A. & M. H. MAKMAN. 1972. Mediation by cyclic AMP of hormone-stimulated glycogenolysis in cultured rat astrocytoma cells. Biochem. Biophys. Res. Commun. **46**: 1140-1145.

28. SHAIN, W., K. L. SMITH & D. L. MARTIN. 1983. Receptor-stimulated release of taurine by glial cells in culture. J. Cell Biol. **97**: 244A.

29. SHAIN, W. & D. L. MARTIN. 1984. Activation of β-adrenergic receptors stimulates taurine release from glial cells. Cell. Mol. Neurobiol. **4**: 191-196.

30. MADELIAN, V., D. L. MARTIN, R. LEPORE, M. PERRONE & W. SHAIN. 1985. β-Receptor-stimulated and cyclic adenosine 3',5'-monophosphate-mediated taurine release from LRM55 glial cells. J. Neurosci. **5**(12): 3154-3160.

31. SCHWARTZ, J. P. & E. COSTA. 1977. Regulation of nerve growth factor content in C6 glioma cells by α-adrenergic receptor stimulation. Naunyn-Schmiedeberg's Arch. Pharmacol. **300**: 123-129.

32. MOONEN, G. 1975. Variability of the effects of serum-free medium, dibutyryl cyclic AMP or theophylline on the morphology of cultured newborn rat astroblasts. Cell Tissue Res. **163**: 365-372.

33. POLITIS, M. J. & J. D. HOULE. 1985. Effect of cytosine arabinoside (AraC) on reactive gliosis *in vivo:* An immunohistochemical and morphometric study. Brain Res. **328**: 291-300.

34. BILLINGSLEY, M. L. & H. G. MANDEL. 1982. Effects of DNA synthesis inhibitors on post-traumatic glial cell proliferation. J. Pharmacol. Exp. Ther. **2**: 765-770.

35. NIETO-SAMPEDRO, M., S. R. WHITTEMORE, D. L. NEEDELS, J. LARSON & C. W. COTMAN. 1984. The survival of brain transplants is enhanced by extracts from injured brain. Proc. Natl. Acad. Sci. USA **81**: 6250-6254.

36. ISACSON, O., P. BRUNDIN, P. A. T. KELLY, F. H. GAGE & A. BJÖRKLUND. 1984. Functional neuronal replacement by grafted striatal neurons in the ibotenic acid-lesioned rat striatum. Nature **311**: 458-460.

37. BREMER, A. M., K. YAMADA & C. R. WEST. 1980. Ischemic cerebral edema in primates: Effects of acetazolamide, phenytoin, sorbitol, dexamethasone, and methylprednisolone on brain water and electrolytes. Neurosurgery **6**(2): 149-154.

38. ARTRU, A. A. & J. D. MICHENFELDER. 1980. Cerebral protective, metabolic, and vascular effects of phenytoin. Stroke **11**(4): 377-382.

39. ALDRETE, J. A., F. ROMO-SALAS, V. D. B. MAZZIA & S. L. TAN. 1981. Phenytoin for brain resuscitation after cardiac arrest. Crit. Care Med. **9**(6): 474-477.

40. LUST, W. D., H. J. KUPFERBERG, W. D. YONEKAWA, J. K. PENRY, J. V. PASSONNEAU & A. B. WHEATON. 1978. Changes in brain metabolites induced by convulsants or electroshock: Effects of anticonvulsant agents. Mol. Pharmacol. **14**: 347-356.

41. PALMER, G. C., D. J. JONES, M. A. MEDINA & W. B. STAVINOHA. 1979. Anticonvulsant drug actions on *in vitro* and *in vivo* levels of cyclic AMP in the mouse brain. Epilepsia **20**: 95-104.

42. McCANDLESS, D. W., G. K. FEUSSNER, W. D. LUST & J. V. PASSONNEAU. 1979. Metabolite levels in brain following experimental seizures: The effects of maximal electroshock and phenytoin in cerebellar layers. J. Neurochem. **32**: 743-753.

43. CULVER, B. & A. VERNADAKIS. 1979. Effects of anticonvulsant drugs on chick embryonic neurons and glia in cell culture. Dev. Neurosci. **2**: 74-85.

44. HARBISON, R. D. & B. A. BECKER. 1972. Diphenylhydantoin teratogenicity in rats. Toxicol. Appl. Pharmacol. **22**: 193-200.

45. VORHEES, C. V. 1985. Fetal anticonvulsant syndrome in rats: Effects on postnatal behavior and brain amino acid content. Neurobehav. Toxicol. Teratol. **7**(5): 471-482.

DISCUSSION OF THE PAPER

B. E. LEVIN (*Veterans Administration Medical Center, East Orange, NJ*): It was not clear to me whether you thought the response to dilantin was beneficial or not. It obviously could have profound implications.

WHITAKER-AZMITIA: I would say it is not part of the migration formation of the border, that it is the early phase that is inhibited. So if the border is what arrests the maturation and development and the astrocytes becoming reactive is where we get growth factors such as laminin, then in theory the dilantin would inhibit the beneficial part of the astrocytic response.

L. KROMER (*Georgetown University, Washington, DC*): It looks as though all your transplants are cell suspension injection transplants.

WHITAKER-AZMITIA: Right. They are mainly injections of dissociated cells.

KROMER: Have you looked at other transplantation procedures and other sources of transplant tissue? When I do aspiration lesions and solid transplants, quite often there is no glial scarring in various areas of aposition between hippocampal transplants and the host hippocampus. That would go along with regional variation, but also could be due to different transplantation procedures.

WHITAKER-AZMITIA: This is something that we considered. We never aspirate tissue before we transplant into it, and that may be why we get a greater astrocytic response than other people do. We might simply be increasing the whole volume within the area.

R. M. LINDSAY (*Sandoz Institute for Medical Research, London*): You said in your serial lesion transplants that the ingrowth of astrocytes seems to be greater than otherwise. Did this affect survival of the transplants for the long term?

WHITAKER-AZMITIA: We have not done it yet. The latest time point we have in the serial lesions is one week. I do not think we have gone beyond that, but certainly it is something we will look into.

C. B. JAEGER (*New York University Medical Center, New York, NY*): Can you distinguish intrinsic astrocytes from the extrinsic ones? You give the impression you get migration of astrocytes into the transplants.

WHITAKER-AZMITIA: No.

JAEGER: How do you know?

WHITAKER-AZMITIA: We haven't done it yet. We are going to start the thymidine labeling of our cultures before we do the transplants so we can answer your question.

C. SOTELO (*INSERM U106, CMC Foch, Suresnes*): What is the meaning of having a gliosis around something you put in the brain? We know that when you just make a lesion or whatsoever with a pipette or with a transplant, you always have a reactive gliosis. What is the significance for transplantation experiments? Does it mean that it is bad? Does it mean that it is a good substrate for growth? Or does it mean that the neurons cannot migrate out because of the gliosis?

WHITAKER-AZMITIA: I think the fact that the astroglial reaction appears to be bimodal, or to have two stages, signifies that astrocytes can be both beneficial and detrimental. It might be that the host astrocytes recognize that the transplanted neurons are in a sense beneficial and belong in the brain, but they are still foreign tissue. So we might see both responses from the astroglial cells, initially the reactivity, followed by production of growth factors and then finally the formation of the border, the sealing off of the region as though it was some sort of invasive substance not beneficial to the brain.

M. SHELANSKI (*New York University, New York, NY*): Do you know the answer Constantino?

SOTELO: Yes sir.

SHELANSKI: Listen to what I have to say, Constantino, and then you can decide. Several years ago, we did a study with nerve growth factor injections into the caudate nucleus to look at the reactive astrocyte reaction. To make a long story short, what we found was that a single injection of nerve growth factor after caudate nucleus injury increased the number of reactive astrocytes as well as their size. Interestingly enough, we did a lot of behavioral work in looking at spatial reversal learning in these animals. The time of their increase and migration into the damaged zone correlated very nicely with the time it took to observe behavioral recovery following bilateral caudate nucleus injury.

Transplantation of Mouse Astrocyte Precursor Cells Cultured *in Vitro* into Neonatal Cerebellum[a]

S. FEDOROFF[b] AND L. C. DOERING[c]

Department of Anatomy
University of Saskatchewan
Saskatoon, Saskatchewan S7N 0W0, Canada

INTRODUCTION

The last decade has seen considerable development of the intracerebral transplantation of fragments of neural tissue or disaggregated neural cells. The survival of such transplants and the possibility of successful integration with the tissue of the host depends to a large extent on the age of the donor. The younger the cells the better they survive (see the review by Gage *et al.*[1]). Tissue fragments and suspensions of disaggregated neural cells usually consist of live cells and cells that have been injured and cells that have died as a result of manipulation during their isolation. The ideal situation would be to know the exact composition of cells in the transplant, to be able to alter this at will, and, most importantly, to have only healthy, viable cells, with no cell debris. Preparations of fetal cells grown in tissue culture approach this ideal. Using *in vitro* techniques, the identity of the cell type can be determined and immature proliferative cells can be preferentially selected. Thus, various cell types can be isolated from appropriate tissue culture preparations and used for transplantation.

In this paper we describe a procedure that can be used for the isolation of astrocyte precursor cells and their transplantation into newborn mouse brain. In addition, we show that the stage of astrocyte development at the time of transplantation is the crucial factor in determining whether or not the cells will transform into reactive astrocytes following transplantation.

MATERIALS AND METHODS

Tissue Cultures

Pregnant DBA/1J females were used to obtain staged E14 (Theiler stage 22) and E17 (Theiler stage 27) embryos.[2] Newborn DBA/1J mice were obtained within a 24-

[a]This research was supported by Grant MT4235 from the Medical Research Council of Canada.

[b]Address for correspondence: Department of Anatomy, College of Medicine, University of Saskatchewan, Saskatoon, Saskatchewan S7N 0W0, Canada.

[c]Present address: Neurosciences Unit, Research Institute, Montreal General Hospital, 1650 Cedar Avenue, Montreal, Quebec H3G 1A4, Canada.

hr period after birth; the brains were removed and transferred to modified Eagle's minimal essential medium (mMEM).

The neopallia were dissected from the brains and freed from basal ganglia, thalamus, and hippocampus and disaggregated by passing the tissue through a 75-μm mesh (Nitex) with mMEM containing 5% (v/v) horse serum.[3] The cultures were kept in a humidified (95%) incubator at 37° C in an atmosphere of 5% carbon dioxide and 95% air.

Metrizamide Density Step Gradients

Four-step gradients were prepared consisting of a bottom cushion of 19.0% metrizamide (Sigma) in mMEM, followed by decreasing steps of 13.6, 9.3, and 6.4% metrizamide.[4] The metrizamide solutions were kept on ice, and the four concentrations of metrizamide were loaded with fine-bore pasteur pipettes into 15-ml test tubes (Pyrex).

Cells were removed from the culture dishes with a 0.025% trypsin solution containing 0.05 mg of DNase I (Sigma) per ml. The cell suspensions were centrifuged at 200 g for 2 min, washed in mMEM, layered on top of the chilled metrizamide gradient, and centrifuged at 2500 g for 10 min at 4° C.

Cell fractions were removed from the metrizamide gradient interfaces with Pasteur pipettes, suspended in mMEM, centrifuged, and used immediately for transplantation and assessment of cellular composition.

Composition of the cell types in the various fractions was determined by plating dispersed cells on poly-L-lysine-coated, 35-mm tissue culture dishes (Falcon). The cells were grown for 24 hr in the conditioned medium obtained from the original cultures and scored according to their type with phase-contrast microscopy. Cells with spherical somas and long thin processes were classified as neurons; flattened cells with abundant cytoplasm, as astrocytes; and cells with spherical somas with short broad processes, as oligodendrocytes. A total of 1000 cells was counted, and the frequency of appearance of each cell type was expressed as a percentage.

Transplantation of Cells

Glass tuberculin syringes (.25-ml luer tip) fitted with capillary tubing (outside tip diameter: 0.2 to 0.5 mm) were used to transplant the cells.

Neonatal mice (DBA/1J), 1 to 2 weeks old, were anesthetized with diethyl ether, and the backs of their heads were swabbed with 70% alcohol. A coronal skin incision was made between the ears, the neck musculature was gently retracted from the occipital surface of the skull, and the parietal-interparietal suture was incised with a scalpel blade to allow entry of the needle tip into the cerebellum. Incisions made through the parietal-interparietal suture avoided the major blood vessels and minimized bleeding during the transplantation procedure.

Approximately 1 μl of the centrifuged cell pellet was aspirated into the tip of the syringe. The cells were slowly injected into the cerebellum of each neonate host, and the incision was closed with a 6.0% solution of celloidin. Approximately 30 min after the last animal was injected the entire litter of injected animals was returned to their mother.

Light and Electron Microscopy of Transplants

The host mice were anesthetized with diethyl ether and perfused intracardially with phosphate-buffered (0.1 M) 2.0% paraformaldehyde. The brains were dissected and immersed in phosphate-buffered (0.1 M) 2.0% paraformaldehyde overnight at room temperature. The brains were then dehydrated and infiltrated with paraffin (Paraplast) using an alcohol-xylene series of solutions. Coronal sections (8 μm thick) of the cerebellums containing the transplants were cut, mounted on glass microscope slides, and used for immunocytochemistry and histology.

For examination of transplants by electron microscopy, the animals were anesthetized with ether and perfused intracardially with a phosphate-buffered (0.1 M) solution of 1.0% glutaraldehyde and 2.0% paraformaldehyde containing 0.005% calcium chloride. The brains were dissected and placed in fresh fixative for a 24-hr period at 4° C. The cerebellums were separated from the brains and infiltrated with an Epon-Araldite mixture. Coronal sections (1.0 μm thick) of the cerebellums were cut and stained with methylene blue-Azure B to locate the transplants. The blocks were then trimmed around the transplants; thin sections were cut and examined by electron microscopy.

Immunocytochemistry of Cells in Culture and Transplants

The three-step peroxidase-antiperoxidase procedure of Sternberger[5] was used to visualize glial fibrillary protein (GFP) immunoreactivity in the cultures and in the transplants. The GFP antibodies were donated by Dr. V. I. Kalnins. Their properties have been described by Fedoroff et al.[6] The cells in culture were fixed in phosphate-buffered (0.1 M) 2.0% paraformaldehyde. Paraffin sections of transplants fixed with phosphate-buffered paraformaldehyde were used for immunocytochemistry.

For detecting GFP, cultures and sections were treated with a 1:20 dilution of normal goat serum for 10 min. The cultures or sections were then incubated for 15 min with a 1:150 dilution of antibodies to GFP, followed by incubation for 15 min with a 1:20 dilution of goat antirabbit immunoglobulin G (Boehringer Mannheim). A final 15-min incubation was made with a 1:50 dilution of rabbit peroxidase-antiperoxidase (Boehringer Mannheim). The peroxidase was visualized in the cultures with a solution of 0.01% hydrogen peroxide and 0.05% of 3,3'-diaminobenzidine tetrahydrochloride (Aldrich) in Tris (Sigma) buffer. This solution was applied for 10 min, and the cultures were rinsed with phosphate-buffered saline and air dried.

Control cultures and sections of transplants were treated as described above except that the primary antibodies were either omitted or replaced by preimmune serum. In addition, occasional sections were placed in 3,3'-diaminobenzidine solution to check for endogenous peroxidase activity.

Morphometry of Cell Nuclei in Culture and in Transplants

To determine nuclear dimensions, a Zeiss (IBAS I) semiautomated image analyzer was used. The cells were displayed through a television camera adapted to a microscope. Cells in culture were fixed with 2.0% paraformaldehyde and stained with celestine blue. Paraffin sections of transplants were stained with hematoxylin and eosin.

The nuclear perimeters of cells in cultures and in transplants were traced out with a television overlay system, the values of nuclear area (NA) and maximum nuclear diameter (MND) were compiled, and the averages were computed. The nuclear dimensions of 300 GFP-positive cells both in transplants and in normal cerebral cortices of 45-day-old mice were determined.

[³H]Thymidine Labeling of Cells and Autoradiographic Procedure

To label cells and assess possible cell migration from the transplants, 1.0 μCi of [³H]thymidine with a specific activity of 5.0 μCi/mmole (Amersham) was added to the medium on the third day of culturing. After 24 hr, the cells were collected and transplanted. Paraffin sections (8 μm thick) of the cerebellums containing transplants of the cultured cells were stained with carbofuschin, dried, and coated with liquid photographic emulsion (Kodak NTB2). The slides were then exposed for 4 days, developed in D19 (Kodak) for 2 min, mounted in Permount, and examined by light microscopy.

RESULTS

We isolated astroglia from E14, E17, and PO neopallia using colony culture techniques and, after 1 week of culturing, transplanted the cell colonies into the cerebellums of neonatal mice. Astrocytes were identified by immunostaining with antibodies to GFP.

Three- to 4-week-old transplants were usually localized within the folia of the cerebellums close to the middle or directly within the vermis. Occasionally transplants were located on the surfaces of the cerebellums partially wedged between the superficial folia.

As a result of the growth and differentiation of the neopallial precursor cells, the transplants could be recognized as discrete islands of cells within the cerebellums in sections stained with hematoxylin and eosin. Blood vessels and capillaries of various sizes were observed in all transplants. There was no inflammation or gliosis at the interfaces between the transplants and the host cerebellum.

Transplants of E14 Neopallial Astroglia

The 7-day-old cultures of E14 neopallia used for transplantation contained a predominance of epithelial-like cells, which are GFP negative and may contain a low concentration of vimentin. Also present were small refractile cells, which use the epithelial cells as a substratum. It has been shown that the epithelial cells in culture form GFP-positive astroglia. Some of these astroglia have been described as mature fibrous astrocytes.[6,7] Transplants of such E14 neopallial cultures contained GFP-positive cells with small oval nuclei. GFP immunoreactivity was strong in the perinuclear regions and gradually decreased in intensity toward the cell periphery and in the cell processes. The positive cells were randomly dispersed within the transplants and sometimes occurred in small groups of three or four cells. The GFP staining patterns of astrocytes in the transplants were similar to the GFP staining patterns of astrocytes in sections of the cerebral white matter of normal adult mice.

In cresyl-violet-stained sections of the transplants, numerous groups of small and large neurons with perikarya containing Nissl substance were seen. Silver-impregnated sections of the transplants had argentophilic neurites throughout the transplant neuropil and at the interface with the host cerebellum.

GFP-positive cells had an average MND of 8.07 ± 1.08 μm and an average NA of 35.35 ± 6.08 μm^2 (TABLE 1). The MND and NA values for the smaller neurons were 10.7 ± 1.17 μm and 67.29 ± 15.64 μm^2, respectively. The larger neurons had an MND of 13.55 ± 1.18 μm and an NA of 122.90 ± 17.03 μm^2.

In semithin sections of the E14 transplants stained with methylene blue-Azure B, cells with and cells without Nissl substance could be recognized. The former were identified as neurons and the latter were identified as astrocytes by electron microscopy. Astrocytes were identified as having a moderately electron-dense nucleus, a somewhat irregular shape, and a cytoplasm containing bundles of linearly arranged intermediate filaments. The organelle content was sparse, but the occasional Golgi apparatus was seen among the ribosomes, as were short strands of rough endoplasmic reticulum.

Cells from E14 neopallial cultures could be separated on the metrizamide density gradients into enriched fractions containing small refractile cells and epithelial-like cells. Centrifugation of the cells from 7-day-old cultures through the metrizamide gradients produced four fractions of cells, one at each interface of the gradient. Examination of the fractions (F1 through F4) plated on poly-L-lysine substrate after 20 hr of culturing indicated that the F2 fraction contained the highest percentage (87 $\pm$ 3%) of the small refractile cells. The F3 and F4 fractions were found to contain predominantly epithelial-like cells, but no detailed assessments of enrichment were made on these fractions. Transplants of the F2 fraction consisted mainly of neurons and very few astrocytes, indicating that the small refractile cells are proliferative neuronal precursor cells.[8] Transplants of F3 and F4 fractions, however, were composed of typical fibrous astrocytes and some neurons.

Transplants of E17 Neopallial Astroglia

Cells from E17 neopallia maintained *in vitro* for 7 days were used for transplantation. Such cultures were composed mainly of cells of the pleomorphic epithelial-like type; some cells were GFP positive and some GFP negative, but all cells were vimentin positive.

The transplants of E17 neopallium cultures were seen as islands of cells within the cerebellums. The boundaries of the E17 transplants were clearly distinguishable in all cases, since the neuropil staining densities of the transplants were different from those of the cerebellum. Transplantation of the cells resulted in minimal disturbance of the trilaminar cerebellar structure, primarily in the region of insertion of the needle.

Antibodies to GFP identified numerous astrocytes in the E17 transplants. The astrocyte density in these transplants was higher than that in the E14 transplants.

The pattern of GFP staining of individual astrocytes was similar to the pattern obtained in the E14 transplants as indicated by the staining of the perinuclear cytoplasm and gradual diminishing of reaction product in the distal processes. Frequently the astrocyte processes could be traced to their ends, or feet, which often contacted neighboring blood vessels, other astrocytes, or neurons.

No inflammation or reactive gliosis at the interfaces of the transplants and host cerebellums were apparent in sections of the transplants immunostained with GFP antibodies. Nuclear measurements of the GFP-positive cells in paraffin sections were calculated. The MND was 8.07 ± 0.85 μm and the NA was 34.95 ± 5.03 μm^2 (TABLE 1).

Neurons were identified by cresyl violet staining of Nissl substance and silver impregnation of neuronal processes. The neuronal density was noticeably reduced when compared with the neuronal density in the E14 neopallial transplants.

TABLE 1. Nuclear Morphometric Measurements of Astrocytes[a]

Area Analyzed	NA (μm^2)	MND (μm)
E14 (transplants)	35.35 ± 6.08	8.07 ± 1.08
E17 (transplants)	34.95 ± 5.03	8.07 ± 0.85
PO (transplants)	53.18 ± 11.50[b]	10.74 ± 1.69[b]
Adult mice (neopallial white matter)	36.45 ± 6.66	8.08 ± 0.97

[a] A total of 300 cells were evaluated for each age. Each value represents a mean $\pm$ 1 SD.
[b] Significantly different ($p < .001$) when compared with astrocytes in cerebral white matter, E14 transplants, or E17 transplants.

Transplants of PO Neopallial Astroglia

Seven-day-old cultures from PO neopallia were used for transplantation. They consist of pleomorphic epithelial-like cells, the majority of which are GFP and vimentin positive. They also have a complex arrangement of actin-containing filaments.[9] When these cells are cultured for 10 days or longer, small stellate cells appear on top of the pleomorphic epithelial-like cells. The stellate cells are strongly GFP and vimentin positive and have been considered to be similar to fibrous astrocytes *in vivo*.

The transplants of newborn neopallium cultures were smaller than the transplants of either E14 or E17 neopallia. The transplants could easily be recognized as discrete islands of cells located in either the granular, molecular, or white matter layer of the cerebellums. Occasionally, transplants were wedged between the folia.

In sections stained with cresyl violet or impregnated with silver, no cells within the transplants could be identified as neurons. Cultures initiated from the neopallium of PO mice contain only a few, if any, neurons or their precursors. At this stage of development *in vivo*, the majority of neurons in the neopallium are postmitotic, and hence culture procedures select against them. Although in silver-impregnated sections no argentophilic processes were seen within the transplants, many argentophilic processes were present at the interfaces of the transplants.

Immunocytochemistry of paraffin sections of the PO transplants indicated that astrocytes were the predominating cells that stained intensely with the GFP antibodies. The astrocyte processes were of various sizes and lengths and were arranged in interlacing networks in most regions of the transplants. Especially large pale nuclei in the transplants were associated with intense GFP staining of the perikarya. The GFP-positive processes of such cells were thick at their origins, and the GFP staining remained intense throughout the processes. This GFP immunoreactivity was in sharp contrast to the GFP immunoreactivity of astrocytes in the E14 and E17 neopallial transplants, which had shorter, tapered processes. Focusing through the sections was required to follow the GFP-positive processes in their entirety within the PO transplants. The astrocyte processes could be traced for distances up to 150 μm in these transplants.

Nuclear morphometric measurements of the astrocytes in the transplants were computed. The MND was 10.74 $\pm$ 1.69 μm, and the NA was 53.18 $\pm$ 11.50 μm^2 (TABLE 1). A t-test indicated that the NA and MND of the astrocytes in the PO transplants were both significantly ($p < .001$) larger than the corresponding nuclear measurements of astrocytes in the E14 and E17 transplants, and in the white matter fiber tracts of P45 mouse neopallium (TABLE 1).

Further examination of the PO transplants revealed a few astrocytes with GFP immunoreactivity similar to that of astrocytes in the E14 and E17 neopallial transplants. These cells had an MND of 8.01 $\pm$ .69 μm and formed less than 20% of the total population of astrocytes.

As expected, electron microscopy revealed that the PO neopallial transplants consisted predominantly of astrocytes. The astrocyte nuclei were electron lucent and showed homogeneous nuclear chromatin staining patterns. Nuclei of the smaller astrocytes in the micrographs were slightly oval in shape and had ultrastructural features similar to the astrocytes in the E14 transplants.

Nuclei of the larger astrocytes were predominantly oval and elongated. Thse nuclei were very electron lucent and had a thin rim of heterochromatin attached beneath the nuclear membrane. Bundles of intermediate filaments were the predominant cytoplasmic feature of these astrocytes. The intermediate filaments formed extensive networks that encircled the nuclei and radiated into the perikaryal cytoplasm and processes of the cells.

DISCUSSION

The isolation, enrichment, and transplantation techniques utilized in this laboratory provide the framework for studying neuronal, astrocytic, and oligodendrocytic precursor cells.[8,10] Tissue culture is used to select proliferative neural cells; metrizamide density gradients enrich the desired cell types for transplantation; and transplantation of the cells into a heterotypic central nervous system (CNS) location permits their identification and subsequent analysis. Morphological differences between the transplanted cells and the cerebellar cells, as well as differences in cell densities and neuropil staining provide the criteria for identifying the transplants in the cerebellums.

The neural cell composition is defined before transplantation; hence the procedures differ from the transplantation techniques employing the injection of solid pieces of embryonic nervous tissue in which the precise cellular composition of the transplanted tissue is unknown. Transplants of cultured neural cells are clearly identifiable in the cerebellums of mice, and the cells have been proven to be derived from the cultures in which the disaggregated neopallial cells were pulse labeled with [³H]thymidine. Autoradiography indicates that only cells within the transplants had grains over their nuclei: therefore these cells originated from the cultures. The transplanted cells remained aggregated and did not appear to migrate.

It has been reported that granule cells in the cerebellum will anomalously migrate into transplants of adult superior cervical ganglia[11] and into transplants of embryonic cerebral cortex[12] when placed on the cerebellar surfaces of neonatal rats. Rosenstein and Brightman[11] showed that small groups of granule cells will migrate through tissue bridges that form between transplants of superior cervical ganglia and the cerebellar surfaces of 1-2-week-old rats. There was no evidence in the present study, however, of granule cell migration into the transplants of neopallial cell cultures. In fact, there was very little disruption of the cerebellar architecture and no arresting of granule cell migration from the external granule layer toward the internal granule cell layer as reported by Rosenstein and Brightman[11] and by Jaeger and Lund.[12]

No host reaction toward the transplants was detected; it should be stressed, however, that we used a syngeneic system. The GFP immunoperoxidase procedures indicated no reactive gliosis at the boundaries of the transplants. The fact that argentophilic neuronal processes passed across the interfaces of the transplants and cerebellums indicates that there were no glial barriers at the interfaces. These observations indicate acceptance of the transplants in the host cerebellums with no observable pathologic reaction.

Proliferating undifferentiated neural cells of the neopallium seem to complete their lineage of differentiation in transplants despite the *in vitro* procedures, density gradient centrifugation, and transplantation procedures to which they were exposed. The precursors of neurons, astrocytes, and oligodendrocytes have all been isolated in culture and transplanted into the cerebellums of neonatal mice, and all these precursor cells could differentiate in the transplants.[8,10,13]

Since the discovery of GFP, its presence has been generally accepted as a specific marker for astrocytes. The presence of GFP in astrocytes, however, does not necessarily mean that the cells are normal. GFP is present in astrocyte-derived tumor cells (astrocytomas) and in reactive and abnormal astrocytes in various neurological disorders. In addition, various amounts of GFP are detected in various types of astrocytes with differing morphology *in vitro*.[14–17]

Cultures of E14 and E17 neopallia contained both neuroblasts and astroblasts, and the transplants consisted of neurons and astrocytes. The neurons in the transplants (identified by Nissl substance staining with cresyl violet) have been previously shown to correspond to pyramidal cells and interneurons of the mature cerebral cortex.[8] The astrocytes in the E14 and E17 transplants had GFP immunoreactivity and nuclear dimensions similar to those of astrocytes in the white matter fiber tracts of the mature neopallium, and astrocyte processes were seen to end as perivascular foot plates when located near blood vessels, indicating a normal affinity toward vascular surfaces. We have therefore considered the astrocytes in the E14 and E17 transplants as normal fibrous astrocytes.

Cultures of PO disaggregated neopallium contain pleomorphic flat cells (astroblasts), which form large stellate cells upon the addition of Bt_2cAMP, and senescent cells, but contain few or no preneurons.[3,18,19] The nuclei of the flat astroblasts and Bt_2cAMP-induced astrocytes in cultures are considerably larger than the nuclei of astrocytes in the cerebral white matter of adult mice and of stellate cells that form in culture without the addition of Bt_2cAMP. Transplants of PO cultures were composed mainly of astrocytes, but also contained a few cells that did not have Nissl substance and that were negative for GFP. These cells could be oligodendrocytes.

Two populations of astrocytes were identified on the basis of nuclear morphometry in the transplants of PO cultures. The population with small nuclei (20%) was identified as consisting of normal fibrous astrocytes. The second population (80%) of the astrocytes had nuclear measurements significantly larger than those of astrocytes within the cerebral white matter. The nuclear measurements of the large stellate cells with large nuclei in the PO transplants corresponded to those of nuclei in reactive astrocytes in the vicinity of brain wounds in mice.[7] Because reactive astrocytes are characterized by a hypertrophied nucleus and an increase in glial filament content, we consider that the astrocytes with large nuclei, with intense GFP immunoreactivity, and containing large numbers of intermediate filaments, in the PO transplants, are not normal astrocytes, but rather belong to a group of reactive astrocytes stimulated by as yet unidentified factors.

It is especially interesting that astroblasts in cultures of E14 and E17 neopallia, grown under identical conditions and in the same medium as astroblasts of PO neopallium, did not form reactive astrocytes after transplantation. This could be a reflection of the presence of neuroblasts and neurons in the E14 and E17 cultures and transplants, or an indication of maturation of astroblasts and aquisition of the property to respond to adverse conditions by forming reactive astrocytes.

Neurons may modulate the differentiation and function of astrocytes. The absence of such a modulation because of a lack of neuron-astrocyte interactions may lead to the formation of reactive astrocytes. Björklund and Dahl[20] observed intense GFP immunostaining of astrocytes in intraocular transplants of cerebral cortex. This was in contrast to combined transplants of cerebral cortex and locus ceruleus in which the astrocyte immunostaining with GFP antibodies was considerably reduced. They suggested that the presence of neurons may have a modulatory effect on GFP synthesis by way of trophic factors.

Alternatively, astrocytes may react differently to physical disruption according to their developmental age. Kozak et al.[21] have reported an intense gliosis in aggregating cultures of neonatal mouse cerebellum in contrast to an absence of gliosis in aggregating cultures of fetal mouse cerebellum. Similarly, Kromer[22] reported the absence of glial scarring at the interfaces of embryonic CNS transplants in contrast to adult CNS transplants, which are associated with reactive gliosis at their interfaces when examined with the electron microscope.

We have observed that when Bt_2cAMP is added to cultures of astroblasts from fetuses of various ages and astroblasts at various times of their in vitro life, large reactive astrocyte-like cells form only from astroblasts that have been isolated from perinatal animals and cultured for at least 2 weeks. We concluded that during astrocyte differentiation there is a stage at which the cells respond to Bt_2cAMP by forming large stellate astrocytes with increased amounts of GFP. These cells, according to their morphology and morphometry, appear more like reactive astrocytes than normal fibrous astrocytes. We also observed that such reactive astrocyte-like cells form from astroblasts rather than from normal fibrous astrocytes.[7,23] It should be noted that reactive gliosis in response to cerebral cortical injury begins to appear in rats at about the second postnatal week,[24] and in humans the capacity to respond by reactive gliosis appears only late in gestation.[25,26] These in vivo observations support our notion, in principle.

These observations indicate that there are differences in astrocytes according to the developmental age of the CNS at the time of their isolation. Whether the differences in the developmental expression of astrocytes are a result of physical trauma, death or absence of neurons, or some as yet unidentified factor remains to be determined.

REFERENCES

1. GAGE, F. H., S. B. DUNNETT, P. BRUNDIN, O. ISACSON & A. BJÖRKLUND. 1984. Intracerebral grafting of embryonic neural cells into the adult host brain: An overview of the cell suspension method and its application. Dev. Neurosci. **6:** 137-151.
2. THEILER, K. 1972. Development and Normal Stages from Fertilization to 4 Weeks of Age: The House Mouse: 168. Springer-Verlag. Berlin.
3. FEDOROFF, S. 1978. The development of glial cells in primary cultures. *In* Dynamic Properties of Glial Cells. E. Schoffeniels, G. Franke, L. Hertz & D. B. Tower, Eds.: 83-92. Pergamon Press. New York, NY.
4. SCHNAAR, R. L. & A. E. SCHAFFNER. 1981. Separation of embryonic CNS cell types using metrizamide density gradient centrifugation. *In* New Approaches in Developmental Neurobiology: Short Course Syllabus: 59-73. Society of Neuroscience. Bethesda, MD.
5. STERNBERGER, L. A. 1979. The unlabeled antibody peroxidase-antiperoxidase (PAP) method. *In* Immunochemistry. L. A. Sternberger, Ed.: 104-169. John Wiley & Sons. New York, NY.
6. FEDOROFF, S., R. V. WHITE, J. NEAL, L. SUBRAHMANYAN & V. I. KALNINS. 1983. Astrocyte cell lineage. II. Mouse fibrous astrocytes and reactive astrocytes in cultures have vimentin- and GFP-containing intermediate filaments. Dev. Brain Res. **7:** 303-315.
7. FEDOROFF, S., W. A. J. MCAULEY, J. D. HOULE & R. M. DEVON. 1984. Astrocyte cell lineage. V. Similarity of astrocytes that form in the presence of dBcAMP in cultures to reactive astrocytes *in vivo*. J. Neurosci. Res. **12:** 15-27.
8. DOERING, L. C. & S. FEDOROFF. 1982. Isolation and identification of neuroblast precursor cells from mouse neopallium. Dev. Brain Res. **5:** 229-233.
9. FEDOROFF, S., I. AHMED, V. I. KALNINS & M. OPAS. 1986. Microfilament organization in reactive astrocytes in culture. Neuroscience. In press.
10. DOERING, L. C., S. FEDOROFF & R. M. DEVON. 1983. Fibrous astrocytes and reactive astrocyte-like cells in transplants of cultured astrocyte precursor cells. Dev. Brain Res. **6:** 183-198.
11. ROSENSTEIN, J. M. & M. W. BRIGHTMAN. 1978. Intact cerebral ventricle as a site for tissue transplantation. Nature (London) **276:** 83-85.
12. JAEGER, C. B. & R. D. LUND. 1982. Influence of grafted glial cells and host mossy fibers on anomalously migrated host granule cells surviving in cortical transplants. Neuroscience. **7:** 3069-3076.
13. DOERING, L. C. & S. FEDOROFF. 1984. Isolation and transplantation of oligodendrocyte precursor cells. J. Neurol. Sci. **63:** 183-196.
14. ENG, L. F. & L. J. RUBINSTEIN. 1978. Contribution of immunohistochemistry to diagnostic problems of human cerebral tumors. J. Histochem. Cytochem. **26:** 513-522.
15. VELASCO, M. E., D. DAHL, U. ROESSMANN & P. GAMBETTI. 1980. Immunohistochemical localization of GFAP in human glial neoplasms. Cancer **45:** 484-494.
16. ENG, L. F. & S. J. DEARMOND. 1981. Glial fibrillary acidic (GFA) protein immunocytochemistry in development and neuropathology. *In* Glial and Neuronal Cell Biology. Vidrio & S. Fedoroff, Eds.: 65-79. Alan R. Liss. New York, NY.
17. ENG, L. F. 1980. The glial fibrillary acidic (GFA) protein. *In* Proteins of the Nervous System. R. A. Bradshaw & D. M. Schneider, Eds.: 88-117. 2nd edit. Raven Press. New York, NY.
18. FEDOROFF, S. 1980. Tracing the astrocyte cell lineage in mouse neopallium *in vitro* and *in vivo*. *In* Tissue Culture in Neurobiology. E. Giacobini, A. Vernadakis & A. Shahar, Eds.: 349-372. Raven Press. New York, NY.
19. MOONEN G., Y. CAM, M. SENSENBRENNER & P. MANDEL. 1975. Variability of the effects of serum-free medium dibutyryl cyclic AMP or theophyline on the morphology of cultured newborn rat astroblasts. Cell Tissue Res. **163:** 365-372.
20. BJÖRKLUND, H. & D. DAHL. 1982. Glial disturbances in isolated neocortex: Evidence from immunochemistry of intraocular grafts. Dev. Neurosci. **5:** 424-435.

21. KOZAK, L. P., D. DAHL & A. BIGNAMI. 1978. GFAP in reaggregating and monolayer cultures of fetal mouse cerebral hemispheres. Brain Res. **150:** 631-637.
22. KROMER, L. F. 1980. Glial scar formation in the brain of adult rats is inhibited by implants of embryonic CNS tissue. Soc. Neurosci. Abstr. **6:** 688.
23. FEDOROFF, S. & L. C. DOERING. 1980. Colony culture of neural cells as a model for the study of cell lineages in the developing CNS: The astrocyte cell lineage. Curr. Top. Dev. Biol. **16:** 283-304.
24. SUMI, S. M. & H. HAGER. 1968. Electron microscopic study of the reaction of the newborn rat brain to injury. Acta Neuropathol. **10:** 324-335.
25. DAMSBKA, M. 1968. Encephalic necrosis and inflammatory reaction in fetuses and newborn. Pol. Med. J. **7:** 404-434.
26. GILLES, F. H. 1983. Neural damage: Inconstancy during gestation. *In* The Developing Human Brain. F. H. Gilles, A. Leviton & E. C. Dooling, Eds.: 227-243. John Wright. Boston, MA.

DISCUSSION OF THE PAPER

P. M. WHITAKER-AZMITIA (*SUNY, Stony Brook, NY*): That was a very elegant presentation. One of the questions I had concerns the survival of neurons. You showed some neuronal grafts in your presentation. Many people have observed that there is age dependency for the survival of grafted neurons, and we have always speculated on some of the factors that make this time requirement for grafts. How would you speculate reactive astrocytes might influence the survival of neurons and in some way influence its time window for survival of fetal neuronal grafts?

FEDOROFF: This is an extremely difficult question. There may be no answer. It seems that astrocytes can do very many things—particularly reactive astrocytes. I do not think that there is any question that they can synthesize or secrete many favorable components that would act on survival and the sprouting of neurons, etc., but at the same time there are probably some other things they can do. They may be inhibitory when they contact connective tissue elements or other elements. This still has to be analyzed, so I do not have a reply. My personal feeling is that reactive astrocytes do more things than we know about today.

Application of Tissue Culture and Cell-marking Techniques to the Study of Neural Transplants

RONALD M. LINDSAY,[a] CAROLINE EMMETT,
GEOFFREY RAISMAN, AND P. JOHN SEELEY

Laboratory of Neurobiology
National Institute for Medical Research
London NW7 1AA, England

INTRODUCTION

Although grafting of neural tissue in invertebrates and birds has been used with great success in developmental neurobiology since the turn of the century, it is only in the last decade that neural grafting in the mammalian central nervous system (CNS) has been considered to have potential as both a research tool and as an approach with therapeutic potential.[1-3] Within basic research the experimental questions that are currently being addressed through studies of neural grafting in the mammalian CNS can be divided into two broad categories: 1) those that pursue a more detailed understanding of the limited regenerative capacity of the adult nervous system and 2) those that explore the plasticity of the developing nervous system. In practical terms, these two categories cover, respectively, studies of fetal neural tissue transplanted to adult brain and studies of fetal neural tissue transplanted to neonatal brain. For the most part, grafting studies in the mammalian CNS have been carried out using rodents, where small pieces of solid tissue have been dissected from embryos in intermediate or late stages of gestation and implanted directly into neonatal or adult recipients.[3-5] Although the results obtained from analyses of solid tissue grafts have demonstrated that most regions of the embryonic CNS survive well and undergo a considerable degree of normal development and maturation within adult or neonatal recipients, the diversity of neuronal and glial cell types inherent in even a small piece of embryonic tissue has made it difficult to identify which specific cellular and molecular interactions are important in promoting survival of the grafted tissue and in eliciting host-donor-host connections.

After a series of studies of the connections formed between grafted embryonic hippocampal primordia and adult host brain,[6-8] we embarked on a set of experiments to reduce the heterogeneity of cell types within the graft. Given the detailed information available on the pattern of neurogenesis in the rodent hippocampus and dentate gyrus,[9] we initially tried to eliminate either dentate granule cells or CA3 pyramidal cells from E18 hippocampal primordia while maintaining the tissue as an explant in culture

[a] Present address: Department of Cell Biology, Sandoz Institute for Medical Research, 5 Gower Place, London WC1E 6BN, England.

before transplantation. Mitotic inhibitors were employed in attempts to eliminate dividing granule cells or their precursors; the neurotoxin kainic acid was employed in attempts to selectively eliminate CA3 pyramidal cells. Although neither of these approaches were entirely successful in themselves, we determined that an intermediate stage in tissue culture was not detrimental to the survival of fetal tissue when subsequently transplanted to adult brain.[10]

SOLID TISSUE GRAFTS

Fate of Neurons

If, before transplantation, hippocampal primordia from E16–E18 embryos are maintained in culture medium containing [3H]thymidine, cells that undergo DNA synthesis during the culture period become radiolabeled and can later be identified by autoradiography of sections of host brain. Using such a procedure, we have observed[10–12] that neuroblasts or neurons of donor origin largely remain at the site of implantation and undergo a relatively normal pattern of differentiation and maturation. As shown in the camera lucida drawing in FIGURE 1, many labeled granule and CA1 pyramidal cells and a few labeled CA3 pyramidal cells were found within the transplant, but not within the host neuropil. Given that in this case E17 donor tissue was incubated with [3H]thymidine-containing medium for 1 day, the labeling pattern within the graft is consistent with the donor neurons having continued normal development during the culture period and after implantation; that is, 1) the absence of labeled nuclei among the CA3 pyramidal cells (FIG. 1B) and 2) the heavy labeling of the smaller CA1 pyramidal cells is consistent with the fact that the latter undergo their final division between E17 and E18, while the former are already postmitotic at this stage in development. The light labeling of nuclei of dentate granule cells in FIGURE 1C is consistent with the observation that the period of neurogenesis of dentate granule cells is more protracted than that of pyramidal cells. Thus, although some granule cells or their precursors incorporated [3H]thymidine during the period in explant culture, the radiolabel was subsequently diluted from these cells by further mitotic divisions after transplantation. In addition to remaining at the site of implantation within the host, it is evident that there is little random migration of neurons within the transplant, otherwise the distribution of cell types and sizes within the transplant might be expected to be more uniform.

FIGURE 1. (A) Camera lucida drawing of an E17 donor hippocampal transplant (1 month survival) labeled with [3H]thymidine for 1 day in culture. The transplant (area with bold outline) lies in the host alveus (alv) and stratum oriens (so). Within the transplant, dentate granule cells (dg), CA1 pyramids (t1), giant CA3 pyramids (t3), and glia were labeled. (dots, glia; filled triangles, pyramids; filled circles, dentate granule cells). The majority of labeled glia are in the host: external capsule (ec), fimbria (fb), stratum oriens, alveus, and CA1 and CA3 pyramidal cell layers. Scale bar: 100 μm. (B) Photograph from the region of the star in A. Heavily labeled CA1 pyramids (tp-CA1) adjacent to essentially unlabeled and larger CA3 pyramids (tp-CA3). Scale bar: 20 μm. (C) Photograph of labeled dentate granule cells (tp-dg) (from the region of the asterisk in A). Scale bar: 20 μm.

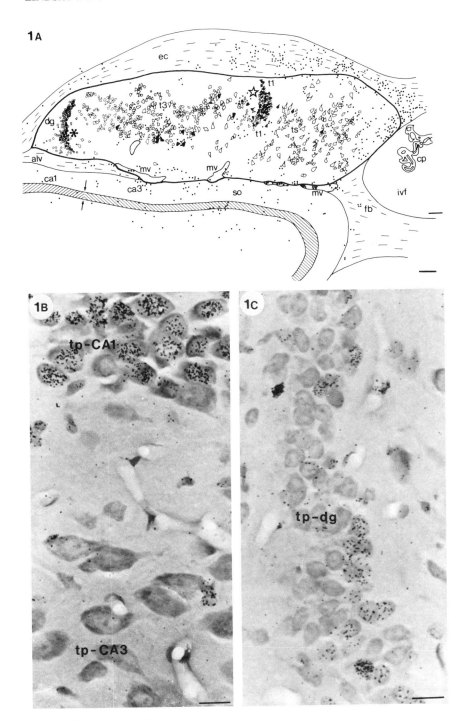

Fate of Nonneuronal Cells

We have observed that there is, in contrast to the static behavior of the grafted neurons, very prominent migration of nonneuronal cells from donor tissue into host neuropil.[10,11] As shown by the distribution of labeled nuclei (black dots) in the camera lucida drawing in FIGURE 2, it is evident that donor nonneuronal cells can migrate for up to 2-3 mm into intact host brain. As yet we have not identified the precise composition of macroglia (astrocytes and oligodendrocytes) and microglia within this migrating population of nonneuronal cells, but we have identified, on morphological criteria alone, labeled astrocytes, labeled endothelial cells, and other labeled small dark and large light cells.[10] The significance of the migration of nonneuronal cells from donor to host is still uncertain, but we believe that the migration of endothelial cells into host tissue, which results in the formation of a mosaic of donor and host endothelial cells in the blood vessels, may influence the rapidity of vascularization of the grafts.[8] This may be a critical factor in determining the size of the viable graft. At the moment the importance of glial migration is less clear. Although the migration of glial cells is widespread, there do seem to be certain restricted routes of migration through the host neuropil. Labeled cells observed at the farthest distance (2-3 mm) from the transplant are most often found in myelinated fiber tracts or in a perivascular position. To some degree this may be due to degeneration of host fiber bundles as a result of surgery. Many labeled glial cells have been observed, however, in parts of the host alveus and external capsule that show no evidence of any degeneration.

At shorter distances from the graft, labeled glia were observed as perineuronal satellite cells in both granule cell and pyramidal cell layers of the host. The positions occupied by these migrant cells (FIG. 2B) are in conformity with the glial-neuronal relationships observed in normal tissue. In some cases of this shorter distance migration, the routes occupied by labeled glial cells parallel fiber projections from donor granule cells to host pyramidal cells,[6,7,10] although a consistent relationship has not been demonstrated. These pathways may represent specific trophic or tropic interactions.

To exclude the possibility that labeled cells observed in sections of host brain were not of donor origin but arose through adult cells becoming labeled by acquisition of [³H]thymidine (either free or incorporated into DNA) released from dying cells within the transplant, we made control experiments in which 1) donor cells were freed, before transplantation, of any cytoplasmic radiolabel by incubation for 2 days in a vast excess (10 mM) of unlabeled thymidine; 2) radiolabeled donor tissue was lethally X-irradiated before transplantation such that all label would eventually be released into host tissue; and 3) postnatal donor tissue, which does not survive in adult brain under the conditions used, was implanted after radiolabeling such that again all label was released into host brain. In none of these controls was there any indication that host nonneuronal cells could become labeled either in the nucleus or in the cytoplasm by transfer of [³H]thymidine from donor cells.

FIGURE 2. (A) Camera lucida drawing of the location of labeled glial cells (dots) derived from a transplant lying in the host hippocampus. The transplant (gray area with bold outline) was from an E16 donor and was labeled for 2 days in culture with [³H]thymidine. Hippocampal strata: sm, moleculare; so, oriens; sp, pyramidale; sr, radiatum; sg, granulosum. Scale bar: 500 μm. (B) Labeled glial cells in the host hippocampal field CA3 (h-sp, host stratum pyramidale). The transplant was from an E17 donor, and was labeled for 1 day in culture. Scale bar: 10 μm. (C) Labeled glia migrating through host fiber bundles. The transplant was from an E16 donor and was labeled for 2 days in culture. Scale bar: 10 μm.

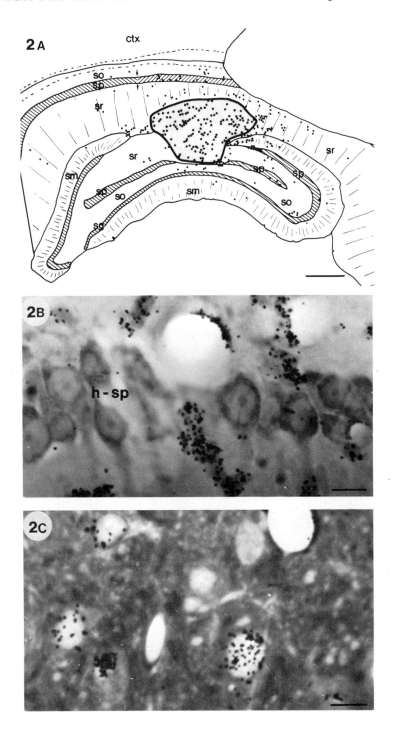

Double-labeling of Cells Migrating from Solid Grafts

Although morphological criteria have given us an indication of the spectrum of glial cell types and other nonneuronal cells that migrate from fetal grafts into adult recipients, it is important that these cell types are more definitively identified and categorized before we can draw further conclusions as to the mechanism and possible importance of migration of glial cells from graft to host. To this end, we have begun a series of studies (Zhou, Lindsay, and Raisman, unpublished results) using immunocytochemical staining to try and identify by double-labeling the types of nonneuronal cells that migrate from donor to transplant. In the first instance, we have used antisera to glial fibrillary acidic protein (GFAP) to identify astroglial cells. As shown in the example in FIGURE 3A, indirect immunoperoxidase labeling with GFAP antiserum revealed astrocytic processes throughout the host brain, but the most intense staining was seen within the transplant and at the host-transplant interface. Within the transplant mass, the majority of nonneuronal cells were radiolabeled, and a large proportion of these were intensely stained with anti-GFAP. Of the [^{3}H]thymidine-labeled cells at the graft-host interface or that had migrated for short distances (100-200 μm) into host brain, the majority were found to be astrocytes, not only because of their intense staining for GFAP (FIG. 3B), but because of the typical stellate morphology revealed by the GFAP staining (FIGS. 3C & 3D). At distances of 1-2 mm from the transplant, however, very few of the [^{3}H]thymidine-labeled cells were positive for GFAP. Such cells occurred in all regions, but were particularly prevalent in the corpus callosum. Although these cells are negative for GFAP, we cannot rule out that they may also be astrocytes, but in view of the paucity of cytoplasm and the small dark nuclei of these GFAP-negative cells, it is more probable that they are undifferentiated glial precursors, oligodendrocytes, or microglia.

Migration of Glia from Grafts of Adult Tissue

Although it is generally true that neither neurons nor glia from adult mammalian CNS can be transplanted or maintained in culture, we have taken advantage of a previous finding[13] to determine 1) whether reactive astrocytes from injured adult brain can be successfully transplanted to another adult brain and 2) whether in this situation reactive astrocytes migrate from the site of implantation with any of the characteristics previously observed with migration of fetal nonneuronal cells.

In these experiments the donor tissue was taken from the lateral or medial cut edges (asterisks, FIG. 4A) at a lesion site in adult animals in which the corpus callosum had been transected 5 days previously. The dissected tissue was labeled in explant culture with [^{3}H]thymidine for 24 hr; any free label in the cytoplasm was then washed out by incubation for a further 24 hr (four changes of medium) with an excess of unlabeled thymidine (10 mM). For comparative purposes such grafts were implanted in the hippocampal formation of adult recipients (FIG. 4B). Such grafts of adult corpus callosum survived as well as fetal grafts, although there were occasional signs of necrosis and more evidence of macrophages within the adult transplant than seen with embryonic donor tissue. At survival times of 1 and 2 months, heavily labeled cells were found both within the transplant itself and within the host brain. The greatest concentration of labeled cells was observed at the graft-host interface (FIG. 4C), but just as with fetal transplants, labeled nonneuronal cells were found 1-2 mm

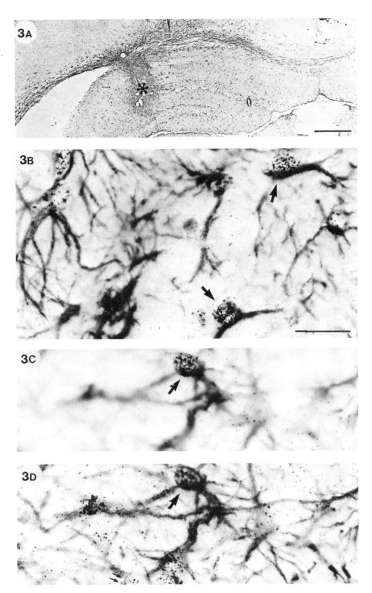

FIGURE 3. Identification of migratory donor cells as astroglial cells by double labeling with [³H]thymidine and antibodies to glial fibrillary acidic protein. (A) Location of an E18 donor mouse embryo hippocampal primordia graft (asterisk) in the hippocampal formation of the host. Strong immunoperoxidase staining with anti-GFAP was seen in the transplant and in the overlying host corpus callosum. Donor tissue was labeled for 2 days in culture and survived for 8 weeks. Scale bar: 500 μm. (B) Donor astroglial cells located in host brain 100-200 μm from the transplant in **A**. Coincidence of silver grains and anti-GFAP staining of processes (arrows) verifies the donor origin of these astrocytes. Scale bar: 20 μm. (C & D) The same field photographed at different levels of focus to show the heavy concentration of silver grains over the cell body (C) and the GFAP staining of the stellate processes (D) of a single donor astrocyte located in the host brain. Large arrow indicates the same cell perikaryon in C and D. Small arrows in **D** indicate a GFAP-negative migratory cell. Scale bar: 20 μm.

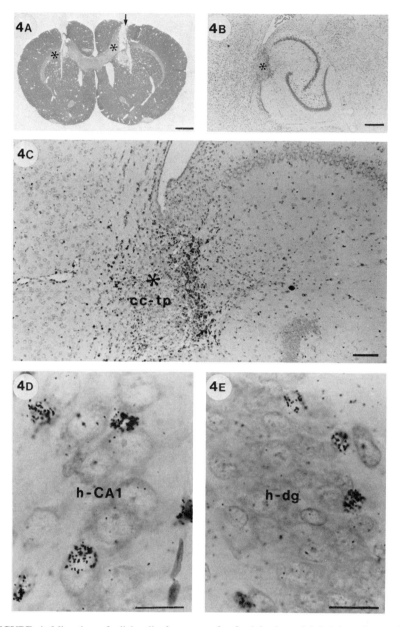

FIGURE 4. Migration of glial cells from a graft of adult tissue labeled in culture with [³H]thymidine for 1 day. (**A**) Donor tissue taken from an adult rat brain, which had been lesioned 5 days earlier by bilateral transection of the corpus callosum. The areas from which tissue was taken is shown with asterisks; the arrow shows where the lesion was made. Scale bar: 2 mm. (**B**) Photograph of an adult callosal transplant (asterisk) within the hippocampal formation of an adult host. The survival time of the transplant was 2 months. Scale bar: 500 μm. (**C**) Higher magnification of **B** showing the dense concentration of labeled nonneuronal cells at the interface between the host tissue and the corpus callosum transplant (cc-tp). Scale bar: 100 μm. (**D & E**) Perineuronal or satellite glial cells of transplant origin located in host CA1 pyramidal layer (h-CA1) and host dentate granule cell layer (h-dg). Scale bar: 10 μm.

from the graft. Heavily labeled glial cells were found as perineuronal satellite cells in the host hippocampal pyramidal and dentate granule cell layers (FIGS. 4D & 4E). Labeled perivascular glia and small dark glia were also found in the host neurophil. Although we have not made detailed comparisons of the relative distribution of cells that migrate from fetal hippocampal as opposed to adult corpus callosal donor tissue, we have seen no obvious differences in the pattern of migration of labeled cells from these two types of grafts. Double-labeling studies, using cell-type-specific antigenic markers, will be carried out to determine the exact types of glia present within and migrating from these adult callosal grafts.

DISSOCIATED CELL GRAFTS

Reaggregation and Grafting of Cultured Cells in a Plasma Clot

As indicated in the introduction, one of our recent objectives has been to devise procedures that will permit enrichment of specific cell types, thus allowing transplantation of particular subpopulations of neurons or glia. Having previously established that an intermediate period in explant culture had no deleterious effect on the survival of fetal neurons or glia, we have now determined that embryonic neurons and perinatal glia maintained in dissociated culture can be successfully reaggregated and grafted to adult hosts. The long-term objective in establishing such procedures is based on the belief that enrichment or purification of desired subpopulations of cells will be best achieved with dissociated cells in culture. With dissociated cells, cell-type-specific antibodies can be used either to eliminate unwanted populations (such as immunocytolysis) or to directly select the specific subpopulations required (such as fluorescent-activated cell sorting).

In contrast to the failure of mitotic inhibitor or kainic acid treatment to enrich hippocampal primordia for either pyramidal cells or granule cells, respectively, we have recently established (Lindsay, Raisman, and Seeley, unpublished results) that low-level γ-irradiation of E18 hippocampal explants followed by a period in dissociated culture leads to enrichment of pyramidal cells. This enrichment is achieved at this age (E18) because of the much greater radiation sensitivity (and consequent death) of mitotic cells (granule cells and glial cells or their precursors) compared to postmitotic cells (all CA3 pyramids and most CA1 pyramids). Although several possible methods of implanting dissociated cells have been described, we considered these—especially the simple injection of a cell suspension[14–16]—to be unsuitable for our purposes, where we wished to keep the grafted cells localized as much as possible in a compact transplant at the site of implantation. We have therefore devised a procedure[17] whereby dissociated cells growing in monolayer culture are harvested from the culture dish, suspended in bovine plasma, gently centrifuged to form a dense suspension, and finally entrapped in the matrix of a plasma clot. Clot formation is induced by the addition of thrombin to a small drop of the cells suspended in plasma. This reaggregated cell graft can be handled and transplanted in a cannula using the same procedures employed for solid tissue grafts. In an initial series of experiments, the bovine plasma proteins were coupled with fluorescein isothiocyanate such that the graft could be readily identified by fluorescence microscopy of sections of host brain (FIG. 5A). In addition, by examining a series of fluorescent plasma clot grafts at survival times between 1 day and

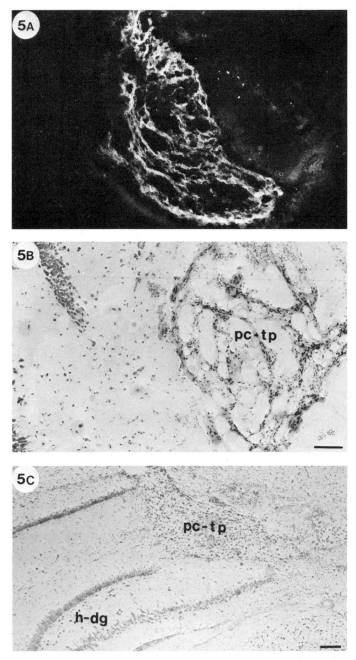

FIGURE 5. Grafts of dissociated hippocampal cells reaggregated in a plasma clot. (A) Photograph taken under fluorescent optics to show the plasma clot matrix (the plasma proteins were labeled with fluorescein isothiocyante) after the graft had survived for 5 days. (B) Similar graft to the one in **A**. After surviving for 5 days, this graft was counterstained to show donor cells trapped within the matrix of the plasma clot transplant (pc-tp). Scale bar: 100 μm. (C) Plasma clot transplant after a 17-day survival period. Scale bar: 100 μm.

6 weeks, we were able to determine that the plasma cot matrix was completely degraded by the host tissue within 10-20 days and did not at all interfere with fusion of graft and host. The plasma clot matrix initially maintained the cells in an open sponge-like structure (FIGS. 5A & 5B), which presumably (*cf.* solid grafts or pelletted cell suspensions) aids the maintenance of the donor cells before establishment of a continuous vasculature with the host. After 2-3 weeks, there was little indication of any remaining fluorescence or plasma clot matrix, and the donor cells appeared as a clearly identifiable compact graft that had fused totally with the host neuropil (FIG. 5C) and, although obviously lacking internal organization, was otherwise indistinguishable from a solid tissue graft.

Fate of Cultured Neurons Reaggregated and Transplanted in a Plasma Clot Graft

After the technique was established, the potential of the plasma clot method was tested by applying it to the grafting of fetal pyramidal cells that had been enriched by irradiation (see above) and maintained for 5 days in monolayer culture before implantation. A typical graft of such cells examined after 2 months of survival is shown in FIGURE 6. In this case, the graft retained a rather spherical appearance in which large CA3-type pyramidal cells were clearly predominant and evenly dispersed throughout. By staining alternate sections with Nissl and Timm stains (FIGS. 6A & 6B, respectively), it was observed that the location of the graft was such that it had severed host mossy fibers during the grafting procedure and thus elicited a substantial host-to-donor mossy fiber projection, as seen at higher power in FIGURES 6C & 6D. The donor CA3 pyramidal cell bodies are seen to lie in a cluster surrounded by a wide dendritic field, and the host mossy fibers are seen to form terminals selectively in and around the CA3 cell body cluster, ignoring the peripheral dendritic field. Verification of the donor origin of the pyramidal cells receiving the host mossy fiber terminals was obtained from a third series of sections from the same brain (not shown) that were processed for autoradiography. As the donor embryo had been labeled with [³H]thymidine *in utero* at gestational days E15 and E16, many labeled pyramidal cells were found within the graft.[17] No labeled neurons were found outside the immediate proximity of the graft, and thus, in agreement with our observations with solid tissue grafts, implanted neurons remain at the site of implantation and are not migratory, even though their axons can project into the host brain. Further evidence that transplanted neurons do not migrate out of a plasma clot comes from our studies[17,18] of transplants between A/Thy-1.1 and A/Thy-1.2 mice, where immunohistochemical staining with Thy-1.1 antisera was used to detect the neuronal cell surface antigen Thy-1.1, which was present only on the donor neurons and not in the host tissue, which bore the distinct allelic form Thy-1.2.[19]

Fate of Cultured Glial Cells Reaggregated and Transplanted in a Plasma Clot Graft

In parallel with plasma clot transplants from neuron-enriched cultures, preliminary studies (Emmett, Seeley, and Raisman, unpublished results) have been carried out

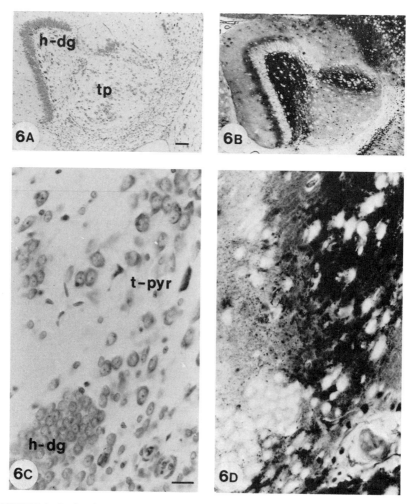

FIGURE 6. Grafts of dissociated and enriched cultures of pyramidal cells reaggregated in a plasma clot. (**A & B**) Nissl- and Timm-stained adjacent sections show the projection of host dentate granule cell (h-dg) mossy fibers into the transplant (tp). Scale bar: 100 μm. (**C & D**) Higher magnification of the transplant in **A & B** showing mossy fiber terminals of host granule cells (h-dg) among clusters of the donor pyramidal cells (t-pyr). Scale bar: 50 μm.

using material from glia-enriched cultures. In this case, cultures enriched in astroglia were prepared from the corpus callosum of postnatal day 5 rats. The cells were maintained in culture for 1 month and were determined to be 95% positive for the astroglial marker GFAP, and virtually negative for neurofilament protein and for the fibroblast and meningeal cell marker fibronectin. Before reaggregation and implantation, the astroglial cultures were incubated with [³H]thymidine (7 days) followed by a cold chase in 10 mM unlabeled thymidine to eliminate any free cytoplasmic tracer. At survival times of 1 month, sections of host brain were stained for GFAP by an indirect immunoperoxidase method and then exposed for autoradiography to detect [³H]thymidine-labeled cells. As shown in FIGURE 7, strong GFAP reactivity was found within the graft, and many of the cells were heavily radiolabeled. The majority of labeled cells were observed at the host-transplant interface, but, as in the previous cases with solid grafts of embryonic hippocampus or adult corpus callosum, many labeled nonneuronal cells were found to have migrated into the host brain. Although the majority of radiolabeled migratory cells were GFAP negative (FIG. 7B), double-labeled cells with typical stellate astrocyte morphology were found up to 200-300 μm from the host-transplant boundary.

It would thus appear that within plasma clot grafts of enriched neurons or glia the same pattern of events occurs as with solid tissue grafts; that is, 1) grafted embryonic neurons remain at the site of implantation and undergo normal differentiation and maturation and 2) grafted nonneuronal cells are invasive and can penetrate for considerable distances through host neurophil. In future studies, combinations of different types of neurons and nonneuronal cells will be incorporated into a single plasma clot, and thus the influence of glial cells upon donor neuron survival and integration with host circuitry can be investigated.

Other Cell-marking Possibilities

Although we consider that [³H]thymidine labeling of donor cells and their subsequent identification in host brain sections by autoradiography is unambiguous, and despite an extensive series of control experiments, the objection has been raised that some of the radiolabeled cells we observe may not be of donor origin but may be host cells that have incorporated radiolabel released from grafted cells. To clarify this situation, we have searched for a more universally useful and more stable biological marker ([³H]thymidine does not label postmitotic cells and is lost from those cells that undergo several further mitotic divisions after the initial labeling period). Unfortunately, there is no known parallel in rodents of the quail-chick transplant paradigm, which has been used so successfully in elucidating the development of the peripheral nervous system. In such transplant chimeras, quail cells are easily recognized by their distinctive "clumpy" heterochromatin pattern. By turning to cross-strain transplants in mice, however, we have found a promising paradigm in transplants between Mus musculus (any laboratory mouse strain) and Mus caroli (a mouse subspecies indigenous to Thailand). As reported by Rossant et al.,[20] there are distinct base sequence differences between the two species in areas of repeat sequence satellite DNA such that a genomic DNA probe, pMR196, can be used with great specificity to detect single Mus musculus cells against a background of Mus caroli cells. So far this probe has only been used in early development studies, where chimeras of Mus musculus-Mus caroli may offer great opportunities in the study of cell lineage. Although there is some problem with rejection that must be overcome in future studies, we

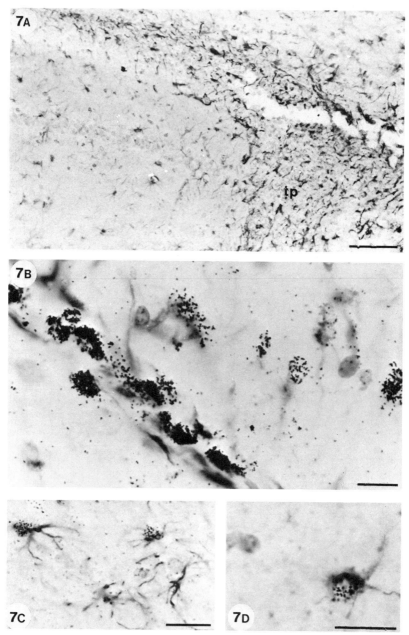

FIGURE 7. Grafts of astroglial cells (postnatal day 5 rat corpus callosum) labeled in culture with [³H]thymidine and reaggregated and implanted in a plasma clot. (**A**) Photograph of a glial cell graft (tp) within the hippocampal formation of an adult host after a survival time of 1 month. The section was stained with anti-GFAP antiserum. Note the prominent staining within the graft. Scale bar: 200 μm. (**B**) Heavily labeled nonneuronal cells in the region of the host-graft interface. Scale bar: 10 μm. (**C & D**) Stellate astrocytes of donor origin in the host neuropil. The donor origin is indicated by silver grains over the cell nuclei and the GFAP staining of the cellular processes. Scale bar: 20 μm.

have made several successful transplants of embryonic *Mus musculus* (Balb c) hippocampal primordia to adult *Mus caroli* hosts, as shown in FIGURE 8A. The host animals are much smaller (10 g) than laboratory mice, and the correspondingly smaller skull and brain size limits donor tissue to smaller grafts than we have used with laboratory strains of rats or mice. The effectiveness of the pMR196 probe for detection of *Mus musculus* cells by *in situ* hybridization is shown in FIGURES 8B & 8C, where a control section and a probe-labeled section of adult Balb c brain are compared. Although the resolution is not as yet optimal, because of some destruction of morphology during the harsh processing involved in *in situ* hybridization, the distribution of silver grains in FIGURE 8C brings out a pattern of dentate granule cell nuclei that is more or less identical to that observed in the adjacent stained section shown in FIGURE 8B. Use of this methodology to detect donor cells that have migrated into host brain is shown in FIGURE 8D where heavily labeled nonneuronal cells (large arrows) indicate detection via the DNA probe of *Mus musculus* cells in the hippocampal formation of the *Mus caroli* recipient. We hope that refinement of this technique coupled with double-labeling with cell-type-specific markers will circumvent possible objections raised to the interpretation of the origin of [³H]thymidine-labeled cells in transplant studies.

CONCLUSIONS

Grafting in the mammalian CNS is no longer a bizarre notion; it is a practical reality. Studies in the last decade that have used (for the most part) solid tissue grafts have concentrated 1) on the basic anatomical description of graft development and integration with recipient brain and 2) on examining the feasibility of using grafted tissue to restore functional or behavioral deficits arising through injury, disease, or aging.[21] To some degree, the future of intracerebral grafting as a research tool must lie in its utilization to understand the underlying cellular and molecular mechanisms that result in the very limited regenerative capacity of the adult mammalian CNS. To elucidate specific aspects of this mechanism through grafting studies, it is clear that the complexity of the donor tissue must ultimately be reduced to specific subpopulations of neurons or glia. Our preliminary studies outlined here, along with other studies using cell suspensions,[15–17] indicate that manipulation of the donor tissue in dissociated cell culture is compatible with the subsequent survival of grafted neurons or glia, and thus manipulation of embryonic tissue in an intermediate stage in culture shows promise as a method for enriching for specific cell types before transplantation. The plasma clot technique we have recently described[17] for the reaggregation and implantation of dissociated cells provides a simple method for implanting purified cells as a relatively compact graft, thus avoiding the dispersion of cells that occurs if cell suspensions are injected directly into host brain. The incorporation of donor cells within a small plasma clot does not appear to affect their survival or integration with the host, but advantageously localizes the cells (apart from migratory nonneuronal cells) at the site of implantation. This localization simplifies identification of the donor cells in histological sections, slice preparations, etc.

Finally, as we have described here, tissue culture manipulations and the plasma clot technique are readily combined with cell-labeling ([³H]thymidine) and cell-marking techniques (immunocytochemical staining with GFAP and for Thy-1 alleles) and can also be used with specific mRNA and DNA probes for *in situ* hybridization on tissue sections.

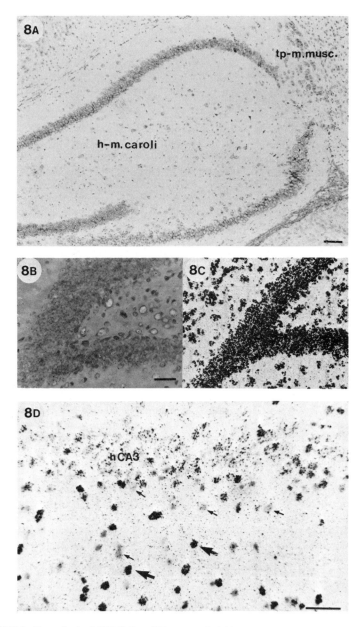

FIGURE 8. Transplant of E18 Balb c (*Mus musculus*) hippocampus to the hippocampal formation of an adult *Mus caroli* host. The transplant survived for 6 months. (**A**) Nissl-stained section showing the location of the transplant (tp-m.musc.) in the pyramidal layers of the recipient (h-m.caroli). Scale bar: 100 μm. (**B & C**) Control and hybridized sections, respectively, of Balb c mouse dentate gyrus. The *in situ* hybridization with the pMR196 probe (**C**) detects a pattern of nuclei similar to that observed with the histological stain. Scale bar: 50 μm. (**D**) Photograph of a section from the transplant in **A** after incubation of the section with the pMR196 probe. Large arrows indicate nonneuronal cells of graft origin (*Mus musculus*) that have migrated into host brain (*Mus caroli*). Host nuclei are unlabeled (small arrows). Scale bar: 50 μm.

ACKNOWLEDGMENTS

The authors gratefully acknowledge the expert work of Dr. C.-F. Zhou in much of the surgery with mice, and Mr. M. R. C. Sherwood with many of the other transplants. The histological expertise of Dr. J. M. Lawrence and Miss U. Starega was invaluable in these studies. R. M. L. thanks Drs. J. Rossant, B. Chapman, and N. Hastie for encouragement, advice, mice, and the pMR196 probe to undertake the *Mus caroli* experiments. Dr. B. Ely and Mrs. N. S. Lindsay are thanked for the help and advice they gave during our preliminary *in situ* hybridization studies.

REFERENCES

1. STENEVI, U., A. BJÖRKLUND & N.-A. SVENDGAARD. 1976. Transplantation of central and peripheral monoamine neurons to the adult rat brain: Techniques and conditions for survival. Brain Res. **114:** 1-20.
2. BJÖRKLUND, A. & U. STENEVI. 1984. Intracerebral neural implants: Neuronal replacement and reconstruction of damaged circuitries. Annu. Rev. Neurosci. **7:** 279-308.
3. BJÖRKLUND, A. & U. STENEVI, Eds. 1985. Neural Grafting in the Mammalian CNS. Elsevier. Amsterdam.
4. KROMER, L. F., A. BJÖRKLUND & U. STENEVI. 1983. Intracephalic embryonic neural implants in the adult rat brain. I. Growth and mature organization of brainstem, cerebellar, and hippocampal implants. J. Comp. Neurol. **218:** 433-459.
5. ZIMMER, J. & N. SUNDE. 1984. Neuropeptides and astroglia in intracerebral hippocampal transplants: An immunohistochemical study in the rat. J. Comp. Neurol. **227:** 331-347.
6. RAISMAN, G. & F. F. EBNER. 1983. Mossy fiber projections into and out of hippocampal transplants. Neuroscience **9:** 783-801.
7. RAISMAN, G. 1983. Formation of mossy fiber connections between hippocampal transplants and the brain of adult host rats. Acta Neurochir. **32**(Suppl.): 55-59.
8. LAWRENCE, J. M., S. K. HUANG & G. RAISMAN. 1984. Vascular and astrocytic reactions during establishment of hippocampal transplants in adult host brain. Neuroscience **12:** 745-760.
9. BAYER, S. A. 1980. Development of the hippocampal region in the rat. I. Neurogenesis examined with [³H]thymidine autoradiography. J. Comp. Neurol. **190:** 87-114.
10. LINDSAY, R. M. & G. RAISMAN. 1984. An autoradiographic study of neuronal development, vascularization and glial cell migration from hippocampal transplants labelled in intermediate explant culture. Neuroscience **12:** 513-530.
11. RAISMAN, G., J. M. LAWRENCE, C.-F. ZHOU & R. M. LINDSAY. 1985. Some neuronal, glial and vascular interactions which occur when developing hippocampal primordia are incorporated into adult host hippocampal. *In* Neural Grafting in the Mammalian CNS. A. Björklund & U. Stenevi, Eds.: 125-149. Elsevier. Amsterdam.
12. LINDSAY, R. M., G. RAISMAN & P. J. SEELEY. 1987. Neural tissue transplants: Studies using tissue culture manipulations, cell-marking techniques and a plasma clot method to follow development of grafted neurons and glia. *In* Glial-Neuronal Communication in Development and Regeneration. H. H. Althaus & W. Seifert, Eds.: 585-603. NATO ASI Series. Vol. 42. Springer. Heidelberg.
13. LINDSAY, R. M., P. C. BARBER, M. R. C. SHERWOOD, J. ZIMMER & G. RAISMAN. 1982. Astrocyte cultures from adult brain: Derivation, characterization, and neurotrophic properties of pure astroglial cells from corpus callosum. Brain Res. **243:** 329-343.
14. SCHMIDT, R. H., A. BJÖRKLUND & U. STENEVI. 1981. Intracerebral grafting of dissociated CNS tissue suspensions: A new approach to neuronal transplantation to deep brain sites. Brain Res. **218:** 347-356.
15. BRUNDIN, P., O. ISACSON & A. BJÖRKLUND. 1985. Monitoring of cell viability in sus-

pensions of embryonic CNS tissue and its use as a criterion for intracerebral graft survival. Brain Res. **331**: 251-259.

16. BRUNDIN, P., O. ISACSON, F. GAGE, U. STENEVI & A. BJÖRKLUND. 1985. Intracerebral grafts of neuronal cell suspensions. *In* Neural Grafting in the Mammalian CNS. A. Björklund & U. Stenevi, Eds.: 51-60. Elsevier. Amsterdam.

17. LINDSAY, R. M., G. RAISMAN & P. J. SEELEY. 1987. Intracerebral transplantation of cultured neurons after reaggregation in a plasma clot. Neuroscience. In press.

18. ZHOU, C.-F., G. RAISMAN & R. J. MORRIS. 1985. Specific patterns of outgrowth from transplants to host mice hippocampi, shown immunohistochemically by the use of allelic forms of Thy-1. Neuroscience **16**: 819-833.

19. CHARLTON, H. M., A. N. BARCLAY & A. F. WILLIAMS. 1983. Detection of neuronal tissue from brain grafts with anti-Thy-1.1 antibody. Nature **305**: 825-827.

20. ROSSANT, J., M. VIJH, L. D. SIRACUSA & V. M. CHAPMAN. 1983. Identification of embryonic cell lineages in histological sections of *M. musculus-M. caroli* chimeras. J. Embryol. Exp. Morphol. **73**: 163-178.

21. GAGE, F. H., A. BJÖRKLUND & U. STENEVI. 1984. Intrahippocampal septal grafts ameliorate learning impairments in aged rats. Science **255**: 533-536.

DISCUSSION OF THE PAPER

B. S. BREGMAN (*University of Maryland School of Medicine, Baltimore, MD*): Do you see any difference in either the extent or the pattern of migration in the adult callosal versus the hippocampal glial cells? And does that lead to a difference in the axonal interaction?

LINDSAY: We really have not analyzed that in detail yet, but I noticed the glial cells travel. In either case, we see double-labeled cells deposited close to the transplant, as well as small dark cells that have migrated farther distances.

L. KROMER (*Georgetown University, Washington, DC*): On some of your slides you have shown that the glial migration seems to be in sheets, almost. Are there fracture planes that you cause when you inject along the granule cell layer, that you can get preferential glial migration? If that is indeed the case, can you correlate axons along these glial planes?

LINDSAY: Certainly, in many cases the corpus callosum is damaged, and one sees a preference of glia to take a route like that. But in certain other areas, we have seen that there is no obvious degeneration of any kind, and you see many glia that are following different fiber bundles. So I do not think opening up the structure itself or degeneration is the only reason for astrocytic migration.

R. MIAO (*Hanna Biologics, Berkeley, CA*): On the most distant glial cells from the injection, do you find that there is a decrease in the number of silver granules per cell?

LINDSAY: I would say no. There are very densely labeled cells that have migrated a long way from the transplant. We have done a lot of controls where we have washed out the thymidine and where we have killed the transplant, and I think the idea that the host cells pick up thymidine is really not tenable.

Neural Transplantation in Normal and Traumatized Spinal Cord

GOPAL D. DAS

Department of Biological Sciences
Purdue University
West Lafayette, Indiana 47907

In recent years, there has been an overwhelming surge in research on neural transplantation as related to functional or clinically related issues. This kind of research requires appropriate animal models for neurological abnormality or deficiency. Models involving experimentally induced lesion or trauma to the nervous system are found to be the most valuable animal models for such investigations. In such preparations, the severity of trauma can be defined precisely in terms of anatomical structures, and the severity of immediate pathological reactions, such as hemorrhaging, can be noticed and controlled. These pathological conditions, no matter how well controlled, pose numerous problems for successful neural transplantation in a traumatized brain structure. Progress in neural transplantation in such preparations will require thorough basic research, in particular, analyses of the immediate and lasting pathological changes following a trauma, the relationship between the trauma and the neurological syndrome, and the interaction between pathological changes and the transplants. In the following, some findings are presented in relation to the surgical trauma to the spinal cord of the adult rat, and neural transplantation at the site of the trauma.

NEURAL TRANSPLANTATION IN A NORMAL SPINAL CORD

Transplantation of neural tissues in a normal spinal cord involves exposing the spinal cord by following an appropriate surgical procedure, inserting a needle carrying the transplant, and injecting the tissue within the spinal cord parenchyma.[1] This approach involves minimal trauma to the host neural structure. Even this minimal trauma, which is associated with the insertion of the needle and the injection of the transplant into the spinal cord, is seen to result in a small amount of hemorrhaging and edema immediately surrounding the path of the needle and the site of deposition of the transplant. The zone of the pathological reaction in the host spinal cord is restricted, and the pathological changes follow a short time course before they completely subside (FIG. 1). The neurons in this zone become necrotic and eventually die. The neural transplants, surrounded by this zone of pathological reaction, undergo some degree of initial necrosis, and then show phases of recovery and growth. Generally, the pathological conditions of hemorrhaging and edema in the host spinal cord subside 4-6 days after the surgery, and right around this time the neural transplants show their phase of growth. The outward growing surface of transplants gradually comes in close apposition to the exposed surface of the spinal cord parenchyma, and achieves the initial parenchymal attachment. This matching of time course between the two events is of great importance for the transplants to grow through the spongy tissue effectively and reach the normal and viable spinal cord tissue before glial scar formation sets in. The achievement of initial parenchymal attachment between the transplant and the host spinal cord is important as this provides the anatomical substratum for the development of a neural interface between the two. These conditions of rapid recovery and growth of neural transplants and maximum possible interface between the transplants and the host spinal cord are best achieved by employing neural transplants of high growth potential. If the time course between the two events, namely pathological conditions in the spinal cord and the recovery and growth of the transplants, is mismatched, the host spinal cord shows a glial reaction that develops into a glial scar formation at the exposed surface of the spinal cord parenchyma. As a result, the transplants that have followed a slow time course of recovery and growth become apposed to the glial scar formation and not the normal parenchyma of the spinal cord. This is observed when neural tissues of low growth potential, such as brain stem and spinal cord tissues from old donor embryos, are used as the transplants.

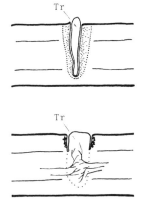

FIGURE 1. Schematic drawings to show neural transplantation in a normal, or nontraumatized, spinal cord. After the neural transplant is injected, a small zone of edema is left surrounding the transplant (Tr). The transplant becomes fully grown, fills the zone of edema, and becomes integrated with the spinal cord parenchyma.

Such transplants may survive as long as extraparenchymal transplants, and may show very tight apposition to the spinal cord but remain separated by a thin band of glial scar formation.[2] In some instances, where neonate animals are used as hosts, it is possible to see a small and fragmentary interface between transplants and the host spinal cord. In these preparations, however, where neural tissues of high growth potential are used and the transplants are seen to be maximally integrated with the host tissue, the true interface is seen primarily in the region of apposition to the gray matter of the spinal cord. It is through this interface that the transplants receive afferents from the host brain and project their efferents into it. Generally, at the region of apposition to the white matter of the spinal cord, a thin and compact glial scar formation is seen to intervene between the transplants and the spinal cord.

It is significant that these animals with minimal trauma do not show any readily detectable somatic abnormalities or deficiencies. Therefore, it is difficult to determine the nature of the functional role of these transplants. In order to investigate their functional role, it is essential to make large lesions in the spinal cord that produce permanent motor abnormalities or deficiencies, and then transplant neural tissues at the site of the trauma.[3,4] Some details on this are given in the following section.

NEURAL TRANSPLANTATION IN A TRAUMATIZED
SPINAL CORD

There are various models of inducing trauma to the spinal cord, such as weight-dropping, knife lesions, and surgical lesions involving ablation of tissue. Each model has its own advantages and disadvantages. The observations described below were made on animals that received surgical lesions and had tissue ablated at the lower thoracic level (T8-T9 or T9-T10) of the spinal cord. These lesions are far more extensive than those made with a knife, they bring about pathological conditions similar to those seen in weight-dropping trauma, and they can be defined precisely in anatomical terms at the time of surgery. Threshold-subtotal lesions that yield permanent paraplegic syndrome can be produced with a high degree of consistency, and the nature of pathological events following such lesions can be determined carefully; furthermore, the nature of the interaction between the pathological events and growing transplants can be investigated.[4]

Pattern of Pathological Changes

Pathological changes following a severe laceration type of trauma to the spinal cord can be broken down into three categories: direct or primary changes, secondary traumatic changes, and progressive degenerative changes. The order of these pathological conditions indicates their direction of spread from the site of trauma, and the time course they follow.

Primary Pathological Changes

The primary pathological changes are seen at the time of surgery. They include loss of neural tissue that is excised, physical trauma to the tissue close to the site of lesion, and damage to the vasculature (Fig. 2). A loss of neural tissue due to ablation is irreparable; that is, the loss of a mass of gray matter containing neurons and glial elements, as well as segments of axons coursing through that region, is permanent. Such a loss of tissue leaves behind a cavity in the spinal cord. The neural tissue along the borders of the cavity is also affected by the surgical lesion. Here, neurons are traumatized and are dislocated; axons are pulled and left frayed; and dendrites and synaptic structures are left damaged. Although immediately after the surgery this tissue may appear parenchymally an integral part of the intact spinal cord, it becomes necrotic within a few hours and is seen to be eventually phagocytized. The necrosis and loss of neural tissue along the borders of the lesion is the earliest pathological event that contributes to the enlargement of the cavity left behind by the lesion. Damage to the vasculature refers to the severing of blood vessels at the time the lesion was made. This damage leads to cutting open the arterioles, venules, and capillaries, which results in immediate bleeding at the site of the lesion. In the spinal cord, lesions of this severity invariably lead to extensive hemorrhaging—this is discussed below. It is important to remember that damage to major subdural and subpial arteries and veins invariably proves fatal. Unlike neural tissue, however, damaged blood vessels, after a certain period of recovery, show regenerative changes, which have an important bearing on the integration of the transplants.

Secondary Traumatic Changes

The secondary traumatic changes following a severe lesion include hemorrhaging, edema, ischemia, and vasoconstriction.[4-7] Hemorrhaging is the first reaction observed when a lesion is made. In the spinal cord, which has a rich vascular system, a lesion causes severe damage to numerous arterioles and venules. The resulting hemorrhage is always seen to be extensive, and extends into the spinal cord tissue a considerable distance from the site of the trauma. Generally, after reaching a peak, a hemorrhage is seen to slow down in about 5-10 minutes, and then subsides soon after. The blood cells, erythrocytes, and leukocytes that have infiltrated the spinal cord parenchyma

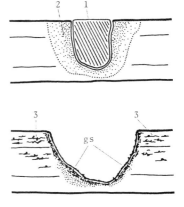

FIGURE 2. Schematic drawings to show the nature and development of pathological conditions after a severe trauma in the spinal cord of adult animals. The conditions are as follows: 1) primary traumatic changes: loss of tissue and damage to blood vessels by lesion; 2) secondary traumatic changes: hemorrhaging, edema, ischemia, and massive vasoconstriction in the tissue surrounding the lesion; and 3) progressive degenerative changes: persistent changes away from the site of the lesion. The loss of tissue because of primary and secondary traumatic changes results in cavitation. The cavity is bounded by glial scar (gs) formation.

remain in large patches, giving it the characteristic hemorrhagic appearance. If the hemorrhage continues for long, it invariably proves fatal. It is interesting to note that those animals that do survive severe hemorrhaging at the time of surgery become hypothermic: they lose the ability to achieve normal body temperature and, more often than not, fail to recover from anesthesia, and die. The few that recover from anesthesia remain hypothermic and die after a few days. Following a hemorrhage in close step is edema. It is characterized by sponginess of the tissue. Generally, an edema spreads into the spinal cord tissue far beyond the limits of the hemorrhage that preceded it. Unlike a hemorrhage, an edema continues to extend, reaching its peak 4-7 days after the lesion. At this stage, it becomes stationary and then slowly subsides. All the neuronal and glial elements in this edematous region become necrotic and die. Following this, the edematous tissue gradually shrinks, and the necrotic cells may be lysed away or phagocytized by macrophages. Loss of tissue in the edematous region is the main cause of enlargement of the cavity created by the lesion. It is important to note that the region of edema extending into the spinal cord is not uniform. As it comes close to the normal spinal cord, it shows a transition from fully edematous tissue containing a necrotic mass to partially edematous tissue containing a mixture of necrotic and viable cells, and finally to viable and normal spinal cord tissue. It is in this zone of partially edematous tissue that most of the interactions among the pathological tissue, normal spinal cord tissue, and growing transplants take place. It is here that the glial reaction, which appears in the form of glial proliferation; the emergence of glial scar formation; the regeneration and proliferation of damaged blood vessels; and the early signs of parenchymal attachment eventually leading to the development of an interface between the growing transplants and the spinal cord tissue are seen. Ischemic reaction of neurons and glial cells is seen not only throughout the region of the edematous reaction, but in the normal spinal cord. This pathological reaction develops fast, and lingers for a long time. Finally, of great importance is vasoconstriction. Strictly speaking, it should be considered as a collapse of the vasculature, including arterioles, venules, and capillary beds. It appears to be initiated by the direct trauma to the blood vessels themselves caused during the lesion, but extends rapidly into the region of the secondary traumatic changes. Many endothelial cells become necrotic. Collapsed blood vessels are generally confined within the region of the secondary traumatic reaction. Moreover, it is here that the subsequent vascular regenerative changes are seen. These secondary traumatic changes appear soon after the lesion is made. At first, they are close to the borders of the lesion; they then gradually extend deep into the spinal cord parenchyma. These pathological events may progress for some days before they eventually stop and slowly regress. Furthermore, these secondary pathological changes, following such extensive lesions of the spinal cord, are seen to extend for a distance of about one segment both rostrally and caudally. Since the necrotic tissue of the spinal cord in this region of secondary pathological changes lingers for a few days, it actually serves to slow down and inhibit the penetration of meningeal and mesenchymal tissue from outside. The glial proliferation in the zone of partially edematous tissue in the spinal cord, during these few days, is held at abeyance from precipitating into a glial scar formation by the protracted presence of this necrotic mass. This, as a matter of fact, proves to be favorable for the transplants so that they can grow through this disorganized mass easily and reach the intact spinal cord as fast as possible before the glial scar formation sets in as a barrier.[8–13]

Progressive Degenerative Changes

In addition to the above-mentioned primary and secondary traumatic changes, which are found in and around the site of the lesion, there are other pathological changes in the spinal cord, which are far removed from the region of trauma. They are known as progressive degenerative changes, and are seen to progress at a slow rate in the spinal cord as far as 8-10 segments away from the site of the lesion and to persist for many months. Of the various changes, the most striking ones are retrograde degeneration of neurons; enhanced glial density indicating glial reaction; presence of swollen and atrophied axons; vacuolation in the white matter region associated with the breakdown of myelin; and hypotrophy of astrocytes, particularly in the white matter. In the literature, there is no adequate information available on these progressive degenerative changes in the spinal cord. Experimental studies have shown that they are more extensive in control animals that have only received lesions than in the experimental animals that have received neural transplants in addition to lesions. Overall, the neural transplants seem to play a role in the reduction of these progressive degenerative changes, but only to a limited extent. The nature of these progressive degenerative changes indicates that even when neural transplants are fully grown and are maximally integrated with the host spinal cord, the traumatized spinal cord continues to undergo progressive degeneration, albeit at a slow rate. This finding has an important bearing on the functional or clinical significance of the neural transplants. It helps one to pose many relevant questions. To what extent is the observed clinical syndrome attributable to the primary changes, secondary traumatic changes, or progressive degenerative changes? Can a neural transplant arrest these pathological changes? Does a neural transplant truly compensate for the lost neural tissue both structurally and functionally, or does it merely support the spared structures of the spinal cord from progressive degeneration? These questions require thorough experimental analyses and, more importantly, provide a different perspective of viewing neural transplantation in relation to the trauma in the spinal cord.

Neural Transplants and Pathological Changes

Transplantation of neural tissues in a traumatized spinal cord requires an analysis of the influence of pathological events on the growth and integration of the neural transplants, and, reciprocally, an analysis of the effects of growing neural transplants on the course and intensity of pathological changes.[2,3,4,14] During the first few days after transplantation, the neural transplants are known to undergo some degree of necrosis; they then show recovery and growth.[15] The initial necrosis of transplants is minimal when the tissues are transplanted in a normal spinal cord, but this necrosis appears to be highly enhanced in a traumatized spinal cord. Then, during the later stages of development, as the secondary pathological changes become stabilized and start to regress, the neural transplants are seen to play a dominant role and aid in slowing or arresting some of the secondary traumatic changes and in containing the progressive degenerative changes.

Initially, after the primary trauma, the pathological changes follow an independent course and are influenced in no way by the transplants. Some of these changes—hemorrhaging, edema, and ischemia—appear to progress entirely on their own. They are related to the severity of the trauma. The transplants do not seem to have any influence on arresting these pathological changes or retarding their severity. Continued hemorrhaging and edema are seen to affect the initial survival of the transplants. Another external factor that affects the initial survival of the transplants is the penetration of loose connective tissue and interstitial fluid. Under such conditions, the mass of the transplanted neural tissues undergoing initial necrosis is seen to be very large; the mass of surviving transplants is very small. It is this small surviving mass of transplants that must recover and grow at a very fast rate if it is to grow, fill in the expanding cavity, push through the edematous tissue, and reach the normal spinal cord. These demands for recovery and growth are met only by the neural tissues that are characterized by high growth potential, such as neocortical tissue obtained from 15- or 16-day-old rat embryos.[16,17] This tissue contains neuroepithelial cells, which after their recovery following transplantation proliferate extensively at a high rate. Proliferation of neuroepithelial cells contributes to the growth in volume by increasing the number of cells, and this aids in the rapid growth of the transplants, in pushing through the edematous tissue, and in reaching the viable spinal cord tissue. Tissues with low growth potential, such as spinal cord or brain stem tissues from 15- or 16-day-old rat embryos fail to meet these developmental requirements. These tissues do not grow fast enough or produce masses of tissue large enough to fill the enlarging cavity. As a matter of fact, under these pathological conditions, large amounts of these transplants become necrotic and die. What remains is a small mass of tissue containing a small number of undifferentiated and partially differentiated neuroblasts in the transplants. They do not proliferate to yield more cells. As they differentiate, they yield only small and sluggishly growing transplants. They may survive as extra-parenchymal transplants, but are incapable of pushing through the edematous tissue and achieving the parenchymal attachment with the spinal cord tissue.[18] Under these conditions the secondary pathological changes progress unhindered and uninhibited at their own pace just as they do in control animals that receive only lesions. Thus, the secondary pathological conditions during the initial period have an effect on all types of neural transplants irrespective of their growth potential: transplants with high growth potential recover and grow rapidly to overcome these adverse conditions; transplants with low growth potential, however, fail to do so and undergo the secondary degenerative changes.

Goals of Neural Transplantation

At later stages, after the edema has reached its peak and shows signs of gradual decline, the neural transplants (neocortical transplants showing high growth potential)

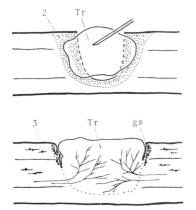

FIGURE 3. Schematic drawings to show the development of a neocortical transplant (Tr) after it has been intraparenchymally injected into a traumatized spinal cord. The top drawing shows the lesion site filled by the transplant, which must grow rapidly and push through the edematous tissue (2) and reach the spinal cord before glial scar (gs) formation sets in. The bottom drawing shows the transplant fully grown, filling the cavity, and integrated with the spinal cord parenchyma. The transplant has established an interface with the gray matter, but is separated from the white matter by glial scar formation (see FIG. 7 as well). Some progressive degenerative changes still persist.

are seen to have grown and extended into this edematous region. At this point, they seem to push through the necrotic tissue in the edematous region. By this process the necrotic tissue is broken down and pushed out. When the transplants reach the normal spinal cord and establish the initial parenchymal attachment, the first important goal of neural transplantation is achieved. In all likelihood the rapid growth of a neural transplant through the edematous region helps prevent the further spread of edema into the spinal cord. The region of initial parenchymal attachment between the transplant and the spinal cord eventually develops into a viable neural interface between the two. Furthermore, once the transplant has established an interface, development of glial scar formation in that region is arrested. As a rule, no glial scar formation as a morphological barrier is seen at the region of the interface. This indicates that the second major objective of neural transplantation in a traumatized spinal cord has been achieved (FIG. 3).

A neural transplant that has established a viable neural interface with the spinal cord tissue is generally seen to be anatomically integrated with it. Anatomical integration is achieved when afferents from the spinal cord, which are the axonal collaterals that have grown or sprouted from the partially damaged axons, have been received by the transplant and efferents from the transplant have been projected into the spinal cord.[1,3] Receiving axonal collaterals from the spinal cord and sustaining them permanently indicates that the third major goal of neural transplantation has been achieved. Fully grown and integrated transplants provide a neural milieu for the ingrowth of the collateral sprouts, which otherwise would have meandered through the edematous tissue and glial scar formation and would have remained as an abortive phenomenon. By this process, the neural transplants aid in preserving the spared axons or partially traumatized axons that would have otherwise degenerated during the course of progressive degeneration. The neural transplants thus seem to retard to some extent the progressive degeneration in a traumatized spinal cord.[4] This indicates that the fourth major goal of neural transplantation in a severely traumatized spinal cord has been achieved.

Persistent Pathological Conditions

Although successful neural transplantation in a traumatized spinal cord is seen to contribute to retardation and arrest of some pathological conditions, there are some pathological changes that are seen to remain permanently and, in some way, to affect the complete integration of the transplants with the spinal cord. Of the various persisting pathological changes only three will be discussed here: the penetration of perivascular fibers into the transplants, the presence of some glial scar formation, and the hypertrophy of astrocytes in the host spinal cord.

One primary traumatic change wrought by lesion on the spinal cord is damage to the blood vessels. The role of damaged blood vessels in some secondary pathological changes is considered to be important.[19] As the secondary traumatic conditions subside, however, the damaged blood vessels show active regeneration.[20] During the course of this regeneration, the perivascular fibers surrounding the blood vessels also show an extensive growth and arborization.[21-23] They essentially follow the blood vessels, but along the way they branch out profusely and penetrate into the neural transplants (FIG. 4). Since the blood vessels proliferate extensively while growing into the transplants and into the developing glial scar formation, the perivascular fibers are seen to grow largely in these regions (FIGS. 5 & 6). The perivascular fibers are characterized by their fine caliber, close juxtaposition to the blood vessels, and wavy or spiral pattern of coursing.[24,25] They are also characterized by a tendency to proliferate and arborize extensively—they often form dense meshworks in response to trauma.[26,27] As they penetrate into the transplants and glial scar formation they maintain these histological characteristics. The perivascular fibers in the transplants are seen to grow deep and terminate in the form of fine endings around the neurons. Although these observations are based upon Bodian-stain preparations, it is possible that they may indeed have synaptic endings on the neurons. If so, they would represent an additional source of afferents to the transplants. It is also possible to find some perivascular fibers growing into the white matter of the host spinal cord close to the glial scar formation and the transplant (FIG. 6). These findings based upon fiber stains may not reveal the full extent of growth of the perivascular fibers, but, with appropriate histochemical techniques, it may be possible to observe far more extensive ingrowth of these fibers. It is significant that these perivascular fibers remain permanently, provide fine terminations around the somata of the neurons, and represent afferents in addition to those from the spinal cord. The above morphological observations on perivascular fibers indicate that if these fibers are not analyzed adequately, it is highly probable that they may be misidentified as regenerating axons or axonal collaterals, particularly when they are near the site of trauma and near glial scar formations. Furthermore, various histochemical studies have shown that these fibers may be cholinergic,[28] adrenergic,[29,30] or both.[31,32] Irrespective of their histochemical differences, the perivascular fibers are autonomic, and they are capable of extensive regeneration and penetration into the parenchyma of the central nervous system.

The second lasting pathological condition is the presence of glial scar formation. It has been noted earlier that at the regions of apposition between the transplants and the damaged white matter a dense glial scar formation is seen (FIG. 7). It is primarily composed of hypertrophied astrocytes, oligodendroglial cells, macrophages, and a dense network of blood vessels (FIGS. 8 & 9). The network of blood vessels seems to be the scaffolding into which the neuroglial elements, macrophages, and perivascular

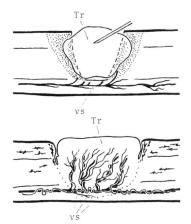

FIGURE 4. Schematic drawings to show how blood vessels (vs) of the spinal cord are damaged when lesions are made and how these blood vessels and the perivascular fibers surrounding them regenerate profusely and penetrate the transplant (Tr). The top drawing shows how the lesion damages arterioles and venules and how close the transplant is to the damaged blood vessels. The bottom drawing shows the transplant fully grown. Damaged blood vessels have regenerated and penetrated the transplant; perivascular fibers have also regenerated. These fibers follow the blood vessels and penetrate the transplant, where they remain permanently. It should be noted that many blood vessels are damaged during surgery, and that they grow into the transplant in varying degrees.

fibers are embedded. It does seem to be an insurmountable barrier for the late-arising fine collaterals of damaged axons, which represent an abortive regenerative phenomenon.[33] No fibers are seen to penetrate the transplants through this scar formation. In some cases, it may be very thin; in others, very dense. In some cases, the scar formation and the transplant may be tightly apposed: still, no afferent fibers are seen to penetrate the transplant.[1,3,4] These observations indicate that a neural transplant growing in a pathological environment of traumatized spinal cord is able to achieve anatomical integration only with the gray matter region, and not with the damaged white matter regions of the spinal cord. In the literature, it is generally assumed that because of glial scar formation the damaged axons do not regenerate. This prevalent notion does not take the following into consideration: that glial scar formation does not emerge immediately after the lesion to stand as a barrier against the damaged axons, that it has its own developmental history, that it develops gradually as the secondary pathological conditions subside, and that it actually serves as a barrier to the invading pathological conditions in the spinal cord. It is an important protective mechanism for the preservation of the spared and normal neural tissue; it remains

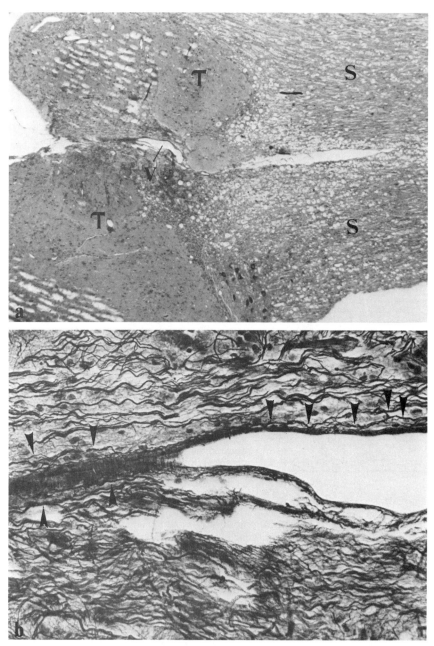

FIGURE 5. Sections showing a neocortical transplant in the spinal cord 6 months following extensive lesion (Bodian-Protargol stain). (a) Horizontal view of the transplant (T) and the host spinal cord (S). A venule (V) is seen, from the ventral aspect, to enter the transplant. (b) High-power view of the venule. Arrowheads indicate some perivascular fibers closely related to the venule. Other fibers, wavy and spiral in appearance, are also perivascular fibers. These fibers are related to other blood vessels but have branched out to penetrate the parenchyma. The original magnifications for **a** and **b** were ×25 and ×250, respectively; the figure was enlarged to 102% of its original size.

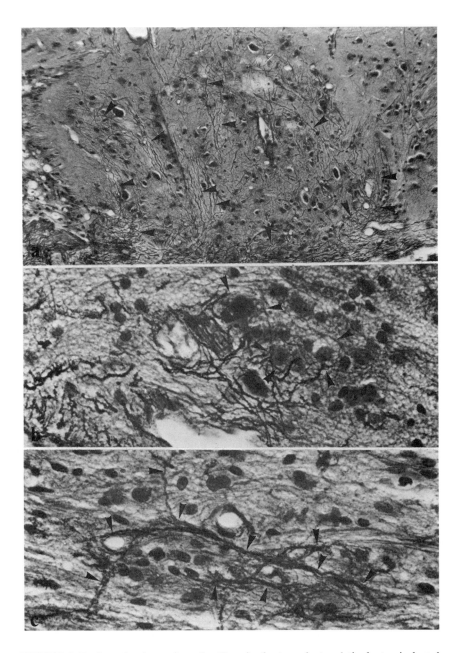

FIGURE 6. Sections showing perivascular fibers in the transplant and the host spinal cord (Bodian-Protargol stain). (a) Fine-caliber perivascular fibers are seen to break away from the blood vessels and to penetrate the transplant (arrowheads). (b) Perivascular fibers are found to enwrap the neurons of the transplant (arrowheads), thus, very likely, providing synaptic endings on them. (c) Perivascular fibers (arrowheads) very close to the glial scar formation between the transplant and the host spinal cord penetrating into a fiber tract of the host spinal cord. Instead of running straight and parallel to the host fibers, they are seen to form a meshwork. The magnifications for **a**, **b**, and **c** are ×100, ×400, and ×400, respectively.

permanently. Neural transplants, even those with high growth potential, are not seen to penetrate it. These two lasting pathological changes, among others, indicate that the neural transplants, although histologically normal and well integrated with the damaged host spinal cord, do not obliterate all the pathological changes. They interact during their development with pathological changes surrounding them in such a manner that they aid in the reduction and containment of the pathological reactions. The final outcome is a neural transplant surrounded by some residual pathological conditions that manages to maintain anatomical integration with the host spinal cord.

There are various other pathological changes that seem to linger for a long time in the host spinal cord, and the most striking one is the presence of hypertrophied astrocytes in the white matter regions subjected to trauma. It is one of the charac-

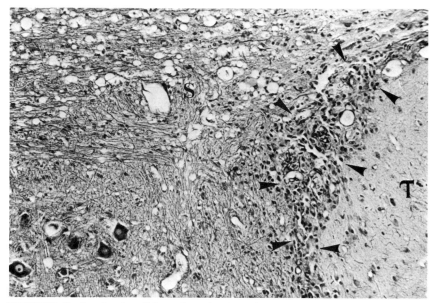

FIGURE 7. Section showing glial scar formation (arrowheads) between the transplants (T) and the white matter of the host spinal cord (S) (Bodian-Protargol stain). Note that in the white matter region some necrotic mass is still seen close to the glial scar formation, and that vacuoles of different sizes are seen within the fiber tract. Original magnification: ×130; enlarged to 102% of original size.

teristics of progressive degeneration in the spinal cord. The mechanism that induces such a reaction is unknown. The hypertrophied astrocytes can be seen 8-10 segments away rostrally as well as caudally from the site of the lesion. They are located within the vacuolated white matter that has atrophied axons. These astrocytes have very long processes that extend for more than 100 μm parallel to atrophying axons. These long processes are readily observed in Golgi-Cox preparations (FIGS. 10 & 11). They might, however, remain unnoticed or, if noticed, be misinterpreted in routine histological and histochemical preparations. Their exact role in the failure of damaged axons to regenerate, in the continued breakdown of myelin, and in the slow and gradual atrophy of axons is unknown. Their presence, however, indicates that even with the best possible neural transplantation, low-level degenerative changes in the host spinal cord remain for a long time.

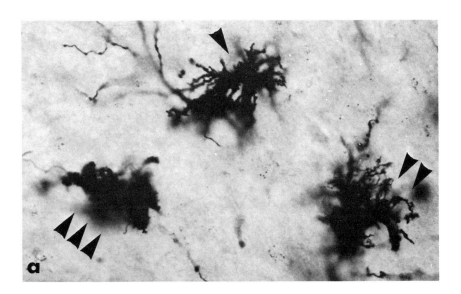

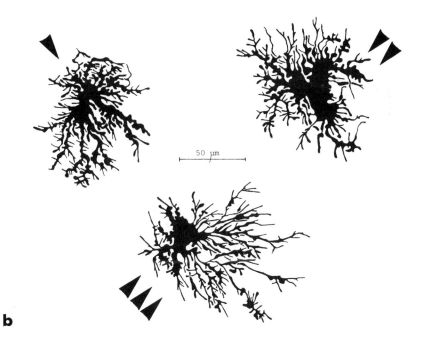

FIGURE 8. (a) Section showing hypertrophied astrocytes in the glial scar formation (Golgi-Cox impregnation). The astrocytes, which are marked with arrowheads, are drawn in **b**. Original magnification: ×330; enlarged to 102% of original size. (b) Drawings of the hypertrophied astrocytes. The astrocyte indicated with three arrowheads was out of the plane of focusing in **a**. Note the large size of the astrocytes and the extensive arborization of their processes.

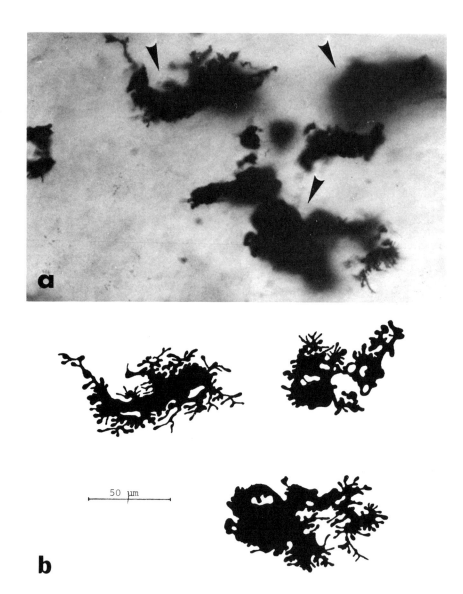

FIGURE 9. (a) Section showing macrophages in the glial scar formation (Golgi-Cox impregnation). Detailed drawings of those macrophages marked with arrowheads are shown in **b**. Original magnification: $\times 330$; enlarged to 130% of original size. **(b)** Drawing of the macrophages. Note their large size, the presence of vacuoles, and the various forms of pseudopodia extending out from their somata.

A General Comment

The pathological findings presented above are not unique to the traumatized spinal cord. They are also observable when severe trauma is caused to other neural structures in an attempt to deposit neural transplants in surgically prepared cavities. Pathological changes following severe trauma to brain structures rostral to brain stem have effects not only on the survival, growth, and integration of neural transplants, but on various

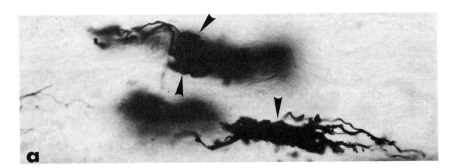

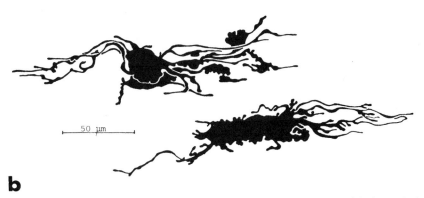

FIGURE 10. (a) Section showing hypertrophied astrocytes in the white matter of the host spinal cord, 8-10 segments away from the site of lesion and transplantation (Golgi-Cox impregnation). The three astrocytes marked with arrows are shown in greater detail in the drawing in **b**. Original magnification: ×330; enlarged to 102% of original size. (b) Drawing of the three astrocytes. Note their large size and long processes running parallel to the host axons. The processes of upper two astrocytes show flower-like expansions.

other telencephalic and subtelencephalic structures of the host brain. In researches addressing the trauma to the telencephalic and subtelencephalic structures, it is important to ask the following questions: To what extent do such generalized pathological changes, an aspect of progressive degenerative changes, have a bearing on the functional repertoire of the animals and the functional compensation following such a severe trauma? To what extent can such functional changes, particularly improvements, be directly attributed to the neural transplants? Histopathological analyses of host brain and transplants are essential if experimental findings are to be correctly interpreted and the true underlying causal relationships revealed.

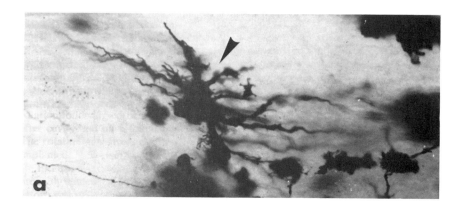

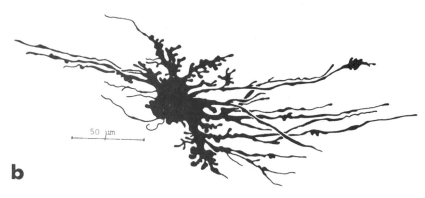

FIGURE 11. (a) Section showing a hypertrophied astrocyte embedded in the white matter of the spinal cord (Golgi-Cox impregnation). It is shown in detail in the drawing below. Original magnification: ×330; enlarged to 103% of original size. (b) Drawing of the astrocyte. Note its large size, the extensive branching of its processes, the long processes running parallel to the axons of the host spinal cord, and the irregular expansions along its processes.

CONCLUDING COMMENTS

1. It is possible to obtain fully grown and well-integrated neural transplants in a traumatized spinal cord only when neural tissues with high growth potential are used for transplantation, and only when they are injected intraparenchymally.[34,35]
2. Growing transplants are capable of pushing through the region of secondary pathological conditions, which is characterized by hemorrhaging, edema, and ischemia.
3. The absence of vascular supply during the first few days after the surgery does not affect the initial survival and growth of the transplants.
4. Neural transplants readily establish a neural interface with the normal gray matter of the spinal cord, but they are unable to establish an interface with

damaged white matter. A glial scar formation is seen to intervene in this region.

5. If a neural transplant is of moderate or low growth potential, it is unable to grow and push through the region of edematous spinal cord tissue: it is thus unable to establish an interface with the spinal cord. In such a case, glial scar formation covers the entire surface of the cavity in the spinal cord and keeps the transplant totally isolated from the spinal cord parenchyma.

6. Progressive pathological changes, such as protracted degeneration of the severed and the partially damaged axons and gradual necrosis of neurons near and far away from the site of the lesion, seem to persist for a long time—even after a transplant has grown and become integrated. Neural transplants do not stop or obliterate pathological conditions completely. At best, these transplants slow them and thus retard their effects.

7. One of the permanent changes is the extensive growth of perivascular fibers into the transplants, into the glial scar formation, and into the host spinal cord.

8. Hypertrophy of astrocytes, as a lasting pathological condition, is commonly seen in the traumatized spinal cord. Its effects on the integration and on the functional role of transplants are not known.

9. The collateral sprouts that penetrate transplants as afferents are seen to arise mainly from partially damaged axons and axons severed close to their terminations. Such axons are found near and in the gray matter of the spinal cord. Axons severed in their midcourse, which are found in the dorsal and lateral fasciculi, do not show new sprouts emerging from their cut ends; they simply atrophy and gradually degenerate.

10. The functional or clinical significance of neural transplants should always be viewed in the context of the nature of their integration with the spinal cord, the lasting pathological conditions, and the growth of perivascular or autonomic fibers into the transplants.

REFERENCES

1. DAS, G. D. 1983. *In* Reconstruction of the Spinal Cord. C. C. Kao, R. P. Bunge & P. J. Reier, Eds.: 367-396. Raven Press, New York, NY.
2. DAS, G. D. 1983. *In* Neural Tissue Transplantation Research. R. B. Wallace & G. D. Das, Eds.: 1-64. Springer-Verlag. New York, NY.
3. DAS, G. D. 1983. J. Neurol. Sci. **62:** 191-210.
4. DAS, G. D. 1986. *In* Neural Transplantation and Regeneration. G. D. Das & R. B. Wallace, Eds.: 1-61. Springer-Verlag. New York, NY.
5. TATOR, C. H. 1972. Can. Med. Assoc. J. **107:** 143-150.
6. OSTERHOLM, J. L. 1974. J. Neurosurg. **40:** 5-33.
7. DUCKER, T. B. 1976. *In* Handbook of Clinical Neurology. Injuries of the Spine and Spinal Cord. Part I. Vol. 25. P. J. Vinken & G. W. Bruyn, Eds.: 9-26. Elsevier/North-Holland. Amsterdam.
8. PENFIELD, W. 1927. Brain **50:** 499-517.
9. BROWN, J. O. & G. P. McCOUCH. 1947. J. Comp. Neurol. **87:** 131-137.
10. LAMPERT, P. W. & M. CRESSMAN. 1964. Lab. Invest. **13:** 825-839.
11. MATHEWS, M. A., M. F. ST. ONGE, C. L. FACIANE & J. B. GELDERD. 1979. Neuropathol. Appl. Neurobiol. **5:** 161-180.
12. MATHEWS, M. A., M. F. ST. ONGE, C. L. FACIANE & J. B. GELDERD. 1979. Neuropathol. Appl. Neurobiol. **5:** 181-196.

13. LUDWIN, S. K. 1985. Lab. Invest. **52:** 20-30.
14. DAS, G. D. 1986. Exp. Brain Res. **13**(Suppl.): 88-106.
15. DAS, G. D., K. G. DAS, J. BRASKO & J. ALEMAN-GOMEZ. 1983. Neurosci. Lett. **41:** 73-79.
16. DAS, G. D., B. H. HALLS & K. G. DAS. 1980. Am. J. Anat. **158:** 135-145.
17. DAS, G. D. 1986. Exp. Brain Res. **13**(Suppl.): 333-350.
18. DAS, G. D. 1982. Brain Res. **241:** 182-186.
19. BALENTINE, J. D. & D. U. PARIS. 1978. Lab. Invest. **39:** 236-253.
20. CANCILLA, P. A., S. P. FROMMES, L. E. KAHN & L. E. DEBAULT. 1979. Lab. Invest. **40:** 74-82.
21. LOY, R. & R. Y. MOORE. 1977. Exp. Neurol. **57:** 399-411.
22. STENEVI, U. & A. BJÖRKLUND. 1978. Neurosci. Lett. **7:** 219-224.
23. MILNER, T. A. & R. LOY. 1980. Anat. Embryol. **161:** 159-168.
24. RICHARDSON, K. C. 1960. J. Anat. (London) **94:** 457-472.
25. ITAKURA, T. 1983. J. Neurosurg. **58:** 900-905.
26. LEE, F. C. 1929. Physiol. Rev. **9:** 575-623.
27. CLARK, E. R., E. L. CLARK & R. G. WILLIAMS. 1934. Am. J. Physiol. **212:** 1081-1085.
28. D'ALECY, L. G. & C. J. ROSE. 1977. Circ. Res. **41:** 324-331.
29. OGUSHI, N. 1968. Arch. Jpn. Chir. **37:** 294-303.
30. MCNICHOLAS, L. F., W. R. MARTIN, J. W. SLOAN & M. NOZAKI. 1980. Exp. Neurol. **69:** 383-394.
31. MEYLING, H. A. 1953. J. Comp. Neurol. **99:** 495-535.
32. IWAYAMA, T., J. B. FURNESS & G. BURNSTOCK. 1970. Circ. Res. **26:** 635-646.
33. RAMON Y CAJAL, S. 1928. Degeneration and Regeneration of the Nervous System. R. M. May, Trans. and Ed. Oxford University Press. London.
34. DAS, G. D. 1974. TIT J. Life Sci. **4:** 93-124.
35. DAS, G. D., B. H. HALLS & K. G. DAS. 1980. Experientia **35:** 143-153.

DISCUSSION OF THE PAPER

C. B. JAEGER (*New York University Medical Center, New York, NY*): It seems these perivascular fibers may be autonomic. Have you done any experiments removing input from the autonomic nervous system to the central nervous system?

DAS: No, we are not doing anything of the kind.

Transplantation of Human Embryonic Oligodendrocytes into Shiverer Brain[a]

M. GUMPEL,[b,c] F. LACHAPELLE,[c] A. GANSMULLER,[c]
M. BAULAC,[d] A. BARON VAN EVERCOOREN,[c]
AND N. BAUMANN[c]

[c]Laboratoire de Neurochimie
Institut National de La Santé
et de la Recherche Médicale Unité 134
and
[d]Laboratoire Charles Foix
Hôpital de la Salpêtrière
Paris, France

INTRODUCTION

In previous papers, we described experiments in which fragments of newborn mouse (normal or mutant) olfactory bulb were implanted into newborn mouse brain in such experimental conditions that the myelin formed by transplanted oligodendrocytes could be distinguished from the myelin of the host. Under these conditions, transplanted oligodendrocytes have been shown to survive in the host brain, to migrate over very long distances, and to myelinate host axons.[1-7]

The use of human embryonic brain tissues appeared interesting from at least three points of view.

1) The myelination process is much longer in man than in mouse. By using intracerebral transplantation techniques, it is possible to create a situation in which human oligodendrocytes at a premyelinating stage *in situ* are placed in a myelin-forming mouse brain. The differentiation of human oligodendrocytes could thus be studied in a very heterochronic environment.

2) Primates and rodents, although both mammals, are phylogenetically divergent and different regarding brain anatomy. It might be interesting to compare the respective behaviors of mouse and human oligodendrocytes and their interactions with the mouse brain cells and structures. It should also be interesting to know whether human grafts are rejected.

3) Myelination by transplanted oligodendrocytes could be considered as a possible

[a]This work was supported by ARSEP, INSERM, and Grant 1773 A1 from the National Multiple Sclerosis Society.

[b]Address for correspondance: Laboratoire de Neurochimie, INSERM U134, Hôpital de la Salpêtrière, 47 Boulevard de l'Hôpital, 75651 Paris Cedex 13, France.

approach to repair demyelination diseases. Thus, among many other problems, it seemed worthwhile to study the conditions of transplantability of human brain material during development.

MATERIALS AND METHODS

Shiverer Model

The shiverer model makes it possible to distinguish, in mature animals, between the myelin formed by transplanted oligodendrocytes and the myelin of the host. The shiverer model has been described in detail elsewhere.[1-6] Very briefly, the shiverer mutant mouse[8] is hypomyelinated, and its myelin is chemically deprived of myelin basic protein (MBP) (FIGS. 1A & 1B).[9-12] In these conditions, MBP$^+$ myelin from implanted oligodendrocytes appears clearly in immunohistology using the antiserum anti-MBP. Moreover, the shiverer myelin presents a defect of compaction of the myelin lamellae at the level of the major dense line. Thus the presence of myelin formed by transplanted oligodendrocytes in shiverer brain can be confirmed by electron microscopy studies. Such studies reveal more details on the host reaction at the level of MBP$^+$ myelinated axons.[6] The host was always a newborn shiverer mouse (0-24 hr after birth).

Grafts

The graft was always a solid fragment of human embryonic brain. Even at the late stage of 20 weeks, no signs of myelination was ever detected (FIG. 1C). It is necessary, however, to divide the grafts into three main groups.

First Series

During the last 3 years, we obtained three 20-week-old human embryos by cesarian operation. We also transplanted tissues from seven embryos obtained 14, 19, and 20 weeks after expulsion provoked by prostaglandins. In these 10 embryos, we were able to dissect any region of the brain. We could then transplant periventricular layer removed at any rostrocaudal level.

Immediately after expulsion, the embryonic tissues were placed on ice, dissected, and transplanted within the next 3 hr. It must be noted here that we never obtained survival of grafts dissected from embryos obtained by expulsion provoked by prostaglandins. In all of these cases, the embryo was probably dead several hours before expulsion: the brain cells appeared necrotic even at first examination. The dissected fragments of CNS tissue (1-2 mm^3) were placed in saline on ice. Finally, charcoal powder was added. The powder adhered to the tissues and allowed the detection of the grafted tissues in the host brain after fixation.

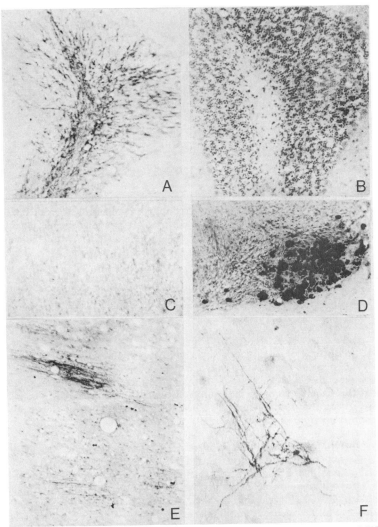

FIGURE 1. Each section in this figure was treated immunohistologically to detect MBP and was colored with methyl green. Original magnifications shown in parentheses; figure reduced to 60% of original size. (**A**) Section from the cerebellum of a control adult mouse. Note the PAP$^+$ reaction of the myelin ($\times 180$). (**B**) Section from the cerebellum of a shiverer adult brain. The cells were made visible by the use of a red filter. There was no MBP reaction in the myelin ($\times 180$). (**C**) Human embryo (16 weeks old). Periventricular zone of the telencephalon. Columnar organization with probable presence of radial glia. No MBP$^+$ reaction. The same result was obtained with a 20-week-old embryo. No positive myelinated fibers were ever detected at this stage ($\times 120$). (**D**) Graft of 6-week-old human CNS tissue in the brain of a newborn shiverer. Sixty days after grafting, the tissues heavily marked with charcoal were well integrated into the host tissues ($\times 100$). (**E**) Graft from a 16-week-old human embryo in the anterior thalamus of a newborn shiverer. Thirty days after grafting, MBP$^+$ myelin was found in the spinal cord ($\times 180$). (**F**) Graft from an 8-week-old human embryo in the rostral thalamus of a newborn shiverer. Thirty days after grafting, MBP$^+$ myelin patches were found in the brain stem ($\times 450$).

Second Series

An 16-week-old embryo was obtained by fragmentation followed by suction abortion. The skull was partially preserved with the left hemisphere and a part of the cerebellum. From this embryo, we transplanted only periventricular tissue from the left hemisphere. According to neuromorphologists, the immature oligodendroblasts are supposed to be present as free cells in the periventricular layer.[13]

Third Series

Embryos in this series were 6-8 weeks old and were obtained by suction abortion. Although the integrity of these embryos could not be preserved, fragments of central nervous system (CNS) could be easily recognized. It was not possible, however, to specify their anatomical origin inside the brain. Spinal cord tissue was always avoided by taking nervous tissues still attached to the skull.

Transplantation and Sample Preparation

The transplantation was performed under cold anesthesia according to a procedure already described,[2] by means of a micropipette connected to a peristaltic pump. The tissue to be grafted was placed at the extremity of the pipette to prevent saline from entering the brain. If even a small quantity of liquid was introduced, it was immediately expulsed. Because it has now been demonstrated that migration of oligodendrocytes can occur from any location in the brain,[7] the graft was placed at various transplantation sites.

Ten to 130 days after grafting (most of the shiverer mice die between 90 and 120 days), the host animals were anesthetized with Imalgen G500 (Mérieux) and Vetranquil (Clin Midi). For immunocytochemistry, the animals were intracardially perfused with a fixative, which was a solution of 4% paraformaldehyde and 1% glutaraldehyde in 0.1 M sodium phosphate buffer, pH 7.3, at 20° C. After perfusion, the brains were dissected out and immersed in the same fixative for 24 hr at 4° C. Finally, the brains were washed overnight in 0.1 M sodium phosphate buffer, pH 7.3, and immersed for 24 hr in the same buffer with 10% sucrose.

Then the brains were embedded and frozen in OCT (Miles Laboratories). The grafted hemisphere was sagitally sectioned on a cryostat, and the 6-μm-thick sections were collected at the level where the graft was localized.

This technique does not provide a view of the distribution throughout the whole brain of myelin formed by implanted oligodendrocytes. In the positive cases that were studied, however, including those in which the whole brain was sectioned,[7] at least a few MBP+ myelin fibers could always be found around the graft. Thus, it is most probable that we were able to detect all the cases with myelination by implanted oligodendrocytes by studying only those tissues directly surrounding the graft.

However, serial horizontal sections from brains that had received a graft were collected. It was possible to appreciate, after preparing the material for immunohistological study, the dispersion of the myelin with respect to the different structures of the brain and the location of the graft.[7]

Immunohistology

In the immunohistological studies, the peroxidase-antiperoxidase (PAP) labeling technique[14] was used instead of the FITC labeling technique.[2] The sections were first immersed for 5 min in 100% ethanol at 20° C, then treated for 30 min in a 1:100 to 1:1000 solution of anti-MBP rabbit antiserum (according to the origin of the serum) containing 10% of normal sheep serum in phosphate-buffered saline (PBS). After washing, the tissues were incubated with a 1:20 solution of antirabbit sheep antiserum in PBS and with a 1:100 solution of rabbit PAP-complexed serum (Miles Laboratories). After rinsing in PBS, the PAP-labeled complex was revealed after being immersed for 20 min in a 0.005% solution of diaminobenzidine with 0.02% H_2O_2. Sections from adult normal mice and shiverer mice brains were submitted to the same treatment in each experiment to serve as positive and negative controls.

Electron Microscopy

It has been possible to study the graft or the host-graft interactions or even the myelin formed by grafted oligodendrocytes in host tissues surrounding the graft by using classical electron microscopy fixation and embedding. But, as myelin formed by implanted oligodendrocytes was very dispersed in the host brain, it did not seem possible to study the patches of myelin formed by oligodendrocytes far from the graft without a prelocalization of these patches by immunohistology.

Thus, after the fixation described above, the hemispheres containing the graft marked with charcoal were immersed for 6 hr at 4° C in the fixative, washed for 24 hr in PBS, and immersed for 24 hr in the same buffer with 10% sucrose and 10% glycerol. The samples were embedded and frozen in OCT and sectioned on a cryostat so as to obtain alternating 10- and 60-μm-thick sections. The 10-μm-thick sections were tested for immunocytochemistry as described above. The MBP$^+$ areas were dissected out from the adjacent 60-μm-thick sections, and these dissected areas were prepared for electron microscopy. The MBP$^+$ tissue was immersed for 1 hr at 4° C in 2% osmic acid. Serial dehydration and embedding in epon were followed by semithin sections stained with toludine blue. These sections were then observed to determine the location and density of the MBP$^+$ fibers, which were usually clearly defined because of the thickness of human myelin compared to shiverer myelin. Finally, 600-Å-thick sections of the most interesting areas were contrasted with uranyl acetate and lead citrate and observed in a JEOL 100 CX microscope at 80 kV.[6]

RESULTS

We studied 83 shiverer brains transplanted with fragments of human embryonic material that were obtained and subsequently maintained on ice for a maximum of 3 hr.

Myelination and the Length of the Experiment

First Series

We had the whole brain for each of the 20-week-old embryos, and were thus able to design an experiment to study the myelinating properties of different regions of the donor brain. The fragments to be transplanted were excised in the periventricular region of the telencephalon, diencephalon, cerebellum, and rhombencephalon. We killed the host animals 60, 70-75, and 115-130 days after grafting. The total number of animals showing MBP$^+$ myelination after grafting in this series did not seem to be significantly different from that in either of the other two series. The most important result was that oligodendrocytes from any part of the brain were able to survive and myelinate in the host brain. Vertically, it appeared that healthy immunoreactive myelin was present for at least 130 days (TABLE 1).

TABLE 1. Myelination from 20-week-old Human Embryo Tissue with Respect to Origin of the Graft

	Number of Animals with MBP$^+$ Myelination/ Number of Animals Tested			
	Days after Grafting			
Origin of the Graft	60	70–75	115–130	Total
Rostral telencephalon	1/1	8/15	2/3	11/19 (58)
Diencephalon	2/3	3/3	1/3	6/9 (67)
Cerebellum	1/3	0/3	3/3	4/9 (44)
Rhombencephalon and cervical cord	1/1	1/3		2/4 (50)
Total	5/8(63)	12/24(5)	6/9(66)	

NOTE: Percentages shown in parentheses.

It must be noted that this series was the first one that we performed with human tissue, and that we sometimes transplanted fragments of CNS that were too large. In these conditions, some grafts became necrotic in the middle. This is probably the reason for the relatively low percentage of animals myelinated by the graft, compared to series 1 and 2.

Second Series

This second series of experiments was performed with 16-week-old embryos. We did not have the complete brain, but we did have one hemisphere and a part of the cerebellum. The material we implanted was always a fragment of the telencephalon periventricular area. Taking advantage of our experience in the first series, we transplanted very small fragments of CNS (FIGS. 1E, 2A, 2C & 2F).

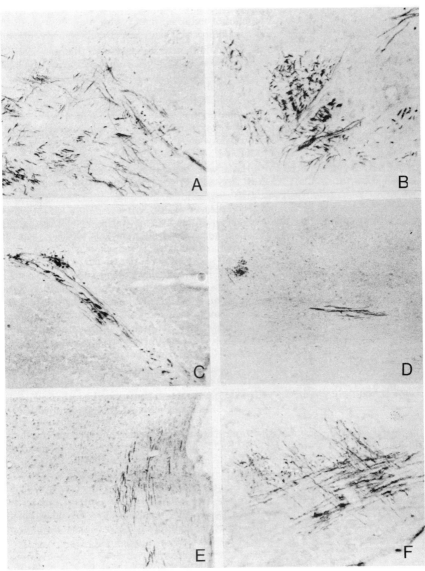

FIGURE 2. (A) A 16-week-old human embryo 50 days after grafting. Note the patch of MBP⁺ myelin at the level of the brain stem. The graft was in the internal capsule (×40). (B) An 8-week-old human embryo 22 days after grafting. Note the zone of MBP⁺ myelin in the brain stem. The graft was in the rostral thalamus (×180). (C) A 16-week-old human embryo 50 days after grafting. Note the MBP⁺ myelin in the cerebellum (×150). (D) An 8-week-old human embryo grafted into the brain of a newborn shiverer. Twenty-two days after grafting, myelination was found in the hippocampus (×150). (E) An 8-week-old human embryo grafted into the brain of a newborn shiverer. Twenty-two days after grafting, MBP⁺ myelination was found in the spinal cord. (F) A 16-week-old human embryo grafted into the brain of a newborn shiverer. Note the MBP⁺ myelination in the spinal cord (×180). Original magnifications shown in parentheses; figure reduced to 65% of original size.

TABLE 2. Myelination from 16-week-old Human Embryo Tissue with Respect to the Length of the Experiment

	Days after Grafting						
	5	10	17	19	25	35	50
Number of animals with MBP$^+$ myelination/ Number of animals tested	0/5	0/5	1/5	2/2	5/6	1/1	5/7

NOTE: Combined figures for days 5 and 10: 0/10; for days 19, 25, 35, and 50: 13/16 (81%).

Animals were sacrificed 6, 10, 17, 19, 28, 35, and 50 days after grafting. TABLE 2 summarizes the results. Five to 10 days after grafting, the implant appeared healthy, but no MBP$^+$ myelin was present.

The first signs of MBP$^+$ myelination appeared at day 17. We noted at this stage a long-distance migration and myelination in the cerebellum. From day 19 to day 50, 13 grafted brains out of 16 (81%) showed numerous patches of MBP$^+$ myelin. It should be noted that the age of transplanted oligodendrocytes 17 days after grafting is 16 weeks plus 17 days (nearly 5 months) (FIGS. 1D, 1F, 2B, 2D & 2E).

According to Yakovlev and Lecours,[15] myelination is detected in man at this stage only at the level of the motor roots in the spinal cord. In the brain, myelination starts later on. This experiment, however, does not seem convincing enough. Nobody knows exactly where the myelinating oligodendrocytes are located in the spinal cord during their premature stage. We have demonstrated that myelination is possible in the spinal cord from a graft placed in the anterior brain.

Third Series

In this series we grafted tissue from 6-8-week-old human embryos into newborn shiverer brain. It was not possible to identify a specific brain structure because of the dilaceration of the embryo. Spinal cord tissue, however, was avoided.

We studied 11 host animals, and animals were killed after 22, 30, 45, and 60 days (TABLE 3). Seventy-two percent were myelinated by human oligodendrocytes. Three out of 3 were positive at day 22 with a large extent of MBP$^+$ myelin and a long migration, which probably means that implanted oligodendrocytes myelinate before day 22. It should be noted that the oligodendrocytes from the grafts in this series are

TABLE 3. Myelination from 6-8-week-old Human Embryo Tissue with Respect to the Length of the Experiment

	Days after Grafting			
	22	30	45	60
Number of animals with MBP$^+$ myelination/ Number of animals tested	3/3	1/2	1/3	3/3

NOTE: Combined figures for the whole experiment: 8/11 (73%).

3 months old 22 days after grafting. Myelination in human brain *in situ* has been described as starting at least 3 months later.

These experiments demonstrated that the internal clock of human oligodendrocytes can be clearly modified by the maturation of the environment. In fact, the environment appeared to be so important that whatever the age of the maturation of the implanted human oligodendrocytes, myelination from implanted oligodendrocytes started around 15-20 days after grafting.

Distribution of MBP⁺ Myelin throughout the Brain

Two animals, each of which had received a graft, had their brains horizontally semiserially sectioned and studied in immunohistology to appreciate the distribution of MBP⁺ myelin throughout the brain.

The grafts in both cases were so well integrated in the host tissues that their limits were not defined.

Concerning the formation of MBP⁺ myelin in the brain, the scheme was comparable to that obtained after grafting newborn mouse tissues.[7] Myelin appeared in the graft region and was widely dispersed in patches of various sizes in both hemispheres.

TABLE 4 gives one example of the MBP⁺ myelin formed from a graft implanted at the level of the left anterior thalamus. The dispersion of MBP⁺ patches involved mainly the large myelinated fascicles, such as the corpus callosum, internal capsule, medial lemniscus, cerebellar peduncles, and white matter. MBP⁺ fibers radiated in several directions from the thalamic area (as was observed when the graft was of mouse origin). Migration occurred in the caudal and rostral directions, and contralaterally as well.

Essentially, we showed that the behaviors of newborn mouse and embryonic human oligodendrocytes were comparable after transplantation. The mechanisms involved in the migration of oligodendrocytes, attachment to the axons, and myelination appeared to be the same in phylogenetically divergent species.

Electron Microscopy

The prelocalization by immunohistology allowed us to evidence the patches of human myelin in the shiverer brain. Human myelin appeared much thicker than shiverer myelin, and was rather densely packed around oligodendrocytes (FIG. 3C). On ultrathin sections and at electron microscopy observations, deposits of human myelin appeared dispersed among deposits of shiverer myelin and nonmyelinated axons. Although the brain tissues and the axons were always very well preserved, the human myelin appeared dislocated (FIG. 3A). At higher magnification, however, it was obvious that the human myelin presented the major dense line (FIG. 3B), which is missing in the shiverer myelin. We think that the dislocation of the human myelin observed at the ultrastructural level after sectioning on a cryostat is due to freezing. Single oligodendrocytes or groups of oligodendrocytes were frequently seen near the human myelin. We never saw a continuity of myelin between a single oligodendrocyte and the human myelin sheath. At the ultrastructural level, no gliotic reaction was ever observed at the level of the patches of MBP$^+$ myelin. We never saw necrotic cells or an invasion of macrophages. By contrast, if, at the same stage (130 days after grafting), we observed the graft at the point it was implanted (FIG. 4A), it appeared to be healthy but packed and enveloped in a very dense astrocytic reaction. This reaction included enormous filamentous processes that isolated the graft from the surrounding tissues (FIG. 4C). Between the astrocytic process and the cells of the graft, a continuous or interrupted basal lamina was often visible (FIG. 4B).

CONCLUSION AND DISCUSSION

Oligodendrocytes taken from any region of a 20-week-old human embryo seem to have the same ability to survive, migrate, and myelinate host axons when transplanted

TABLE 4. Localization of MBP$^+$ Patches in the Host Brain

Left[a]	Right
Corpus callosum	Corpus callosum
Caudate nucleus	Caudate nucleus (+ + +) and putamen
Thalamus: ventral and lateral nuclei radiations	Thalamus: ventral and lateral nuclei radiations
Medial lemniscus (+ + +)	Medial lemniscus
Internal capsule	
Forel's field	
Pretectal area	Pretectal area
Superior colliculus	
Corticotectal fibers	
Central gray (mesencephalon)	Red nucleus and rubrospinal fasciculus
Longitudinal dorsal fasciculus	
Mesencephalic tegmentum	Mesencephalic tegmentum
Middle cerebellar peduncle	Decussation of superior cerebellar peduncle
Cerebellum (+ + + +): white matter of vermis and hemisphere	Cerebellum: white matter of vermis and hemisphere
Dentate nucleus	

[a] Graft position: rostral thalamus.

in a mouse brain. The migration depends much more on the site of implantation than on the origin of the oligodendrocytes. Migration may also depend on the time of implantation, but we have no results that would confirm this.

The results presented in this paper confirm those obtained with newborn mouse olfactory bulb, cerebellum, and spinal cord grafted in newborn shiverer brain.[4] In fact, the results obtained in these different studies—newborn normal mouse CNS or embryonic human CNS—are very comparable. The following were observed in both: migration of the myelin-forming cells over long distances (up to the spinal cord), patches of myelin dispersed throughout the brain, and enhanced dispersion for those grafts placed in structures that could be considered as "crossroads" structures. The mechanisms involved in these migrations are significant for both species, however phylogenetically divergent and anatomically different they may be.

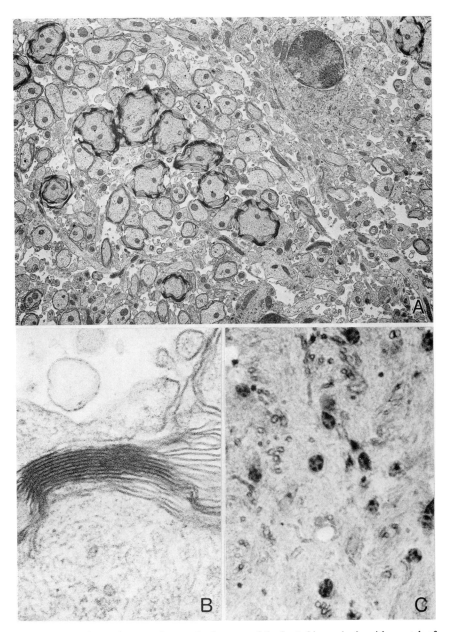

FIGURE 3. (**A**) An electron micrograph of a zone of the host shiverer brain with a patch of human myelin. No gliotic reaction was visible 130 days after grafting (×6000). (**B**) Same sample. Ultrastructure of the human myelin. The major dense line is clearly visible (×10 000). (**C**) Same sample. Even in the semithin sections, human myelin was so thick compared to shiverer myelin that it was possible to detect human myelin or to have a more general view of the patch (×1000). Original magnifications in parentheses; figure reduced to 73% of original size.

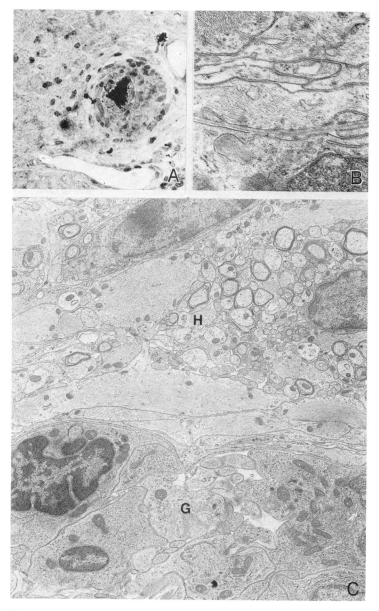

FIGURE 4. (A) An electron micrograph taken 130 days after grafting. Optic aspect of the graft in semithin sections. This particular graft was marked with charcoal and appeared to be clearly limited (×400). (B) Same sample. The limit between the graft (G) and host parenchyma (H). The graft is completely surrounded by large astrocytic processes. The cells of the graft were healthy. It was possible to recognize some oligodendrocytes, astrocytes, and neurons (×26 000). (C) Between astrocytic processes and graft cells a clear basal lamina is visible. It could be rather continuous or interrupted (×9000). Original magnifications in parentheses; figure reduced to 69% of original size.

It appeared that 16-week-old human oligodendrocytes transplanted in newborn shiverer were able to myelinate in host brain around 17 days after grafting. If newborn mouse tissue was transplanted in newborn shiverer mouse, the myelination by implanted oligodendrocytes appeared 15 days after implantation.[2]

Moreover, if the transplanted oligodendrocytes are much younger (6-8 weeks), normal human myelination appears in the shiverer brain, probably less than 22 days after grafting. This suggests that the differentiation of the transplanted oligodendrocytes is much more dependant upon the stage of maturation of the surrounding tissues than on an internal clock. It is particularly impressive that the younger (6-8-week-old) oligodendrocytes become able to differentiate at the age of 3 months (8 weeks and 22 days). Myelin fibers normally appear in the human brain after about 6 months.[15]

The internal clock of oligodendrocyte differentiation in culture was found to be determined by type 1 astrocytes.[16,17] In culture, conditions are such that heterochronic factors cannot play an important role. In our experiments, mouse type 1 astrocytes might be able to change the developmental clock of very immature human oligodendrocytes.

Transplantation of oligodendrocytes purified in culture was performed by Doering and Fedoroff.[18] In the absence of markers, the authors could not have discerned any movement of implanted oligodendrocytes, but they noted that the transplant attracted host axons and myelinated them. Thus, oligodendrocytes are able to myelinate after culture, and this could be one technique to obtain pure functional oligodendrocytes.

ACKNOWLEDGMENTS

We are very grateful to Dr. Tournaire and his co-workers. Without their comprehensive help, this work would not have been possible. We are also grateful to Dr. Jacque and Dr. Campagnoni for their kind gift of anti-MBP antisera.

Thanks to C. Burté for typing the manuscript.

We are indebted to Dr. J. J. Hauw, who kindly provided us the use of an electron microscope.

REFERENCES

1. GUMPEL, M., N. BAUMANN, M. RAOUL & C. JACQUE. 1983. Survival and differentiation of oligodendrocytes from neural tissue transplanted into newborn mouse brain. Neurosci. Lett. **37:** 307-312.
2. LACHAPELLE, F., M. GUMPEL, M. BAULAC, C. JACQUE, P. DUC & N. BAUMANN. 1983/ 1984. Transplantation of fragments of CNS into the brain of shiverer mutant mice: Extensive myelination by implanted oligodendrocytes. Dev. Neurosci. **6:** 326-334.
3. GUMPEL, M., F. LACHAPELLE, C. JACQUE & N. BAUMANN. 1985. Central nervous tissue transplantation into mouse brain: Differentiation of myelin from transplanted oligodendrocytes. *In* Neural Grafting in the Mammalian CNS. A. Björklund & U. Stenevi, Eds.: 151-158. Elsevier. Amsterdam.
4. GUMPEL, M., F. LACHAPELLE, A. BARON VAN EVERCOOREN, C. LUBETZKI, A. GANSMULLER, P. LOMBRAIL, C. JACQUE & N. BAUMANN. 1987. Myelination in the mouse by transplanted oligodendrocytes. *In* Neuronal Communication in Development and Regeneration. H. H. Althaus & W. Seifert, Eds. In press.

5. GUMPEL, M., F. LACHAPELLE, M. BAULAC, A. BARON VAN EVERCOOREN, A. GANS-
MULLER, C. JACQUE & N. BAUMANN. 1987. Intracerebral transplantation as a model
for studying the myelination process. *In* Model Systems of Development and Aging of
the Nervous System. A. Vernadakis, Ed. In press. Martinus Nijhoff. The Hague.

6. GANSMÜLLER, A., F. LACHAPELLE, A. BARON VAN EVERCOOREN, J. J. HAUW, N.
BAUMANN & M. GUMPEL. 1986. Transplantation of newborn CNS fragment into the
brain of shiverer mutant mouse. II. Long-distance myelination by implanted oligodendrocytes. Dev. Neurosci. **8:** 197-204.

7. BAULAC, M., F. LACHAPELLE, O. GOUT, B. BERGER, N. BAUMANN & M. GUMPEL. 1987.
Transplantation of oligodendrocytes in the mouse brain: Anatomical studies on the sites
of myelination by transplanted myelin-forming cells. Brain Res. In press.

8. BIRD, T., D. F. FARRELL & S. M. SUMI. 1977. Genetic developmental myelin defect in
shiverer mouse. Trans. Am. Soc. Neurochem. **8:** 153.

9. JACQUE, C., A. PRIVAT, P. DUPOUEY, J. M. BOURRE, T. BIRD & N. BAUMANN. 1978.
Shiverer mouse: A dysmyelinating mutant with absence of major dense line and basic
protein in myelin. Proc. Eur. Soc. Neurochem. **1:** 131.

10. DUPOUEY, P., C. JACQUE, J. M. BOURRE, F. CESSELIN, A. PRIVAT & N. BAUMANN.
1979. Immunochemical studies of myelin basic protein in shiverer mouse devoid of major
dense line of myelin. Neurosci. Lett. **12:** 113-118.

11. PRIVAT, A., C. JACQUE, J. M. BOURRE, P. DUPOUEY & N. BAUMANN. 1979. Absence of
the major dense line in the mutant mouse shiverer. Neurosci. Lett. **12:** 107-112.

12. DELASALLE, A., C. JACQUE, J. DROUET, J. C. LEGRAND & F. CESSELIN. 1980. Radioimmunoassay of the myelin basic protein in biological fluids: Conditions improving sensitivity and specificity. Biochimie **62:** 159-165.

13. PRIVAT, A. 1975. Postnatal gliogenesis in the mammalian brain. Int. Rev. Cytol. **40:**
281-323.

14. STERNBERGER, L. A., P. H. HARDY, J. J. CUCULUS & H. G. MEYER. 1970. The unlabeled
antibody enzyme method of immunohistochemistry: Preparation and properties of soluble
antigen-antibody complex (horseradish peroxidase-antihorseradish peroxidase) and its
use in identification of spirochetes. J. Histochem. Cytochem. **18:** 315-333.

15. YAKOVLEV, P. I. & A. R. LECOURS. 1967. *In* Regional Development of the Brain in Early
Life. A. Minkowski, Ed. Blackwell. Oxford.

16. RAFF, M. C. & L. T. MILLER. 1984. Glial cell development in the rat optic nerve. TINS:
469-472.

17. RAFF, M. C., E. R. ABNEY & J. FOK SEANG. 1985. Reconstitution of a developmental
clock *in vitro:* A critical role for astrocytes in the timing of oligodendrocyte differentiation.
Cell **42:** 61-69.

18. DOERING, L. C. & S. FEDOROFF. 1984. Isolation and transplantation of oligodendrocyte
precursor cells. J. Neurol. Sci. **63:** 183-186.

DISCUSSION OF THE PAPER

I. D. DUNCAN (*University of Wisconsin, Madison, WI*): If you irradiate the neonatal
rat spinal cord there is quite marked migration and proliferation of Schwann cells.
Therefore, I was surprised that your rat Schwann cells did not migrate away from
the graft. Do you have any explanation for this?

GUMPEL: No, I do not have an explanation, but I think it is very good for us.
Do not forget that these experiments are done during development, and if during
development Schwann cells were able to enter the central nervous system, you would
see a terrible mixture of glial cells everywhere. These experiments are performed

during the myelination process, and it seems that the astrocytes are very much against Schwann cells during the myelination process. I agree that in experiments done by others in adult animals they seem to penetrate very easily. Although this is a problem, I do not have an explanation, but I think there is a necessary system of protection.

DUNKAN: Before Dr. Aguayo intervenes, are you sure that mature oligos can migrate, or is this not an undifferentiated population of glioblasts?

GUMPEL: This is a very good question. I am sure of nothing because I told you that in the case of adult rat oligodendrocytes I had an oligo population that was 90% pure. That means 90% of the cells had positive characteristics of differentiated oligodendrocytes. In the optic nerve there are precursor cells of oligodendrocytes. So of course I can have precursor cells of oligodendrocytes in my cell preparations, especially in the case of embryonic human transplantation.

P. BRUNDIN (*University of Lund, Sweden*): I was very interested to hear the last bit you said about freezing tissue. Could you mention anything about how you did it? A lot of people have tried to do it. It is tricky to get the tissue to survive after being deep-frozen.

GUMPEL: We tried several techniques. We had success with a technique that involved placing tissue in minimal essential medium plus 20% fetal calf serum. Just before freezing, we add a buffer solution plus 20% DMSO. That means that the final solution contains 10% fetal calf serum and 10% DMSO. This is a preliminary result, but it works very well.

BRUNDIN: Did you freeze the tissue slowly or was it frozen rapidly?

GUMPEL: We go to 4° slowly, and from 4° rapidly.

A. J. AGUAYO (*Montreal General Hospital, Montreal, Quebec, Canada*): I was very impressed by some of the figures you gave as to where you actually found the cells that you had inserted in the newborn animals. One, is it possible that the migration may not have been as extensive as it appears in the grown animal? That, perhaps all it did, is migrate for a very short distance, and with the growth of the animal there has been a wide separation between source and site of retrieval? Two, and if this is so, can you find them in association with some of the projections that are still growing? For instance, the ones in the spinal cord as they associate with the dorsal columns where the decending projections from the motor cortex come from.

GUMPEL: Of course this is not solely migration from a point to another: the brain is growing and neurons are projecting during this time. What is very important is what electron microscopy reveals about the interactions between hosts and grafts. After 3 days, 4 days, 5 days, we see around the graft a ring of cell processes coming from the host and from the graft. This ring of tissue is not compact at all, and we can see oligodendrocytes within it. The oligodendrocytes in the brain seem to try to adhere immediately to axons. So of course they could be transported passively by the axon projections.

If this is indeed the case, it can be completely impossible for oligodendrocytes to migrate in adults.

C. SOTELO (*INSERM U106, CMC Foch, Suresnes*): Are oligodendrocytes moving along from the graft, or are there some other cells that can accompany the oligodendrocytes? In other words, you use only one marker, that is, the basic protein of the myelin, so with this marker alone it is probably difficult to answer the question. But now I see that you have new experiments in which you have followed sequential events using electron microscopy to probe the semithin sections where you can see which type of population is moving.

GUMPEL: Of course, probably many cells are moving, and where we see oligodendrocytes in this ring of very smooth tissue formed by the transplant we recognize only oligodendrocytes, but this is not a proof they are alone.

Vascular and Glial Alterations after Autonomic Tissue Grants into the Brain[a]

JEFFREY M. ROSENSTEIN[b]

Department of Anatomy
George Washington University Medical Center
Washington, DC 20037

INTRODUCTION

It is now fairly well established that neural transplantation can provide an important experimental direction for the study of questions in several neurobiological disciplines. Transplant experiments have been useful in the amelioration of anatomical and physiological deficits[1-3] and in studying changes in functional behavior.[4,5] Although the observed functional restorations might be due to axonal connectivity between host and graft in many systems, anatomical evidence for such connections is limited.[6-8] The accommodation of the new grafted tissue that necessitates some destruction of host brain tissue probably produces significant cellular and vascular changes, particularly at the host-donor interface. In the absence of newly formed projections, a fluid-borne dissemination between host and graft of potential neuroactive compounds in the blood or cerebrospinal fluid compartment could occur. Previous studies[9,10] have shown that the presence of an autonomic graft within the cerebral ventricle changes the character of the blood-brain barrier (BBB) at the site of transplantation. Normally, the BBB plays a major role in homeostasis of the brain fluid environment by preventing most blood-borne compounds from entering the parenchyma and the extracellular fluid compartment. The extracellular fluid surrounding neurons and glia is in dynamic and controlled equilibrium with the cerebrospinal fluid. Solutes thus freely exchange across the internal (ependymal) or external (glial) linings of the brain. At least transiently, a breakdown of the BBB must occur following the trauma of graft placement such as that which occurs after mechanical lesion to the central nervous system.[11,12]

The barrier changes after transplantation could be produced by anatomical and physiological confluences between the extracellular fluid of the host and that of the graft.[9,10] The potential significance of this pathway underscores the importance of studying cellular dynamics. The connections between host and graft, if not axonal, are limited to cellular elements that stand between the two or serve as the intermediary conduit for vascularization or both. Neural transplantation as a dynamic cellular

[a] This work was supported by Grant NS-17468 from the National Institutes of Health.

[b] Address for correspondence: George Washington University Medical Center, 2300 I Street, N.W., Washington, DC 20037.

process must involve the growth of new blood vessels (angiogenesis) and concurrent changes in reactive cells at the interface; the cells involved are the endothelial cell and the astrocyte.

In the present studies, autonomic tissue was grafted into the brain. The considerations from a cellular viewpoint for studying these foreign neural tissues are as follows: 1) endothelial linings of capillaries are fenestrated and permeable lacking any blood-neuronal barrier, 2) astroglia are not normally present, and 3) connective or supporting cell types are within. Using the fourth ventricle as a transplant site where there is minimal trauma and the direct approach of graft insertion into the brain substance allows for comparison of morphologic and physiologic perturbations in these transplantation models.

MATERIALS AND METHODS

The superior cervical ganglion (SCG) or the dissected adrenal medulla was removed from outbred strains of young adult Sprague-Dawley rats and transplanted into the fourth ventricle, with minimal damage to the surrounding brain, as described previously.[13,14] The 1.00-1.25-mm³ fragment of autonomic tissue, after being immersed briefly in Earle's balanced salt solution and then in biologically inert Pelikan ink to delineate its borders after fixation, was placed in normal recipient rats ranging in age from 6 days to young adult (allografts). In addition, some SCG grafts were autotransplanted in young adults (autografts).

Autonomic transplants were also placed traumatically into areas of the central nervous system such as cerebral cortex or spinal cord. The surgical placement was made either by direct insertion using a needle and stylet under visual control or immediately after the preparation of a small resection cavity. Both allografts and autografts were given to recipient animals that were at least 3 weeks old. Because the BBB is mechanically disrupted after direct brain damage, postoperative periods for both the ventricular and the traumatic intraparenchymal transplants were at least 4 weeks long and ranged for periods to over 1 year.

The recipient animals first were perfused with an aldehyde mixture to determine changes in host astroglia to the placement of the autonomic grafts. The graft and surrounding host brain were dissected as a single block and placed in 1% osmium for 3-4 hr. The tissue was next dehydrated and embedded in epon resin. Sequential 1-μ sections were immunostained with glial fibrillary acidic protein (GFAP) antiserum (kindly provided by Dr. B. Trapp) using the postembedding technique of Trapp et al.[15] Using this method, the same block could then be thin sectioned for electron microscopy.

A single bolus of horseradish peroxidase (HRP) solution (Sigma Type VI; .35 ml of a 5% solution/100 g body weight) was injected into the femoral vein to determine the effects of the autonomic grafts on the host BBB. The glycoprotein circulated for periods between 2 and 90 min. After an appropriate circulation time, the animals were perfused with the balanced salt solution to clear the vasculature and then with an aldehyde mixture. The transplant and surrounding brain were serially sectioned on a vibratome and processed for HRP histochemistry.[16,17] Some sections were further processed for electron microscopy.

RESULTS

Astroglia

Because autonomic ganglia under normal conditions (and in our control preparations) do not contain classical astrocytes, it was relatively easy to detect the reactive nature of these cells at the site of transplantation. Immunocytochemical staining for GFAP, the major filament protein in astrocytes, revealed that astroglia responded vigorously to the foreign allograft, even in the intraventricular transplant model where there is minimal trauma.[13,14] This response consisted of proliferating and enlarging GFAP-positive processes, which originated just beneath the host outer (glial) or inner (ependymal) limiting membranes, and was followed temporally by a directed migration into the autonomic graft. The initiation of migration could not be detected in the autonomic grafts until about 3-4 weeks after transplantation. After this time, "gliosis" in the grafts proceeded rapidly with enlarged astrocyte processes being the major component; relatively few cell bodies actually migrated into the allografts (FIG. 1A). The directed migration continued at least until the latest time examined (16 months), where in some specimens GFAP and processes filled much of the graft.

An interesting phenomenon was investigated in this study, and continues to be investigated: the nearly complete lack of astrocyte migration in autografted SCG specimens under identical transplant experimental conditions. Allografts contain an extensive glial population 6 months after transplantation, but autografts remain free of glial infiltration (FIG. 1B).

GFAP staining also provided important information with regard to the revascularization process of the transplants. Microvessels in the central nervous system are contacted by astrocytic end feet, which in GFAP staining appear to stud their circumference (FIG. 1B). Even after several months, when glial processes had mostly infiltrated the SCG allografts, the patent blood vessels had not been contacted by glial end feet (FIG. 1C).

At the ultrastructural level, astrocytic processes that have invaded allografts take up residence in very close proximity to autonomic neurites much as a Schwann cell might (FIG. 2A). These processes are packed with filaments and form gap junctions—two hallmarks that Schwann cells lack. At later survival periods, astroglia take on an interesting configuration essentially replacing what were autonomic neurite bundles, which are normally isolated by fibroblasts (FIG. 2B).

Vascular Alterations and the BBB

Under normal conditions, blood-borne protein will not cross cerebral endothelial cells and enter the interstitial space of the central nervous system. This is due to the presence of tight junctions between these cells and a lack of pinocytotic vesicular transport. On the other hand, endothelial cells within autonomic tissue are not only fenestrated but have significant vesicular transport; they are freely permeable to protein. How might these differences in cellular physiology translate to changes in the barrier properties in host and graft? After systemic administration of the glycoprotein HRP (M_r: 40 000), all autonomic tissue grafts contained exuded HRP after even just 1 min

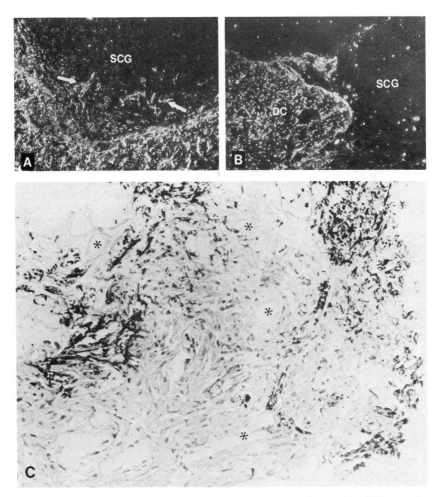

FIGURE 1. (A) An SCG allograft (SCG) rests within the fourth ventricle. GFAP-positive processes (arrows) have begun to migrate into the graft. Dark-field microscopy. (B) An SCG autograft (SCG) lies against host dorsal column (DC). There is only a minimal GFAP-positive (astroglial) migration into the transplant. The apparently labeled structures at the edge of the graft are not astroglial but are marker carbon ink grains. Dark-field microscopy. Postoperative times for **A** and **B**: 3 weeks and 6 months, respectively. Original magnification for **A** and **B**: × 60; reduction: 84% of original size. (C) An SCG allograft that has GFAP-positive processes coursing throughout. Note that blood vessels do not have glial end feet (∗). Postoperative time: 4 months. Original magnification: × 100; reduction: 97% of original size.

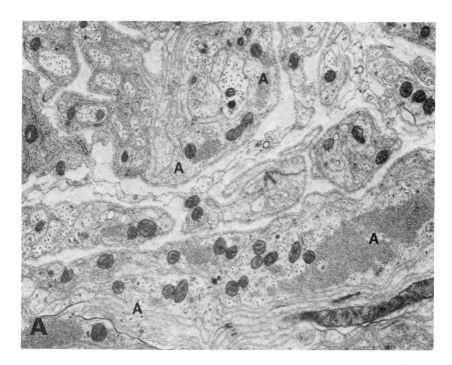

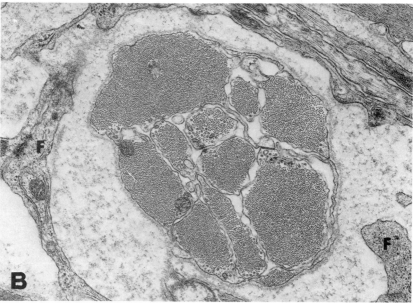

FIGURE 2. (A) An electron micrograph showing reactive astrocytic processes (A) infiltrating an SCG graft in close proximity to autonomic neurites. (B) Reactive astrocytic bundles appear to have replaced autonomic neurite bundles within a fibroblast (F) framework. Postoperative times for **A** and **B**: 2 and 14 months, respectively. Original magnifications for **A** and **B**: × 7200 and × 20 000, respectively; enlargement: 109% of original size.

of vascular circulation. Using the very sensitive chromagen tetramethylbenzidine added greatly to the description of protein dissemination within the host brain. After 15 min of circulation, not only was the graft completely inundated significantly, the protein traversed through the interstitial spaces of the graft and entered and circulated in the cerebrospinal fluid (FIG. 3A). The circulating protein in the cerebrospinal fluid entered the perivascular spaces of surface vessels and infiltrated to the level of the capillary bed, thus outlining the entire microvasculature. The exogenous protein borne in the cerebrospinal fluid can also leak through the ependymal lining of the ventricle. Glycoprotein was also detected within the adjacent host brain parenchyma. In plastic sections, HRP-laden vessels could be seen traversing the host-graft interface (FIG. 3B). Within the ganglion transplant at the ultrastructural level, all extracellular spaces surrounding regenerating neurites were filled with reaction product (FIG. 4A). Interestingly, massive astroglial processes that migrated into the graft sometimes contained HRP (FIG. 4B).

After adrenal medullary tissue was transplanted into the brain, a similar pattern of protein exudation was observed. The adrenal graft, which invariably contains some cortical tissue, was completely inundated with protein. The exudation into the adjacent host brain tissue, however, was far greater than that for the SCG. Often the entire breadth of the cerebellar vermis or the bilateral dorsal column area was filled with disseminated protein (FIG. 5A). Vessels within the flooded medulla neuropil appeared to be rimmed by HRP (FIG. 5B). The endothelial cells of these vessels have been shown to contain abnormally high numbers of transporting organelles.[9] At the ultrastructural level, surviving chromaffin cells were surrounded by HRP, which was adherent to cell surfaces (FIG. 6B). Some chromaffin cells sequestered the exogenous protein into dense bodies within 20 min (FIG. 6B).

When adrenal medulla was placed traumatically into the brain parenchyma, in as little as 5 min of HRP circulation, the graft was filled with reaction product. The systemic protein, as in the intraventricular model, traversed the graft and entered the adjacent brain tissue (FIG. 6A). At longer periods, there was a progressive increase in the amount of exudated protein into the host brain and the cerebrospinal fluid. Macrophages, which react strongly with diaminobenzidine, were invariably found to cover the graft in the wound cavity (FIG. 6A).

DISCUSSION

The transplantation of autonomic tissue into the brain can provide information about specific cellular interrelationships between host and graft. Autonomic, SCG, or adrenal medullary tissue, having different cellular constituents than cerebral tissue, are useful models to study alterations in the host to the imposition of foreign grafts. The two cell types that are prominent at the important host-graft interface, the astrocyte and the endothelial cell, are shown to play important roles in transplant integration.

Astroglia

Astroglia in the host brain respond vigorously to the presence of autonomic transplants. In the intraventricular model, where there is minimal trauma, the response

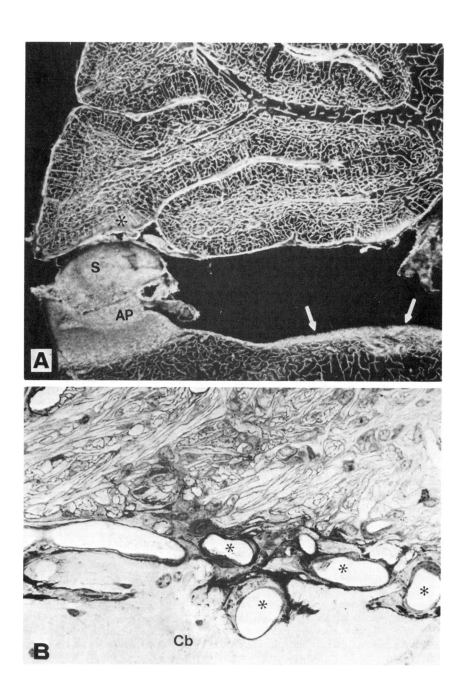

FIGURE 3. (A) An SCG (S) graft rests on the area postrema (AP). After 20 min of HRP circulation, the protein fills the graft and enters the cerebrospinal fluid where it fills perivascular spaces and thus outlines the entire microvasculature. Some HRP leakage is seen in the adjacent cerebellum (*) and beneath the ependyma (arrows). Tetramethylbenzidine reaction; dark-field microscopy. **(B)** A 1-μ-thick plastic section shows HRP delineating a neurite bundle in an SCG graft. HRP-laden vessels (*) traverse the interface between graft and host cerebellum (CB). Postoperative time for **A** and **B**: 3 months. Original magnifications for **A** and **B**: × 20 and × 100, respectively; enlargement: 105% of original size.

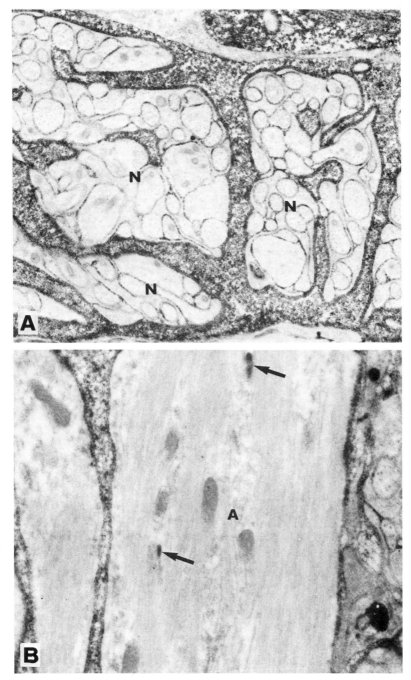

FIGURE 4. (A) An electron micrograph showing neurite bundles (N) in an SCG graft surrounded by HRP in extracellular space. (B) Reactive astroglial process (A) within an HRP-filled SCG graft. The astroglial process appear to have taken up small amounts of HRP (arrows). Postoperative times for A and B: 3 months and 8 weeks, respectively. Original magnifications for A and B: × 8000 and × 24 000, respectively; enlargement: 102% of original size.

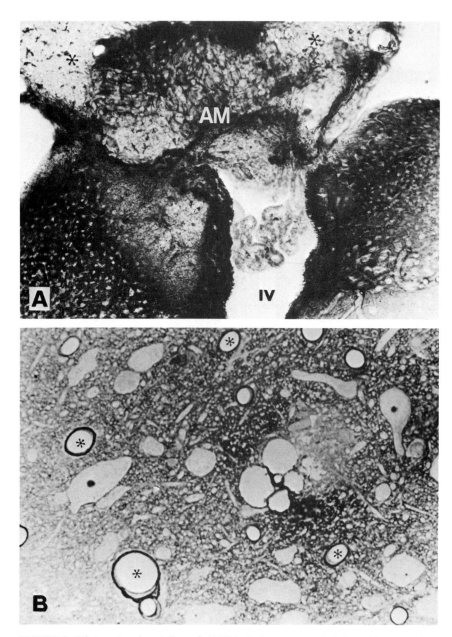

FIGURE 5. (A) An adrenal medulla graft (AM) including some cortical tissue (∗) rests against dorsal columns in the caudal region of the fourth ventricle (IV). After 30 min of HRP circulation, the protein has infiltrated both the graft and the entire dorsal column region. (B) A 1-µ-thick plastic section of dorsal column neuropil from the specimen in A. HRP fills the neuropil outlining neurons and blood vessels (∗). Postoperative time: 10 weeks. Original magnifications for A and B: × 90 and × 200, respectively; enlargement: 106% of original size.

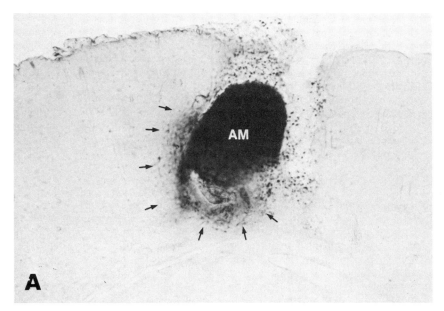

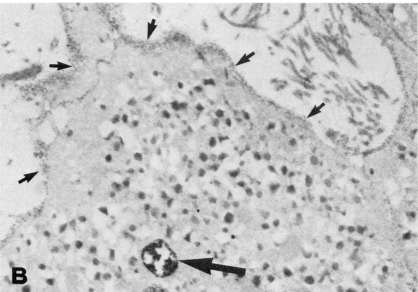

FIGURE 6. (A) An adrenal medulla graft (AM) within the cerebral cortex. After 10 min of HRP circulation, the protein has exuded from the graft into the surrounding host brain (arrows). Note the numerous macrophages surrounding the graft. (B) A chromaffin cell from an adrenal medullary graft. HRP adheres to the cell surface (small arrows), and some has been taken up in a dense body (large arrows). Postoperative times for **A** and **B**: 10 weeks and 4 months, respectively. Original magnifications for **A** and **B**: $\times$ 40 and $\times$ 8500, respectively; enlargement: 106% of original size.

takes the form of a proliferation and migration of reactive astrocytic processes. As shown by GFAP immunohistochemistry, the directed movement into the foreign graft occurs in the relative absence of mechanical damage in which an astroglial scar invariably forms.[18,19] As the autonomic graft apposes the brain surfaces, the reactive astroglia, which at the ultrastructural level are packed with filaments, migrate out of their normal confines and freely enter the graft. The lack of injury stimulus indicates that the host astrocytes might be susceptible to diffusible factors emanating from the graft that might stimulate their reaction. Such "growth-promoting" factors might be derived from either regenerating ganglion cells or products of degeneration, which are, in turn, believed to induce regeneration.[20] The delivery of transplant-produced compounds could reach the host either through pericellular clefts or through the blood.

The glial migratory activity appears to be both cumulative and temporal. Astrocytes do not appear to respond until 1-2 weeks after grafting. After this time, astroglial processes progressively accumulate within the graft. Because autonomic neurons and processes decrease over time,[10] presumably more space would become available for astrocytes to invade. Although the astrocytic response may be to exclude the foreign graft or, conversely, to incorporate it, the astrocytes do not appear to have a detrimental effect on surviving neurons. Astroglial processes take up residence in very close association with ganglion cells and neurites in a manner similar to that observed with Schwann cells. Whether they in fact provide support to neural tissue or compete with Schwann cells to provide such support is unclear.

An aspect of astroglial involvement with blood vessels associated with the central nervous system is the presence of glial processes or end feet upon the perimeter of capillaries. Originally believed to be responsible for the BBB, they have been suggested as having a supportive role.[21] Their complete absence around vessels in the autonomic graft further supports the mechanism of direct anastomotic connections between host and graft.[9,22,23] Invariably, there is an abrupt transition in GFAP material between central nervous system vessels studded with end feet and graft vessels that have none. It would seem unlikely that both host vessels and astroglia would co-migrate into a transplant without at least some forming their normal association.

A final point concerns the lack of glial migration into SCG autografts. This observation raises interesting questions about glial behavior and is still under study. It has been shown recently that astrocytes can act as accessory cells and present antigen to T lymphocytes *in vitro*.[24] If there exists a comparable situation *in vivo*, then host astrocytes might readily perceive foreign allografts through surface antigens but not autografts. Lymphocytes and macrophages only are seen very early in intraventricular grafts. Autonomic allografts may not be sufficiently strong antigens to mount a complete rejection. It appears that only after lymphocytes are no longer in the graft that astrocytes mount a directed migration. Whether astrocytes have an immunological involvement after neural transplantation remains to be determined.

BBB

The results of these studies elucidate a potentially important effect of transplanting autonomic neural tissue into the brain. At sites of transplantation, there appears to be a permanent alteration of the BBB such that systemically administered protein can reach the interstitial space of the host brain. Moreover, the blood-borne protein freely traverses the permeable transplant and enters and circulates in the cerebrospinal fluid where it can be detected in perivascular spaces and beneath ependymal linings. Normally, only lipid-soluble compounds and glucose are permitted access to brain parenchyma across the endothelial cell linings of brain capillaries. Endothelial cells are connected by tight junctions that effectively limit passage of large polar compounds, such as the foreign HRP, into the brain. Thus, the interstitial space of the brain and the cerebrospinal fluid are normally inaccessible compartments. The placement of an autonomic, or even a fetal central nervous system graft[25] produces alterations in both capillaries and the tightly controlled homeostatic fluid milieu of the brain. It appears that the newly formed and directly continuous extracellular channels[9] between host and graft are largely responsible for the permanent barrier dysfunction.

Foreign protein, after a single vascular injection, rapidly fills the permeable autonomic transplant and then floods the adjacent host brain where it fills even the synaptic clefts. It is conceivable that a smaller injected compound such as a neurotransmitter[10] could have the same potential to affect synaptic sites of graft and host. As demonstrated in the study by Rennels et al.,[26] in which tetramethylbenzidine methodology was used, HRP passes into perivascular spaces and outlines the microvasculature after it is injected into the lateral ventricle. The autonomic graft acts like a pump or a portal that permits the comparable dissemination of HRP after a vascular injection. The lack of anatomical[27] or physiological[28] barriers between the cerebrospinal fluid and the brain extracellular space could allow systemically administered compounds to affect brain regions some distance from the graft. The compound at the perivascular basement membrane would spread widely through the central nervous system and could exchange with interstitial fluid.[26] The observed distribution of HRP probably represents only 20-25% of the total concentration that was injected (the figure is the approximate blood flow to the brain), and much of the injected protein would be lost to the body tissues. Over time, less protein would be available to leak at the transplantation site, and, moreover, the foreign protein would be "washed" from the brain by the continuous bulk flow of cerebrospinal fluid.

An interesting observation concerns the greater leaking that occurs after adrenal medullary grafts than after SCG grafts.[29] Although the cellular content of these grafts is dissimilar and neurotransmitter production is probably dissimilar as well, a physical factor might be involved. Unlike the SCG, the adrenal medulla contains large sinusoidal vessels and lacks a distinct fibroblast capsule or matrix. HRP may thus flow more freely through the adrenal medulla.

In summary, the placement of an autonomic graft in the mammalian brain appears to cause a permanent BBB dysfunction. Transplant-induced vascular growth causes irreversible changes in the tightly controlled fluid environment of the brain. Through vascular and pericellular confluence between host and graft, the increased BBB permeability might facilitate the passage of neuroactive compounds to adjacent brain regions where they would normally be excluded. On a cellular level, these studies may be useful to determine blood vessel alterations in certain neurovascular disorders where the BBB is affected.

REFERENCES

1. BJÖRKLUND, A., M. SEGAL & V. STENEVI. 1979. Functional reinnervation of rat hippocampus by locus coeruleus implants. Brain Res. **170:** 409-426.
2. PERLOW, M. J., W. FREED, B. HOFFER, A. SEIGER, L. OLSON & R. WYATT. 1979. Brain grafts reduce motor abnormalities produced by destruction of nigrostriatal dopamine system. Science **204:** 643-645.

3. GASH, D., J. R. SLADEK & C. D. SLADEK. 1980. Functional development of grafted vasopressin neurons. Science 210: 1367-1369.
4. BJÖRKLUND, A., S. B. DUNNETT, V. STENEVI, M. E. LEWIS & S. D. IVERSEN. 1980. Reinnervation of the denervated striatum by substantia nigra transplants: Functional consequences as revealed by pharmacological and sensorimotor testing. Brain Res. 199: 307-333.
5. FREED, W. J., J. M. MORIHISA, E. SPOOR, B. HOFFER, L. OLSON, A. SEIGER & R. WYATT. 1981. Transplanted adrenal chromaffin cells in rat brain reduce lesion-induced rotational behavior. Nature (London) 292: 351-352.
6. REIER, P. J., M. J. PERLOW & L. GUTH. 1983. Development of embryonic spinal cord transplants in the rat. Dev. Brain Res. 10: 201-219.
7. McLOON, S. C. & R. D. LUND. 1983. Development of fetal retina, tectum and cortex transplanted to the superior colliculus of adult rats. J. Comp. Neurol. 217: 376-389.
8. JAEGER, C. B. 1985. Cytoarchitectonics of substantia nigra grafts: A light and electron microscopic study of immunocytochemically identified dopaminergic neurons and fibrous astrocytes. J. Comp. Neurol. 231: 121-135.
9. ROSENSTEIN, J. M. & M. W. BRIGHTMAN. 1983. Circumventing the blood-brain barrier with autonomic ganglion transplants. Science 221: 879-881.
10. ROSENSTEIN, J. M. & M. W. BRIGHTMAN. 1984. Some consequences of grafting autonomic ganglion to brain surfaces. In Neural Transplants: Development and Function. J. Sladek & D. Gash, Eds.: 423-443. Plenum. New York, NY.
11. KLATZO, I. 1967. Neurological aspects of brain edema. J. Neuropathol. Exp. Neurol. 26: 1-12.
12. BEGGS, J. L. & J. D. WAGGENER. 1975. Vasogenic edema in the injured spinal cord: A method of evaluating the extent of blood-brain barrier alteration to horseradish peroxidase. Exp. Neurol. 49: 86-96.
13. ROSENSTEIN, J. M. & M. W. BRIGHTMAN. 1978. Intact cerebral ventricle as a site for tissue transplantation. Nature (London) 275: 83-85.
14. ROSENSTEIN, J. M. & M. W. BRIGHTMAN. 1979. Regeneration and myelination in autonomic ganglia transplanted to intact brain surfaces. J. Neurocytol. 8: 359-380.
15. TRAPP, B., L. McINTYRE, R. QUARLES, N. STEINBERGER & H. WEBSTER. 1979. Immunocytochemical localization of rat peripheral nervous system myelin proteins. Proc. Natl. Acad. Sci. USA 76: 3552-3556.
16. GRAHAM, R. C. & M. J. KARNOVSKY. 1966. The early stages of absorption of injected horseradish peroxidase in the proximal tubules of the mouse kidney: Ultrastructural cytochemistry by a new technique. J. Histochem. 14: 291-299.
17. MESULAM, M. M. 1978. Tetramethylbenzidine for horseradish peroxidase neurohistochemistry: A noncarcinogenic blue reaction with superior sensitivity for visualizing neural afferents and efferents. J. Histochem. Cytochem. 26: 106-117.
18. KONIGSMARK, B. & R. SIDMAN. 1963. Origin of brain macrophages in the mouse. J. Neuropathol. Exp. Neurol. 22: 643-676.
19. ANDERS, J. J. & M. W. BRIGHTMAN. 1980. Assemblies of particles in the cell membranes of developing, mature and reactive astrocytes. J. Neurocytol. 8: 777-795.
20. CAJAL, S. R. 1928. Degeneration and Regeneration of the Nervous System. R. May, Ed. Oxford Press. London.
21. BECK, D. W., H. V. VINTERS, M. N. HART & P. A. CANCILLA. 1984. Glial cells influence polarity of the blood-brain barrier. J. Neuropathol. Exp. Neurol. 43: 219-224.
22. KRUM, J. M. & J. M. ROSENSTEIN. 1985. Temporal sequence of angiogenesis in neural transplant models. Soc. Neurosci. Abstr. 15: 1149.
23. ROSENSTEIN, J. M. & M. W. BRIGHTMAN. 1986. Alterations in the blood-brain barrier after transplantation of autonomic ganglion into the mammalian central nervous system. J. Comp. Neurol. 250: 339-351.
24. FONTANA, A., W. FIERZ & H. WEKERLE. 1984. Astrocytes present myelin basic protein to encephalitogenic T-cell lines. Nature (London) 307: 273-276.
25. ROSENSTEIN, J. M. 1987. Neocortical transplants in the mammalian brain lack a blood-brain barrier to macromolecules. Science 235: 772-774.
26. RENNELS, M. L., T. F. GREGORY, O. R. BLAUMANIS, K. FUJIMOTO & P. A. GRADY. 1985. Evidence for a "paravascular" fluid circulation in the mammalian central nervous

system, provided by the rapid distribution of tracer protein throughout the brain from the subarachnoid space. Brain Res. **326:** 47-63.

27. BRIGHTMAN, M. W. 1965. The distribution within the brain of ferritin injected into cerebrospinal fluid compartments. II. Parenchymal distribution. Am. J. Anat. **117:** 193-220.
28. BRADBURY, M. W. 1979. The Concept of a Blood-Brain Barrier. John Wiley & Sons. New York, NY.
29. ROSENSTEIN, J. M. 1985. The blood-brain barrier is permanently altered by transplants of adrenal medulla. Soc. Neurosci. Abstr. **15:** 840.

DISCUSSION OF THE PAPER

B. E. LEVIN (*Veterans Administration Medical Center, East Orange, NJ*): Could you speak to the issue of immunologic privilege of the brain in this setting since you went to the trouble of using immunoglobulin G?

ROSENSTEIN: The question that is involved here, especially in neural transplants, is if there is no blood-brain barrier, why is the transplant not rejected? I do not know the answer. It may be that neural tissue itself is not highly antigenic. In fetal brain grafts, I have found that there is no blood-brain barrier, either. Immediately after transplantation—1 or 2 days—the transplant will be loaded with lymphocytes and macrophages, but, over time, they disappear without any particular detrimental effect on the graft.

D. GOLDOWITZ (*Thomas Jefferson University, Philadelphia, PA*): Your finding of some semipermanent or long-term broaching of the traditional blood-brain barrier in transplants is fascinating. Svengard and co-workers have indicated that when central nerve fibers have access to peripheral molecules they may undergo degeneration. In your material, do you see degenerative events around your transplants?

ROSENSTEIN: Hardly ever, other than initial transplant shock. And, as I said, fetal transplants that do not have a barrier exhibit no degeneration, either. I think there is a hypothesis proposed by Kiernan about a lack of a barrier causing degeneration. I think that Kiernan transplanted skin. I do not see much degeneration at all: these grafts have lived 30 months. The neurons decrease over time, probably because of the lack of contact with synaptic fibers—not because of outright degeneration or immunological rejection.

P. PASIK (*Mount Sinai School of Medicine, New York, NY*): I understand that the effect is not specific for autonomic grafts, that if you implant other pieces of brain not related to the autonomic nervous system you would also find an opening of the barriers.

ROSENSTEIN: What we think is happening is that after transplantation there is angiogenesis or neovascularization. It has been shown a while ago in the neuropathology literature that if you wound the spinal cord or wound anywhere else in the central nervous system, the new vessels that form will leak but will become impermeable in 2 to 3 weeks. It might be that the placement of a graft and the connection of vessels somehow obscures that. Also, it might be an immunological effect that lymphocytes that are circulating in the blood stream may pass through the endothelial cells, leaving them permeable. That is another possibility that we are investigating.

PASIK: Have you ever seen fenestration of the capillaries at the electron microscopic level?

ROSENSTEIN: No, not in fetal brain grafts.

PASIK: Or disappearance of tight junctions?

ROSENSTEIN: Well, in the autonomic graft, there are fenestrations because the original, intrinsic vessels remain. In fetal brain grafts, although I have not observed fenestrated vessels, a number of vessels have extensive astroglial investments or are cuffed by leucocytes. It may be that these vessels are responsible for barrier permeability.

Summary

M. SHELANSKI (*New York University, New York, NY*): What is most striking about these presentations is the complexity and the number of events we have been shown. Certain things, however, leap out at me. Dr. Aguayo very clearly pointed out that we can dissect out the mechanism of axon regrowth. The axons will follow an appropriate and hospitable pathway to a target that you have chosen for them, even if you take them around an extraordinary detour.

One thing that comes out of Dr. Aguayo's work, which he did not emphasize but must be aware of, is that when you use this system you also clean up your transplant's system; that is, when you reimplant the end of this graft, you have the fibers growing out of and into the appropriate region where you have put them free of their cell bodies. This allows you to look at a little bit of the graft-host response without the problem of the insertion of the cell body.

In many of the experiments, things were transplanted from region A to region B, not to mention from strain A to strain B or from species A to species B. The assumption in all of these things is that the glial response that one looks at somehow creates a barrier. Even though Dr. Whitaker-Azmitia pointed out that there were beneficial things that one might attribute to glia, what we saw time and time again was a glial wall.

We have to look at the glia in a much deeper fashion, and consider what astrocytes might do outside of releasing odd substances or outside of making this barrier. The first thing that we must face is that the glial filament staining and its intensity may be a marker of reaction, but it really does not tell us a lot about what that astrocyte might be doing. It is a marker for astrocytes and a marker for their extent, but it tells us nothing about the business end of the astrocyte—its surface, which is what is producing the things we have to look at. So we know, in addition to what we know about the barrier function, that the astrocyte can produce various enzymes, various substrates, and various growth factors. There are other things that the astrocyte does remarkably well. One thing, which Rakic has very elegantly shown, and which has also been shown by Hatten in his tissue culture work, is that the astrocyte provides a matrix on which the neuron may move and send out processes.

The guidance of migration is very clear. The extent to which the guidance of process growth is important is unclear. What is also clear is that there is a reciprocity between the neurons and the glia: you cannot look at one without the other. Neurons arrest astroglial cell proliferation.

Glial cells appear, at least in the embryonic neonatal cerebellar cultures, to be required for neuronal survival. So again you must look at this.

Finally, of course, you have to look at the work Prochiantz has reported: different glial cells support very different differentiations of the same neurons. To push this a little further, Prochiantz and I have done some experiments over the past year that indicate you can make highly specific antibodies, antibodies that will differentiate between a mesencephalic astrocyte and a striatal astrocyte. In all of these things, we are only looking at the tip of the iceberg.

An extremely interesting tool was discussed by Dr. Whitaker-Azmitia. She raised the possibility that diphenylhydantoin might block the glial response. If it does, one might be able to do transplants and get rid of what is probably a red herring.

Overall, we have been shown some wonderful phenomena. The implications for extensive grafting and transplantation regeneration in the central nervous system are encouraging.

CNS Tissue Culture Analyses of Trophic Mechanisms in Brain Transplantation

STANLEY M. CRAIN

Departments of Neuroscience and Physiology
Albert Einstein College of Medicine
and
Rose F. Kennedy Center for Research in
Mental Retardation and Human Development
Yeshiva University
New York, New York 10461

Many of the papers presented in this part have utilized cell and tissue culture techniques to facilitate critical analyses of some of the putative trophic factors and substrata that appear to be produced by transplanted brain cells as they interact with the host central nervous system (CNS) and vice versa. These studies provide elegant demonstrations of the significant insights that can be obtained by *in vitro* manipulation and analysis of CNS cells before transplantation, as well as by assays of trophic factors derived from experimentally altered host brain tissues on the growth and development of specific types of neurons in culture. The exciting progress in this field during the past decade was undoubtedly stimulated by the pioneering nerve growth factor (NGF) studies by Levi-Montalcini during the previous two decades.[1,2] Certain types of sarcoma tissues had been reported to elicit dense neuritic projections when transplanted near dorsal root ganglia.[3] Levi-Montalcini discovered that transplantation of these tissues onto the chorio-allantoic membrane around the chick embryo resulted in marked enhancement of the growth of sympathetic, as well as dorsal root ganglion, neurons all along the neuraxis, similar to the results of intraembryonic transplants.[4] This critical experiment indicated that a diffusible trophic factor, rather than a local neurotrophic factor,[5] was evidently released by the sarcoma tissue and circulated to the chick embryo nervous system.[6] Systematic *in vitro* bioassays of extracts from these sarcoma tissues, and subsequently from salivary gland tissues, on the outgrowth of neurites from explants of chick embryo dorsal root ganglia greatly accelerated the isolation and characterization of this important neuronotrophic factor.[2] The crucial role of NGF in the development and maintenance of peripheral ganglion neurons[2,7,8] has recently been extended to the CNS, following demonstrations of NGF-enhanced choline acetyltransferase levels in certaina types of central cholinergic neurons[9–13] and NGF rescue of these CNS neurons after injury.[14–16] Additional types of neuronotrophic factors have been recently demonstrated,[15,17–19] including a factor that appears to enhance the maturation (but not survival) of serotonergic neurons—but not noradrenergic neurons.[20]

The studies by Kromer and Cornbrooks[16] and by Smith *et al.*[21] provide valuable new data indicating that laminin may play an important role in the substrata that support projections of neurites following transplantation into host CNS as well as during normal development of the CNS.[cf.22–24] These studies of neurite growth on laminin-containing substrata may help to clarify the dramatic growth of CNS axons through long lengths of transplanted peripheral nerve,[25] in contrast to the poor growth within optic nerve (which contains relatively little laminin in the adult mammal, but not in the adult fish optic nerve, which regenerates more successfully[22]).

In addition to the use of tissue cultures for analytical bioassays of specific trophic factors and substratum components, it should be emphasized that electrophysiologic and morphologic analyses of organotypic CNS tissue cultures have provided crucial evidence that fetal rodent (and even human) brain and spinal cord tissues can, indeed, continue to develop a remarkable degree of mature structure and function during many months of complete isolation from the organism.[26–31] Our demonstrations that cultures of fetal CNS neurons could establish organotypic synaptic networks with many characteristic physiologic and pharmacologic properties certainly stimulated attempts by Olson and co-workers to maintain similarly isolated CNS tissues as transplants in the anterior eye chamber,[32–35] as a prelude to the exciting transplantation studies reviewed in this volume.

Furthermore, in more recent tissue culture studies, we have shown that fetal mouse dorsal root ganglion neurons can make preferential projections to specific CNS target regions within separate explants and establish functional synaptic connections with appropriate neurons in these dorsal spinal cord and dorsal column nuclei tissues.[36–39] Similarly, fetal mouse retinal ganglion neurons can make preferential projections, characteristic arborizations, and functional connections with co-cultured tectal explants—but not with co-cultured spinal cord.[40–45] These studies demonstrate the capacity of fetal CNS neurons to establish appropriate interneuronal relationships with "host" CNS tissues under rigorously controlled conditions in vitro,[cf.46,47] and they may help to guide and interpret analogous studies of CNS transplants into host brain in situ. The formation of synaptic connections between fetal neurons introduced near CNS target explants that had been allowed to mature for weeks in vitro before co-culture[48,49] provides an even more useful model to supplement studies of CNS transplants into adult brain.[30] Finally, manipulation of the physico-chemical environment and the tissue combinations in organotypic cultures permits analyses of trophic requirements and target-tissue dependencies of specific types of neurons during normal development and after various experimental treatments.[31,50–52] These in vitro studies may be relevant to problems associated with the complex alterations in trophic factors that occur during transplantation of neural tissue into the adult brain.

REFERENCES

1. LEVI-MONTALCINI, R. 1966. The nerve growth factor: Its mode of action on sensory and sympathetic nerve cells. Harvey Lect. **60:** 217-259.
2. LEVI-MONTALCINI, R. & P. U. ANGELETTI. 1968. Nerve growth factor. Physiol. Rev. **48:** 534-569.
3. BUEKER, E. D. 1948. Implantation of tumors in the hind limb field of the embryonic chick and the developmental response of the lumbrosacral nervous system. Anat. Rec. **102:** 369-389.
4. LEVI-MONTALCINI, R. 1952. Effects of mouse tumor transplantation on the nervous system. Ann. N.Y. Acad. Sci. **55:** 330-343.
5. SOTELO, C. & R. M. ALVARADO-MALLART. 1987. Cerebellar transplantations in adult mice with heredo-degenerative ataxia. Ann. N.Y. Acad. Sci. This volume.

6. LEVI-MONTALCINI, R. & V. HAMBURGER. 1953. A diffusible agent of mouse sarcoma, producing hyperplasia of sympathetic ganglia and hyperneurotization of viscera in the chick embryo. J. Exp. Zool. **123:** 233-287.

7. GREENE, L. A. & E. M. SHOOTER. 1980. The nerve growth factor: Biochemistry, synthesis and mechanism of action. Annu. Rev. Neurosci. **3:** 353-402.

8. THOENEN, H. & Y. A. BARDE. 1980. Physiology of the nerve growth factor. Physiol. Rev. **60:** 1284-1335.

9. GNAHN, H., F. HEFTI, R. HEUMANN, M. E. SCHWAB & H. THOENEN. 1983. NGF-mediated increase of choline acetyltransferase (ChAT) in the neonatal rat forebrain: Evidence for a physiological role of NGF in the brain? Dev. Brain Res. **9:** 45-52.

10. HEFTI, F., A. DRAVID & J. HARTIKKA. 1984. Chronic intraventricular injections of nerve growth factor elevate hippocampal choline acetyltransferase activity in adult rats with partial septo-hippocampal lesions. Brain Res. **293:** 305-311.

11. HEFTI, F., J. HARTIKKA, F. ECKENSTEIN, H. GNAHN, R. HEUMANN & M. SCHWAB. 1985. Nerve growth factor increases choline acetyltransferase but not survival or fiber outgrowth of cultured fetal septal cholinergic neurons. Neuroscience **14:** 55-68.

12. MARTINEZ, H. J., C. F. DREYFUS, G. M. JONAKEIT & I. B. BLACK. 1985. NGF specifically enhances development of brain cholinergic neurons in culture. Soc. Neurosci. Abstr. **11:** 660.

13. MOBLEY, W. C., J. L. RUTKOWSKI, G. I. TENNEKOON, K. BUCHANAN & M. V. JOHNSTON. 1985. Choline acetyltransferase activity in striatum of neonatal rats increased by nerve growth factor. Science **229:** 284-287.

14. HEFTI, F. 1985. Nerve growth factor (NGF) promotes survival of septal cholinergic neurons after injury. Soc. Neurosci. Abstr. **11:** 660.

15. BJÖRKLUND, A. & F. H. GAGE. 1987. Grafts of fetal septal cholinergic neurons to the hippocampal formation in aged or fimbria-fornix-lesioned rats. Ann. N.Y. Acad. Sci. This volume.

16. KROMER, L. F. & C. J. CORNBROOKS. 1987. Identification of trophic factors and transplanted cellular environments that promote CNS axonal regeneration. Ann. N.Y. Acad. Sci. This volume.

17. THOENEN, H. & D. EDGAR. 1985. Neurotrophic factors. Science **229:** 238-242.

18. NIETO-SAMPEDRO, M., J. P. KESSLAK, R. GIBBS & C. W. COTMAN. 1987. Effects of conditioning lesions on transplant survival, connectivity, and function: Role of neuro-trophic factors. Ann. N.Y. Acad. Sci. This volume.

19. CUNNINGHAM, T. J., C. B. SUTILLA & F. HAUN. 1987. Trophic effects of transplants following damage to the cerebral cortex. Ann. N.Y. Acad. Sci. This volume.

20. ZHOU, F. C., S. B. AUERBACH & E. C. AZMITIA. 1987. Stimulation of serotonergic neuronal maturation after fetal mesencephalic raphe transplantation into the 5,7-DHT-lesioned hippocampus of the adult rat. Ann. N.Y. Acad. Sci. This volume.

21. SMITH, G. M., R. H. MILLER & J. SILVER. 1987. Astrocyte transplantation induces callosal regeneration in postnatal acallosal mice. Ann. N.Y. Acad. Sci. This volume.

22. HOPKINS, J. M., T. S. FORD-HOLEVINSKI, J. P. MCCOY & B. W. AGRANOFF. 1985. Laminin and optic nerve regeneration in the goldfish. J. Neurosci. **5:** 3030-3038.

23. SCHWAB, M. E. & H. THOENEN. 1985. Dissociated neurons regenerate into sciatic but not optic nerve explants in culture irrespective of neurotrophic factors. J. Neurosci. **5:** 2415-2423.

24. SMALHEISER, N., S. M. CRAIN & L. REID. 1984. Laminin as a substrate for retinal axons *in vitro.* Dev. Brain Res. **12:** 136-140.

25. AGUAYO, A. J., M. VIDAL-SANZ, M. P. VILLEGAS-PÉREZ & G. M. BRAY. 1987. Growth and connectivity of axotomized retinal neurons in adult rats with optic nerves substituted by PNS grafts linking the eye and the midbrain. Ann. N.Y. Acad. Sci. This volume.

26. CRAIN, S. M. & M. B. BORNSTEIN. 1964. Bioelectric activity of neonatal mouse cerebral cortex during growth and differentiation in tissue culture. Exp. Neurol. **10:** 425-450.

27. CRAIN, S. M. & E. R. PETERSON. 1963. Bioelectric activity in long-term cultures of spinal cord tissues. Science **141:** 427-429.

28. CRAIN, S. M. & E. R. PETERSON. 1964. Complex bioelectric activity in organized tissue cultures of spinal cord (human, rat and chick). J. Cell. Comp. Physiol. **64:** 1-13.

29. CRAIN, S. M. 1966. Development of "organotypic" bioelectric activities in central nervous tissues during maturation in culture. Int. Rev. Neurobiol. **9:** 1-43.
30. CRAIN, S. M. 1976. Neurophysiologic Studies in Tissue Cultures. Raven Press. New York, NY.
31. CRAIN, S. M. & E. R. PETERSON. 1974. Development of neural connections in culture. Ann. N.Y. Acad. Sci. **228:** 6-34.
32. HOFFER, B., A. SEIGER, T. LJUNGBERG & L. OLSON. 1974. Electrophysiological studies of brain homografts in the anterior chamber of the eye: Maturation of cerebellar cortex *in oculo.* Brain Res. **79:** 165-184.
33. OLSON, L. & A. SEIGER. 1972. Brain tissue transplanted to the anterior chamber of the eye. I. Fluorescence histochemistry of immature catecholamine and 5-hydroxytryptamine neurons reinnervating the rat iris. Z. Zellforsch. **135:** 175-194.
34. OLSON, L. & A. SEIGER. 1973. Development and growth of immature neurons in rat and man *in situ* and following intraocular transplantation in the rat. Brain Res. **62:** 353-360.
35. OLSON, L., R. FREEDMAN, A. SEIGER & B. HOFFER. 1977. Electrophysiology and cytology of hippocampal formation transplants in the anterior chamber of the eye. I. Intrinsic organization. Brain Res. **119:** 87-106.
36. CRAIN, S. M. & E. R. PETERSON. 1975. Development of specific sensory-evoked synaptic networks in fetal mouse cord-brainstem cultures. Science **188:** 275-278.
37. CRAIN, S. M. & E. R. PETERSON. 1982. Selective innervation of target regions within fetal mouse spinal cord and medulla explants by isolated dorsal root ganglia in organotypic co-cultures. Dev. Brain Res. **2:** 341-362.
38. PETERSON, E. R. & S. M. CRAIN. 1982. Preferential growth of neurites from isolated fetal mouse dorsal root ganglia in relation to specific regions of co-cultured spinal cord explants. Dev. Brain Res. **2:** 363-382.
39. SMALHEISER, N. R., E. R. PETERSON & S. M. CRAIN. 1982. Specific neuritic pathways and arborizations formed by fetal mouse dorsal root ganglion cells within organized spinal cord explants in culture: A peroxidase labeling study. Dev. Brain. Res. **2:** 383-395.
40. SMALHEISER, N. R. & S. M. CRAIN. 1978. Formation of functional retinotectal connections in co-cultures of fetal mouse explants. Brain Res. **148:** 484-492.
41. SMALHEISER, N. R., E. R. PETERSON & S. M. CRAIN. 1981. Neurites from mouse retina and dorsal root ganglion explants show specific behavior within co-cultured tectum or spinal cord. Brain Res. **208:** 499-505.
42. BONHOEFFER, F. & J. HUF. 1985. Position-dependent properties of retinal axons and their growth cones. Nature **315:** 409-410.
43. CRAIN, S. M. 1980. Development of specific synaptic networks in organotypic CNS tissue cultures. *In* Current Topics in Developmental Biology. R. K. Hunt, Ed. Vol. **16:** 87-115. Academic Press. New York, NY.
44. CRAIN, S. M. 1982. Role of CNS target cues in formation of specific afferent synaptic connections in organotypic cultures. *In* Neuroscience Approached through Cell Culture. S. E. Pfeiffer, Ed. Vol. **2:** 1-32. CRC Press. Boca Raton, FL.
45. CRAIN, S. M. 1985. Development and plasticity of specific sensory synaptic networks in fetal mouse spinal cord cultures. *In* Perspectives of Neuroscience: From Molecule to Mind. Y. Tsukada, Ed.: 105-131. University of Tokyo Press. Tokyo.
46. DREYFUS, C. F., M. D. GERSHON & S. M. CRAIN. 1979. Innervation of hippocampal explants by central catecholaminergic neurons in co-cultured fetal mouse brain stem explants. Brain Res. **161:** 431-445.
47. GAHWILER, B. H. & F. HEFTI. 1984. Guidance of acetylcholinesterase-containing fibers by target tissue in co-cultured brain slices. Neuroscience **13:** 681-689.
48. CRAIN, S. M. & E. R. PETERSON. 1973. A tissue culture model for studies of regeneration and formation of new functional connections in adult CNS. Paper read at 3rd Annual Meeting of the Society for Neuroscience. San Diego, CA.
49. PETERSON, E. R. & S. M. CRAIN. 1973. CNS regeneration and formation of new functional connections *in vitro* after transfer of mature spinal cord cultures. Anat. Rec. **175:** 411-412.
50. CRAIN, S. M. & E. R. PETERSON. 1974. Enhanced afferent synaptic functions in fetal mouse spinal cord-sensory ganglion explants following NGF-induced ganglion hyper- trophy. Brain Res. **79:** 145-152.

51. CRAIN, S. M. & E. R. PETERSON. 1984. Enhanced dependence of fetal mouse neurons on trophic factors after taxol exposure in organotypic cultures. *In* Cellular and Molecular Biology of Neuronal Development. I. B. Black, Ed.: 177-200. Plenum. New York, NY.
52. PETERSON, E. R. & S. M. CRAIN. 1982. Nerve growth factor attenuates neurotoxic effects of taxol on spinal cord-ganglion explants from mice. Science **217:** 377-379.

Effects of Conditioning Lesions on Transplant Survival, Connectivity, and Function

Role of Neurotrophic Factors

MANUEL NIETO-SAMPEDRO, J. PATRICK KESSLAK,
ROBERT GIBBS, AND CARL W. COTMAN

University of California at Irvine
Irvine, California 92717

Are there mechanisms intrinsic to the brain that can be drawn upon to promote functional repair after central nervous system (CNS) injury? Brain transplants provide a powerful approach for investigating this question. The successful grafting of neurons into damaged brain depends not only on the type of neurons transplanted but on the ability of the host brain to support and integrate these cells. In cell culture, for example, neurons will grow only if provided the proper medium and substrate. Similarly, the mature brain must provide the proper environment and be sufficiently adaptable to incorporate fetal neurons into its circuits. One of the first clues to the nature of intrinsic mechanisms came from the observation that introducing a delay between the time of injury and transplantation could significantly enhance the survival and integration of grafted neurons. This effect is correlated with the production and accumulation of trophic factors in the brain in response to injury. Thus, transplanted neurons may depend upon the establishment of proper "conditions" to enhance survival, integration, and behavioral function.

NEUROTROPHIC FACTORS INDUCED BY BRAIN INJURY

Neurotrophic (neuron survival) and neurite promoting (sprouting) factors increase in the brain following injury. These data have been reviewed recently[1] and will only be summarized here. In brief, CNS injury induces the production of factors that support the survival of both peripheral and central neurons maintained in cell culture. Survival- and neurite-promoting activities begin to increase a few days after injury, reach a maximum at 1-2 weeks (in adults), and decline thereafter.[2,3] These activities are highest within tissues surrounding the wound, but are also high within denervated areas distal from the lesion.

EFFECT OF DELAY ON TRANSPLANT SURVIVAL

Some tissues survive poorly when transplanted to a wound cavity at the time the cavity is made. For example, grafts of striatal cholinergic neurons fail to survive when transplanted to the entorhinal region immediately after producing a retrohippocampal lesion. Survival of these cells is greatly enhanced by conditioning lesions, that is, by introducing a delay of several days between the lesion and implant surgeries.[3,4] Cholinergic septal neurons appear less dependent on conditioning lesions, whereas cholinergic habenular neurons are intermediate between striatal and septal.[5] Therefore, dependence on environment appears to be contingent, at least in part, on the type of neuron transplanted. One possible explanation is that specific trophic factors are more beneficial for some cells than for others, and that factors produced at the site of injury are most beneficial to cells that normally reside within the injured area. Therefore, we have recently examined the effect of delay on the transplantation of entorhinal cortical neurons into the damaged entorhinal cortex.

Animals received a unilateral knife cut through the angular bundle[6] to destroy native entorhinal projections to the hippocampal formation. Embryonic (E17-E18) entorhinal tissues (0.5-1.0 mm^3) were placed into the cavity either immediately after severing the angular bundle or after a delay of 8-10 days. In addition, some animals received entorhinal implants injected directly into the angular bundle without producing any prior lesion. Grafts were examined 2 months after surgery for size and connectivity.

Grafts transplanted with a delay (ECX-delay) survived well and were severalfold larger than those transplanted with no delay (ECX-no delay)(FIGS. 1 & 2).[7] Grafts injected into the brain without producing any prior lesion also survived well and were intermediate in size. In the ECX-no delay group, cavitation was often observed in the transplant area, suggesting that the majority of the transplant had degenerated. Such cavities were never observed when the ECX-delay paradigm was used. These data suggest that the delay has beneficial effects for two reasons: 1) introducing a delay avoids the detrimental effects of events that take place immediately after producing the lesion (for example, bleeding, gliosis, and degeneration); and 2) the survival-promoting activity of the local environment increases after injury. Once again, the effectiveness of the delay correlates with the brain's ability to produce trophic factors in response to injury. Also, the time course for the production and accumulation of these factors closely parallels that for axon sprouting in the partially denervated target, suggesting that these factors may facilitate the formation of new functional connections after injury. If so, we reasoned that such factors might also enhance outgrowth from entorhinal transplants.

EFFECT OF DELAY ON TRANSPLANT-DERIVED INNERVATION
OF THE HOST

As previously mentioned, introduction of a delay between the lesion and transplant surgeries significantly enhanced the survival of entorhinal grafts; survival was probably enhanced because of the induction and accumulation of trophic factors by the lesion. In addition, graft-derived innervation of the hippocampal formation was examined by injecting wheat germ agglutin-horseradish peroxidase (WGA-HRP) into the hippo-

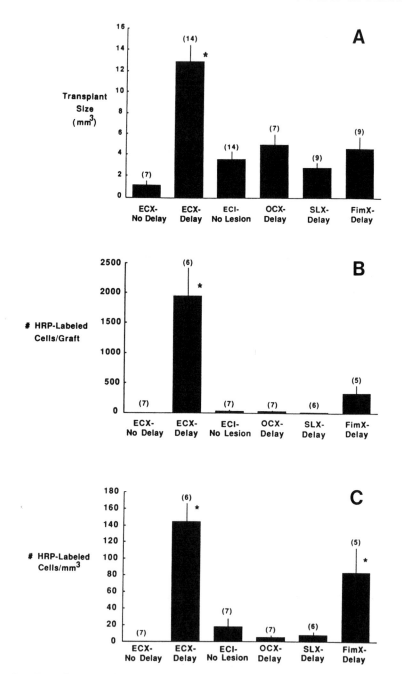

FIGURE 1. The effects of using a delay, and the effects of different lesions on transplant size and connectivity (see the text for details). Error bars represent SEMs; asterisks indicate statistically significant differences ($p < .02$). Taken from Gibbs *et al.*[7]

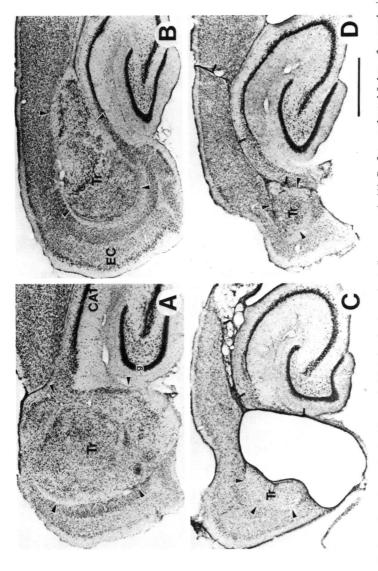

FIGURE 2. Horizontal sections stained with cresyl violet showing transplants (large arrows). (**A**) Graft transplanted 8 days after producing an angular bundle lesion (ECX-delay). (**B**) Graft injected into the angular bundle without producing any prior lesion (ECI-no lesion). This is also representative of grafts transplanted 8–10 days after producing a lesion in occipital cortex, medial septum, or fimbria fornix. (**C** and **D**) Grafts transplanted immediately after producing an angular bundle lesion (ECX-no delay). Note the poor survival of the grafts in comparison with **A** and the cavitation in **C** (small arrows point to the knife cuts). Tr: transplant; EC: entorhinal cortex; g: dentate granule cells. Scale bar: 0.5 mm. Taken from Gibbs *et al.*[7]

campus ipsilateral to the transplant (FIG. 2). Grafts in the ECX-delay group contained an average total of about 1940 HRP-labeled cells per graft.[7] In contrast, grafts in the ECX-no delay group contained essentially no labeled cells, even when reasonable survival was observed (FIGS. 1 & 3).[7] Therefore, in addition to promoting graft survival, introduction of a delay can also enhance the development of connectivity between transplant and host.

EFFECT OF DIFFERENT LESIONS ON TRANSPLANT-DERIVED INNERVATION OF THE HOST

As previously mentioned, entorhinal grafts transplanted without severing the angular bundle were smaller than those in the ECX-delay group (FIG. 2). Little graft-derived innervation of the hippocampal formation was observed when grafts were transplanted in the absence of a prior lesion (ECI-no lesion) or following lesions of occipital cortex (OCX-delay) or medial septum (SLX-delay) (FIG. 3).[7] This was true even though grafts integrated well with the host tissues and, in some cases, were in direct contact with the hippocampus or dentate gyrus. All of the grafts received acetylcholine esterase-positive innervation from the host, demonstrating that no physical barrier separated the grafts from the rest of the brain.

Considerably more innervation was obtained when grafts were transplanted after transecting the fimbria-fornix (FimX-delay).[7] Because of the variability in the size of the grafts, this increase was significant only when expressed in terms of the number of HRP-labeled cells per cubic millimeter of graft tissue (FIG. 1C). In these cases, in addition to septal deafferentation, some damage of entorhinal fibers was produced that was due to partial destruction of the dorsal psalterium.

These data suggest that the specific removal of entorhinal projections significantly enhances outgrowth from the entorhinal grafts. Similarly, innervation of the hippocampal formation by septal cholinergic grafts is greatly facilitated by the removal of native cholinergic projections.[4]

NATURE OF ENDOGENOUS CONTRIBUTIONS OF THE HOST TO TRANSPLANT

Thus, introduction of a delay between the lesion and implant surgeries significantly enhances graft survival and appears to be beneficial for the establishment of transplant-to-host projections. Growth factors that accumulate for several days around the site of injury may contribute to the survival and growth of the grafts. In support of this hypothesis, we have previously shown that supplements of exogenous factors improved survival of transplants when grafted immediately after a brain wound.[3] In addition to a possible role of growth factors, an enhanced rate and extent of vascularization may also contribute to transplant viability.[8]

New capillary growth around the lesion site begins after about 1 day and reaches its near maximal levels about 10 days postlesion (FIG. 4). Thus, transplants placed into the lesion cavity come into contact with a well-vascularized surface. It is unlikely, however, that vascular effects alone account for the enhanced survival; after all, it

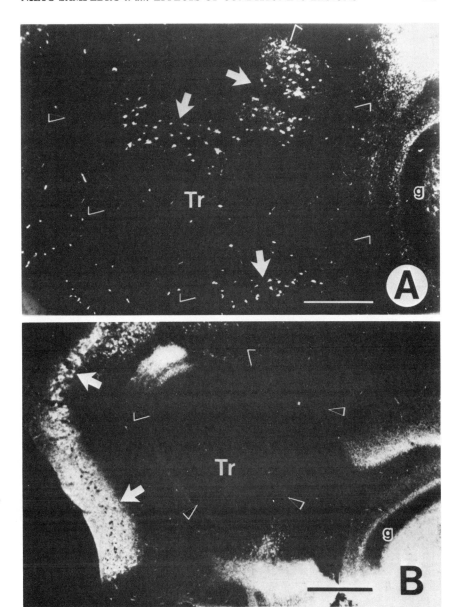

FIGURE 3. Horizontal sections showing transplants (outlined by small arrows) and HRP-labeled cells following an injection of WGA-HRP into the hippocampal formation. (A) Graft injected 8 days after producing an angular bundle lesion. Note the presence of many HRP-labeled cells in the transplant (large arrows). (B) Graft injected directly into the angular bundle without producing any prior lesion. Note the absence of HRP-labeled cells in the transplant. Also note that many cells are labeled in the host entorhinal cortex (large arrows), demonstrating that few native entorhinal projections were severed during the transplantation procedure. Tr: transplant; g: dendate granule cells. Scale bars: 0.5 mm. Taken from Gibbs *et al.*[7]

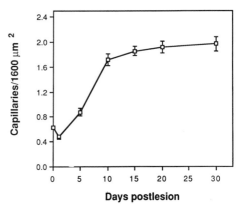

FIGURE 4. Density of capillaries surrounding a wound cavity at various times after damage.

has been demonstrated that tissue growth is also dependent upon the location where the tissue is placed. Other location-dependent interactions are critical, such as the existence of specific growth factors and a compatible environment for synapse formation.

CREATING A FAVORABLE ENVIRONMENT: PIVOTAL ROLE OF ASTROCYTES

What cells produce growth factors and "condition" the environment? Astrocytes *in vitro* secrete factors that promote neuronal survival and process outgrowth.[9] Furthermore, astrocytes provide a unique substrate for neuron attachment and guidance of neurite extension.[10,11] Following injury to the adult rat CNS, the conditions that lead to the production of neurotrophic and neurite-promoting factors *in vivo,* and the time course for their increase, parallel those of astrocytosis and astrogliosis.[3] Suppression of glial proliferation causes suppression of trophic factor production.[12] Thus, there is evidence both *in vitro* and *in vivo* indicating that astrocytes provide trophic support to central neurons.

It was noted previously that transplants performed in the absence of a delay frequently produced a cavity adjacent to part of the perimeter of the transplant. Such cavitation may be due to toxins released by the injury. As a result of trauma, for example, excessive amounts of glutamate (up to eight times the normal level) are released into the extracellular space.[13] Cell death results if glutamate levels remain elevated for periods beyond several minutes, or if excitatory amino acids are injected directly into the CNS.[14] Astrocytes have powerful transport systems that can accumulate excess glutamate released after injury and convert it into nonneuroactive glutamine.[15,16] Thus, glial cells may provide a natural protective mechanism against glutamate toxicity.

ASTROCYTES AND RECOVERY OF FUNCTION

These facts suggest that astrocytes may play an active and beneficial role after brain injury. The question then arises whether glial transplants can be used to facilitate functional recovery. The use of behavioral measures provides a generalized assay of the functional significance of transplants. Bilateral ablation of the mediofrontal cortex of adult rats causes severe deficits in learning spatial tasks. Typically, cortically damaged animals require at least twice as many trials as sham-operated controls to learn a simple reinforced alternation task in a T-shaped maze. Previously, Labbe and co-workers[17] found that transplants of embryonic frontal cortex accelerated recovery of this behavior. Recovery was observed within 6 days after transplantation. It seemed likely that such rapid recovery was too fast to involve the formation of neuronal connections between host and transplant and was possibly due to other factors associated with the presence of astrocytes. Accordingly, we examined whether transplants of primary astrocytes grown in culture would facilitate recovery following frontal cortex lesions and examined behavioral recovery.

Purified astrocytes transplanted into in a wound cavity immediately after injury accelerated the rate of learning a reinforced alternation task to sham-operated levels (FIG. 5). The efficiency of such astrocyte transplants did not differ from that of delayed transplants of embryonic frontal cortex or unlesioned controls.[18]

These data suggest that transplant of cultured, purified astrocytes could have therapeutic usefulness in the treatment of certain types of CNS injury. The essential role played by astrocytes in the natural repair mechanisms after minor CNS injury indicates that they could be used in the treatment of major lesions to prevent cytotoxic reactions and stimulate growth. In this way and others, astrocytes may provide a more favorable environment. If a high density of astrocytes can be supplied at the time of injury, their response mechanisms to trauma can act faster, much like a conditioning lesion.

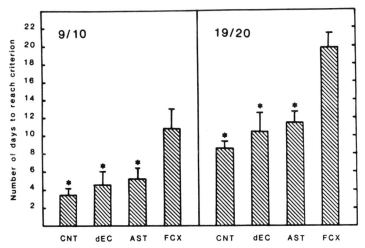

FIGURE 5. Number of days required to attain criterion after frontal cortex ablation. Means and SEMs for groups at two performance criteria (∗: $p < .05$). The groups are as follows: CNT-undamaged control ($N = 8$); dEC-delayed transplant of embryonic frontal cortex ($N = 9$); AST-purified astrocytes grown in culture and transplanted immediately after ablation ($N = 7$); and FCX-frontal cortex ablation ($N = 9$). Data from Kesslak *et al.*[18]

THE INFLUENCE OF CONDITIONING LESIONS ON
TRANSPLANTS AND BEHAVIORAL RECOVERY

If a delay mobilizes intrinsic reactions that promote functional recovery, then transplants should be more effective in behavioral restoration when introduced with a delay. In fact, this appears to be the case. Recently, Kesslak and co-workers[18] studied the effect of conditioning lesions on the ability of transplants to restore the learning deficits in animals with frontal cortex lesions. Embryonic tissues grafted immediately after frontal cortex ablation produced a transient increase in the rate of learning, but it quickly declined to levels of lesions alone. This correlated to the poor survival of embryonic transplants placed immediately after the lesion. Only 20% of those transplants survived, and those were only of moderate size. In contrast, animals that received a transplant 10 days after frontal cortex ablation learned the reinforced alternation task significantly faster than the no-delay transplant and frontal cortex lesion groups. These transplants showed a higher rate of survival (80%) and stained for acetylcholine esterase, illustrating that they were innervated by the host fibers.

In order to further evaluate the effect of conditioning lesions on behavioral recovery, a more stringent transplant paradigm is needed. Transplants of adult tissues have not been shown to enhance behavioral recovery after injuries. It is generally believed that few, if any, adult cells can survive. Adult brain has higher basal levels of trophic activity, possibly indicating that higher endogenous levels are necessary for survival. If so, a conditioning lesion might facilitate survival of transplanted adult tissue.

Surprisingly, animals with transplants of adult frontal cortex placed after a conditioning lesion performed very similarly to animals with embryonic transplants (FIG. 6). Animals that received transplants of adult CNS tissues learned the task in fewer trials than those with frontal cortex lesions and no transplants ($p < .05$). The adult tissue transplants contained many apparent glial cells, but adult cells having neuronal-like morphology also appeared to be present. Studies are still in progress to quantitate the relative number of neurons in these transplants and their properties. At present, we prefer to be very cautious about the prospect that some adult neurons will survive transplantation. Nonetheless, transplants of adult frontal cortex did accelerate the rate of behavioral recovery.

CONCLUSIONS

Our results, and those of other groups, suggest that after injury the brain mobilizes healing reactions that favor the survival and integration of transplants, even those of adult tissues. These are probably some of the same mechanisms involved in the regrowth of circuitry after partial denervation (reactive synaptogenesis) and possibly in the cessation of secondary cell death around the injury site (see reference 1 for discussion). The induction of neurotrophic factors and vascularization are prominent among the mechanisms. Vascularization, no doubt, is necessary for survival of large transplants, but it cannot account for the dependence of transplant survival and integration on host site and the type of cell transplanted. In our studies, entorhinal neurons survived and integrated best when placed in their native site, but only when most of the normal hippocampal innervation was destroyed. This suggests that normal homotypic synaptic interactions are competitive with transplanted neurons. It may be that they compete for the same trophic support, that selective growth inhibitors are produced, or that adequate synaptic space is simply unavailable.

Astrocytes play an apparently paradoxical role in the recovery of functions and rebuilding of circuits after injury. Astrocyte transplants can mediate behavioral recovery, which illustrates that under select circumstances their net effect can be beneficial. They may protect against toxicity by excitatory amino acids, and they appear to produce growth factors that can aid neurons. Yet they are generally regarded as being detrimental to regeneration. It is not possible to determine which of their many properties are most advantageous nor, unfortunately, can we identify those features that limit recovery. Taken together, it seems that these cells play a key role in supporting the essential steps necessary to achieve more significant functional recovery. Clearly, the series of reactions mobilized by conditioning lesions is of benefit to transplant survival and integration and the ability of transplants to promote functional recovery.

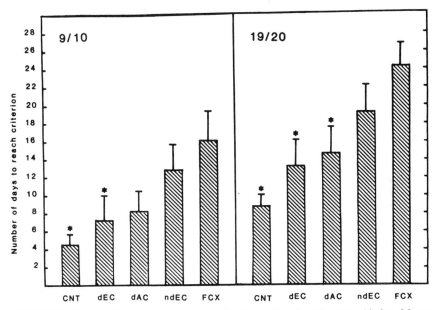

FIGURE 6. Number of days required to attain criterion after frontal cortex ablation. Means and SEMs for groups at two performance criteria (*: $p < .05$). The groups are as follows: CNT-undamaged control ($N = 17$); dEC-delayed transplant of embryonic frontal cortex ($N = 7$); dAC-delayed transplant of adult frontal cortex ($N = 7$); ndEC-no delay frontal cortex transplant placed immediately after ablation ($N = 6$); and FCX-frontal cortex ablation ($N = 16$).

REFERENCES

1. NIETO-SAMPEDRO, M. & C. W. COTMAN. 1985. Growth factor induction and temporal order in CNS repair. *In* Synaptic Plasticity and Remodeling. C. W. Cotman, Ed.: Chapter 14. Guilford Press. New York, NY.
2. NEEDELS, D. L., M. NIETO-SAMPEDRO & C. W. COTMAN. 1986. Induction of a novel neurite-promoting activity in rat brain following injury. Neuroscience **18**: 517-526.

3. NIETO-SAMPEDRO, M., M. MANTHORPE, G. BARBIN, S. VARON & C. W. COTMAN. 1983. Injury-induced neuronotrophic activity in adult rat brain: Correlation with survival of delayed implants in the wound cavity. J. Neurosci. **3:** 2219-2229.

4. LEWIS, E. R. & C. W. COTMAN. 1982. Mechanisms of septal lamination in the developing hippocampus revealed by outgrowth of fibers from septal implants. III. Competitive interactions. Brain Res. **233:** 29-44.

5. GIBBS, R. B., K. J. ANDERSON & C. W. COTMAN. 1986. Factors affecting innervation in the CNS: Comparison of three cholinergic cell types transplanted to the hippocampus of adult rats. Brain Res. **383:** 362-366.

6. GIBBS, R. B., E. W. HARRIS & C. W. COTMAN. 1985. Replacement of damaged cortical projections with transplants of entorhinal cortex. J. Comp. Neurol. **26:** 47-65.

7. GIBBS, R. B. & C. W. COTMAN. 1986. Factors affecting survival and outgrowth from transplants of entorhinal cortex. Neuroscience. In press.

8. STENEVI, U., A. BJÖRKLUND & N.-A. SVENDGAARD. 1976. Transplantation of central and peripheral monoamine neurons to the adult rat brain: Techniques and conditions for survival. Brain Res. **114:** 1-20.

9. BANKER, G. A. 1980. Trophic interactions between astroglial cells and hippocampal neurons in culture. Science **209:** 809-810.

10. NOBLE, M., J. FOK-SEANG & J. COHEN. 1984. Glia are a unique substrate for the *in vitro* growth of central nervous system neurons. J. Neurosci. **4:** 1892-1903.

11. FALLON, J. R. 1985. Neurite guidance by non-neuronal cells in culture: Preferential outgrowth of peripheral neurites on glial as compared to nonglial cell surfaces. J. Neurosci. **5:** 170-174.

12. HEACOCK, A. M., A. R. SCHONFELD & R. KATZMAN. 1984. Relation of hippocampal trophic activity to cholinergic nerve sprouting. Neurosci. Abstr. **10:** 1052.

13. BENEVISTE, H., J. DREJER, A. SCHOUSBOE & N. H. DIEMER. 1984. Elevation of the extracellular concentrations of glutamate and aspartate in rat hippocampus during transient cerebral ischemia monitored by intracerebral microdialysis. J. Neurochem. **43:** 1369-1374.

14. ROTHMAN, S. M. & J. W. OLNEY. 1986. Glutamate and the pathology of hypoxic/ischemic brain damage. Ann. Neurol. In press.

15. NICKLAS, W. J. 1986. Glia-neuronal interrelationships in the metabolism of excitatory amino acids. *In* Excitatory Amino Acids. P. J. Roberts, J. Storm Mathisen & H. F. Bradford, Eds. Macmillan. London.

16. SHANK, R. P. & M. H. APRISON. 1981. Present status and significance of the glutamine cycle in neural tissue. Life Sci. **28:** 837-842.

17. LABBE, R., A. FIRL, JR., E. J. MUFSON & D. G. STEIN. 1983. Fetal brain transplants: Reduction of cognitive deficits in rats with frontal cortex lesions. Science **221:** 470-472.

18. KESSLAK, J. P., M. NIETO-SAMPEDRO, J. GLOBUS & C. W. COTMAN. 1986. Transplants of purified astrocytes promote behavioral recovery after frontal cortex ablation. Exp. Neurol. **92:** 377-390.

DISCUSSION OF THE PAPER

P. R. SANBERG (*Ohio University, Athens, OH*): What happens if you remove the Gelfoam in a recovered animal?

NIETO-SAMPEDRO: What happens to the Gelfoam?

SANBERG: What happens if you have a recovered animal with Gelfoam in the wound cavities, and then you remove it after it shows recovery of function?

NIETO-SAMPEDRO: We do not know. I could guess that the animal would probably stay recovered, but we have never actually performed such a removal.

R. MIAO (*Hanna Biologics, Berkeley, CA*): How do you extract the Gelfoam?

NIETO-SAMPEDRO: You take it into five volumes of its weight in Hanks' balanced salt solution or any other buffer, and homogenize it in a tight-fitting buffer homogenizer with 20 up-and-down strokes at about 600 RPMs in the cold.

MIAO: And then you put that back into another Gelfoam?

NIETO-SAMPEDRO: And then you put that back into another Gelfoam or test it for activity in tissue culture after sterilizing it.

MIAO: So you have not done any specific extraction for lipid-containing material or for carbohydrates?

NIETO-SAMPEDRO: No. I have been tempted several times to look at things like prostaglandins and leukotrienes, and other odds and ends, but I have never got around to doing it.

G. PAPPAS (*University of Illinois, Chicago, IL*): In our limited experience with Gelfoam, rat brain likes Gelfoam. It becomes vascularized, it is not leaky, it does not leak horseradish peroxidase, it is very nice. As I say, it becomes very well integrated so that we also do not see very much active glia around it after 2 months or so.

NIETO-SAMPEDRO: Yes, Gelfoam is a very good alternative to neurons!

PAPPAS: Yes, it is very good. I recommend it.

NIETO-SAMPEDRO: Probably it is better than some neurons. I think the lack of glial scars happens in the delay transplant paradigm. It has been reported by several workers, particularly by Reier, in transplants in the spinal cord. It is related to something we found: the presence of inhibitors of mitogens. Astrocyte mitogens are inhibited by things contained either in gelfoam or just in brain—particularly neonatal brain, where the mitogens are powerfully inhibited.

Grafts of Fetal Septal Cholinergic Neurons to the Hippocampal Formation in Aged or Fimbria-Fornix-lesioned Rats[a]

ANDERS BJÖRKLUND[b]

Department of Histology
University of Lund
Lund, Sweden

FRED H. GAGE

Department of Neurosciences
University of California at San Diego
La Jolla, California

INTRODUCTION

The role of the basal forebrain cholinergic system in learning and memory processes has attracted considerable attention during recent years. Pharmacological manipulation of central cholinergic transmission has been shown to have profound effects on learning and memory, both in human subjects and in experimental animals.[1-3] Moreover, neuropathological and neurochemical studies on autopsy material from patients with Alzheimer's disease have demonstrated a substantial degeneration or atrophy of the cholinergic neurons in the basal forebrain, including the nucleus basalis, substantia innominata, and septal-diagonal band area.[4-7] This is associated with a loss of the acetylcholine synthetic enzyme choline acetyltransferase (ChAT) in wide areas of the neo- and allocortex,[8-10] and the magnitude of the cortical ChAT reduction post mortem has been reported to correlate with the severity of the dementia in patients with Alzheimer's disease.[9]

In aged rodents, as well, impairments in learning and memory have been associated with an age-dependent decline in the parameters of forebrain cholinergic transmission.[3,11-15] Thus, although there are no data so far to implicate an actual loss of cholinergic forebrain neurons with age in rodents, that is, one that would be similar

[a] This work was supported by Grant 04X-3874 from the Swedish Medical Research Council and by Grants NS-06701 and AG-03766 from the National Institute of Health and Aging.

[b] Address for correspondence: Department of Histology, University of Lund, Biskopsgatan 5, S-223 62, Lund, Sweden.

to that observed in Alzheimer's-type dementia in man, it seems possible that a functional deterioration of the limbic and cortical cholinergic projection systems may contribute to the age-related cognitive impairments in these species, too. This is consistent with experiments in young rats: surgical or excitotoxic damage to either of the two major components of the basal forebrain cholinergic system, that is, the septohippocampal or basalocortical projections, causes marked impairments in a variety of learning and memory tasks.[16-19]

In the present series of experiments, we have studied the ability of grafts of fetal basal forebrain cholinergic neurons to substitute, structurally and functionally, for a lost or age-impaired cholinergic afferent input to the hippocampal formation, and have done so using two experimental models. First, we have transplantated cholinergic-rich tissue from the fetal septal-diagonal band area to the hippocampal formation in young rats with surgical transection of the fimbria-fornix pathways. Second, we have implanted fetal septal-diagonal band neurons into the hippocampal formation of behaviorally impaired aged rats. The combined results show that intrahippocampal grafts of tissue rich in developing cholinergic neurons can compensate at least partly for lesion-induced or age-dependent cognitive impairments in rats, and that this effect may be due to the restoration of cholinergic neurotransmission in the deafferented or dysfunctioning host hippocampal target.

GRAFT SURVIVAL AND FIBER OUTGROWTH

The septal-diagonal band region, which was dissected from 14-17-day-old rat embryos, was grafted either as a solid piece into the cavity formed by an aspirative fimbria-fornix lesion,[20] or in the form of a dissociated cell suspension, which was injected directly into the hippocampal formation of the host.[21,22]

Solid Septal Grafts

The solid septal grafts underwent within the first 2 weeks after grafting a reduction in size, to about half their original volume. Between 1 and 4 months after grafting, however, they grew about threefold to reach a final size that was about 50% larger than that of the initially implanted pieces. Acetylcholinesterase (AChE)-positive fibers were seen to extend from the grafts caudally into the denervated host hippocampus, starting at about 2 weeks after transplantation. By 4 months a new AChE-positive innervation had been established up to a distance of about 6-8 mm from the graft. The laminar pattern established by the newly formed AChE-positive terminal networks was remarkably similar to that of the normal AChE-positive innervation, also with respect to finer details. This suggests that the distribution of the ingrowing fibers from the graft was highly specific. Other experiments, using grafts of different types of monoaminergic neurons, have shown that the patterning of the ingrowing axons is characteristic for each neuron type, and that it is greatly dependent both on graft placement and on the presence or absence of the intrinsic cholinergic innervation.[23-26]

Septal Cell Suspension Grafts

Septal cell suspension grafts were injected, under stereotaxic control, in volumes of 2-5 μl at two or three sites in each hippocampus.[22] The implanted tissue was usually found as several cellular aggregates or tissue masses within the hippocampal or choroidal fissures (FIG. 1), within the overlying ventricle, or embedded in the host hippocampal tissue. It has been estimated that the implanted tissue will grow to about twice its initial volume and that approximately 60% of the potential number of cholinergic neurons will survive, provided the implants are made into a cholinergically denervated (fimbria-fornix-lesioned) hippocampus.[27,28] A new AChE-positive innervation was established from the grafts, starting between 1 and 3 weeks after implantation.[22] Within 3 months, the entire hippocampal formation was reached by the ingrowing fibers and had a terminal density approaching that of the normal hippocampus. As in the fimbria-fornix-lesioned animals with solid septal grafts, the laminar pattern formed by the graft-derived AChE-positive fibers mimicked very closely that of the normal cholinergic innervation (FIG. 2).

Aged Rats

In aged rats, grafting has been performed into the intact hippocampal formation, using the cell suspension technique.[29,30] Graft survival assessed 3-4 months after grafting was comparable to that seen in our previous studies of young adult recipients. Fiber outgrowth into the host brain was evaluated in animals that had their intrinsic septohippocampal pathway removed (by a fimbria-fornix lesion) 6-10 days before being killed. Dense outgrowth of AChE-positive fibers occurred up to about 2 mm away from the septal implants. The overall magnitude of fiber outgrowth was less than that generally seen in the previously denervated hippocampus in young adult recipients, but it appeared to be as extensive as in young recipients when the grafts were placed in the nondenervated hippocampal formation. In addition, the distribution of the AChE-positive fibers from the septal implants in the host hippocampus suggested that the pattern formed in the nondenervated target tissue of the aged recipients was more diffuse than and somewhat different from the normal pattern.

Electron Microscopy

Electron microscopy in combination with ChAT immunocytochemistry has shown that the ingrowing cholinergic axons from the grafts form abundant synaptic contacts with neuronal elements in the host dentate gyrus both in the fimbria-fornix-lesioned young rats as well as in the nondenervated aged rats.[31-33] Although the graft-derived synapses in the aged rats were remarkably similar to normal synapses, both qualitatively and quantitatively, some abnormalities were found in the fimbria-fornix-lesioned young rats with respect to the relative distribution of contacts on dendrites and neuronal perikarya.

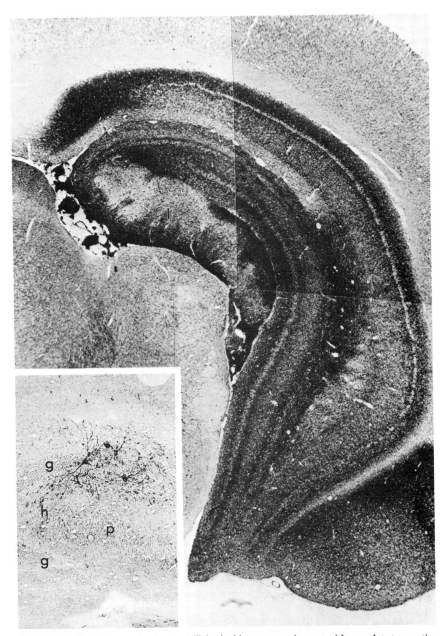

FIGURE 1. Septal suspension implant (I) in the hippocampus in a rat with complete transection of the fimbria-fornix, 9 months survival. The graft, which has grown to destroy part of the dentate gyrus at this level, is rich in AChE staining and has given rise to a new dense AChE-positive fiber network in the host hippocampus. The inset shows examples of AChE-positive (presumably cholinergic) neurons in a graft from a rat pretreated with diisopropyl fluorophosphate, 3 months survival. g: dentate granule cell layer; h: hilus; p: CA3 pyramidal cell layer. Taken from reference 22, with permission.

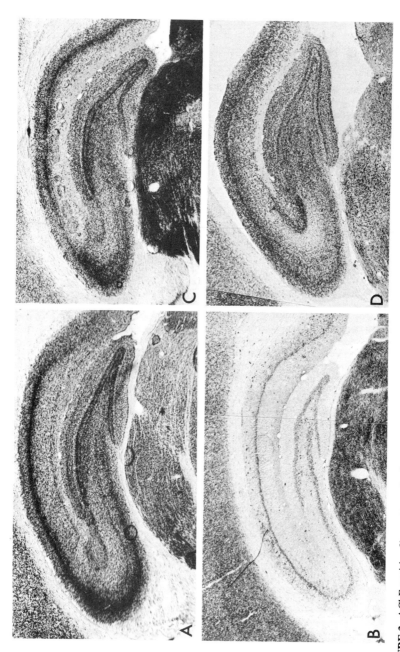

FIGURE 2. AChE-positive fiber patterns in the dorsal hippocampus, rostral to the suspension transplantation site. (**A**) Normal rat. (**B**) Fimbria-fornix-lesioned rat without graft, 3 months survival. (**C**) Fimbria-fornix lesion plus septal suspension grafts, 3 months survival. (**D**) Same as C, but 14 months survival. Taken from reference 22, with permission.

BIOCHEMICAL MEASURES OF GRAFT FUNCTION

The activity of the cholinergic innervation of the denervated hippocampus, derived from solid or suspension grafts of the septal-diagonal band area, has been monitored biochemically by measurements of the acetylcholine-synthesizing enzyme, ChAT, and of acetylcholine synthesis rates *in vitro*.[20,34] Although AChE is a useful anatomical marker in the septohippocampal cholinergic projection system, the AChE enzyme is not a specific marker for cholinergic neurons. The synthetic enzyme, ChAT, by contrast, is an enzyme specifically localized in cholinergic neurons and is therefore a better marker of cholinergic neurotransmission. ChAT enzyme activity has therefore been used to measure the time course and magnitude of fiber outgrowth from both solid and suspended septal grafts. As shown in FIGURE 3, graft-derived ChAT activity was barely detectable the first 10 days after the implantation of cell suspension grafts, but it sharply increased between 10 days and 1 month in the region of the host hippocampus close to the graft. Within 6 months, ChAT activity was restored to nearly normal levels in all segments of the previously denervated hippocampal formation. When the total ChAT activity derived from the solid grafts and the cell suspension grafts were compared (FIG. 4), the cell suspension grafts appeared to be about twice as effective as the solid grafts although the amount of tissue grafted was about the same in each case.

The functional activity of the septal grafts was further assessed by measurements of [14C]acetylcholine synthesis from [14C]glucose *in vitro* in fimbria-fornix-lesioned rats with septal suspension implanted into the depth of the denervated hippocampus.[34] The overall hippocampal [14C]acetylcholine synthesis was restored to normal levels in the grafted animals, and estimates of the acetylcholine turnover rate suggested that the transmitter machinery of the newly established septohippocampal connections operated at a rate similar to that of the intrinsic septohippocampal pathway. Thus, these septal cell suspensions seem capable of maintaining function at a relatively "physiological" level despite their abnormal position.

In a more recent study, Kelly *et al.*[35] investigated the magnitude of lesion-induced functional alterations in different regions of the hippocampal formation, as reflected in the local rates of [14C]2-deoxyglucose (2-DG) utilization, and the degree to which this index of functional activity could be normalized following reinnervation by solid septal grafts. As summarized schematically in FIGURE 5, transection of the septohippocampal pathway by a unilateral fimbria-fornix lesion resulted in a 30-50% reduction in 2-DG utilization throughout the ipsilateral hippocampal formation, and this function remained depressed 6 months after the lesion was made. Interestingly, the areas of depressed 2-DG utilization within the lesioned hemisphere were largely coextensive with the areas of the cingulate cortex and the hippocampal formation that had been substantially cholinergically denervated as a consequence of the fimbria-fornix transection (left panel in FIG. 5). Fimbria-fornix-lesioned rats that had received solid septal grafts displayed a significant recovery in hippocampal 2-DG use, as compared to the rats that had only received a lesion. A significant correlation was found between the graft-induced recovery in 2-DG utilization and the graft-induced recovery in AChE staining density in adjacent sections from the same brains ($r = .84$; $p < .01$); thus there appeared to be a relationship between the cholinergic reinnervation from the septal grafts and the restoration of functional glucose utilization. Indeed, the area of the host hippocampus and dentate gyrus that showed a complete restoration of AChE-positive innervation in these grafted animals was normalized with respect to the 2-DG utilization rate (crosshatching in right panel in FIG. 5), whereas the area with only partial AChE-positive reinnervation showed a partial but incomplete recovery

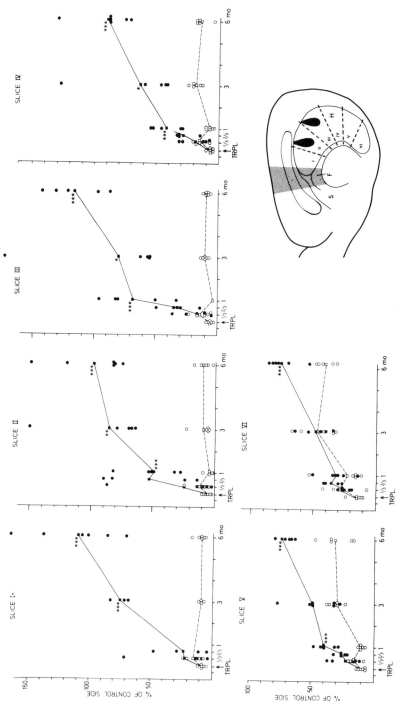

FIGURE 3. Recovery of ChAT activity (expressed as nmoles of ACh formed per mg protein per hour) in the six slices of the host hippocampal formation shown in the insert. Open symbols and dashed lines: animals with fimbria-fornix lesion alone; closed symbols and solid lines: animals with fimbria-fornix lesions and septal suspension grafts (implanted at two sites, as shown in the inset). Differences between grafted and nongrafted groups: * = p < .05; ** = p < .01; *** = p < .001. Taken from reference 34, with permission.

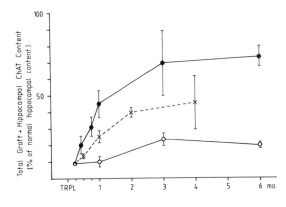

FIGURE 4. Time course of recovery of total ChAT content (expressed as nmoles of ACh formed per hippocampus per hour) in rats with fimbria-fornix lesions only (O); in rats with solid septal grafts placed in the fimbria-fornix lesion cavities (X); and in rats with lesions plus septal suspension grafts, as in FIGURE 3 (●). Taken from reference 34, with permission.

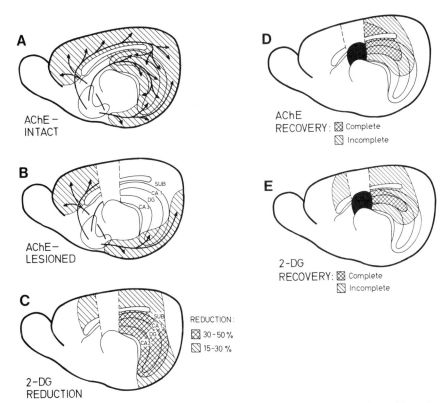

FIGURE 5. Schematic summary of the results obtained in the 2-DG autoradiographic study by Kelly *et al.*[35] (**A**) AChE staining before lesioning. (**B**) Cholinergic denervation induced by the fimbria-fornix lesion. (**C**) Reductions in 2-DG utilization rates accompanying the cholinergic denervation. (**D**) Areas of complete or incomplete graft-induced recovery of AChE-staining. (**D** and **E**) Areas of complete or incomplete graft-induced recovery of 2-DG utilization in rats with solid septal grafts (black areas).

of 2-DG use (hatching in right panel in FIG. 5). Together with the biochemical data quoted above, these results strongly suggest that the cholinergic component of the grafts is functional at the biochemical level and are capable of influencing, or normalizing, the overall functional performance of the deafferented hippocampal formation.

ELECTROPHYSIOLOGICAL STUDIES

A series of studies have applied *in vivo* or *in vitro* electrophysiological techniques to analyze the functional properties of the graft-host connections in the septum-grafted animals, as well as the degree of functional integration of the septal grafts with the host brain.

In the first of these studies,[36] stimulation of solid septal grafts evoked characteristic field potentials in the dentate gyrus, and the depth profile revealed diffuse innervation characteristic of the normal septal afferents. Prepulse stimulation of the septal grafts was found to potentiate the field potentials evoked by perforant path stimulation. This latter effect, which is a characteristic response of the granule cells to septal stimulation also in the intact dentate gyrus, can most probably be attributed to a synaptic cholinergic action, either directly onto the dentate granule cells or indirectly via local interneurons. The electron microscopical-immunocytochemical demonstration of such synapses from the septal grafts[32] is consistent with this interpretation.

Segal *et al.*[37] analyzed the connections of septal suspension implants in fimbria-fornix-lesioned rats by using intracellular recordings in hippocampal slices 4-8 weeks after grafting. Stimulation of the septal graft, which was contained within the slice, produced a slow and long-lasting voltage-dependent depolarization in some host CA1 neurons located up to about 2 mm away from the graft. This was associated with an increase in spontaneous action potential discharges and in spontaneous postsynaptic potentials. These responses were similar to those seen after topical application of acetylcholine. Since topical application of atropine attenuated, and physostigmine potentiated, the graft-induced depolarizing responses, these results are consistent with the formation of functional excitatory cholinergic synapses by the grafted septal neurons onto the host pyramidal neurons.

In a more recent study,[38] electroencephalograms, evoked field responses, and cellular activity were recorded from animals with and without cholinergic grafts. Before the electrophysiological experiment, the rats were trained to run in a wheel for water reward. In animals without transplants, no recovery of rhythmic slow activity (RSA or theta) occurred within the 9-month observation period. RSA is a characteristic electroencephalographic correlate of exploratory behavior in normal rats, and is lost in animals with fimbria-fornix lesions.[39] Instead, sharp waves with large amplitudes and fast activity were present. In all rats with solid septal grafts, but in none of the rats with septal suspension grafts, behavior-dependent RSA reappeared several months after transplantation. The recovered RSA activity showed a strict and constant covariation with behavior; it was present during running in the wheel and absent while the animal was drinking or sitting still. Interestingly, the RSA recorded from the graft-reinnervated hippocampus and the RSA recorded from the contralateral hippocampus occurred in synchrony. In addition, granule cells and interneurons were found to fire rhythmically and phase-locked to the RSA. The rats with septal suspension grafts displayed only short-duration bursts of RSA (not present in the lesioned rats without transplants), and usually did so when immobile.

These findings suggest that at least a portion of the RSA pacemaker cells of the host septum survives the fimbria-fornix transection, and that a solid graft of septal tissue, implanted into the fimbria-fornix lesion cavity, may be capable of relaying this pacemaker activity to the host hippocampus. Alternatively, the grafted septal neurons, in the absence of normal connections, could be providing the pacemaker qualities. This would, however, require that the pacemaker cells in the graft were under the same brainstem control as the host septum. In either case, these data provide strong evidence that the grafts can become at least partly integrated with the host brain and that they are capable of influencing the target neuronal population in a nearly normal manner.

EFFECTS ON LESION-INDUCED OR AGE-DEPENDENT BEHAVIORAL IMPAIRMENTS

Bilateral Fimbria-Fornix Lesions in Young Rats

Bilateral fimbria-fornix lesions in young rats are known to result in severe impairments in learning and memory.[16,18] Several studies have demonstrated the ability of intrahippocampal fetal septal grafts to ameliorate these impairments.

In the eight-arm radial maze,[36] rats with septal grafts (7 months after transplantation) showed a positive linear trend in maze performance over days of testing, but did not differ significantly from nongrafted rats with lesions overall. Potentiation of the cholinergic transmission by pretreatment with the AChE inhibitor physostigmine, however, produced a significant enhancement of maze performance in the grafted group, but not in the lesioned control group, and in some cases the grafted rats performed as well as the nonlesioned control animals. In a more recent study on intrahippocampal septal grafts in rats with medial septal lesions, Pallage et al.[40] obtained significant graft-induced recovery of radial maze performance, also in the absence of AChE inhibition.

In another study,[41] in a T-maze forced-choice alternation test (performed 6 months after transplantation), seven of nine rats with solid septal grafts and four of five rats with septal suspension grafts learned the task, some of them up to the level of control rats. The remaining rats with septal grafts and a separate group of rats with control grafts, which were taken from the brain stem locus ceruleus region, performed at chance level, similar to the rats that only received the fimbria-fornix lesion. The subsequent microscopical analysis showed a significant correlation between performance of the grafted rats and the amount of graft-derived AChE-positive staining in the previously denervated hippocampus ($r = .50$; $p < .02$).

In a more recent study,[42] septal cell suspension grafts (and to a somewhat lesser degree, solid septal grafts) implanted into the hippocampal formation in rats with bilateral fimbria-fornix lesions were also found to improve spatial learning in the Morris water-maze task.[43] This was seen both in rats that had been pretrained in the task before lesioning and grafting, and in rats that had not been exposed to the water-maze before lesioning and transplantation. In the pretrained rats, the bilateral fimbria-fornix lesion completely abolished the acquired performance. Whereas the lesioned rats were able to relearn the task partially using nonspatial strategies, the septally grafted rats were able to reacquire a spatial memory of the platform site.

Interestingly, atropine (50 mg/kg) completely abolished the reacquired spatial memory in the grafted animals. This atropine effect was also seen in the normal control rats, but to a lesser extent. Segal et al.[44] have recently reported similar results in rats with medial septal lesions and intrahippocampal septal suspension grafts.

These various studies show that septal grafts can ameliorate deficits in spatial learning and memory induced by lesions of the septohippocampal projection system, and they strongly suggest that the cholinergic graft-host connections play an important role in the mediation of this effect.

Aged Rats

Aged rats are known to display significant impairments in spatial working memory and spatial reference memory.[45-49] In addition, there is evidence from several laboratories for decrements in parameters of cholinergic synaptic function in the hippocampal formation of aged rats, such as in muscarinic binding sites,[12] in acetylcholine synthesis,[15,50] and in high-affinity choline uptake.[14] These age-dependent cholinergic deficits are further supported by evidence that pyramidal cells of aged rats show a decrease in responsiveness to iontophoretically applied acetylcholine.[51,52] Although no actual cell loss in the cholinergic projection system has been reported so far, a recent study has observed significant atrophy of basal forebrain cholinergic neurons in aged mice.[53] Taken together, these data provide support for the idea that decreases in memory function observed in aged animals may be dependent at least partly upon altered cholinergic function in the hippocampal formation and its associated limbic and cortical structures, and thus that age-dependent decline in function of the septohippocampal cholinergic system may contribute to decreased cognitive function. In analogy with the graft-induced effects seen in young rats with lesions of the septohippocampal pathway, therefore, grafts of cholinergic-rich septal tissue might be capable of compensating for at least some aspects of the learning and memory deficits seen in the aged rats.

Age-dependent learning and memory deficits were assessed in the Morris watermaze task before transplantation.[30,48] This test requires the rat to use spatial cues in the environment to find a platform hidden below the surface of a pool of opaque water. Normal, young rats have no trouble learning this task with speed and accuracy. Because our initial studies showed that only a portion ($\frac{1}{4}$-$\frac{1}{3}$) of our 21-23-month-old Sprague-Dawley rats were markedly impaired in this task, a pretransplant test served to identify the impaired individuals in the aged rat group. Based on the performance of the young controls, we set the criterion for impaired performance in the aged rats such that the mean escape latency (that is, swim time to find the platform) should be above an upper 99% confidence limit of the escape latencies recorded in the young control group. A subgroup of old rats showed mean escape latencies greater than the criterion and were thus allocated to the "old impaired" group, which was used for subsequent transplantation. The remaining subgroup of aged rats constituted the "old nonimpaired" group (left panel in FIG. 6). This latter group and a young control group served as reference groups. A portion of the "old impaired" group received bilateral suspension grafts prepared from the septal-diagonal band area obtained from 14-16-day-old embryos of the same rat strain. Three implant deposits were made stereotaxically into the hippocampal formation on each side. The remaining "old impaired" rats were not operated on and served as the "old impaired" control group. On the posttransplantation test, $2\frac{1}{2}$-3 months after grafting, the nongrafted groups remained impaired, whereas the grafted animals, as a group, showed a significant improvement in performance as indicated by their reduced escape latency (FIG. 6). This improvement of the grafted group was demonstrated by comparisons to its pretransplantation performance as well as to the performance of the nongrafted old controls in the second test.

The ability of the rats to use spatial cues for the location of the platform in the pool was assessed by analyzing their search behavior after removal of the platform on the 5th day of testing. The young rats and rats in the "old nonimpaired" groups focused their search in the quadrant where the platform had previously been placed; the "old impaired" rats failed to do so in the pretransplant test. In the posttransplantation test (FIG. 7A), the grafted rats, but not the nongrafted "old impaired"

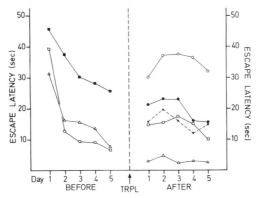

FIGURE 6. Escape latency in seconds in the Morris water-maze test for each day of testing, before and after transplantation, during place navigation (locating a hidden platform). All three groups of rats showed significant acquisition of both tasks during the pretransplantation week of testing. Although the young ($\triangle$; $N = 5$) and the old nonimpaired ($\square$; $N = 5$) rats did not differ from each other, the old impaired rats ($\blacksquare$; $N = 13$) took considerably longer to find both the visible and the hidden platforms. In the posttransplantation test, which was performed 3 months after grafting, the grafted old impaired rats ($\bullet$; $N = 7$) retained the performance level they had reached by the end of the pretransplantation test week, whereas the nongrafted old impaired rats ($\bigcirc$; $N = 6$) performed significantly worse. In the posttransplantation test, the grafted rats no longer differed from the nonimpaired controls. The dashed line indicates the performance of the six grafted rats that had surviving grafts. Taken from reference 48, with permission.

group, showed significantly improved performance. Swim distance in the platform quadrant was increased by 83%, and they swam significantly more in the platform quadrant than in other quadrants of the pool. By contrast, the nongrafted controls showed no significant change over their pretransplant performance.

In a subsequent study,[48] we tried to analyze the septal graft effects pharmacologically. In these experiments, we used a modified water-maze protocol in which the platform was visible ("cue" trials) and invisible ("place" trials) in alternating trials. In this test, it was clear that the "old impaired" rats were severely impaired not only when the platform was hidden (which can be taken as a measure of spatial reference memory), but also in the acquisition of the task when the platform was visible (which can be taken as a measure of nonspatial reference memory). The nongrafted impaired rats remained as impaired on both the "cue" and the "place" tasks when retested $2\frac{1}{2}$ months after the first test, whereas the impaired rats with septal suspension implants in the hippocampal formation were significantly improved on both components of the task. Moreover, although the nongrafted animals showed worse performance during the first 2 days of the second test session, as compared to the last days of the first test session, the grafted animals retained their level of performance from the end of the first test session (FIG. 6). This indicates that the septal grafts can have an effect not only on acquisition but also on retention of the learned performance.

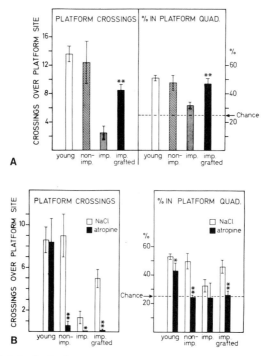

FIGURE 7. Search behavior in the water-maze test after platform removal in the last trial. **(A)** Number of crossings over the former platform site and percentage of total swim distance in the quadrant where the platform had been for all previous trials. The old impaired grafted rats performed significantly better than the old impaired controls (∗∗ = $p < .01$) and about as well as the young rats. **(B)** Effect of atropine (50 mg/kg, i.p.) on the search behavior in the spatial probe trial, as in **A**. Note that atropine totally abolished (∗∗ = $p < .01$) the ability of the grafted rats to locate the former platform site. This effect was present also in the nonimpaired aged, but was only marginal in the impaired aged rats. Taken from reference 48, with permission.

In the pharmacological test (FIG. 7B), atropine (50 mg/kg, i.p.) completely abolished the ability of the grafted animals to find either the visible or the hidden platform. Consistent with this, the ability of the rats to locate the platform site (after platform removal) was eliminated. By contrast, atropine had no significant effect in the "old impaired" rats without grafts and had only a marginal effect in the young control rats. Physostigmine (0.05 mg/kg, i.p.) had no significant effect on either grafted or nongrafted animals when administered during a single day of trials. These observations seem consistent with the idea that the graft-mediated improvements, seen in the aged rats on both spatial and nonspatial learning and memory in the water-maze test, are dependent on a cholinergic mechanism.

DISCUSSION

From the studies conducted in young adult rats with lesions of the cholinergic projection systems, it appears that implanted embryonic cholinergic neurons in some cases can substitute quite well, both morphologically and functionally, for a lost afferent cholinergic input to a denervated brain region. The extent to which the intracerebral implants can be functionally integrated with the host brain is not yet known, however, and remains an interesting question for further investigations. The chances for extensive integration may be greatest for neuronal suspension grafts implanted as deposits directly and deeply into the brain, but even solid grafts inserted as whole pieces have, in several cases (both in adult and developing recipients),[54] been seen to become reinnervated from the host brain. Interestingly, in the above-mentioned study by Buzsaki et al.,[38] rats with solid septal grafts showed much better recovery of behavior-related hippocampal RSA than that shown by rats with suspension grafts. As discussed above, this may be due to the ability of the solid grafts placed in the fimbria-fornix lesion cavity to act as a "bridge" for axons from the host brain, which could serve to synchronize electroencephalographic rhythmicity in the lesioned hippocampus with that on the intact control side.

Whether these observations on grafts in young rats with denervating lesions are valid for the interpretation of the graft-induced functional effects in aged rats (without any preceding experimentally induced brain damage) is unclear. The observations of fiber outgrowth and, ultrastructurally, of synapse formation with neurons in the host hippocampus may support the possibility that also in the nondenervated aged host brain the implanted cholinergic neurons may act via specific efferent connections with the host. As a working hypothesis we propose, therefore, both in aged rats and in young rats with denervating lesions, that the functional effects of implanted septal tissue are exerted by a specific action of selective neuronal elements in the graft onto dysfunctioning neuronal elements of the host hippocampal formation, and that this influence is mediated via the fiber connections established by the implanted neurons. On the assumption that impaired cholinergic neurotransmission contributes to the age-dependent cognitive impairments, we also propose that the ameliorative action of septal grafts in aged rats is at least partly due to a restoration of cholinergic neuro-transmission in the area. Our results suggest, however, that although cholinergic reinnervation of the target may be *necessary* for the behavioral effects of septal grafts in the water-maze task, this may not be *sufficient* for graft function. Several neuronal cell types may participate, and the presence or absence of specific afferent connections to the grafts may also be important.

The basal forebrain cholinergic neurons are commonly conceived of as a modu-latory or level-setting system that tonically regulates the activity or performance of the hippocampal neuronal machinery. Removal of the cholinergic control mechanisms thus results in inhibition or impairment of hippocampal function. It seems possible, therefore, that the functional recovery seen after reinstatement of impaired cholinergic transmission by septal grafts could be interpreted as a relatively nonspecific reactivation of an inhibited, but otherwise intact, hippocampal neuronal machinery.

REFERENCES

1. DRACHMAN, D. A. & B. J. SAHAKIAN. 1979. Effects of cholinergic agents on human learning and memory. *In* Nutrition and the Brain. A. Barbeau, J. H. Growdon & R. J. Wurtman, Eds. Vol. **5**: 351-366. Raven Press. New York, NY.

2. DEUTSCH, J. A. 1983. The cholinergic synapse and the site of memory. *In* The Physiological Basis of Memory. J. A. Deutsch, Ed.: 367-386. Academic Press. New York, NY.

3. BARTUS, R. T., R. L. DEAN, B. BEER & A. S. LIPPA. 1982. The cholinergic hypothesis of geriatric memory dysfunction. Science **217**: 408-416.

4. WHITEHOUSE, P. J., D. L. PRICE, R. G. STRUBLE, A. W. CLARK, J. T. COYLE & M. R. DELONG. 1982. Alzheimer's disease and senile dementia: Loss of neurons in the basal forebrain. Science **215**: 1237-1239.

5. PEARSON, R. C. A., M. V. SOFRONIEW, A. C. CUELLO, T. P. S. POWELL, F. ECKENSTEIN, M. M. ESIRI & G. K. WILCOCK. 1983. Persistence of cholinergic neurons in the basal nucleus in a brain with senile dementia of the Alzheimer's type demonstrated by immunohistochemical staining for choline acetyltransferase. Brain Res. **289**: 375-379.

6. ARENDT, T., V. BIGL, A. TENNSTEDT & A. ARENDT. 1985. Neuronal loss in different parts of the nucleus basalis is related to neuritic plaque formation in cortical target areas in Alzheimer's disease. Neuroscience **14**: 1-14.

7. COYLE, J. T., D. L. PRICE & M. R. DELONG. 1983. Alzheimer's disease: A disorder of cortical cholinergic innervation. Science **219**: 1184-1189.

8. DAVIES, P. & A. J. F. MALONEY. 1976. Selective loss of central cholinergic neurons in Alzheimer's disease. Lancet **ii**: 1403.

9. PERRY, E. K., B. E. TOMLINSON, G. BLESSED, K. BERGMANN, P. H. GIBSON & R. H. PERRY. 1978. Correlation of cholinergic abnormalities with senile plaques and mental test scores in senile dementia. Br. Med. J. **2**: 1457-1459.

10. BOWEN, D. M., C. B. SMITH, P. WHITE & A. N. DAVISON. 1976. Neurotransmitter-related enzymes and indices of hypoxia in senile dementia and other abiotrophies. Brain **99**: 459-496.

11. STRONG, R., P. HICKS, L. HSU, R. T. BARTUS & S. J. ENNA. 1980. Age-related alterations in the rodent brain cholinergic system and behavior. Neurobiol. Aging **1**: 59-63.

12. LIPPA, A. S., R. W. PELHAM, B. BEER, D. J. CRITCHETT, R. L. DEAN & R. I. BARTUS. 1980. Brain cholinergic dysfunction and memory in aged rats. Neurobiol. Aging **1**: 13-19.

13. GIBSON, G. E., C. PETERSON & D. J. JENSEN. 1981. Brain acetylcholine synthesis declines with senescence. Science **213**: 674-676.

14. SHERMAN, K. A., J. E. KUSTER, R. L. DEAN, R. T. BARTUS & E. FRIEDMAN. 1981. Presynaptic cholinergic mechanisms in brain of aged rats with memory impairments. Neurobiol. Aging **2**: 99-104.

15. DRAVID, A. R. 1983. Deficits of cholinergic enzymes and muscarinic receptors in the hippocampus and striatum of senescent rats: Effects of chronic hydergine treatment. Arch. Int. Pharmacodyn. **264**: 195-202.

16. OLTON, D. S., J. T. BECKER & G. E. HANDELMAN. 1979. Hippocampus, space and memory. Behav. Brain Sci. **2**: 313-365.

17. HEPLER, D. J., D. S. OLTON, G. L. WENK & J. T. COYLE. 1985. Lesions in nucleus basalis magnocellularis and medial septal area of rats produce qualitatively similar memory impairments. J. Neurosci. **5**: 866-873.

18. DUNNETT, S. B. 1985. Comparative effects of cholinergic drugs and lesions of nucleus basalis or fimbria-fornix on delayed matching in rats. Psychopharmacology **87**: 357-363.

19. WHISHAW, I. Q., W. T. O'CONNOR & S. B. DUNNETT. 1985. Disruption of central cholinergic systems in the rat by basal forebrain lesions or atropine: Effects on feeding, sensorimotor behavior, locomotor activity and spatial navigation. Behav. Brain Res. **17**: 103-115.

20. BJÖRKLUND, A. & U. STENEVI. 1977. Reformation of the severed septohippocampal cholinergic pathway in the adult rat by transplanted septal neurons. Cell Tissue Res. **185**: 289-302.

21. BJÖRKLUND, A., U. STENEVI, R. H. SCHMIDT, S. B. DUNNETT & F. H. GAGE. 1983. Intracerebral grafting of neuronal cell suspensions. I. Introduction and general methods of preparation. Acta Physiol. Scand. Suppl. **522:** 1-7.

22. BJÖRKLUND, A., F. H. GAGE, U. STENEVI & S. B. DUNNETT. 1983. Intracerebral grafting of neuronal cell suspensions. VI. Survival and growth of intrahippocampal implants of septal cell suspensions. Acta Physiol. Scand. Suppl. **522:** 49-58.

23. BJÖRKLUND, A., U. STENEVI & N.-A. SVENDGAARD. 1976. Growth of transplanted mono-aminergic neurons into the adult hippocampus along the perforant path. Nature **262:** 787-790.

24. BJÖRKLUND, A., L. F. KROMER & U. STENEVI. 1979. Cholinergic reinnervation of the rat hippocampus by septal implants is stimulated by perforant path lesion. Brain Res. **173:** 57-64.

25. BJÖRKLUND, A., M. SEGAL & U. STENEVI. 1979. Functional reinnervation of rat hippo-campus by locus coeruleus implants. Brain Res. **170:** 409-426.

26. BJÖRKLUND, A. & U. STENEVI. 1981. *In vivo* evidence for a hippocampal adrenergic neurotrophic factor specifically released on septal deafferentation. Brain Res. **229:** 403-428.

27. GAGE, F. H. & A. BJÖRKLUND. 1986. Enhanced graft survival in the hippocampus following selective denervation. Neuroscience **17:** 89-98.

28. GAGE, F. H. & A. BJÖRKLUND. 1987. Denervation-induced enhancement of graft survival and growth: A trophic hypothesis. Ann. N.Y. Acad. Sci. This volume.

29. GAGE, F. H., S. B. DUNNETT, U. STENEVI & A. BJÖRKLUND. 1983. Intracerebral grafting of neuronal cell suspensions. VIII. Survival and growth of implants of nigral and septal cell suspensions in intact brains of aged rats. Acta Physiol. Scand. Suppl. **522:** 67-75.

30. GAGE, F. H., A. BJÖRKLUND, U. STENEVI, S. B. DUNNETT & P. A. T. KELLY. 1984. Intrahippocampal septal grafts ameliorate learning impairments in aged rats. Science **225:** 533-536.

31. CLARKE, D. J., F. H. GAGE, O. G. NILSSON & A. BJÖRKLUND. 1986. Grafted septal neurons form synaptic connections in the dentate gyrus of behaviorally impaired aged rats. J. Comp. Neurol. **252:** 483-492.

32. CLARKE, D. J., F. H. GAGE & A. BJÖRKLUND. 1986. Formation of cholinergic synapses by intrahippocampal septal grafts as revealed by choline acetyltransferase immunocy-tochemistry. Brain Res. **369:** 151-162.

33. CLARKE, D. J., F. H. GAGE, S. B. DUNNETT, O. G. NILSSON & A. BJÖRKLUND. 1987. Synaptogenesis of grafted cholinergic neurons. Ann. N.Y. Acad. Sci. This volume.

34. BJÖRKLUND, A., F. H. GAGE, R. H. SCHMIDT, U. STENEVI & S. B. DUNNETT. 1983. Intracerebral grafting of neuronal cell suspensions. VII. Recovery of choline acetyltrans-ferase activity and acetylcholine synthesis in the denervated hippocampus reinnervated by septal suspension implants. Acta Physiol. Scand. Suppl. **522:** 59-66.

35. KELLY, P. A. T., F. H. GAGE, M. INGVAR, O. LINDVALL, U. STENEVI & A. BJÖRKLUND. 1985. Functional reactivation of the deafferented hippocampus by embryonic septal grafts as assessed by measurements of local glucose utilization. Exp. Brain Res. **58:** 570-579.

36. LOW, W. C., P. R. LEWIS, S. T. BUNCH, S. B. DUNNETT, S. R. THOMAS, S. D. IVERSEN, A. BJÖRKLUND & U. STENEVI. 1982. Functional recovery following neural transplan-tation of embryonic septal nuclei in adult rats with septohippocampal lesions. Nature **300:** 260-262.

37. SEGAL, M., A. BJÖRKLUND & F. H. GAGE. 1985. Transplanted septal neurons make viable cholinergic synapses with a host hippocampus. Brain Res. **336:** 302-307.

38. BUZSAKI, G., F. H. GAGE, J. CZOPF & A. BJÖRKLUND. 1987. Restoration of rhythmic slow activity (theta) in the subcortically denervated hippocampus by fetal CNS trans-plants. Brain Res. **400:** 334-347.

39. VANDERWOLF, C. H. 1969. Hippocampal electrical activity and voluntary movement in the rat. Electroencephalogr. Clin. Neurophysiol. **26:** 407-418.

40. PALLAGE, V., G. TONIOLO, B. WILL & F. HEFTI. 1987. Long-term effects of nerve growth factor and neural transplants on behavior of rats with medial septal lesions. Brain Res. In press.

41. DUNNETT, S. B., W. C. LOW, S. D. IVERSEN, U. STENEVI & A. BJÖRKLUND. 1982. Septal transplants restore maze learning in rats with fornix-fimbria lesions. Brain Res. 251: 335-348.
42. NILSSON, O. G., M. L. SHAPIRO, F. H. GAGE & A. BJÖRKLUND. 1987. Spatial learning and memory following fimbria-fornix transection and grafting of fetal septal neurons to the hippocampus. Exp. Brain Res. In press.
43. MORRIS, R. G. M. 1981. Spatial localization does not require the presence of local cues. Learn. Motiv. 12: 239-260.
44. SEGAL, M., V. GREENBERGER & H. W. MILGAM. 1987. A functional analysis of connections between grafted septal neurons and a host hippocampus. Progr. Brain Res. In press.
45. BARNES, C. A., L. NADEL & W. K. HONIG. 1980. Spatial memory defects in senescent rats. Can. J. Psychol. 34: 29-39.
46. INGRAM, D. K., E. D. LONDON & C. L. GOODRICK. 1981. Age and neurochemical correlates of radial maze performance in rats. Neurobiol. Aging 2: 41-47.
47. WALLACE, J. E., E. E. KRAUTER & B. A. CAMPBELL. 1980. Animal models of declining memory in the aged: Short-term and spatial memory in the aged rat. J. Gerontol. 35: 355-363.
48. GAGE, F. H. & A. BJÖRKLUND. 1986. Cholinergic septal grafts into the hippocampal formation improve spatial learning and memory in aged rats by an atropine-sensitive mechanism. J. Neurosci. 6: 2837-2847.
49. GAGE, F. H., P. A. T. KELLY & A. BJÖRKLUND. 1984. Regional changes in brain glucose metabolism reflect cognitive impairments in aged rats. J. Neurosci. 4: 2856-2866.
50. SIMS, N. R., K. L. MAREK, D. M. BOWEN & A. N. DAVISON. 1982. Production of [^{14}C]acetylcholine and [^{14}C]carbon dioxide from [U-^{14}C]glucose in tissue prisms from aging rat brain. J. Neurochem. 38: 488-492.
51. LIPPA, A. S., D. J. CRITCHETT, F. EHLERT, H. I. YAMAMURA, S. J. ENNA & R. T. BARTUS. 1981. Age-related alterations in neurotransmitter receptors: An electrophysiological and biochemical analysis. Neurobiol. Aging 2: 3-8.
52. SEGAL, M. 1982. Changes in neurotransmitter actions in aged rat hippocampus. Neurobiol. Aging 3: 121-124.
53. HORNBERGER, J. C., S. J. BUELL., D. G. FLOOD, T. H. MCNEILL & P. D. COLEMAN. 1985. Stability of numbers but not size of mouse forebrain cholinergic neurons to 53 months. Neurobiol. Aging 6: 275-292.
54. BJÖRKLUND, A. & U. STENEVI. 1984. Intracerebral neural implants: Neuronal replacement and reconstruction of damaged circuitries. Annu. Rev. Neurosci. 7: 279-308.

DISCUSSION OF THE PAPER

M. NIETO-SAMPEDRO (*University of California, Irvine, CA*): How did you do your transplantations? How many days after making an entorhinal cavity did you place the ganglia there?

GAGE: They were made simultaneously with the lesion.

NIETO-SAMPEDRO: Then of course they do not survive.

GAGE: In the presence of fimbria-fornix transection they do survive.

NIETO-SAMPEDRO: Made at the same time.

GAGE: Yes. In the septal lesion situation, there were suspensions that were injected into the hippocampus itself either in the presence of an entorhinal lesion or in the presence of a fimbria-fornix transection. They showed a dramatic increase in survival following a fimbria-fornix transection, but not in the presence of an entorhinal lesion.

NIETO-SAMPEDRO: There are two comments I would like to make. One is that if you follow the time course of action of nerve growth factor (NGF) in an entorhinal cavity, you get NGF in the entorhinal cavity whether you do a fimbria-fornix transection or not. Therefore, if you do a delayed transplantation of superior cervical ganglion, you should get survival.

The other thing is that no matter what you do, if you do not vacate the terminals that are there and if you do not cut the fimbria and therefore make a synaptic space for septal afferents and for monoaminergic afferents, you do not get innervation. Therefore, you do not get increased choline acetyltransferase or monoamines or anything.

GAGE: Precisely. That is why we are trying to find out why this is true. One further comment is that the entorhinal lesions we make are different from the ones you make. Our aspiration results in a ready-made vascular bed on which to place the graft, so we do not have to wait for the vascular bed to form. This may account for some of the differences.

NIETO-SAMPEDRO: My point is the vascular bed early on is not enough.

S. M. CRAIN (*Albert Einstein School of Medicine, New York, NY*): Dr. Gage, do you have any evidence with regard to the types of cholinergic neurons that may be rescued by NGF in the central nervous system?

GAGE: The only situation we have looked at to date is the septal-diagonal band region. There is a better sparing in the vertical aspect of the diagonal band than there is in the median septal area. Median septal cells are less responsive to NGF, but there is no difference in NGF receptors in median septal area and the diagonal band. There is, however, a difference in the number of contacts that diagonal band cells receive versus the number median septal cells receive.

It is true that Mobley has shown that neonatal caudate cells will respond to NGF with direct injections, by an increase in choline acetyltransferase activity.

A. W. DECKEL (*Johns Hopkins University School of Medicine, Baltimore, MD*): Have you done any studies of the time course? If you wait, say, a month, do you still get increased growth? What happens over time to the implants after the fimbria-fornix transection?

GAGE: All of these were done. The data that I showed were for animals that were analyzed 4 to 6 months following grafting.

DECKEL: But I mean making the implant after the transection. You have done these at the same time.

GAGE: We made a fimbria-fornix lesion and left the animals for a year and then went back and grafted sympathetic ganglia. We saw surviving sympathetic ganglia under these conditions. Not all appropriate controls are there, but they were surviving to a lesser extent. I can say from that anecdotal piece of information, as well as from some other things, that it does look as though that elevation of support continues for a while.

M. SEGAL (*Weizmann Institute, Rehovot*): Do you find any change in the size of the hippocampus after performing transection? I wonder if there is any degeneration of hippocampus cells?

GAGE: That study has been done about three times since 1947, where investigators have actually looked in the hippocampus itself to see whether or not a fimbria-fornix transection would change the total number of pyramidal cells or change the number of granular cells. I think Raisman did it most recently, in 1973. There are apparently no changes following the fimbria-fornix transection. There may be smaller changes that have not been detected, but certainly, at the light microscopic level, the volume and number of cells do not decrease. Retrograde degeneration does not occur in the hippocampus, and the argument is that the cells in the hippocampus are so highly collateralized, even within the hippocampus itself, that they are supporting cells that sustain the cells.

Stimulation of Serotonergic Neuronal Maturation after Fetal Mesencephalic Raphe Transplantation into the 5,7-DHT-lesioned Hippocampus of the Adult Rat[a]

F. C. ZHOU,[b] S. B. AUERBACH,[c] AND E. C. AZMITIA[d]

Department of Biology
New York University
New York, New York 10003

INTRODUCTION

Specific lesioning of serotonergic fibers, that is, of fibers releasing 5-hydroxytryptamine (5-HT), in the cingulum bundle triggers homotypic collateral sprouting (sprouting fibers carry the same transmitter as the damaged ones) of the 5-HT fibers afferent to the hippocampus in the fornix-fimbria (FF).[1-3] Fibers releasing norepinephrine (NE) that travel in the same pathways and terminate in an overlapping area in the hippocampus do not seem to respond to the denervation of 5-HT fibers. Other examples of homotypic collateral sprouting are the noradrenergic and cholinergic projections to the hippocampus.[4,5] Thus, the injury of nerve fibers of a single type in a brain region appears to induce homotypic fiber sprouting.

Homotypic collateral sprouting has a slow onset and long duration and correlates closely with the beneficial recuperative mechanisms after brain injury in the central nervous system[1,6] and the peripheral nervous system,[7] whereas heterotypic sprouting (sprouting fibers carry a different transmitter from the damaged ones) often causes functional abnormality, or blockage of the normal reinnervation.[8,9] Furthermore, there is evidence that these two growth responses of undamaged neurons to the damage of neighboring neurons (homotypic and heterotypic) may actually be qualitatively different and regulated by separate sets of factors.[10] For instance, we have shown that

[a] This work was supported by Grants BNS 83-07404 (to E. C. Azmitia) and BNS 83-10869 (to F. C. Zhou and E. C. Azmitia) from the National Science Foundation.

[b] Present address: Mental Retardation Research Center, NPI 58-258, UCLA School of Medicine, Los Angeles, California.

[c] Present address: Department of Biological Sciences, Rutgers University, Busch Campus, Piscataway, New Jersey.

[d] To whom requests for reprints should be addressed.

138

the homotypic collateral sprouting requires the presence of adrenal steroids,[11] whereas others have shown that the heterotypic collateral sprouting is suppressed by this same hormone.[12] Thus, after brain damage, one of the major tasks is to selectively enhance homotypic and suppress heterotypic collateral sprouting.

Current studies were designed to investigate whether the conditions that induced homotypic collateral sprouting by mature 5-HT neurons could similarly enhance the growth of fetal 5-HT neurons. It has previously been shown that transplanted fetal raphe tissue can survive in the normal adult hippocampus of the rat.[13–15] Furthermore, it has been shown that mechanical damage to the brain can result in increased survival of transplanted fetal tissue.[16–21] Our study was aimed at establishing if a specific chemical lesion will selectively enhance a selected population of neurons.

MATERIALS AND METHODS

Animals

Female Sprague-Dawley rats (220-250 g) (Hilltop Labs) were used in this study. They were housed in group cages (two to three per cage) in a quiet room and maintained on a 12-hr light/dark cycle (7:00 hr and 19:00 hr) with standard lab chow and water provided *ad libitum.* Two weeks after lesions or sham lesions, the rats received transplanted raphe or locus ceruleus tissue. Thirty days after transplantation, the rats were killed in various procedures according to the assays to be used.

Lesion and Collection of the Fluid from the Lesioned Hippocampus

Rats were injected intraperitoneally with 10 mg/kg of desipramine (a catecholamine uptake blocker) 45 min before they were anesthetized with 10 mg/kg of chloropent. The microinjection of 0.4 μl (1 mg/10 ml) of ascorbic saline containing 4 μg of 5,7-dihydroxytryptamine (5,7-DHT) was made through a glass micropipette into the FF (coordinates: 15° off vertical, 1.0 mm caudal and 1.3 mm lateral to the bregma suture, and 4.5 mm deep to the skull surface) at a rate of 30 nl/min. The diameter of the tip of the pipette was between 50 and 80 μm to limit mechanical damage and ensure a smooth delivery of the solution. Methods were detailed in our earlier reports.[1,3,11,22–25] Each rat in one group was decapitated 2 weeks after the lesion. The hippocampus of the lesioned side was taken from each rat, and the hippocampi were pooled, weighed, and homogenized in 1:10 (w/v) 0.02 M phosphate buffer (pH 7.4) with 0.14 M saline with a tight-fitting teflon homogenizer. The fluid was then centrifuged at 10 000 $\times$ g at 4° C for 10 min. The supernatant was collected and stored at $-70°$ C before use.

5-HT and Tyrosine Hydroxylase (TH) Immunocytochemistry

A month after transplantation, rats from another group were prepared for immunocytochemistry to evaluate the morphology of transplanted 5-HT and NE neurons.

The intrinsic 5-HT and NE innervations to the hippocampus were removed: a knife cut at the level of the FF and cingulum bundle was made in each rat 3 days before it was perfused. Rats with raphe transplants were pretreated with pargyline (200 mg/kg), and L-tryptophan (200 mg/kg) 90 and 60 min, respectively, before perfusion. All the animals that had undergone transplantation were then perfused with 4% paraformaldehyde and 0.1% $MgSO_4$ in 0.1 M phosphate buffer (pH 7.4). The brains were removed, cut into blocks, and postfixed in same solution overnight at 4° C. Tissue blocks were coronally sectioned at 40 μm with a Vibratome (Oxford). Sections were collected in phosphate buffer (pH 7.4) containing 0.9% NaCl (PBS) and stained with anti-5-HT or anti-TH antiserum using Sternberg's peroxidase-antiperoxidase (PAP) method. The 5-HT antibody was produced and characterized by Dr. Jean Lauder's laboratory and by ourselves. The anti-TH antibody was a gift from Dr. Tong Joh's laboratory. All antibodies were made in PBS containing 0.2% Triton X-100 and 1% normal sheep serum. The PAP reaction was done with 0.003% substrate, H_2O_2 and 0.05% chromogen, 3,3-diaminobenzidine. Morphometric analysis of the areas of the 5-HT neurons was performed from 35-mm slides, each of which was taken from the middle of a transplant. Each slide was projected, and 22 pairs of 5-HT-immunoreactive cells with nuclei were picked from experimental and control groups. The outline of each cell was carefully traced onto paper, the area within the outline was cut out, and the cutout was weighed on a top-loading microbalance to the nearest 0.1 mg.

Transplantation

Pregnant rats of 14-15 days of gestation (E14-15) were operated on under deep ether anesthesia. The fetuses were removed with their placentas and placed in sterile Hanks' solution (GIBCO). Under the dissecting microscope, the fetal brain stem between the mesencephalic flexure and the pontine flexure was dissected out. A midsaggital raphe strip of tissue along the cerebral aqueduct was subsequently trimmed and dissected.[14,26] For locus ceruleus (LC) tissue, the fetal brain stem caudal to the pontine flexure and adjacent to the fourth ventricle was removed. The lateral strips from the block were dissected for transplantation. Tissue blocks from each fetus were minced in 2-5 μl of Hanks' solution immediately before transplantation or were dissociated, and 0.2×10^6 cell/μl suspensions were prepared before transplantation. Fourteen days after the 5,7-DHT lesion, the isogenetic host rat was anesthetized with chloropent (10 mg/kg, i.p.). The raphe strip or LC strips from a "single embryo" was aspirated into a glass micropipette (100-120 μm) and stereotaxically injected over 5 min into the hippocampus of the right hemisphere (coordinates from lambda: 90° from the skull surface; 4.5 mm anterior, 1.5 mm lateral, and 3.7 mm below). The fetal raphe or LC were transplanted into animals either with lesioned or with normal control hippocampi. For biochemical studies, each transplant of 5-HT-raphe and NE-LC tissue was obtained from a "single embryo" of the same gestation day to ensure a roughly equal amount of implanted raphe and LC neurons. For the experiment evaluating the number of surviving 5-HT neurons, a cell suspension of equal volume was injected.

Specific SHAU of [³H]5-HT

A microassay for the specific synaptosomal high-affinity uptake (SHAU) of [³H]5-HT was performed on the dorsal hippocampus.[27] Briefly, the hippocampi from various animal groups were cut into septal and temporal halves midway along their longitudinal axes. (The septal half, which was the half used in the assay, is hereafter taken as the dorsal hippocampus.) The tissue was homogenized in 1 ml of ice-cold 0.32 M sucrose solution and centrifuged at 500 $\times$ g for 10 min. The supernatant was collected and subsequently centrifuged at 12 000 $\times$ g to sediment the synaptosomes in a pellet. After the supernatant was discarded, ice-cold Krebs-Ringer's buffer was added at 10 volumes per original tissue weight. The assay was performed in triplicate in 96-welled plates with a total reaction volume of 300 μl containing 15 μl of the synaptosomal preparation. The reaction was begun by adding 20 μl of tritiated transmitter (final concentration: 5 $\times$ 10^{-8} M) to the reaction mixture at 37° C. After 20 min, the synaptosomes were collected through GF-B Whatman filters using an automatic Titertek cell harvester. The trapped synaptosomes were washed, dried, and counted in a scintillation counter to determine the amount of radioactivity retained. The protein levels were determined using a protein assay kit with reference to a bovine serum albumin standard.

HPLC Analysis of 5-HT and NE

The dorsal hippocampi were removed as described previously, weighed, and homogenized to make a 10% (w/v) solution in 0.1 M perchloric acid containing 100 μM of EDTA. Homogenates were centrifuged at 15 000 $\times$ g for 15 min, and the supernatants were analyzed for 5-HT and NE by HPLC with electrochemical detection (HPLC unit and Catecholamines Analyzer II made by Bas). A 25 cm $\times$ 4.6 mm (inside diameter) stainless steel column packed with C18 reverse-phase resin (particle size: 5 μ) was equilibrated in a mobile phase consisting of 3.5 parts acetonitrile, 1.9 parts tetrahydrofuran, and 96.5 parts 0.15 M monochloroacetate buffer (pH 3.0) containing 200 mg/l sodium octylsulfonic acid and 0.2 μg/l EDTA. The pump rate was 1.7 ml/min. For the detection of tissue monoamines, the voltage applied to the carbon paste (type CP-O) TL3 detection electrode (Bas) was set at +0.70 V relative to the Ag/AgCl reference. Electrode noise fluctuations in our system were reduced to the equivalent of about ± 1 pg of 5-HT and NE. Peak heights were measured and compared to peak heights of standards.[28-30]

RESULTS

Anatomy

5-HT-immunoreactive (5-HT-IR) neurons were observed in all the raphe transplants. Transplants were mainly located in hippocampal parenchyma. In a few cases, small tissue pieces were also scattered in the corpus callosum and in the lateral ventricle adjacent to the rostral hippocampus. In all cases, 5-HT-IR neuronal soma were confined in the transplants. In the case of fetal raphe grafted in normal hippocampus, fibers of 5-HT neurons were mainly confined in the transplants. A few fibers were observed extending outside (FIG. 1). In the case of raphe grafted in lesioned hippocampus, however, the fibers of 5-HT-IR neurons largely extended outside of transplants to reach hippocampal parenchyma (FIG. 2). Varicosities were observed along these fibers, especially in the terminal area immediately adjacent to the granular cell and in the stratum lacunosum moleculare. The 5-HT-IR cells grafted in the lesioned hippocampus were 43% larger than those grafted in the normal hippocampus: the respective sizes, expressed as means ± SEM, were 2.7 ± 0.1 mg ($N = 5$) and 1.9 ± 0.1 mg ($N = 5$) (see the methods section for details).

After the transplantation of dissociated raphe cells, where suspensions of equal amounts were grafted, the number of 5-HT-IR cells observed in the normal hippo-

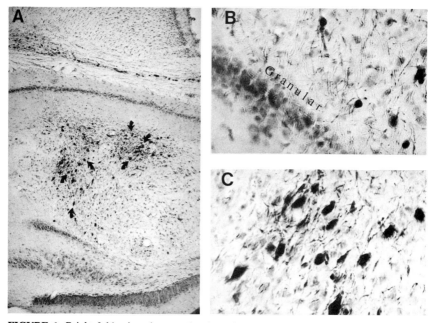

FIGURE 1. Bright-field microphotographs show the 5-HT-IR neuronal profiles in the raphe transplant in normal hippocampus. The cells in the backgrounds were counterstained with methyl green. The 5-HT-IR somas (arrows) and fibers were observed mostly confined in the transplant (**A**); 5-HT-IR neurons may be seen with a few fibers located near granular cells (**B**), and in the stratum oriens and lacunosum-moleculare (**C**).

campus ($N = 6$) was not significantly different from that observed in the lesioned hippocampus ($N = 6$) (FIG. 3).

TH-positive cells were observed in all the LC transplants (FIG. 4). Large multipolar cells with long-branched dendritic profiles were observed. The terminal distribution pattern for these cells was similar to that seen normally and to the 5-HT innervation pattern seen in the adult hippocampus ($N = 6$).

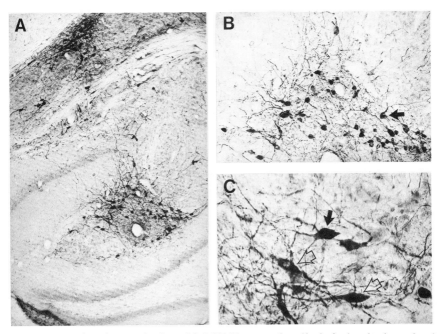

FIGURE 2. Microphotographs show rich 5-HT-IR neuronal profiles in fetal raphe tissue placed in lesioned hippocampus. The cells in the backgrounds were counterstained with methyl green. Neurons had many long processes extending outside of the transplanted tissue into the host brain (**A, B & C**). Highly branched fibers were abundant (solid arrows) and spindle-shaped 5-HT-IR neurons (open arrows) were often discernable (**B & C**). The soma of these 5-HT-IR neurons were 43% larger than those grafted in normal hippocampus.

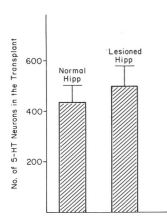

FIGURE 3. Number of 5-HT-IR neurons identified in the transplants of dissociated raphe cells placed in normal-versus-lesioned hippocampus. The number of 5-HT neurons in normal hippocampus is not significantly different from that in the lesioned hippocampus.

Biochemistry

The Normal and 5,7-DHT-lesioned Raphe-Hippocampus System

The 5-HT fibers in the normal dorsal hippocampus have an SHAU of 137 ± 36 pmoles/g [^{3}H]5-HT (mean ± SD) ($N = 5$) (FIG. 5). The 5-HT content in this

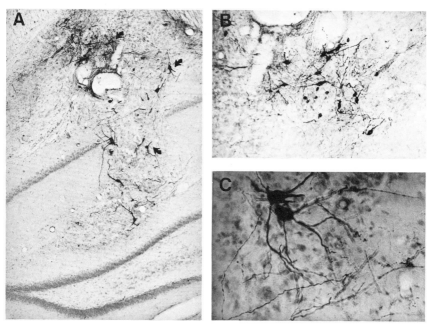

FIGURE 4. Norepinephrine neurons from LC transplants stained with antibody to TH. The TH-positive cells (arrows) have highly branched processes (**A, B & C**). Two multipolar TH-positive cells are shown in **C**. Fibers with many varicosities are shown in lower left of **C**.

same area was 200 ± 40 pg/mg of 5-HT ($N = 8$) (FIG. 6). A week after 5,7-DHT was microinjected into the FF (a midline structure), the 5-HT fibers were selectively and equally depleted from both hemispheres of the hippocampus. The SHAU of [^{3}H]5-HT decreased to 36% of that of the control ($N = 5$) (FIG. 7), and the concentration of 5-HT diminished to 30% of that of the control ($N = 6$) (FIG. 8) in the dorsal hippocampus. Diminished SHAU and 5-HT values indicated that the hippocampus was partially depleted of its serotonergic afferents. No significant effect of 5,7-DHT on the NE levels was detected in the dorsal hippocampus.

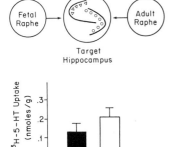

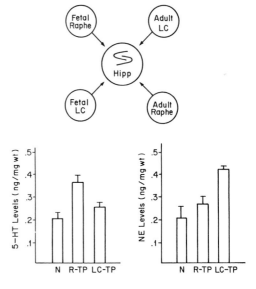

FIGURE 5. SHAU of [^{3}H]5-HT in the hippocampus of the normal and fetal raphe transplant animals. The 5-HT neurons of fetal raphe grafts expressed an increase in SHAU of [^{3}H]5-HT 1 month after transplantation in the host hippocampus.

The Fetal Raphe Transplants in the Adult Normal Hippocampus

Transplants of fetal raphe tissue into the normal dorsal hippocampus produced hyperinnervation by 5-HT fibers within 1 month after transplantation. The SHAU of [^{3}H]5-HT rose 53% ($N = 5$) above normal (FIG. 5); similarly, the concentration of 5-HT rose 80% ($N = 5$) above normal (FIG. 6).

FIGURE 6. The 5-HT and NE levels in the fetal raphe- or LC-transplanted hippocampus. The 5-HT levels are shown on the left side of the figure. One month after transplantation, the raphe transplant (R-TP) has a higher 5-HT level in the hippocampus than both the LC transplant (LC-TP) and the normal hippocampus. The 5-HT level is not significantly different between normal and LC-TP. The NE levels are shown on the right side of the figure. Similarly, the LC-TP in the hippocampus had higher NE levels than the normal and the R-TP. The NE level is not significantly different between normal and R-TP.

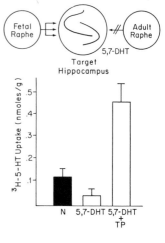

FIGURE 7. SHAU of [^{3}H]5-HT in the hippocampus of the normal, 5,7-DHT-lesioned, and 5,7-DHT-lesioned (with raphe) transplanted animals. One week after the 5,7-DHT lesion in the FF, the animals showed a decrease in uptake in the hippocampus. A fetal raphe transplant made 2 weeks after the 5,7-DHT lesion in the hippocampus exhibited a dramatic increase in SHAU after 1 month as compared to normal, or raphe transplants in the normal (see FIG. 5). The transplants in such conditions show a hyperinnervation with increased, above-normal levels.

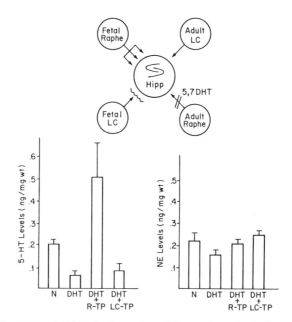

FIGURE 8. The 5-HT and NE levels after raphe or LC transplantation in the 5,7-DHT-lesioned hippocampus. The 5-HT levels are shown on the left side of the figure. The fetal raphe neurons (R-TP) had a greater increase in level of 5-HT when transplanted into a 5,7-DHT-lesioned hippocampus than when transplanted into a normal hippocampus. The LC transplants (LC-TP) do not show increased 5-HT concentration in the 5,7-DHT-lesioned hippocampus. The NE levels are shown on the right side of the figure. There was no difference in NE levels between the normal and 5,7-DHT-lesioned hippocampus, or between LC-TP and R-TP in the 5,7-DHT-lesioned hippocampus as compared to when transplanted into the normal hippocampus.

Fetal Raphe Transplants into the Partially 5-HT-depleted Hippocampus

The transmitter maturation (tissue levels and high-affinity uptake) of 5-HT fetal neurons transplanted into the dorsal hippocampus was stimulated by 5,7-DHT lesions made earlier. When fetal raphe cells were transplanted into the FF-lesioned dorsal hippocampus, the SHAU of [^{3}H]5-HT increased 345% over intact and 946% over FF-5,7-DHT-lesioned hippocampus (FIG. 7). The 5-HT concentration increased 255% over intact and 850% over FF-5,7-DHT-lesioned hippocampus (FIG. 8).

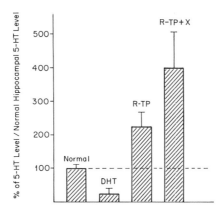

FIGURE 9. The figure shows the 5-HT levels in the hippocampus of four groups of rats. The 5-HT levels seen in the normal animal are shown in column one (Normal). The 5-HT levels 1 week after a 5,7-DHT injection into the FF are shown in column two (DHT). The 5-HT level 1 month after a raphe transplant into a normal hippocampus is shown in column three (R-TP). Finally, the 5-HT levels 1 month after a raphe transplant with addition of the supernatant from a 5,7-DHT-lesioned hippocampus (same condition shown in column two) into a normal hippocampus (compare to column three) is shown in column four (R-TP+X). The level of 5-HT is significantly increased in the R-TP+X and R-TP.

Fetal Raphe and 5,7-DHT Hippocampal Extracts Injected into Normal Hippocampus

In the normal hippocampus, transplantation of fetal raphe tissue in combination with the extracts obtained from lesioned hippocampus ($N = 6$) showed significantly higher 5-HT content than transplantation of fetal raphe without extracts ($N = 5$). A 300% increase in 5-HT content over the normal level with extracts ($N = 4$) as compared to the 100% increase without extracts was observed 1 month after transplantation (FIG. 9).

Fetal LC Transplants in the Normal and Partially 5-HT-depleted Hippocampus

The 5,7-DHT lesions in the FF did not significantly damage the NE fibers. The NE concentrations were 210 ± 40 pg/mg ($N = 16$) in the normal dorsal hippocampus (FIG. 6) and 170 ± 50 pg/ml ($N = 16$) in the 5,7-DHT-FF-lesioned dorsal hippocampus (FIG. 8). When fetal LC tissue was transplanted into the normal hippocampus, a 100% increase of the normal hippocampal NE level ($N = 6$) was observed (FIG. 6). When fetal LC was transplanted into the 5,7-DHT-FF-lesioned hippocampus, however, the concentration of NE after 1 month ($N = 4$) remained at a level similar to that seen in normal nontransplanted hippocampus (FIG. 8).

DISCUSSION

The 5,7-DHT lesions in the FF removed 5-HT fibers from the afferent path to both sides of the hippocampus, while leaving NE fibers relatively intact. Current data are consistent with previous studies showing that, under similar conditions, a subpopulation of 5-HT neurons lost contacts with the hippocampus and that the density of 5-HT fibers as well as the synaptosomal membrane area decreased while the NE-LC hippocampal system remained largely normal.[1,2,11,22,25,31]

The transplantation of minced fetal raphe resulted in a 5-HT innervation in the hippocampus at a level 60-80% above that in the normal hippocampus. These findings suggest that fetal 5-HT neurons of donors of E14-15 can survive, can take up 5-HT, and are committed to the expression of 5-HT in their normal target area in the adult host brain. These results are in agreement with our previous immunocytochemical studies in the intact mouse brain.[14]

The net 5-HT content and SHAU of the fetal raphe transplanted into the lesioned hippocampus after 1 month (the transplanted side minus the contralateral), however, was 3-4 times that of the fetal raphe transplanted in the normal hippocampus. This could be a result of the sprouting of 5-HT fibers through the cingulum bundle in response to the 5,7-DHT lesion in FF or an enhanced increase in the maturation of the 5-HT neurons of the transplant. Since the 5-HT level in the similarly denervated contralateral hippocampus did not increase, the intrinsic 5-HT neurons either did not sprout or postponed their sprouting when extrinsic 5-HT neurons were transplanted in the lesioned area. This large increase after FF-5,7-DHT denervation was previously reported in our raphe transplant study.[28] Thus, the 5-HT fiber denervation apparently provides a trophic environment to enhance the transmitter maturation, synaptosomal membrane formation, and neurite extension of the transplanted 5-HT neurons.

This trophic phenomenon could be a result of the exposure of denervated postsynaptic space. Alternatively, it could be due to the secretion of a growth factor in response to the 5-HT denervation. Current evidence favors the latter case. First, the implanted 5-HT neurons in the lesioned hippocampus can attain or exceed by 2-3 times the normal 5-HT level seen in the adult as measured by levels, SHAU, and immunocytochemistry. Second, the implanted NE neurons in the same condition did not seem to take the advantage of evacuated space in the shared terminal areas occupied in common with 5-HT terminals. Third, *in vivo* and *in vitro* studies have substantiated the existence of a growth factor. A soluble factor extracted from 5,7-DHT-lesioned hippocampus enhanced 5-HT content in a raphe transplant in "normal" hippocampus

(FIG. 9). This factor selectively enhances 5-HT neuron growth in raphe cultures at low dilution.[32] Other workers have reported the existence of nonspecific trophic factors in normal and damaged hippocampal extracts.[33,34] In contrast, the 5,7-DHT-lesion-induced factor we have identified appears to selectively enhance the development of transplanted 5-HT neurons.

Regarding the characteristics of this serotonergic growth factor, current evidence suggests that it affects both the neurite extension and transmitter development but not the survival of 5-HT neurons. The fetal 5-HT and NE neurons survived in both normal and lesioned hippocampal environments. No significant difference in the number of transplanted 5-HT neurons were observed in the two groups after 1 month. Primary raphe cultures also suggested that the outgrowth of fibers rather than the number of surviving 5-HT neurons was stimulated by the extracted serotonergic growth factor.[32] The survival effect and the time course of this hippocampal factor is under investigation.

In conclusion, selective maturational activity can be induced by specific injury to a single chemically identified fiber system. This suspected serotonergic growth factor selectively enhances development of 5-HT neurons. Furthermore, the 5,7-DHT lesion enhances the growth of the immature 5-HT neurons as well as inducing a "homotypic sprouting" of the adult 5-HT neurons in the rat.[1-3,10] Thus, a fundamental question is raised: Can a factor provide a common mechanism both for plasticity of adult neurons and growth of immature neurons in the central nervous system?

SUMMARY

Neurotoxin lesioning of 5-HT fibers selectively induced the homotypic collateral sprouting of spared 5-HT fibers in the hippocampus. We have used this model to investigate the possibility that the neurotoxin-primed hippocampus will enhance the development of transplanted fetal serotonergic neurons in the brain. The neurotoxin 5,7-DHT, when microinjected into the FF, produced a specific and partial depletion of 5-HT in the hippocampus of adult rats. The ability of the 5,7-DHT-primed hippocampus to selectively support the neurochemical maturation of fetal serotonergic cells was tested by assaying the transplanted fetal raphe or LC 1 month after neuronal transplantation.

The neurochemical maturation of fetal 5-HT and NE neurons was dramatically different when they were transplanted in the 5,7-DHT-FF-lesioned hippocampus as compared to the normal hippocampus. The transplanted 5-HT neurons had 480% more SHAU of [^{3}H]5-HT and had a 250% greater content of 5-HT in the partially denervated hippocampus than in the normal hippocampus after 1 month. Furthermore, extracts obtained from lesioned hippocampus enhanced the 5-HT content of 5-HT neurons transplanted in the normal hippocampus, to a level similar to that seen in neurons transplanted in the lesioned hippocampus.

In contrast, the implanted NE neurons of fetal LC had a lower NE level in the 5-HT partially denervated hippocampus than in normal hippocampus after 1 month in the host site. The growth of the NE transplants was not facilitated by the vacant postsynaptic space produced by the 5,7-DHT lesion. These results suggest that the 5-HT denervation triggered a trophic signal selectively enhancing the development of the 5-HT neurons but not the NE neurons. Our results are consistent with previous studies showing homotypic collateral sprouting in 5,7-DHT-primed hippocampus.

ACKNOWLEDGMENTS

The authors wish to thank Dr. Patricia Whitaker-Azmitia for her help in preparing this manuscript and Dr. Robin Fisher for his comments on the manuscript.

REFERENCES

1. AZMITIA, E. C., A. M. BUCHAN & J. H. WILLIAMS. 1978. Structural and functional restoration by collateral sprouting of hippocampal 5-HT axons. Nature (London) **278:** 374-376.
2. ZHOU, F. C. & E. C. AZMITIA. 1984. Induced homotypic collateral sprouting of serotonergic fibers in the hippocampus of rat. Brain Res. **308:** 53-62.
3. ZHOU, F. C. & E. C. AZMITIA. 1986. Induced homotypic sprouting of serotonergic fibers in hippocampus. II. An immunocytochemical study. Brain Res. **373:** 337-348.
4. GAGE, F. H., A. BJÖRKLUND & U. STENEVI. 1983. Reinnervation of the partially deafferented hippocampus by compensatory collateral sprouting from spare cholinergic and noradrenergic afferents. Brain Res. **268:** 27-37.
5. DRAVID, A. R. & E. B. VAN DEUSEN. 1983. Recovery of choline acetyltransferase and acetylcholinesterase activities in the ipsilateral hippocampus following unilateral, partial transection of the fimbria in rats. Brain Res. **277:** 169-174.
6. GAGE, F. H., A. BJÖRKLUND, U. STENEVI & S. B. DUNNETT. 1983. Functional correlates of compensatory collateral sprouting by aminergic and cholinergic afferents in hippocampal formation. Brain Res. **268:** 39-47.
7. DIAMOND, J., E. COOPER, C. TURNER & L. MACINTYRE. 1976. Tropic regulation of nerve sprouting. Science **193:** 371-377.
8. MCCOUGH, G. P., G. M. AUSTIN, C. N. LIU & C. Y. LIU. 1958. Sprouting as a cause of plasticity. J. Neurophysiol. **21:** 205-216.
9. WIKLUND, L. & K. MOLLGARD. 1979. Neurotoxin destruction of the serotonergic innervation of the rat subcommissural organ is followed by reinnervation through collateral sprouting of non-monoaminergic neurons. J. Neurocytol. **8:** 469-480.
10. AZMITIA, E. C. & F. C. ZHOU. 1986. Induced homotypic collateral sprouting of hippocampal serotonergic fibers. *In* Processes of Recovery from Neuronal Trauma. G. M. Gilad, A. Gorio & G. W. Kreutzberg, Eds.: 469-480. Exp. Brain Res. (Suppl. 13).
11. ZHOU, F. C. & E. C. AZMITIA. 1985. The effect of adrenalectomy and corticosterone on homotypic collateral sprouting of serotonergic fibers in hippocampus. Neurosci. Lett. **54:** 111-116.
12. SCHEFF, S. W. & S. T. DEKOSKY. 1983. Steroid suppression of axon sprouting in the hippocampal dentate gyrus of the adult rat: Dose-response relationship. Exp. Neurol. **82:** 183-191.
13. BJÖRKLUND, A., U. STENEVI & N. A. SVENDGAARD. 1976. Growth of transplanted monoaminergic neurons into the adult hippocampus along the perforant path. Nature **262:** 787-790.
14. AZMITIA, E. C., M. J. PERLOW, M. J. BRENNAN & J. M. LAUDER. 1981. Fetal raphe and hippocampal transplants into adult and aged C57BL/6N mice: A preliminary immunocytochemical study. Brain Res. Bull. **7:** 703-710.
15. HOLETS, V. T. & C. W. COTMAN. 1984. Postnatal development of the serotonin innervation of the hippocampus and dentate gyrus: Normal development and reacquisition of normal synaptic density. J. Comp. Neurol. **226:** 457-476.
16. BJÖRKLUND, A. & U. STENEVI. 1981. *In vivo* evidence for a hippocampal adrenergic neurotrophic factor specifically released on septal deafferentation. Brain Res. **229:** 403-428.
17. GAGE, F. H., A. BJÖRKLUND & U. STENEVI. 1984. Denervation releases a neuronal survival factor in adult rat hippocampus. Nature **308:** 637-639.

18. LONGO, F. M., S. D. SKAPER, M. MANTHORPE, L. R. WILLIAMS, G. LUNDBORG & S. VARON. 1983. Temporal changes in neurotrophic activities accumulating in vivo with nerve regeneration chambers. Exp. Neurol. 81: 756-769.
19. NIETO-SAMPEDRO, M., E. R. LEWIS, C. W. COTMAN, M. MANTHORPE, S. D. SKAPER, G. BARBIN, F. M. LONGO & S. VARON. 1982. Brain injury causes a time-dependent increase in neuronotrophic activity at the lesion site. Science 217: 860-861.
20. NIETO-SAMPEDRO, M., M. MANTHORPE, G. BARBIN, S. VARON & C. W. COTMAN. 1983. Injury-induced neuronotrophic activity in adult rat brain: Correlation with survival of delayed implants in the wound cavity. J. Neurosci. 3: 2219-2229.
21. MANTHORPE, M., M. NIETO-SAMPEDRO, S. D. SKAPER, E. R. LEWIS, G. BARBIN, F. M. LONGO, C. W. COTMAN & S. VARON. 1983. Neurotrophic activity in brain wounds of the developing rat: Correlation with implant survival in the wound cavity. Brain Res. 267: 47-56.
22. AZMITIA, E. C. & W. F. MAROVITZ. 1980. In vitro hippocampal uptake of tritiated serotonin ([^{3}H]5-HT): A morphological, biochemical, and pharmacological approach to specificity. J. Histochem. Cytochem. 28: 636-644.
23. CLEWANS, C. & E. C. AZMITIA. 1984. Tryptophan hydroxylase in the hippocampus and midbrain following unilateral injection of 5,7-dihydroxytryptamine. Brain Res. 307: 125-133.
24. WILLIAMS, J. H. & E. C. AZMITIA. 1981. Hippocampal serotonin re-uptake and nocturnal locomotor activity after microinjections of 5,7-DHT in the fornix-fimbria. Brain Res. 207: 95-107.
25. ZHOU, F. C. & E. C. AZMITIA. 1983. Effect of 5,7-DHT on HRP retrograde transport from hippocampus to midbrain raphe nuclei. Brain Res. Bull. 10: 445-451.
26. AZMITIA, E. C. & P. M. WHITAKER. 1983. Formation of a glial scar following microinjections of fetal raphe neurons into the dorsal hippocampus or midbrain of the adult rat: An immunocytochemical study. Neurosci. Lett. 38: 145-150.
27. AZMITIA, E. C., M. J. BRENNAN & D. QUARTERMAN. 1983. Adult development of the hippocampal serotonin system of C57BL/6N mice: Analysis of high-affinity uptake of [^{3}H]5-HT in slices and synaptosomes. Neurochem. Int. 5: 39-44.
28. AUERBACH, S., F. C. ZHOU, B. L. JACOB & E. C. AZMITIA. 1985. Serotonin turnover in raphe neurons transplanted into rat hippocampus. Neurosci. Lett. 61: 147-152.
29. AUERBACH, S. & P. LIPTON. 1985. Regulation of in vitro serotonin release from the rat hippocampus: Effects of alterations in levels of depolarization and in rates of serotonin metabolism. J. Neurochem. 44: 1116-1130.
30. ZHOU, F. C., E. C. AZMITIA, S. AUERBACH & B. L. JACOB. 1985. A specific serotonergic growth factor from 5,7-DHT-lesioned hippocampus: In vivo evidence from fetal transplantation of raphe and locus ceruleus neurons. Soc. Neurosci. Abstr. 11: 1083.
31. MCNAUGHTON, N., E. C. AZMITIA, J. H. WILLIAMS, A. BUCHAN & J. A. GRAY. 1980. Septal elicitation of hippocampal theta rhythm after localized de-afferentation of serotonergic fibers. Brain Res. 200: 259-269.
32. AZMITIA, E. C. & F C. ZHOU. 1985. A specific serotonergic growth factor from 5,7-DHT-lesioned hippocampus: In vitro evidence from dissociated cultures of raphe and locus ceruleus neurons. Soc. Neurosci. Abstr. 11: 1084.
33. CRUTCHER, K. A. & F. COLLINS. 1982. In vitro evidence for two distinct hippocampal growth factors: Basis of neuronal plasticity? Science 217: 67-68.
34. OJIKA, K. & S. H. APPEL. 1984. Neurotrophic effects of hippocampal extracts on medial septal nucleus in vitro. Proc. Natl. Acad. Sci. USA 81: 2567-2571.

DISCUSSION OF THE PAPER

W. LOW (Indiana University School of Medicine, Indianapolis, IN): It has been reported that the serotonin nerve cells seem to survive only for about 6 months after transplantation in the hippocampus. Do you see the difference in the survival rate when you make these lesions versus leaving that pathway intact?

ZHOU: The survival rate does not seem to be affected in the hippocampus 5,7-DHT paradigm.

S. M. CRAIN (*Albert Einstein School of Medicine, New York, NY*): Do you think this factor might have some effect on survival of serotonergic neurons under other experimental conditions? Analogous to the interesting effects of cholinergic denervation having effects on survival of neurons dependent on nerve growth factor, might this be a sign that the sensitivity of these cells to the factor is exaggerated under other circumstances? The serotonergic neurons themselves seem to be stimulated to sprout and to raise transmitter levels as a result of this trophic factor. But yet their survival does not seem to be enhanced in these experimental conditions. The question is whether these test serotonergic neurons, if in a different state of injury, would be rescued by this same trophic factor.

ZHOU: We really need to do a time course study of survival before pursuing this question.

M. SHELANSKI (*New York University, New York, NY*): This is quite a different type of factor than is produced in cholinergic denervation.

ZHOU: We think the normal hippocampus may have different sets of supporting factors for cholinergic and serotonergic neurons. Serotonergic denervation may be stimulating the set of trophic factors that particularly benefit the serotonergic neurons.

Trophic Effects of Transplants Following Damage to the Cerebral Cortex

TIMOTHY J. CUNNINGHAM,[a] CONSTANCE B.
SUTILLA, AND FORREST HAUN

Department of Anatomy
Medical College of Pennsylvania
Philadelphia, Pennsylvania 19129

One of the remarkable differences between developing and mature brains is their response to injury. A specific lesion to developing nervous system pathways usually results in rapid and profound neuron loss while the same lesion in adults may produce only gradual cell loss or no cell death at all.[1-4] This observation is particularly intriguing because of its apparent conflict with the well-known behavioral observation that functional recovery from damage to the central nervous system (CNS) is generally more likely if the damage occurs to developing rather than mature CNS systems.[5,6]

Several explanations have been offered for this difference in the response of different-aged neurons to lesions. First, the fact that younger neurons are less likely to have formed sufficient numbers of sustaining inputs or sustaining collateral axons may make them much more vulnerable when those few inputs or collaterals that have developed are damaged.[1,7] In the CNS, collateral development is likely to be especially important to damaged neurons because these cells often have more widespread connections than neurons in the peripheral nervous system (PNS). A second suggestion relates to the "inherent metabolic capabilities" of younger neurons versus mature neurons.[8] As the neuron matures, so does its protein synthetic machinery, which may allow the cell to maintain itself for longer periods after lesions. Metabolic maturity seems likely to play an important role in the survival of PNS neurons after axotomy because mature synthetic processes appear to be required to support regeneration. A third idea, which may in fact encompass the other two, is that lesions to afferent or target structures separate the cell from sources of specific trophic factors supplied by these connecting cells. Developing neurons may depend more critically on these factors for both survival and continued differentiation. Mature neurons may no longer require such trophic agents,[1] or may have a much lower "rate of utilization" of the factors.[9]

Support for this "trophic hypothesis," at least for developing neurons, has come mainly from studies with nerve growth factor (NGF) in the PNS. NGF is a specific trophic agent for sensory and sympathetic ganglion cells; it is essential for the survival and differentiation of these cells during development. It is unique among the putative trophic factors that have been suggested or even partially isolated because its actions are demonstrable *in vivo.* Exogenous NGF can rescue naturally degenerating ganglion

---

[a]Address for correspondence: Department of Anatomy, Medical College of Pennsylvania, EPPI Division, 3200 Henry Avenue, Philadelphia, Pennsylvania 19129.

cells or ganglion cells degenerating because of axotomy or target deprivation.[10–12] Application of antibodies against NGF during the appropriate developmental period leads to destruction of the ganglia.[13] NGF is therefore the model for most other investigations of neurotrophic interactions and putative trophic agents.

The role of NGF in the maintenance of adult neurons, either normally or after axon damage, is not entirely clear. Antibodies to NGF do not destroy mature ganglion cells and do not accentuate the relatively small but significant loss of cells that occurs after peripheral nerve section in adults.[14] It has been suggested, but not demonstrated, that trophic factors other than NGF operate to maintain the ganglion cells in adults.[15] In the CNS, NGF has also been reported to increase choline acetyltransferase activity in the hippocampus of adult rats with septohippocampal lesions,[16] but the relationship of the finding to cell maintenance after lesions is unclear. Therefore, there is at present little evidence that the cell loss that does occur after damage to mature systems is due to separation from sources of trophic support; that is, it is not clear if the trophic hypothesis can be extended to mature neurons. A reasonable alternative, at least for axotomized neurons, is that the cells die simply from the trauma of amputation of their axon and subsequent loss of cytoplasm—an idea supported by the fact that the amount of cell death is proportional to the amount of axoplasm lost, that is, the proximity of the lesion to the cell body.[3]

Most of the evidence for the trophic hypothesis therefore comes from studies of the developing PNS where a neuron's target structures are well defined and where there are particular developmental periods during which the trophic interactions between neurons and their targets can be readily demonstrated. In the CNS the trophic hypothesis has been more difficult to test, primarily for two reasons. First, the complex interconnections in the CNS make identifying the particular afferent or target neurons that are involved in specific trophic interactions less certain. Second, even when neuron or glial populations can be identified as potential sources of trophic support, the cells must be tested for their ability to rescue damaged or maintain normal neurons *in vivo*. Although there are several *in vitro* models of CNS trophic interactions,[17–23] there is a relative lack of reliable *in vivo* assays.

We are using transplantation methods as part of such an *in vivo* assay for neurotrophic interactions in the visual system of rats. For these studies, transplant cells are used as potential sources of trophic factors in order to effect survival of damaged host neurons following specific lesions. Furthermore, by using different populations of transplant cells and determining their relative effects on the survival of different populations of host neurons, the specificity of the trophic interactions between CNS structures can be studied. Much of this work has focused on the developing visual system because of the prediction (by analogy with the PNS) that neurons are most susceptible to removal of trophic factors at particular stages of their development (see above). More recently, we have begun to test the ability of transplants to support the survival of adult host neurons after lesions, with the aim of determining whether the degeneration of these mature neurons after they are separated from their targets by axotomy may also be attributed to a loss of trophic support.

SPECIFIC NEUROTROPHIC INTERACTIONS IN THE DEVELOPING GENICULO-CORTICAL PATHWAY

In neonatal rats, destruction of the cortical visual areas results in rapid and massive degeneration of the ipsilateral dorsal lateral geniculate nucleus (dLGN).[cf.24,25] Our experiments have been based on the assumption that in undamaged animals this cortical tissue is an important source of trophic factors for the dLGN neurons; removal of this trophic support during critical periods of the neurons' development is therefore responsible for the death of these cells following the lesion. We have used embryonic posterior cortex cells as a potential source of these agents and have studied the effects of transplanting the cells into the cavity created by the lesion in newborn hosts.[26,27] We will first review our particular evidence for the trophic action of these cortical transplants in neonatal rats, with special emphasis on the specificity of the trophic interactions in this pathway. We will also include some recent data indicating that the underlying mechanism for these trophic effects may be diffusible factors derived from the transplant cells.

The host animals are Long-Evans hooded rats that receive a large lesion of the right posterior cortex within 18 hr of birth. Most of the host animals are exposed to [³H]thymidine on gestational days that correspond to particular periods of dLGN neurogenesis. The lesions completely remove all cortical projection areas for neurons of the dLGN and, in rats without transplants, result in near complete degeneration and removal of the nucleus in about 5 days.[cf.24] Donor tissue is obtained from either the posterior third of the cerebral vesicle or the cerebellar plate of day 14 or 15 (E14 or E15) embryos. Each tissue is dissected from the embryo and then cleaned of meninges and large blood vessels. In our initial studies, the tissue was dissociated with trypsin and transplanted directly.[26] More recently, we have cultured the cortical tissue for 5 days either with other pieces of E14 occipital cortex, E14 diencephalon, or E14 optic tectum.[27] These precultured transplants have allowed us to investigate the specificity of the neurotrophic effects of cortical transplants in detail (see below). Precultured transplants are also trypsin-dissociated before transplantation. A fixed volume of the resulting cell suspension is injected into the lesion cavity and then covered with dried collagen. We assay neuron survival in the dLGN 5 or 9 days after the lesion by measuring neuron-occupied volume of the nucleus and by counting thymidine-labeled neurons. For rats with lesions but no transplants, the lesion cavity is filled with gelfoam that has been soaked in fresh culture medium. In some animals, horseradish peroxidase is injected into the eye contralateral to the lesion in order to confirm the boundaries of the dLGN by its characteristic innervation pattern. (Details of all these procedures, including our explant culture techniques appear in reference 27.)

In all groups of animals, the lesions completely remove areas 17, 18a, and 18b in the right hemisphere. The lesions extend laterally to the rhinal fissue, rostrally into the barrel fields of somatosensory cortex, and damage at least some part of the cortical white matter. If the animal receives a transplant, 5 days later the transplant is usually found adhering to the host's hippocampus or subiculum. Transplant cells tend to be smaller and more darkly staining than the host cells, but they are well integrated at the margins, with no glial border or encapsulation. Scattered degenerating cells can be found within the transplant but there are no obvious differences in transplant survival among the various groups of animals.

A significantly greater neuron-occupied volume of the ipsilateral dLGN is found 5 days after the lesions in animals receiving cortical cell transplants, either those transplanted directly or precultured for 5 days (FIG. 1). The results from animals with cerebellar transplants are not significantly different from those of animals with lesions and no transplants. The thymidine labeling studies show that the surviving dLGN volume in cortical transplant animals contains a specific population of geniculate neurons defined by their time of origin. Neurons that are formed during the middle period of geniculate neurogenesis (on embryonic day 14 (E14)) are unaffected by the transplant cells and are almost completely absent in all groups of rats. The numbers of cells that are generated later (E15 and E16) that survive with cortical cell transplants, however, are significantly greater than in rats with cerebellar transplants or rats with lesions only.[26] Neurons of this particular population (and therefore those rescued by the transplant) tend to be concentrated in the medial and caudal parts of the nucleus. These results show that the neuron-supporting—or neurotrophic—effects of the transplants are relatively specific with regard to both the donor origin of transplant cells (cortical versus cerebellar cells) and to the particular population of host neurons affected ("later-generated" versus "earlier-generated" neurons).

We have conducted parallel *in vitro* studies of neurotrophic interactions in the visual pathways,[28] and these experiments have allowed us to test further the specificity of the *in vivo* trophic effects. The *in vitro* studies were designed to investigate the possibility that the survival of specific populations of occipital cortex neurons, developing in culture, depends on diffusible trophic factors derived from specific subcortical visual structures. We cultured explants of E14-15 posterior cortex with explants of either diencephalon or optic tectum harvested from rats of the same age. The explants

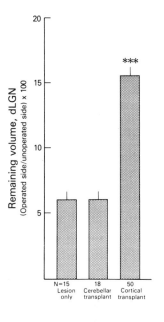

FIGURE 1. A summary of the transplant experiments measuring the neuron-occupied volume of ipsilateral dLGN in P6 rats that have sustained a large right visual cortex lesion at birth. The remaining volume is expressed as a percentage of the dLGN volume on the unoperated side (mean ± SEM). Animals with transplants of cortical cell suspensions placed in the lesion site have significantly more dLGN remaining (15.5 ± 0.7%) compared to rats with cerebellar transplants (6.1 ± 0.6%, $p < .001$ (***)) or rats with lesions only (6.2 ± 0.7%, $p < .001$ (***)). The comparisons were made using the Mann-Whitney U test. The data are from all the animals, irrespective of their transplant treatment (see text).

were grown on a substrate that is not conducive to neurite outgrowth, resulting in no contact between the co-cultured explants. Control cultures consisted of two cortical explants grown on the same substrate. The cultures were terminated after 5 days. To determine if the different co-cultures resulted in preferential survival of different neuron populations in the cortical explants, we used both horseradish peroxidase filling and thymidine labeling techniques. In the cortical explants co-cultured with diencephalon, the cortical neurons that survive after 5 days have small cross-sectional areas, most with a nonpyramidal morphology; furthermore, a significant proportion of the cells are generated late in the culturing period. In contrast, the surviving neurons in the cortex-plus-tectum cultures are larger, many with a pyramidal morphology, and these neurons, according to the labeling studies, are generated earlier in culture. The cortex co-cultured with other cortex gives results that are generally intermediate to the other two conditions. Since there is no contact between the explants, we conclude that there are diffusible molecules derived from different subcortical structures, which support the survival of different cortical neuron populations *in vitro.* The neurons that survive in the presence of diencephalon may represent those later-generated nonpyramidal cells that occupy more superficial cortical layers *in vivo.* Many of these neurons are located in cortical layer IV and are the natural targets for cortically projecting neurons in the thalamus. This result leads to the suggestion that the trophic factors that operate on the cortical tissue in these cultures are derived from those neurons located in the diencephalon that are potential sources of afferent input to the cortical cells. In contrast, the sole relationship between the optic tectum and cortex is the cortico-tectal projection that arises from earlier-generated pyramidal neurons of cortical layer V. This suggests that the factors operating on the cortical explants in these cultures are derived from potential cortical target neurons in the tectum. The composition of the cortical explants co-cultured with other cortex (which in terms of the percentage of pyramid-shaped neurons and time of origin gave intermediate values) may reflect the ability of the different neuron types in the explants to survive in the absence of subcortical tissue. The tectum and diencephalon are suggested to supply trophic factors that bias the explants around this baseline.[28]

The next step was to use these differently biased cortical explants as transplants in order to test the proposition that the *in vivo* trophic effects of the cortical cell suspensions are due to the action of particular cell populations within those transplants. A reasonable prediction is that transplants enriched with dLGN target neurons (later-generated and nonpyramidal neurons) would be the most effective in supporting neuron survival in the geniculate after removal of the posterior cortex. The results of the *in vivo* experiments suggest that this is indeed the case. The most effective transplants, in terms of both remaining dLGN volume and the numbers of surviving dLGN neurons labeled with [³H]thymidine on E15, are those cortical cells that develop in explant culture with diencephalon (FIG. 2). These particular precultured transplants support 50% more dLGN neurons than the direct transplants or transplants first cultured with optic tectum. In order to control for the effects of culturing per se, we also transplanted cerebellar tissue that had been cultured for 5 days, either alone or with a diencephalic explant; the cerebellar tissue is still ineffective after these procedures.

We conclude, therefore, that the trophic interactions in this pathway are highly specific, and may involve specific cortical laminae and those subcortical neurons that ultimately form connections with these laminae.

Regardless of the pretreatment of the transplant cells, however, their survival-promoting properties are only temporary. In all groups of rats, either with or without transplants, precultured or not, the dLGN has virtually disappeared by postnatal day 10. The temporary nature of this trophic effect suggests that the cortical transplants are meeting the survival requirements of some dLGN neurons during a critical period of trophic dependency, but these transplants do not provide a target for permanent, sustaining connections with the dLGN—connections that would be required for continued survival. Such connections do not form even though the transplants remain viable well into adulthood, and are capable of forming connections with both contralateral cortex and thalamic areas not destroyed by the lesion.[29-31] Therefore it is reasonable to suggest that the transplant cells are a source of specific trophic substances, and the survival-promoting properties of these agents are temporally limited (similar to the situation reported for NGF[32,33]).

Recently, we have conducted preliminary experiments to test the proposition that the basis for the transplants' effectiveness is the synthesis of diffusible trophic factors by the transplant cells.[34] Conditioned medium obtained from the cortex-diencephalon co-cultures was concentrated by ultrafiltration or lyophilization and then mixed in equal parts with solutions of either 25% polyacrylamide or 2% sodium alginate so

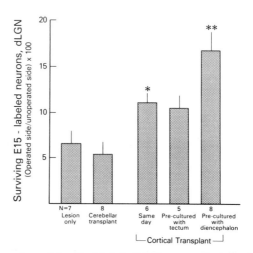

FIGURE 2. The numbers of heavily labeled dLGN neurons (≥ 15 grains/nucleus) on the ipsilateral side of P6 rats that have sustained large right visual cortex lesions at birth. Host animals are [³H]thymidine labeled *in utero* at E15; neuron counts are corrected by the method of Abercrombie[45] and expressed as a percentage of the number of labeled neurons on the unoperated side (mean ± SEM). Transplants of cell suspensions derived from either posterior cortex or cerebellum (harvested from E14/15 donors) are placed into the host lesion site. Cortical transplants precultured for 5 days with diencephalon support survival of significantly more host dLGN neurons (17.5 ± 1.5%, $p < .01$ (**)). Transplants taken from E14/15 donors and not precultured ("same day") are also effective (12.5 ± 1.3%, $p < .05$ (*)), but cortical transplants precultured with optic tectum are not (10.6 ± 1.4%, $p > .07$). The comparisons were made with lesion-only animals (6.9 ± 1.3%) using the Mann-Whitney U test.

as to become entrapped in the gel matrix. The gels were made in the form of small beads suitable for implantation into the cavity of a posterior cortex lesion in a newborn rat. To be certain that the beads were capable of supplying the media to the host within the 5-day period of our assay, the time course of elution of known proteins from the beads was measured *in vitro* by spectrophotometry. For example, alginate beads release bovine serum albumin (M_r: 68 000) in about 24 hr. This same time course is obtained when the alginate beads are mixed with culture medium, which contains a variety of proteins of much higher and much lower molecular weights. On the other hand, polyacrylamide appears to have more gradual release properties. So far we have tested the time course of elution of myosin subfragment S-1 (M_r: 120 000) from the acrylamide beads and find it to be released in about 4 days. With both types of beads, we measured dLGN survival 5 days after implanting the beads, which were loaded with either conditioned or unconditioned culture medium, into the posterior cortex lesion cavity. A third group of animals received lesions and gelfoam implants that had been soaked in conditioned or unconditioned medium. Surprisingly (given our preliminary *in vitro* results on its rapid release properties), the alginate bead implants give the best results, followed by the polyacrylamide implants; the gelfoam implants are ineffective (FIG. 3). Regardless of the explanation for the greater effectiveness of the alginate implants, these results strongly suggest that the transplant cells do synthesize diffusible molecules that are capable of supporting dLGN neurons after lesions. Furthermore, these *in vivo* findings, along with our *in vitro* results showing that diffusible factors support the survival of specific populations of cortical neurons,[28] suggest that diffusible molecules derived from target structures or afferent sources play an important role in the development of specific populations of CNS neurons.

NEUROTROPHIC INTERACTIONS IN THE ADULT GENICULO-CORTICAL PATHWAY

The ability of transplants to protect vulnerable populations of adult CNS neurons from degeneration after lesions has received considerably less attention than has their role in promoting the growth or regeneration of specific host axonal projections (see reference 35 for review). The assumption is of course that if the transplant provides an appropriate substrate for regrowth of a damaged projection, then the cells of origin of this projection must still be alive. In most cases, however, it is not clear whether the lesion would have resulted in the death of the involved neurons, or whether the transplant has indeed rescued these particular cells. The geniculo-cortical pathway allows a direct test of the survival-promoting properties of transplants, since it is well established that lesions of area 17 in adult rats result in the degeneration of neurons in the dLGN after a few weeks.[36] Furthermore, the geniculo-cortical projection is strictly topographic; thus small or incomplete lesions of area 17 will produce restricted foci of cell loss in the dLGN. We took advantage of this organization and made incomplete lesions of area 17 that were centered on the cortical representation of the inferior nasal visual field. Such a lesion produces a relatively restricted area of gliosis, cell shrinkage, and cell loss centered in the corresponding representation of the inferior nasal field in the caudomedial portion of the dLGN.[37] It is in this region that many of the cells that are generated later in geniculate neurogenesis normally reside, and it is these cells that are protected by cortical cell transplants into newborn rats. Our aim was thus to determine if the progress of degeneration of this same neuron population would be affected after lesions and transplants in adults.

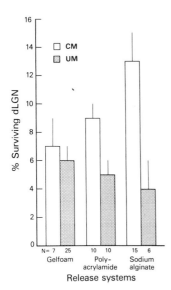

FIGURE 3. The surviving volume of ipsilateral dLGN, expressed as a percentage of the volume on the unoperated side (mean ± SEM), in P6 rats with a gel implant placed in the posterior cortex lesion site on the day of birth. The gel matrix is composed of 25% polyacrylamide or 2% sodium alginate, and contains either unconditioned culture medium (UM) or medium conditioned for 5 days by explant co-cultures of embryonic cortex and diencephalon (CM). Control implants were gelfoam plugs. Both the polyacrylamide and alginate release systems produce significant increases in surviving dLGN when the gel matrix contains CM (polyacrylamide: 9 ± 1%; sodium alginate: 13 ± 2%) compared to UM (polyacrylamide: 5 ± 1%; sodium alginate: 4 ± 2%) ($p < .01$ by the Mann–Whitney U test). CM gelfoam implants are ineffective, relative to UM gelfoam implants.

The host animals in these experiments were also Long-Evans hooded rats that had been exposed to [³H]thymidine on E15 and E16. At 60 days postnatal age, a suction lesion was made in the rostral part of area 17 using the co-ordinates of Espinoza and Thomas[38] as a guide to the representation of the inferior nasal field. The lesion cavity was filled with either a gelfoam plug (saturated with unconditioned culture medium) or a suspension of posterior cortex cells that had been harvested from E14 donors and precultured with diencephalon for 5 days. The transplant was covered with dried collagen or gelfoam, and then a small piece of synthetic dura was placed on the surface of the cortex directly over the lesion cavity. The rats survived for 2 weeks, after which the cortical lesions were reconstructed. Both lesion position and size were recorded. The lesions were all centered in the rostral third of area 17.

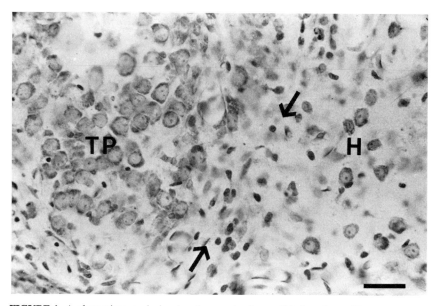

FIGURE 4. A photomicrograph showing the margin of a small lesion of area 17, made 2 weeks earlier in an adult rat (arrow). A group of apparently healthy transplant cells (TP) is evident; the cells adhere to the host's surviving cortex (H). Cresyl violet stain. Bar: 100 μm.

Although there was a range of lesion sizes, the range was similar in the lesion-only and transplant groups; overall there was no significant difference between the groups in either total lesion area or its medial-lateral or rostral-caudal extent (see the legend of FIG. 7).

In all transplant animals, viable transplant cells were seen, usually adhering to adjacent host cortex (FIG. 4). Occasionally, there was degeneration in the center of the transplants; nevertheless, there was no relationship between the amount of transplant seen in the host animal after 2 weeks and its effects on the dLGN. We interpret this lack of correspondence between the trophic action of the transplant (see below) and the extent of permanent transplant survival in the same way we interpret the lack of long-term dLGN survival in animals with neonatal lesions and cortical transplants:

The transplants meet the trophic requirements of some dLGN cells (at least temporarily) but may not provide a permanent target for dLGN-transplant connections.

The area of the geniculate affected by the lesion was the caudomedial portion, as expected. We measured the volume of this affected area (using specific criteria of cell shrinkage and gliosis), as well as the total volume of the nucleus. We found no significant difference between lesion-only and lesion-plus-transplant animals in either the volume of the affected area (see the legend of FIG. 6) or the total volume of remaining dLGN (mean ± SEM in the lesion-only group: 78 ± 7% of the volume on the unoperated side; that for the transplant group: 91 ± 5%). Thus, the lesions resulted in some overall shrinkage of the ipsilateral dLGN, but the amount of this reduction was not significantly affected by the transplant.

The principal and most striking results are found when considering the number of surviving neurons in the dLGN. Qualitatively, more apparently healthy cells are evident in the affected area of the geniculate in rats with transplants, compared to animals with lesions only (FIG. 5). Quantitatively, we confirmed this apparent increase in neuron survival by calculating the density of E15-16 labeled neurons in the affected area of the dLGN, as well as counting the total number of labeled neurons in the entire nucleus (FIG. 6). (The total counts were expressed as percent labeled neurons in the dLGN of the unoperated side; the affected-area densities were normalized to the overall density in the dLGN of the unoperated side. Both procedures are intended to correct for any differences in thymidine uptake or labeling intensities between animals.) In the entire nucleus, the lesion-only animals show a loss of one-third of the labeled neurons, whereas the lesion-plus-transplant animals showed virtually no such neuron loss. The cortical transplants, in other words, rescue all those E15-16 labeled neurons in the ipsilateral dLGN that otherwise would die following the lesion. This overall neuron rescue appears to be accounted for almost entirely by an increase in neuron survival in that portion of the geniculate affected by the lesion. The (normalized) density of labeled neurons in the affected area, expressed as a mean ± SEM, is $9572 \pm 1031/mm^3$ in lesion-only animals, compared to $14\ 130 \pm 243/mm^3$ in lesion-plus-transplant animals, a significant difference identical in size to the difference obtained in the total number of labeled neurons in the entire nucleus (FIG. 6).

In order to completely rule out any relationship between these results and differences in lesion size (even though statistically there is no overall difference in size or location of lesions between the two groups), we plotted the labeled cell densities in the affected area against the percentage of area 17 that was removed in each animal (FIG. 7). The results show that, in the lesion-only group, there is a trend toward decreased neuron survival as the lesion size increases ($r = -.70$). But this trend is entirely absent in the lesion-plus-transplant animals ($r = .26$). Therefore, the presence of the cortical transplant, and not lesion size, is the principal factor that determines the survival of this population of neurons in the dLGN, at least over the somewhat narrow range of lesion sizes used in this study.

Although we have not yet tested the specificity of this trophic effect in the adult, or shown that there are diffusible transplant-derived trophic molecules that give the same results, the rather dramatic trophic action of the transplant cells on adult neurons is somewhat surprising (when compared to their more limited survival-promoting effects on the same population of developing neurons). Our original assumption, and a widely accepted view, is that specific trophic interactions, and the specific agents that are responsible for promoting neuron survival, operate most effectively during critical developmental periods such as the period of naturally occurring neuron death.[39–43] The present results, however, are consistent with the idea that the trophic hypothesis applies as much if not more so to mature CNS neurons; the loss of trophic support contributes to neuron degeneration following CNS damage even when the

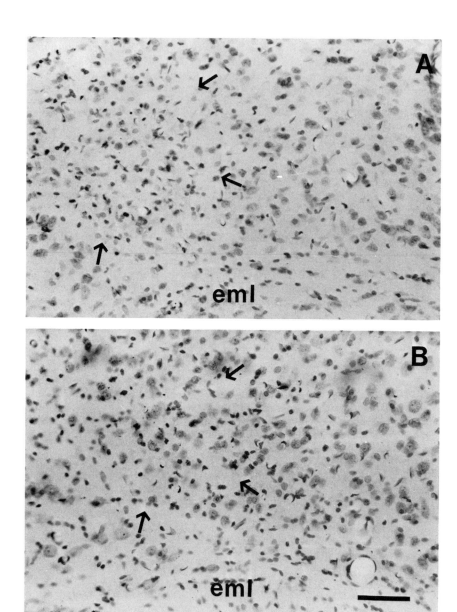

FIGURE 5. Photomicrographs showing the appearance of a region of degenerative changes (arrows) in the dLGN 2 weeks after a small lesion of area 17. (**A**) Lesion-only animal: The region is characterized by marked cell shrinkage and gliosis. (**B**) Lesion-plus-transplant animal: Although some cell shrinkage and gliosis are apparent, many more large apparently healthy neurons are found in this region compared to the lesion-only animal. eml: external medullary lamina. Cresyl violet stain. Bar: 200 μM.

neuron is fully matured at the time of the lesion. Therefore, the difference in the response of immature versus mature neurons to lesions may be related to the relative availability of the trophic agents to cells at different times during their development. Such a view leads to a more comprehensive explanation of lesion-induced neuron death, one that takes into account other factors such as collateralization, metabolic maturity, and, in the case of axotomy, axon amputation and subsequent loss of cytoplasm.

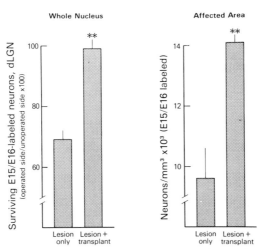

FIGURE 6. The numbers of heavily labeled neurons (≥ 15 grains/nucleus) in the ipsilateral dLGN of adult rats 2 weeks after small unilateral lesion of cortical area 17. Neurons are [³H]thymidine labeled *in utero* at E15 and E16; counts are corrected by the method of Abercrombie.[45] Whole nucleus: the total number of labeled neurons in the nucleus, expressed as a percentage of the number of labeled neurons on the unoperated side (mean ± SEM). Animals with cortical cell transplants in the lesion site have virtually normal numbers of labeled neurons (99 ± 3%); animals with lesions only have significantly fewer labeled neurons (67 ± 3%) ($p < .01$ (∗∗)) by the Mann-Whitney U test). Affected area: the density of labeled neurons in the particular area of the dLGN showing degenerative changes. Affected area densities are normalized to the overall density on the unoperated side (mean ± SEM). Animals with lesions plus transplants have a significantly greater density of labeled neurons in the affected area, compared to animals with lesions only (see text) ($t_{(10)} = 5.63$, $p < .01$ (∗∗)). Affected area measures (defined by cell shrinkage and gliosis criteria) are not significantly different (lesion only: 7 ± 2% of the entire nucleus; lesion plus transplant: 8 ± 1% of the entire nucleus). The percentage difference between the lesion-only ($N = 5$) and lesion-plus-transplant ($N = 7$) groups in the number of labeled neurons is identical in whole nucleus and affected area measures.

For example, the development of collateral axons or diversified inputs would give the mature neuron more access to sustaining trophic agents, so that if one of its collaterals or inputs were damaged, remaining axons or afferents could supply sufficient levels of these agents. The relative concentration of these factors within different inputs or targets may help determine which particular projections are more important to the survival of the neuron. Trophic agents may also trigger the development of mature protein synthetic machinery in the cell, making it metabolically stable and more resistant to the effects of lesions.[8,42] For example, in the case of sympathetic ganglion cells, it is well documented that NGF is involved in the biochemical maturation of the cells.[44] The location of axonal damage may be another important factor in the effectiveness of trophic substances. For example, loss of significant amounts of cytoplasm, which occurs when the lesion is close to the cell body, may drastically deplete the stores of factors in the cytoplasm, with the gap between the proximal stump of the axon and its target being too wide for replenishment via diffusion.

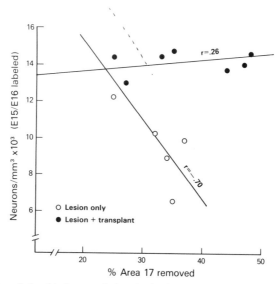

FIGURE 7. The relationship between lesion size in the visual cortex (area 17) and the number of surviving labeled neurons in the portion of dLGN that undergoes degenerative changes (adult rats, 2 weeks post lesion). Lesion size is expressed as the surface area of the lesion site relative to the total cortical surface of area 17; neuron survival is expressed as the density of E15/16 [³H]thymidine-labeled neurons in the affected portion of dLGN, normalized to the unoperated side (FIG. 6). In lesion-only animals there is a trend toward decreased density of labeled neurons in affected dLGN as the surface area of the cortical lesion increases ($r = -.70$); there is no such effect of lesion size on neuron survival in the lesion-plus-transplant animals ($r = .26$). (Boundaries of area 17 are determined from coronal sections by the strict use of the cytoarchitectonic criteria of Krieg[46]; in so doing the caudal pole of area 17 is most likely not included, thereby underestimating the total area and overestimating the percentage removed.) The mean percentage ($\pm$ SEM) removed in the two groups is not significantly different (lesion only: 33 $\pm$ 2%; lesion plus transplant: 37 $\pm$ 4%). Similarly, the lesion extent in area 17, expressed in μm (mean $\pm$ SEM), is not different in the two groups: 1) all lesions extend to rostral border of area 17; 2) the distance to the medial boundary of area 17 is not significantly different (lesion only: 710 $\pm$ 200 μm; lesion plus transplant: 890 $\pm$ 140 μm); and 3) the distance to the defined caudal boundary of area 17 is not significantly different (lesion only: 660 $\pm$ 120 μm; lesion plus transplant: 570 $\pm$ 150 μm).

The validity of these ideas awaits more direct experimentation, especially for neurons in the CNS. The technique of CNS transplantation may be an important part of such experiments because the action of potential sources of trophic support can be tested *in situ*. In other words, if the underlying cause of neuron degeneration after lesions is the lack of appropriate concentrations of specific trophic agents, then the relative concentration of such agents can be manipulated by transplanting cells from different areas of the nervous system (which are more or less enriched with the specific appropriate factors), or by transplanting potent trophic sources into different locations in the host (making diffusible factors more or less available to the damaged neurons). Since these substances can actually be collected from culture medium conditioned by the transplant cells, ultimately they could be chemically isolated and purified, which should lead to even more direct tests of their survival promoting properties *in vivo* and help clarify the nature of neurotrophic interactions in the CNS. Finally, a trophic interpretation of CNS transplant effects has an important implication for the potential therapeutic value of CNS transplants: their functional effectiveness may well depend not only on providing appropriate substrates for the outgrowth of axons in damaged pathways, but also on their ability to enhance the viability of the damaged host neurons that may give rise to those axons.

REFERENCES

1. COWAN, W. M. 1970. Anterograde and retrograde transneuronal degeneration in the central and peripheral nervous system. *In* Contemporary Research Methods in Neuroanatomy. W. J. H. Nauta & S. O. E. Ebbesson, Eds.: 217-251. Springer-Verlag. New York, NY.
2. CUNNINGHAM, T. J. & F. A. HAUN. 1984. Trophic relationships during visual system development. *In* Development of Visual Pathways in Mammals. J. Stone, B. Dreher & D. Rapaport, Eds.: 315-327. Alan R. Liss. New York, NY.
3. LIEBERMAN, A. R. 1974. Some factors affecting retrograde neuronal responses to axonal lesions. *In* Essays on the Nervous System. R. Bellairs & E. G. Gray, Eds.: 71-105. Clarendon Press. Oxford.
4. MISANTONE, L. J., M. GERSHENBAUM & M. MURRAY. 1984. Viability of retinal ganglion cells after optic nerve crush in adult rats. J. Neurocytol. **13:** 449-465.
5. GOLDMAN, P. S. 1974. An alternative to developmental plasticity: Heterology of CNS structures in infants and adults. *In* Plasticity and Recovery of Function in the Central Nervous System. D. G. Stein, J. J. Rosen & N. Butlers, Eds.: 149-174. Academic Press. New York, NY.
6. KENNARD, M. 1942. Cortical reorganization of motor function: Studies on series of monkeys of various ages from infancy to maturity. Arch. Neurol. Psychiatry **47:** 227-240.
7. BLIER, R. 1969. Retrograde transsynaptic cellular degeneration in mamillary and central tegmental nuclei following limbic decortication in rabbits of various ages. Brain Res. **15:** 365-393.
8. LAVELLE, A. & F. W. LAVELLE. 1984. Neuronal reaction to injury during development. *In* Early Brain Damage. S. Finger & C. R. Almli, Eds.: Vol. **2:** 3-15. Academic Press. New York, NY.
9. JACOBSON, M. 1970. Developmental Neurobiology. Holt, Rinehart & Winston. New York, NY.
10. HAMBURGER, V., J. K. BRUNSO-BECHTOLD & J. W. YIP. 1981. Neuronal death in the spinal ganglia of the chick embryo and its reduction by nerve growth factor. J. Neurosci. **1:** 60-71.
11. HENDRY, I. A. & J. CAMPBELL. 1976. Morphometric analysis of rat superior cervical ganglion after axotomy and NGF treatment. J. Neurocytol. **5:** 351-360.
12. YIP, H. K. & E. M. JOHNSON. 1984. Developing dorsal root ganglion neurons require trophic support from their central processes: Evidence for a role of retrogradely transported nerve growth factor from the central nervous system to the periphery. Proc. Natl. Acad. Sci. USA **81:** 6245-6249.
13. JOHNSON, E. M., P. D. GORIN, L. D. BRANDEIS & J. PEARSON. 1980. Dorsal root ganglion neurons are destroyed by exposure *in utero* to maternal antibody to nerve growth factor. Science **210:** 916-918.

14. RICH, K. M., H. K. YIP, P. A. OSBOURNE, R. E. SCHMIDT & E. M. JOHNSON. 1984. Role of nerve growth factor in the dorsal root ganglia neuron and its response to injury. J. Comp. Neurol. 230: 110-118.

15. JOHNSON, E. M. & H. K. YIP. 1985. Central nervous system and peripheral nerve growth factor provide trophic support critical to mature sensory neuronal survival. Nature 314: 751-752.

16. HEFTI, F., A. DRAVID & J. HARTIKKA. 1984. Chronic intraventricular injections of nerve growth factor elevate hippocampal choline acetyltransferase activity in adult rats with partial septo-hippocampal lesions. Brain Res. 293: 305-311.

17. CARNOW, T. B., M. MANTHORPE, G. E. DAVIS & S. VARON. 1985. Localized survival of ciliary ganglionic neurons identifies neuronotrophic factor bands on nitrocellulose blots. J. Neurosci. 5(8): 1965-1971.

18. DRIBIN, L. B. & J. N. BARRETT. 1982. Two components of conditioned medium increase neuritic outgrowth from rat spinal cord explants. J. Neurosci. 8: 271-280.

19. KLIGMAN, D. 1982. Neurite outgrowth from cerebral cortical neurons is promoted by medium conditioned over heart cells. J. Neurosci. Res. 8: 281-287.

20. McCAFFREY, C. A., M. R. BENNETT & B. DREHER. 1982. The survival of neonatal rat retinal ganglion cells in vitro is enhanced in the presence of appropriate parts of the brain. J. Comp. Neurol. 177: 519-528.

21. MIZRACHI, Y. & M. SCHWARTZ. 1982. Goldfish tectal explants have a growth-promoting effect on neurites emerging from co-cultured regenerating retinal explants. Dev. Brain Res. 3: 502-505.

22. TURNER, J. E., Y.-A. BARDE, M. E. SCHWAB & H. THOENEN. 1983. Extract from brain stimulates neurite outgrowth from fetal rat retinal explants. Dev. Brain Res. 6: 77-83.

23. WHITTEMORE, S. R., M. NIETO-SAMPEDRO, D. L. NEEDELS & C. W. COTMAN. 1985. Neuronotrophic factors for mammalian brain neurons: Injury induction in neonatal, adult and aged rat brain. Dev. Brain Res. 20: 169-178.

24. CUNNINGHAM, T. J., C. HUDDLESTON & M. MURRAY. 1979. Modification of neuron numbers in the visual system of the rat. J. Comp. Neurol. 184: 423-424.

25. PERRY, V. H. & A. COWEY. 1979. Changes in the retino-fugal pathways following cortical and tectal lesions in neonatal and adult rats. Exp. Brain Res. 35: 97-108.

26. HAUN, F. A. & T. J. CUNNINGHAM. 1984. Cortical transplants reveal CNS trophic interactions in situ. Dev. Brain Res. 15: 290-294.

27. HAUN, F. A. & T. J. CUNNINGHAM. 1987. Specific neurotrophic interactions between cortical and subcortical visual structures in developing rat: In vivo assay. J. Comp. Neurol. In press.

28. REPKA, A. & T. J. CUNNINGHAM. 1987. Specific neurotrophic interactions between cortical and subcortical visual structures in developing rat: In vitro assay. J. Comp. Neurol. In press.

29. HAUN, F. A., L. A. ROTHBLAT & T. J. CUNNINGHAM. 1985. Visual cortex transplants in rats restore normal learning of a difficult visual pattern discrimination. Invest. Ophthalmol. Vision Sci. 26(3)(Suppl.): 288.

30. CHANG, F.-L., J. G. STEEDMAN & R. D. LUND. 1984. Embryonic cerebral cortex placed in the occipital region of newborn rats makes connections with the host brain. Dev. Brain Res. 13: 164-166.

31. FLOETER, M. K. & E. G. JONES. 1985. Transplantation of postmitotic neurons to rat cortex: Survival, early pathway choices and long-term projections of outgrowing axons. Dev. Brain Res. 22: 19-38.

32. BANKS, B. E. C. & S. J. WALTER. 1977. The effects of postganglionic axotomy and nerve growth factor on the superior cervical ganglia of developing mice. J. Neurocytol. 6: 287-297.

33. BARDE, Y. A., D. EDGAR & H. THOENEN. 1980. Sensory neurons in culture: Changing requirements for survival factors during embryonic development. Proc. Natl. Acad. Sci. USA 77: 1199-1203.

34. CUNNINGHAM, T. J., F. A. HAUN, M. E. McGUIRE & P. D. CHANTLER. 1986. Diffusible trophic factors delay lesion-induced neuron death in developing rat visual system. Anat. Rec. 214: 28A.

35. NIETO-SAMPEDRO, M. & C. W. COTMAN. 1985. Growth factor induction and temporal order in central nervous system repair. *In* Synaptic Plasticity. C. W. Cotman, Ed.: 407-455. Guilford Press. New York, NY.
36. LASHLEY, K. S. 1941. Thalamo-cortical connections of the rat's brain. J. Comp. Neurol. **75:** 67-121.
37. MONTERO, V. M., J. F. BRUGGE & R. E. BEITEL. 1968. Relation of the visual field to the lateral geniculate body of the albino rat. J. Neurophys. **31:** 221-236.
38. ESPINOZA, S. G. & H. C. THOMAS. 1983. Retinotopic organization of striate and extrastriate visual cortex in the hooded rat. Brain Res. **272:** 137-144.
39. BERG, D. K. 1984. New neuronal growth factors. Annu. Rev. Neurosci. **7:** 149-170.
40. COWAN, W. M., J. W. FAWCETT, D. D. M. O'LEARY & B. B. STANFIELD. 1984. Regressive events in neurogenesis. Science **225:** 1256-1258.
41. COWAN, W. M. 1978. Aspects of neuronal development. *In* International Review of Physiology and Neurophysiology III. R. Porter, Ed. Vol. 17. University Park Press. Baltimore, MD.
42. CUNNINGHAM, T. J. 1982. Naturally occurring neuron death and its regulation by developing neural pathways. *In* International Review of Cytology. G. H. Bourne & J. F. Danielli, Eds. Vol. **72:** 163-186. Academic Press. New York, NY.
43. OPPENHEIM, R. W. 1981. Neuronal cell death and some related regressive phenomena during neurogenesis: A selective historical review and progress report. *In* Studies in Developmental Neurobiology. W. M. Cowan, Ed.: 74-133. Oxford University Press. New York, NY.
44. BLACK, I. B., I. A. HENDRY & L. L. IVERSON. 1972. Effects of surgical decentralization and NGF on the maturation of adrenergic neurons in a mouse sympathetic ganglion. J. Neurochem. **19:** 1367-1377.
45. ABERCROMBIE, M. 1946. Estimation of nuclear population from microtome sections. Anat. Rec. **94:** 238-248.
46. KRIEG, W. J. S. 1946. Connections of the cerebral cortex. I. The albino rat. A. Topography of the cortical areas. J. Comp. Neurol. **84:** 277-284.

DISCUSSION OF THE PAPER

C. SOTELO (*INSERM U106, CMC Foch, Suresnes*): I have two questions. The first one is about the immature cerebellar transplants. What happened with the cerebellar cells from the transplant? They probably degenerate.

CUNNINGHAM: No, they do not degenerate. In fact, transplant viability appears equivalent regardless of the origin of the tissue.

SOTELO: All right. My second question is about the mechanism. We should try peroxidase methods to try to see if the transplants, instead of only having this trophic factor, have some other anatomical basis of synergistic interaction between the cells, so that by putting peroxidase in transplants . . .

CUNNINGHAM: We have not yet investigated whether there is invasion of the transplant by thalamocortical axons. We do want to test this, especially in adults, because we recently obtained data that suggests dLGN neuron rescue is permanent after transplantation into adult cortex. We first want to test for the possibility that there are transplant-derived factors that can give the same result.

P. PASIK (*Mount Sinai School of Medicine, New York, NY*): On the basis of your culture data, you suggested that the source of the factor you are finding may be neurons that actually receive the geniculate input. Could you entertain a possibility that the thalamo-cortical source is important since it would be presynaptic to the geniculate cells?

CUNNINGHAM: Yes, it is possible. All we can say now is that the majority of cells contained in cortical explants co-cultured with diencephalon, that is, the tissue which is most effective when used as a transplant, are nonpyramidal and generated later. Cells providing different input to the geniculate are generated early in cortical neurogenesis.

PASIK: It is difficult because in your cultures it is difficult to say which is pyramidal and which is not. And with respect to the size of the neurons that project from cortex to thalamus—these are considerably smaller than those that project to the tectum, so . . .

CUNNINGHAM: Yes, but that is why you cannot go on morphology alone. You have to show that these cells are generated at different times.

PASIK: Are you getting a significant amount of developmental cell death in the geniculate nucleus?

CUNNINGHAM: Yes. Others have looked at this problem. It occurs within the first 30 postnatal days.

PASIK: So have you taken this extract as an example to see whether or not you can prevent the developmental cell death by grafting directly to the target area or to the cell body.

CUNNINGHAM: We certainly want to do that. We would, however, like to get a cleaner molecular weight fraction before we start testing. We can inject the extract into ventricles and see if it rescues the naturally degenerating cells.

F. H. GAGE (*University of California, La Jolla, CA*): Even your graft to the cortex of the neonate should survive.

CUNNINGHAM: Without making a lesion?

GAGE: Yes, in a developing system.

CUNNINGHAM: We have had difficulty getting good transplant survival without a lesion in cortex.

J. P. MCALLISTER (*Temple University School of Medicine, Philadelphia, PA*): Have you done any time studies on when either the transplants or the trophic factor has to be available? Is it just a short period of time or does it have to be there continually in order to promote the survival of your cells?

CUNNINGHAM: We do not know much about the time course of delivery of the factor *in vivo*. *In vitro*, the polyacrylamide chips release proteins over about 4 days while the alginate beads have much more rapid release properties. It looks as though fast delivery of the factors may be important because the beads are more effective.

Functional Activity of Raphe Neurons Transplanted to the Hippocampus and Caudate-Putamen

An Immunohistochemical and Neurochemical Analysis in Adult and Aged Rats

HARRY W. M. STEINBUSCH,[a,b] ALMA BEEK,[b]
ABRAHAM L. FRANKHUYZEN,[b] JEROEN A. D. M.
TONNAER,[c] FRED H. GAGE,[d] AND
ANDERS BJÖRKLUND[e]

[b]Department of Pharmacology
Faculty of Medicine
Vrije Universiteit
Amsterdam, the Netherlands

[c]Department of Central Nervous System Pharmacology
Organon International Bv.
Oss, the Netherlands

[d]Department of Neurosciences
University of California at San Diego
La Jolla, California 92037

[e]Department of Histology
University of Lund
Lund, Sweden

INTRODUCTION

It is now well established that grafted neuronal cell suspensions can survive, differentiate, and make new synaptic contacts in the adult and aged mammalian central nervous system.[1-6] These studies were focused on monoaminergic and cholinergic systems, using histochemical, electrophysiological, and behavioral techniques. Moreover, Schultzberg et al.[7] and Foster et al.[8] have recently shown that peptidergic neurons taken from the embryonic rat brain are able to withstand the process of suspension and subsequent grafting into a host recipient.

[a]Address for correspondence: Department of Pharmacology, Faculty of Medicine, Vrije Universiteit, Van der Boechorststraat 7, NL 1081 BT Amsterdam, the Netherlands.

169

The present study can be divided into two parts. The first part is an immunocytochemical study that focuses on the use of mesencephalic raphe (MR) and rhombencephalic raphe (RR) cell suspensions injected into the hippocampus and caudate-putamen of the adult and aged rats. It was our aim to test if fiber outgrowth is influenced by its target and by the age of the host recipient. In addition, we were interested to see if other transmitter systems will grow out of the same cell suspension and follow the same pattern of innervation. The second part is a combined neurochemical and morphological study in which we show additional evidence for the functionality of grafted cell suspensions. The recent study by Auerbach et al.[9] showed that the newly formed serotonin-immunoreactive fibers also synthesize serotonin (5-hydroxytryptamine (5-HT)), which is reflected in the amount and strength of the immunocytochemical staining. In our study, we want to address the functional activity of these sprouts and present evidence that the newly formed fibers spontaneously release 5-HT and, moreover, that this release can be potentiated with K^+. In addition, and of equal importance, we show that immunocytochemistry can be performed on *in vitro* slices and that the combination with neurochemical studies reveals a meaningful correlation between the number of the newly formed serotonergic fibers and the K^+-induced release of 5-HT.

MATERIALS AND METHODS

Twelve adult female Wistar rats (3 months old; 140-160 g) and two aged female rats (28 months old; 480-520 g) were used as hosts. Grafts were taken from fetuses of the same inbred strain with a crown-to-rump length (CRL) of 10-18 mm. One hour before the 5,7-dihydroxytryptamine (5,7-DHT) lesion, the host received an injection of desimipramine (DMI) (25 mg/kg, i.p.) to prevent uptake of the neurotoxin into noradrenergic neurons.[10] After 150 μg 5,7-DHT was dissolved in 20 μl of saline with 0.2 mg/ml ascorbic acid, the solution was injected over a period of 10 min into one of the lateral ventricles, using a stereotaxic apparatus during the 10 min. The rats were not used for grafting until at least 12 days after lesioning. All surgery was conducted under ketamine (Ketalar, 50 mg/kg) and xylazine (Rompun, 5 mg/kg) anesthesia (i.m.).

Transplant Suspension Preparation and Injections

For the description of the preparation of intracerebral grafts of neuronal cell suspensions, we refer to Björklund et al.,[1] Gage et al.,[11] Steinbusch et al.,[12] and Brundin et al.[13]

Pregnant Wistar rats at 13-17 days gestation were anesthetized, and fetuses were removed one at a time by cesarean section.

The brain was excised and serotonergic cells were taken from the ventral surface between the mesencephalic and pontine flexure (MR) and from the ventral surface at the pontine flexure (RR) as indicated in FIGURE 1.[14]

The tissue pieces were kept in 500 μl of saline containing 0.6% D-glucose at room temperature. The tissue was disrupted by repeated pipetting with a fire-polished Pasteur pipette. The resulting suspension was kept at room temperature for a maximum of 4 hr.

Stereotaxic suspension injections were made with a 10-μl Hamilton syringe. Each graft consisted of a 4-μl cell suspension that contained 80 000 cells; each suspension was injected over a 4-min period. The needle was left *in situ* for an additional 6 min before it was slowly retracted.

The injection coordinates (anterior, caudal to the bregma; lateral; and ventral, below the dura) were 3.0, 1.8, and 2.6 mm for the hippocampus and 0, 3.0, and 3.5 mm for the caudate-putamen.

All possible combinations of injection sites (hippocampus and caudate-putamen) and cell suspensions (MR and RR cells) were made.

Tissue Preparation

After 10 weeks graft survival, the hosts were prepared for immunohistochemistry. Two hours before perfusion, the animals received a pargyline injection (150 mg/kg, i.p.). The animals were anesthetized with sodium pertobarbital (Nembutal, 90 mg/

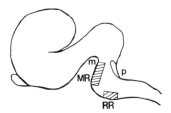

FIGURE 1. Lateral view of a dissected brain that was taken from a fetus on embryonic day 15. The CRL was 13 mm. m: mesencephalic flexure; MR: mesencephalic raphe area; p: pontine flexure; RR: rhombencephalic raphe area.

kg) and perfused through the ascending aorta reached via the left ventricle of the heart. The blood was washed out with ice-cold, oxygen-enriched, Ca^{2+}-free Tyrode's buffer (for 2 min) followed by 500 ml of ice-cold 4% (w/v) paraformaldehyde in 0.1 M sodium phosphate buffer (pH 7.4) at a pressure of 90 mm Hg. The brains were quickly removed and immersed in fresh fixative at 4° C for 2 hr. After fixation, they were rinsed in 20% sucrose dissolved in 0.1 M sodium phosphate buffer (pH 7.4) (for free-floating frozen microtome sections) or in 5% sucrose dissolved in the same buffer (for cryostat sections) for at least 1 day. Tissue pieces were then frozen with dry ice and serially sectioned at 50 μm for microtome sections and 16 μm for cryostat sections. Free-floating frozen microtome sections were collected in Tris-buffered saline (TBS). Cryostat sections were mounted on glass slides coated with chrome alum gelatine. The sections were used for immunohistochemistry or immunofluorescence.

Immunohistochemical and Immunofluorescence Procedures

The indirect immunohistochemical procedure was used. All primary antisera used were raised in rabbits. The sections were first washed with TBS at room temperature for 3 × 10 min (that is, three times, 10 min each time). They were then incubated with antiserum diluted in TBS containing 0.5% Triton X-100 (TBS-T) for 18 hr at room temperature or for 72 hr at 4°C. For immunofluorescence, a dilution of 1:500 for anti-5-HT was used; for immunohistochemistry, dilutions of 1:2000 (for anti-5-HT), 1:9000 (for antinoradrenaline), and 1:500 (for antisubstance P) were used. Details about the production of antibodies to 5-HT and noradrenaline have been published elsewhere.[14,15] Hereafter, the sections were washed alternately with TBS and TBS-T for 3 × 15 min.

Cryostat sections were treated with fluorescein isothiocyanate-conjugated sheep antirabbit immunoglobulin G (IgG), diluted 1:20 with TBS-T, for 1 hr at room temperature. After this final incubation, they were alternately washed in TBS-T and TBS for 3 × 10 min and mounted under a coverslip in a 1:3 mixture of TBS and glycerin (v/v). The sections were examined in an Olympus Vanox microscope equipped for epifluorescence.

Microtome sections were incubated for 2 hr with goat-antirabbit IgG (Fc specific) diluted in TBS-T 1:60 and washed alternately in TBS and TBS-T for 3 × 15 min at room temperature. They were then treated with rabbit peroxidase-antiperoxidase complex diluted in TBS-T 1:600 for 1 hr at room temperature and washed for 2 × 15 min in TBS and for 15 min in 0.05 M Tris-HCl (pH 7.6). Hereafter, the sections were incubated with 0.05% (w/v) diaminobenzidine dissolved in Tris-HCl containing H_2O_2 (0.01 wt%). The sections were mounted on glass slides coated with chrome alum gelatine and dried. They were fixed in 2% glutaraldehyde; diluted in Tris-HCl for 10 min; dehydrated in five steps, beginning with three steps in alcohol and water (70, 90, and 96% alcohol) and ending with two steps in xylol, 2 min each step; and mounted in Entellan.

Kodak Tri-X film was used for taking photomicrographs of immunofluorescent sections, and Agfapan 25 film was used for taking photomicrographs of immunohistochemically stained sections.

Preparation, Labeling, and Superfusion of Slices

Host (10 weeks graft survival) and normal female Wistar rats (200-240 g) were sacrificed by decapitation, and their brains were kept in ice-cold Krebs-Ringer bicarbonate medium before use.

The hippocampi (or neocortices) were dissected, and 300-μm-thick slices were prepared by transverse cuts using a McIllwain tissue chopper. Each hippocampus was divided into four successive groups (as indicated in FIG. 2), and each group contained five slices. The third slice in each group was fixed for 1 hr and prepared for cryostat sectioning and immunofluorescence. The remaining four slices in each group were subsequently cut in a longitudinal direction.

The slices (wet tissue weight: ~10 mg) were incubated with radiolabeled transmitter and superfused as described previously.[17] In short, after a 10-min preincubation, the slices were incubated for 15 min at 37° C with 5 μCi of [³H]5-HT (final concentration: 0.08 μM) and 2 μCi of [¹⁴C]choline (final concentration: 0.016 μM) in 2.5 ml of Krebs-Ringer bicarbonate medium in a 95% O_2-5% CO_2 atmosphere. After incubation, the slices were washed and medium was removed; 15 μl of the slice suspension (wet tissue weight: ~3 mg) was transferred to each of 24 chambers (volume: 0.2 ml) of a superfusion apparatus. The separate areas of the hippocampus were superfused at a rate of 0.25 ml/min with oxygenated Krebs-Ringer bicarbonate medium containing 10^{-5} M fluvoxamine to prevent reuptake of 5-HT in serotonergic neurons. After 30 min of superfusion, successive 10-min fractions were collected; 10 min later, depolarization of the tissue was effected by superfusion with medium containing 20 mM K^+. Separate chambers contained normal or 5,7-DHT-lesioned hippocampus slices that were not exposed to high-K^+ medium; these slices were used to determine spontaneous [^{3}H]5-HT and [^{14}C]choline efflux. The basel efflux course was used to calculate the basal efflux in the stimulated chambers from the first 10-min fraction (t = 30-40 min). The tissue was stimulated continuously with high-K^+ medium until the end of the experiment at t = 90 min. At the end of the experiment, the radioactivity remaining in the tissue was extracted with 0.1 M hydrochloric acid. Radioactivity was determined by liquid scintillation counting.

Labeling and Superfusion of a Cell Suspension

Freshly prepared cell suspension was also used for superfusion. The cell suspension was prepared as described above from fetuses with a CRL of 20 mm. A 500-μl cell

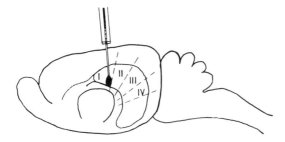

FIGURE 2. Schematic illustration of the position of the raphe suspension implants in the hippocampal formation. The levels I-IV denote the four frontal planes, which are spaced at approximately 1.5-mm intervals.

suspension that contained approximately 10^7 cells (counted after Evans-Blue vital staining) was incubated with 5 μCi of [^{3}H]5-HT (0.08 μM) in 2.5 ml of Krebs-Ringer solution at 37° C in a 95% O_2-5% CO_2 atmosphere. Subsequently, the cell suspension was centrifuged for 2 min and the supernatant was removed. The pellet was resuspended in 1 ml of Krebs-Ringer medium. A 50-μl cell suspension (5 × 10^5 cells) was immobilized in the superfusion chambers on small layers of Sephadex as described previously for synaptosomes.[18] The cell suspension was superfused as described above and depolarized by superfusion. The latter superfusion was carried out in three successive media: the first contained 20; the second, 40; and the third, 56 mM K^+. The release was compared with the release of slices from the neocortex of a normal rat that was labeled with [^{3}H]5-HT and superfused in parallel.

The efflux of radioactivity collected in each 10-min fraction was expressed at the mean fractional rate as percentage (Fr%) of the total radioactivity present at each time of the superfusion. The K^+-induced release of radioactivity in excess of the basal efflux was calculated by subtracting the fractional rate of the basal efflux (B) during each 10-min fraction of the corresponding fractions collected from slices continuously exposed to the elevated K^+ concentration (S) (see reference 19 for details).

The statistical significance of differences was determined by the two-tailed Student's *t* test.

The total amount of transmitter uptake was expressed as the total extraction (dpm), which is all radioactivity present at the beginning of fraction collection (t = 30 min).

RESULTS AND DISCUSSION

Raphe Cell Suspension in the Adult and Aged Hippocampus and Caudate-Putamen: Morphology

Suspensions, taken from MR or RR taken from fetuses with a CRL of 10-18 mm, were injected into the adult and aged hippocampus and caudate-putamen, which had been depleted of 5-HT innervation. Eight weeks to 3 months after transplantation, we observed a large number of 5-HT-positive cells that had survived the grafting process. In the hippocampus, most of these cells had migrated away from the transplantation site into the bordering tissue, whereas the cells in the caudate-putamen were situated at the outer boundaries of the grafted tissue. In the hippocampus, outgrowth of varicose fibers from the 5-HT-immunoreactive cells into the surrounding host tissue was equally extensive from the RR and MR grafts. In the caudate-putamen, on the other hand, little outgrowth from the RR serotonergic cells extended beyond the boundaries of the transplant proper, whereas MR serotonergic cells developed dense networks of serotonergic varicose fibers into the surrounding caudate-putamen.

Immunohistochemical analysis of the grafted cells revealed that many exhibited 5-HT immunoreactivity. In addition, as revealed by antibodies to noradrenaline, a few noradrenergic cells were present in the RR cell suspension grafts in the caudate-putamen. These cells have never been seen after RR cell suspension into the hippocampus, or after an MR cell suspension into either the hippocampus or the caudate-putamen. It should be noted, however, that although these cells survived, little fiber outgrowth was observed, and the transplantation site was not innervated (FIG. 3).

The same RR and MR cell suspensions were also studied for their ability to elicit substance P-containing fibers. We found newly formed substance P-immunoreactive fibers originating from the RR as well as from the MR cell suspensions. The innervations of the caudate-putamen and hippocampus by the serotonin- and substance P-positive fibers were not identical (FIGS. 4 & 5).

With regard to the age of the donor and the age of the recipient, we made the following observations. The extent of fiber outgrowth depended on the age of the donor. We observed the largest outgrowth with donors that had a CRL of 10-12 mm. Larger donors, which had a CRL of 12-18 mm, normally provided a poor outgrowth, although the cell survival was comparable. We did not find differences between recipients of different ages. In both the young adult (3-month-old) and the aged (28-month-old) rats, we were able to obtain the same pattern and extent of outgrowth from the same MR and RR cell suspensions.

Immunohistochemistry of Slices of Host Hippocampus

Cryostat sections of hippocampus slices of normal rats showed many 5-HT-positive fibers, whereas sections of slices of 5,7-DHT-lesioned hippocampus and caudate-putamen showed very few fibers (FIG. 6).

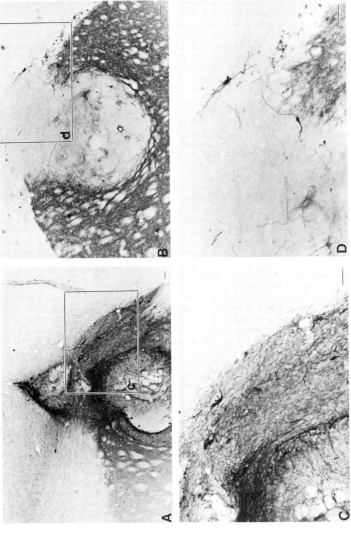

FIGURE 3. Photomicrographs of two transverse Vibratome sections through the dorsal part of the caudate-putamen of a 5,7-DHT-pretreated adult rat, 8 weeks after transplantation of an RR cell suspension taken from fetuses with a CRL of 15 mm. Sections were stained with antibodies to 5-HT (A & C) and noradrenaline (B & D). Several 5-HT-immunoreactive cells are demonstrated in C, as is a network of varicose fibers emanating from the grafted cells into the bordering caudate-putamen complex. Two noradrenaline-positive cells are visualized in D. The area that received the graft has received only a few newly formed noradrenergic fibers, whereas the remaining caudate-putamen complex still bears a moderate to dense noradrenergic innervation, revealing the specificity of the 5,7-DHT treatment. Bars: 50 μm.

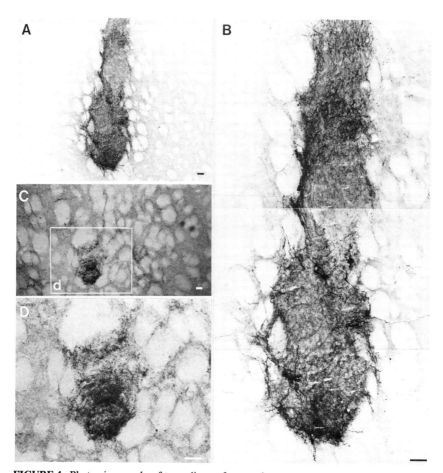

FIGURE 4. Photomicrographs of two adjacent frozen microtome sections through the caudate-putamen of an adult rat, 10 weeks after transplantation of an RR cell suspensions taken from fetuses with a CRL of 13 mm. Adjacent sections of a rat pretreated with 5,7-DHT were stained with antibodies to 5-HT ($\mathbf{A}$ & $\mathbf{B}$) and substance P ($\mathbf{C}$ & $\mathbf{D}$). A large number of grafted serotonergic neurons have migrated toward the borderline of the graft. Some newly formed fibers have started to grow into the serotonergic, denervated caudate-putamen. Note in $\mathbf{C}$ and $\mathbf{D}$ that there are to a much lesser extent newly formed substance P-immunoreactive fibers. They are only observed in the most ventral part of the graft. Little outgrowth into the host tissue occurs, however. Bars: 50 μm.

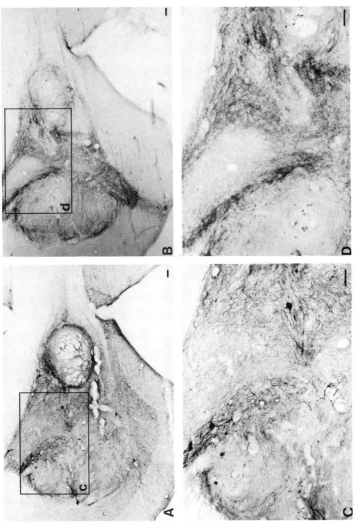

FIGURE 5. Photomicrographs of two adjacent sections through the anterior part of the hippocampus of an aged (31-month-old) rat, 3 months after transplantation of an MR cell suspension taken from fetuses with a CRL of 10 mm. Adjacent sections of a nondenervated rat were stained with antibodies to 5-HT (**A** & **C**) and substance P (**B** & **D**). A large number of serotonergic neurons have migrated into the hippocampal formation. No 5-HT-positive cells were observed at the injection site itself. No substance P-positive cells were found because the rat was not pretreated with colchicine. Note the difference in patterns of outgrowth of serotonergic and substance P-immunoreactive fibers in the hippocampus. Bars: 50 μm.

In the hippocampus of 5,7-DHT-treated rats that contained the transplant, serotonergic fibers were clearly evident (FIG. 7). In area I, close to the injection site, a dense fiber network was visible with some surviving transplanted serotonergic cells. In area II, 5-HT-immunoreactive cells were visible, too, but less than in area I, and the fiber network was as dense as the fiber innervation in the normal hippocampus.

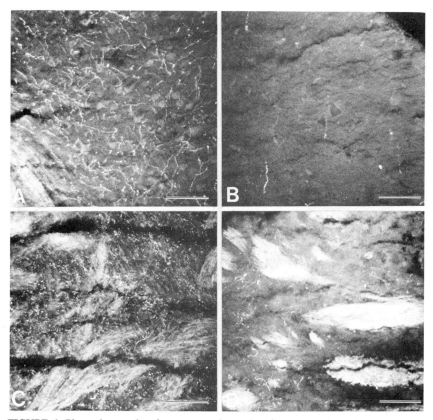

FIGURE 6. Photomicrographs of cryostat sections taken from brain slices through the hippocampus (**A & B**) and caudate-putamen (**C & D**) of a normal (**A & C**) and a 5,7-DHT-denervated (**B & D**) adult rat. Sections were stained with antibodies to 5-HT. Note that the 5,7-DHT treatment results in a strong reduction of the 5-HT immunoreactivity in the hippocampal formation; this effect in the caudate-putamen is not so pronounced under these circumstances. Bars: 50 μm.

In area III, the fiber network was still present, but much less than in areas I or II, and no cells were seen. In area IV, neither a fiber network nor cells were visible.

In the hippocampus, contralateral to the transplant, no 5-HT-immunoreactive fiber outgrowth was observed. The pattern was similar to that of nongrafted 5,7-DHT-lesioned control animals.

Superfusion of Raphe Cell Suspension

The initially high spontaneous efflux of [^{3}H]5-HT from both preloaded raphe cell suspension and cortex slices at the start of the superfusion rapidly declined to a value of about 4% at the beginning of the collection period (that is, at t = 45 min). In contrast with the efflux from cortex slices, which remained almost constant during the next 50 min of the superfusion, the spontaneous efflux from the raphe cell suspension continued to decline, reaching a value of about 2% at the end of the superfusion (that is, at t = 90 min). Moreover, the amount of radioactivity left in the cortex slices continued to decline as well.

Exposure of the cortex slices to depolarization with high K$^+$ (20–56 mM) resulted in a concentration-dependent increase of the [^{3}H]5-HT release: a maximum of 20% was reached. Superfusion of raphe cell suspension with medium containing high K$^+$ concentrations, however, only slightly increased (2%) the release of [^{3}H]5-HT, which in addition appeared not to be Ca^{2+}-dependent (FIG. 8).

Superfusion of Hippocampus Slices

The spontaneous efflux of [^{3}H]5-HT from hippocampus slices of rats pretreated with 5,7-DHT was about 90% of the spontaneous efflux from slices of rats not pretreated with 5,7-DHT. The amount of radioactivity in slices from 5,7-DHT-lesioned rats at the start of the collection period (t = 45 min), however, amounted to only about 40% of control. Moreover, the release of [^{3}H]5-HT induced by K$^+$ (20 mM) was almost completely abolished, being only about 10% of the [^{3}H]5-HT release from the controls (FIG. 9). The same held true with respect to the values of these three parameters for slices prepared from hippocampi contralateral to the 5,7-DHT injection site.

In order to determine the selectivity of the 5,7-DHT lesion, the slices were labeled with [^{14}C]choline as well. Pretreatment with 5,7-DHT did not affect the amount of radioactivity taken up by the tissue or the spontaneous efflux and K$^+$-induced release of [^{14}C]choline from the tissue. When hippocampus slices were used from host rats pretreated with 5,7-DHT, the effectiveness of the outgrowth of the transplant from area I into the other areas of the hippocampus (FIG. 2) was evaluated by studying the K$^+$-induced, Ca^{2+}-dependent release of [^{3}H]5-HT. Using a parallel experimental setup, a direct comparison could be made between the release of 5-HT from the host hippocampus containing the transplant, and the release from the contralateral hippocampus of the same host rat.

The release of [^{3}H]5-HT from slices of host hippocampus was, except for area IV, significantly higher than from slices of corresponding areas of the hippocampus contralateral to the injection side. The highest release of [^{3}H]5-HT was obtained from slices of area I containing the transplant, being about 60% of the release from the untreated control animals (FIG. 9). The release from slices of areas more remote from the injection site gradually decreased to a value of about 4%, obtained from slices of area IV, during the first 10-min collection period. This value was not significantly different from the release from 5,7-DHT-treated control animals. Although the release from areas I, II, and III of the contralateral hippocampus of the host rats was significantly lower than that from the corresponding areas of the ipsilateral hippocampus bearing the transplant, the release of [^{3}H]5-HT from the contralateral side

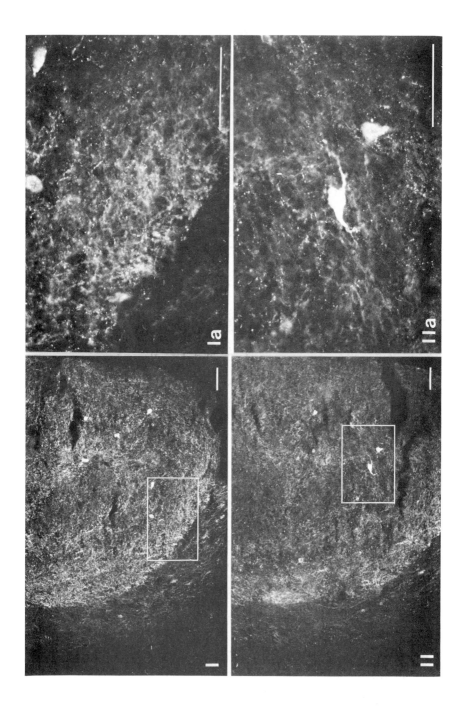

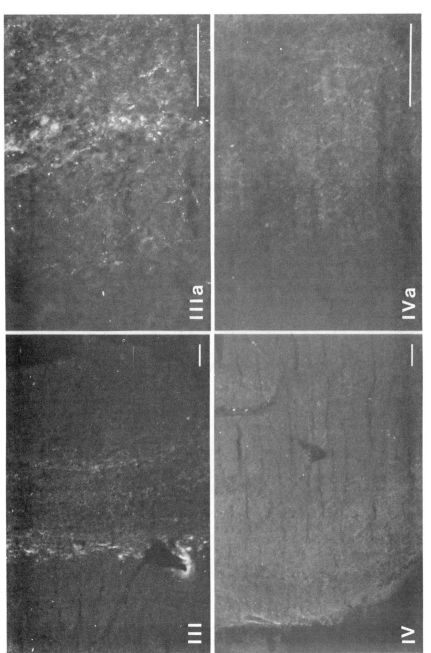

FIGURE 7. Photomicrographs of cryostat sections taken from hippocampus slices. The levels I–IV are indicated in FIGURE 2. Sections from level I were taken from the anterior part of the raphe cell suspension. The remaining four 300-μm-thick slices were collected for neurochemical purposes (FIG. 9). There is a good correspondence between the distance to the injection site and the decrease of newly formed serotonergic fibers. Bars: 50 μm.

FIGURE 8. [³H]5-HT release from a raphe cell suspension, compared to [³H]5-HT release from cortex slices. Raphe cell suspension and cortex slices labeled with [³H]5-HT were superfused with Krebs-Ringer medium. After 40 min of superfusion, stimulated [³H]5-HT release was effected with medium containing 20, 40, or 56 mM K⁺. X-----X: Graft cell suspension (about 4×10^5 raphe cells/chamber of the superfusion apparatus). The total [³H]5-HT content amounted to 8.79 ± 0.4 × 10^3 dpm/chamber. The spontaneous efflux of [³H]5-HT at t = 40 min was 3.74 ± 0.23% (Fr). ●——●: Cortex slices. The total [³H]5-HT content was 46.32 ± 2.79 × 10^3/chamber. The spontaneous efflux of [³H]5-HT at t = 40 min was 4.26 ± 0.05% (Fr).

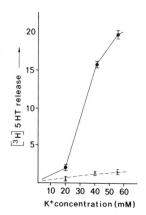

from the hippocampus bearing the transplant was not significantly different from slices obtained from 5,7-DHT-treated control rats.

From the results, it is evident that many types of neurons survive in the cell suspension grafts. To establish the proportion of a specified transmitter system from the total number of newly formed fibers, we are currently exploring the combination of anterograde tracing using lectins with immunohistochemistry on transplanted rats. The present observations on grafts implanted into the aged brain are consistent with those reported by Azmitia et al.[20] and Gage et al.[2,3] The former authors demonstrated survival of fetal grafts of brain stem 5-HT neurons placed into the hippocampus, whereas the latter authors showed this in their studies on nigral and septal grafts. We have presented additional evidence for the outgrowth of MR cell suspensions taken from fetuses with a CRL of only 10 mm into aged rats.

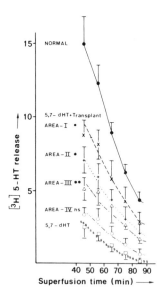

FIGURE 9. [³H]5-HT release induced by continuous K⁺ (20 mM) stimulation from normal, from 5,7-DHT-lesioned, and from 5,7-DHT-lesioned and transplanted hippocampus slices. Hippocampus slices labeled with [³H]5-HT were superfused with medium containing 10^{-5} M fluvoxamine. After 40 min of superfusion, [³H]5-HT release was effected with medium containing 20 mM K⁺. Areas I-IV are areas of the hippocampus from host rats as indicated in FIGURE 2. The spontaneous [³H]5-HT efflux at t = 40 min amounted to 6.77 ± 0.21% (Fr) in normal hippocampus slices and 5.08 ± 0.34% (Fr) in 5,7-DHT-lesioned hippocampus slices. In 5,7-DHT-lesioned rats with a transplant, the spontaneous [³H]5-HT efflux at t = 40 min amounted to 5.62 ± 0.11% (Fr) in slices from the hippocampus containing the graft and 6.11 ± 0.07% (Fr) in slices from the hippocampus contralateral to the transplant. Data represent the mean of three experiments ± SEM. Significantly different release ipsilateral to the graft as from the release in slices from the hippocampus contralateral to the graft: *: $p < .001$; **: $p < .01$ or $p < .02$; ns: not significant.

We attempted to demonstrate the functionality of newly formed serotonergic fibers. We combined superfusion of brain slices and immunohistochemistry. The main advantage of this procedure is that outgrowth of fibers and stimulation-induced release of 5-HT can be studied on adjacent slices from the same host structure (for example, the hippocampus) while the contralateral side serves as an internal control. A general disadvantage of immunocytochemical techniques, however, is that only the number of newly formed fibers can be measured semiquantitatively. It is hoped that this will change in the near future with the use of the newly developed laser scan microscope. The K^+-evoked release of radiolabeled 5-HT showed that 5-HT can be taken up by the newly formed fibers released in a dose-dependent manner. Further studies, however, are needed to indicate the presence and functional activity of presynaptic autoreceptors on these new fibers and to determine whether released 5-HT can induce postsynaptic receptor-mediated effects.

SUMMARY

Adult (3-month-old) and aged (28-month-old) rats that had been pretreated with 5,7-DHT in both lateral ventricles received grafts of cell suspensions taken from the RR or MR regions taken from the embryonic stages E12-21. These cell suspensions were implanted unilaterally into the rostral part of the hippocampus or the caudate-putamen for immunohistochemical and neurochemical studies. MR and RR cell suspensions have the potency to regenerate serotonergic fibers in the previously denervated adult and aged hippocampus and caudate-putamen. The RR cell suspension, however, also showed outgrowth of other transmitter-specific neuronal systems, specifically noradrenaline and substance P.

To evaluate the functional activity of the serotonergic reinnervation, we have combined immunohistochemistry and neurotransmitter release studies on adjacent hippocampus slices of adult rats. Results showed that after a survival time of 10 weeks, the serotonergic innervation of the hippocampus was greatly restored and, moreover, that the K^+-induced Ca^{2+}-dependent release of 5-HT amounted to about 80% of normal values. There appeared to be a striking similarity between the immunohistochemical and neurochemical data regarding the increase in the number of newly formed serotonergic fibers, the increase of the release of radiolabeled 5-HT, and the extent of the outgrowth in the hippocampus.

REFERENCES

1. BJÖRKLUND, A., U. STENEVI, R. H. SCHMIDT, S. B. DUNNET & F. H. GAGE. 1983. Survival and growth of nigral cell suspension implanted in different brain sites. Acta Physiol. Scand. Suppl. **522:** 9-18.
2. GAGE, F. H., A. BJÖRKLUND, U. STENEVI & S. B. DUNNET. 1985. Grafting of embryonic CNS tissue to the damaged adult hippocampal formation. *In* Neural Grafting in the Mammalian CNS. A. Björklund & U. Stenevi, Eds.: 559-574. Elsevier. Amsterdam.
3. GAGE, F. H., A. BJÖRKLUND, U. STENEVI & S. B. DUNNET. 1985. Intracerebral grafting in the aged rat brain: Anatomical and functional characterization. *In* Neural Grafting in the Mammalian CNS. A. Björklund & U. Stenevi, Eds.: 585-594. Elsevier. Amsterdam.
4. CLARKE, D. J., F. H. GAGE & A. BJÖRKLUND. 1986. Formation of cholinergic synapses by intrahippocampal septal grafts as revealed by choline acetyltransferase immunocytochemistry. Brain Res. **369:** 151-162.

5. LUINE, V., K. RENNER, M. FRANKFURT & E. AZMITIA. 1985. Raphe transplants into hypothalamus reverse facilitation of sexual behavior in 5,7-dihydroxytryptamine-treated female rats: Immunocytochemical, neurochemical and behavioral studies. 1985. *In* Neural Grafting in the Mammalian CNS. A. Björklund & U. Stenevi, Eds.: 655-662. Elsevier. Amsterdam.

6. MCRAE-DEGUERCE, A., S. I. BELLIN, A. SERRANO, S. K. LANDAS, L. D. WILKIN, B. SCATTON & A. K. JOHNSON. 1985. Behavioral and neurochemical models to investigate functional recovery with transplants. *In* Neural Grafting in the Mammalian CNS. A. Björklund & U. Stenevi, Eds.: 431-436. Elsevier. Amsterdam.

7. SCHULTZBERG, M., S. B. DUNNET, A. BJÖRKLUND, U. STENEVI, T. HÖKFELT, G. J. DOCKRAY & M. GOLDSTEIN. 1984. Dopamine and cholecystokinin-immunoreactive neurons in mesencephalic grafts reinnervating the neostriatum: Evidence for selective growth regulation. Neuroscience 12: 17-32.

8. FOSTER, G. A., M. SCHULTZBERG, A. BJÖRKLUND, F. H. GAGE & T. HÖKFELT. 1985. Fate of embryonic mesencephalic and medullary raphe neurons transplanted to the striatum, hippocampus or spinal cord of the adult rat: Analysis of 5-hydroxytryptamine-, substance P- and thyrotropin-releasing hormone immunoreactivity. *In* Neural Grafting in the Mammalian CNS. A. Björklund & U. Stenevi, Eds.: 179-189. Elsevier. Amsterdam.

9. AUERBACH, S., F. ZHOU, B. L. JACOBS & E. AZMITIA. 1985. Serotonin turnover in raphe neurons transplanted in the rat hippocampus. Neurosci. Lett. 61: 147-152.

10. BJÖRKLUND, A., H. G. BAUMGARTEN & A. RENSCH. 1974. 5,7-Dihydroxytryptamine: Improvement of its selectivity for serotonin neurons in the CNS by pretreatment with desipramine. J. Neurochem. 24: 833-835.

11. GAGE, F. H., S. B. DUNNET, U. STENEVI & A. BJÖRKLUND. 1983. Survival and growth of implants of nigral and septal cell suspensions in intact brains of aged rats. Acta Physiol. Scand. Suppl. 522: 67-75.

12. STEINBUSCH, H. W. M., F. H. GAGE & A. BJÖRKLUND. 1984. Intracerebral grafting of serotonin-containing neuronal cell suspensions. *In* Modern Techniques in the Study of the Morphology of the Nervous System. H. K. P. Feierabend, Ed.: 23-32. University of Leiden Press. Leiden.

13. BRUNDIN, P., O. ISACSON, F. H. GAGE, U. STENEVI & A. BJÖRKLUND. 1985. Intracerebral grafts of neuronal cell suspensions. *In* Neural Grafting in the Mammalian CNS. A. Björklund & U. Stenevi, Eds.: 51-59. Elsevier. Amsterdam.

14. SEIGER, A. 1985. Preparation of immature central nervous system regions for transplantations. *In* Neural Grafting in the Mammalian CNS. A. Björklund & U. Stenevi, Eds.: 71-77. Elsevier. Amsterdam.

15. STEINBUSCH, H. W. M. & F. J. H. TILDERS. 1987. Immunohistochemical techniques for light microscopical localization of dopamine, noradrenaline, adrenaline, serotonin and histamine in the central nervous system. *In* Monoaminergic Neurons: Light Microscopy and Ultrastructure. IBRO Handbook Series: Methods in the Neurosciences. Vol. 10. H. W. M. Steinbusch, Ed.: 125-166. Wiley. Chichester.

16. STEINBUSCH, H. W. M., J. DE VENTE & J. SCHIPPER. 1986. Antibodies against small neuroactive substances: Immunocytochemistry of monoamines in the central nervous system. *In* Neurology and Neurobiology. Neurohistochemistry: Modern Methods and Applications. Vol. 16. P. Panula, H. Päivärinta & S. Soinila, Eds.: 75-105. Alan R. Liss. New York, NY.

17. MULDER, A. H., A. L. FRANKHUYZEN, J. C. STOOF, J. WEMER & A. N. M. SCHOFFEL-MEER. 1984. Catecholamine receptors, opiate receptors, and presynaptic modulation of neurotransmitter release in the brain. *In* Catecholamines: Neuropharmacology and Central Nervous System. Theoretical Aspects: 47-58. Alan R. Liss. New York, NY.

18. DE LANGEN, C. D. J. & A. H. MULDER. 1980. On the role of calcium ions in the presynaptic α-receptor-mediated inhibition of [^{3}H]noradrenaline release from rat brain cortex synaptosomes. Brain Res. 185: 399-408.

19. FRANKHUYZEN, A. L. & A. H. MULDER. 1982. A cumulative dose-response technique for the characterization of presynaptic receptors modulating [^{3}H]noradrenaline release from rat brain slices. Eur. J. Pharmacol. 78: 91-97.

20. AZMITIA, E. C., M. J. PERLOW, M. J. BRENNAN & J. M. LAUDER. 1981. Fetal raphe and hippocampal transplants into adult and aged C57BL/6N mice: A preliminary study. Brain Res. Bull. 7: 703-710.

Astrocyte Transplantation Induces Callosal Regeneration in Postnatal Acallosal Mice[a]

GEORGE M. SMITH, ROBERT H. MILLER,
AND JERRY SILVER

Department of Developmental Genetics
School of Medicine
Case Western Reserve University
Cleveland, Ohio 44106

INTRODUCTION

Maturation of the vertebrate central nervous system (CNS) is accompanied by its decreasing ability to recover from injury.[1,2] As a result, lesions in embryonic or early postnatal brains are often less functionally detrimental than equivalent lesions in adults.[3–8] In all mammals, functional restoration from CNS injury diminishes significantly and rapidly during early postnatal stages, establishing a "critical period" beyond which axons do not extend through or around the region of the wound.[4,5,8] The lack of axon outgrowth beyond the critical period has previously been attributed to intrinsic factors that may diminish the growth potential of adult axons[9,10] as well as to environmental factors postulated to block axon elongation.[8]

Perhaps the most dramatic experiments designed to test the intrinsic ability for axonal growth are those that have used transplant techniques. The results of these studies show that adult CNS axons have the potential to grow long distances through peripheral nerve grafts,[11–14] Schwann cell bridges,[15] or transplanted pieces of embryonic tissue.[16] The regenerating nerve fibers, however, can only extend a short distance upon reentry into the CNS. Thus, although the injured adult CNS is potentially capable of a considerable amount of regeneration, sprouting is usually abortive and axons fail to reinnervate their appropriate targets.[17–19]

Given the observation that adult axons can grow in transplants, why, then, do they fail to regenerate *in situ?* A fundamental difference in the response of the embryonic and adult brain to injury is the formation of a glial scar. The scar is composed of multiple layers of basal lamina and a variety of cell types, the most predominant of which are astrocytes and fibroblasts. It has been suggested that the loss of functional recovery in animals after the critical period occurs because the scar forms a barrier, inhibiting the regrowth of axons.[17,18,20–23]

Although scars seldom develop after trauma to the embryonic brain,[24] certain embryonic lesions that destroy the normal substrate for axonal elongation do cause

[a]This work was supported by Grant BNS 8218700 from the National Science Foundation and by Grants NS 15731 and EY 05952 from the National Institutes of Health.

185

functional deficits. One particular CNS lesion that has devastating consequences on outgrowing axons is that of mechanically disrupting the presumptive terrain for the developing corpus callosum, the so-called glial "sling." In these animals, the callosal axons fail to cross the midline and instead form neuromas, which are called Probst's bundles[25] and which persist indefinitely in an ectopic location lateral to the cerebral midline.[26-28]

Previous studies have shown that commissure formation can be induced in such acallosal animals by introducing an artificial "sling." In early postnatal acallosal animals, Silver and Ogawa[29] have shown that an untreated, properly shaped nitrocellulose (Millipore) filter, placed adjacent to one or both neuromas and spanning the cerebral midline, can support the migration of glia. The glia attach to the surface of the filter producing a cellular scaffold that, in turn, provides a terrain suitable for the ectopic axons in Probst's bundles to traverse the midline and reform a corpus callosum.[29]

In the present study, we have determined that a critical period also exists for this form of induced callosal axon growth. The critical period for stimulating commissure reformation is similar in length to that established for the lateral olfactory tract, an early spontaneously regenerating CNS fiber pathway in rodents.[8] In addition, we have used the nitrocellulose implant in acallosal animals as a paradigm to analyze the population of cells that interacts with both the prosthesis and newly growing axons. By observing animals that have received implants at successively older ages, we have begun to characterize the variety of cellular and extracellular changes in the environment that may be crucial for determining why axon growth refractory states develop within the mammalian brain. Further, we have transplanted astrocytes from critical period neonates into acallosal adults, and have observed a modulation of the host gliotic response, as well as axonal "regeneration" across the midline.

MATERIALS AND METHODS

Timed pregnant C57BL/6J mice were obtained from the Jackson Labs. The glial sling of day 16 embryos (E16) or the sling and immature corpus callosum of neonates were lesioned by inserting a microneedle into the calvarium approximately 1 mm rostral to the cranial landmark "lambda" to a depth of about 2 mm.[26] The lesioned mice were consistently acallosal. In an experiment to test the efficiency of our technique, 50 animals were acallosal out of 50 lesioned. The lesioned animals were anesthetized and implanted with Millipore bridges on postnatal days (P) 2, 5, 8, 14, and 21 and at 8 months. In the neonates, the skull was still pliable and did not require drilling. An incision through the skin was made horizontally between the eyes and the skin retracted. The surface of the skull was scraped free of tissue in order to minimize contamination of other cell types onto the implant as it was inserted. The prosthesis to be inserted was a specially designed piece of nitrocellulose filter (Millipore) similar in shape and size as that described by Silver and Ogawa.[29] This was then inserted 2 to 5 mm into the stab wound.

In animals receiving transplants, filters plus their cellular coatings were removed from decapitated acallosal mice 48 hr after implantation on P2. The tissue around the transplant was carefully dissected. The transplant was removed with specially designed forceps, which prevent the cells on the surface from being crushed or stripped away when the implant is placed into another animal. Transplants were then dipped in N-2 medium[30] and placed in a humid chamber at 37° C. Host animals (at P17, P34, or 8 months) that were made acallosal in the embryo or on the day of birth were prepared. The transplants were inserted in the same manner as above.

Anesthetized animals were killed 0.5, 1, 2, 3, 5, and 7 days or 2 months after implantation by perfusion through the heart. The perfusion was performed in two steps; first, 2 to 5 ml of a 0.15 M phosphate buffer solution at 37° C was injected into the left ventricle, followed by fixative (0.5% glutaraldehyde/2.0% formaldehyde in the same buffer, with 0.5% dimethyl sulfoxide). The brains were quickly dissected from the cranium and placed in the same fixative overnight at 4° C. The filter and surrounding tissue were subsequently embedded in Spurr's plastic using standard procedures. Serial 1-μm sections were taken through the implant and stained with toluidine blue. Certain regions were sectioned ultrathin, stained with uranyl acetate and lead citrate, and viewed with a Zeiss 109 electron microscope. For specimens examined by scanning electron microscopy, the tissue above the implant was gently dissected away and the specimens osmicated and dehydrated through a graded series of alcohols. The samples were critical point dried in a Balzers CPD 020 and sputter-coated with gold using an Edwards E306 device. After being mounted on aluminum stubs, they were viewed in an Etech scanning electron microscope.

Immunohistochemistry

Postnatal animals were anesthetized and perfused through the heart with 2 to 5 ml of 4.0% formaldehyde in phosphate-buffered saline (PBS) (pH 7.5). The brains were dissected from their calvaria and immersed in fixative for 2 hr, then cryoprotected using a graded series of sucrose PBS solutions (10% sucrose PBS solution for 30 min, 15% for 30 min, and 20% for 2 hr to overnight). Ten-micron sections were taken on a Slee HR Mark II cryostat microtome.

Polyclonal antibodies against purified laminin and fibronectin were received from Dr. G. Martin (National Institutes of Health). The sera were used at dilutions of 1:50. Antibodies against glial fibrillary acidic protein (GFAP) were provided by R. H. Miller. They were diluted 1:1000 and applied for 1 hr at room temperature. Sections were rinsed in PBS (3- to 15-min washes) and incubated with peroxidase-conjugated goat antirabbit immunoglobulin G (Cooper Biomedical) at a dilution of 1:100 for 30 min at room temperature, or goat antirabbit fluorescein isothiocyanate at a dilution of 1:50 for 1 hr. Sections were rinsed again in PBS, and peroxidase conjugates were incubated in a solution containing 15 mg of 3,3-diaminobenzidine tetrahydrochloride (Eastman Kodak) per 100 ml Tris (pH 7.5) for 30 to 45 min at room temperature in the dark.

[³H]Thymidine Autoradiography of Transplants

Acallosal neonates, implanted with filters on P2, were injected intraperitoneally with [³H]thymidine (5 μCi/g body weight) at 6, 18, and 30 hr after implantation. Implants were removed 18 hr after the last injection and transplanted into P23 acallosal animals. Animals were sacrificed 4 days after transplantation and prepared for plastic embedding. Sections 1-μm thick were mounted on slides and coated with Kodak NTB-

2 autoradiographic emulsion. The coated slides were placed in light-proof containers and stored at $-5°$ C for 6 weeks. Slides were processed for photography at $18°$ C.

RESULTS

Axon Elongation over Untreated Implants: Defining the Critical Period

Fifty-nine acallosal animals were implanted with untreated nitrocellulose bridges at various stages (P2, P5, P8, P14, P21, and 8 months). We have found that the glial response between 24 and 48 hr after implantation (see below for a detailed description of the glial phenomena) produces a terrain along the filter that is suitable for axon elongation out of Probst's neuromas, only in animals that are implanted before or on P8. This is shown by the presence of many unmyelinated axons interspersed among the attached glial cells (FIGS. 1, 2a,c, 3b & 4a-c). In animals implanted on P2, with 24-hr survival times, the earliest growing axons tended not to fasciculate. With longer survival times, however, many more fibers crossed the midline, and they now became grouped into multiple fascicles (FIGS. 1 & 3c). The CNS glial response generated by implantation of animals on or later than P14 apparently did not produce a terrain readily suitable for axon elongation. Twenty-seven animals given naked, untreated implants postnatally at 2 and 3 weeks and at 8 months showed little or no growth of axons onto the implant when examined at 1 week and as late as 2 months after implantation (FIGS. 4d, e).

Changes in the Host Glial Reaction to Untreated Nitrocellulose Bridges Implanted at Various Postnatal Ages

Implantation of acallosal animals at various ages was done not only to evaluate the ability of the glial coating to provide an adequate substratum for axonal elongation but to compare age-related changes in the host gliotic response. When implants are placed within the presumptive callosal pathway of acallosal mice at P2 and P8, glial cells rapidly migrate onto the surface of the filter during the first 12 to 24 hr after implantation (FIG. 3a). Cells attach to the implant by extending cytoplasmic processes deep into the system of 0.45-μm pores within the filter (FIGS. 2a & 3a). The glia rapidly incorporate the implant within the brain by interdigitating with each other, the implant, and the surrounding neuropil. The identification of the glial elements on the filter as astrocytes as well as the extensive branching of their processes into both prosthesis and encompassing tissue is dramatically shown in GFAP-stained sections (FIG. 5a). In P2 implants, there were only a few macrophages around the filter 48 hr after implantation, and there was no evidence of tissue necrosis or persistent bleeding (FIGS. 3a-c). The astrocytes that infiltrated the pores of the implant in the neonatal period retained their foothold in the filter for the life of the animal (not shown).

The rapidity of astrocyte movement onto and the attachment with the filter decreased gradually as the age at implantation increased. Thus, in P8 implants examined after 48 hr, many GFAP-positive glia were already attached. There were still some

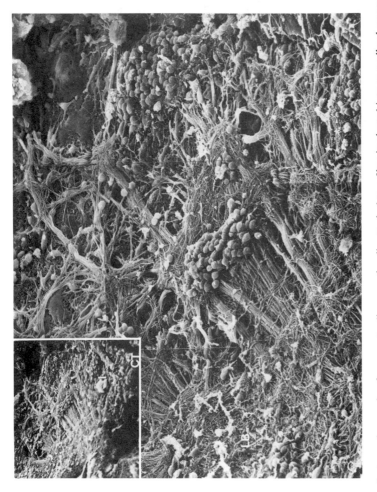

FIGURE 1. Scanning electron micrographs of axons extending over the glia attached to a filter implanted into an acallosal mouse on P2 and examined 48 hr later. The low-power insert shows callosal axons extending from only one hemisphere, out of a neuroma (LB) and across the implant (I). The caudal tip (CT) and borders of the filter are apparent. Higher magnification shows large fascicles of axons traversing the implant toward the opposite hemisphere. However, not all axons retain their orientation and wander in the middle of the filter. The original magnification for the high-power micrograph was ×700, and that for the low-power insert was ×80. The figure has been reduced to 55% of its original size. Reproduced from Smith *et al.*[57] by copyright permission of Allan R. Liss, Inc.

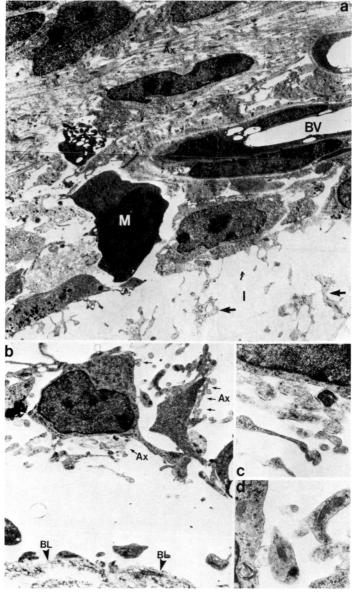

FIGURE 2. Transmission electron micrographs of acallosal mice implanted 8 days after birth and sacrificed 48 hr later. (a) Glia attaching to the implant have a stellate morphology; microglia (M) are also apparent. Among and above the glia that have sent processes into the filter (arrow) are axons (Ax) and blood vessels (BV). (b) The axons (small arrows) that extend into areas where basal lamina (BL; arrowheads) appears are positioned immediately adjacent to the glia, but not the basal lamina. (c & d) Higher magnification shows axons associated with astrocyte processes containing intermediate filaments and glycogen granules. Original magnifications: **a**: ×4500; **b**: ×5000; **c** and **d**: ×12 000. The figure has been reduced to 69% of its original size. Reproduced from Smith *et al.*[57]

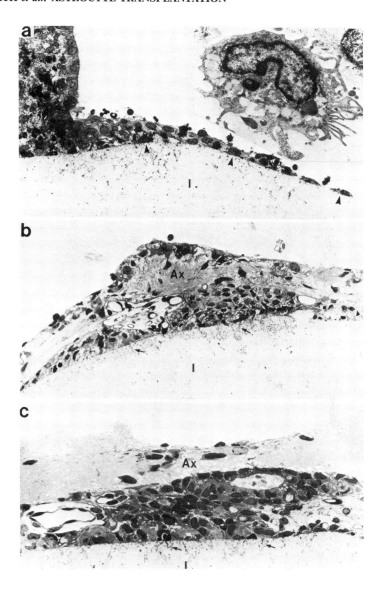

FIGURE 3. Coronal sections through filters implanted into acallosal mice on P2 and examined (a) 24, (b) 48, and (c) 72 hr later. (a) Note that 24 hr after implantation, numerous glia (arrowheads), some which are phagocytotic (insert), have migrated out of the hemisphere and along the implant. As they attach to the implant (I), they extend cytoplasmic processes into the pores of the filter (small arrows); note that the leading glial cell (far right) has extended few processes. (b) Within 48 hr, glia coat the majority of the filter surface, providing a substrate on which axons (Ax) and blood vessels have extended. (c) In some specimens, 72 hr after implantation, the axons fasciculate over the glia above the filter, a configuration similar to that of the normal developing corpus callosum and "sling." Note, however, the absence of a glial-limiting membrane. Original magnifications: **a** and **c**: ×500; **b**: ×400; insert: ×4400. The figure has been reduced to 81% of its original size. Reproduced from Smith *et al.*[57]

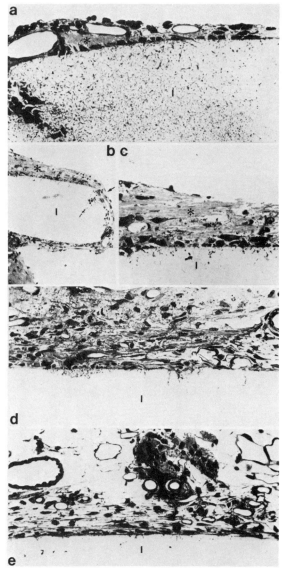

FIGURE 4. Coronal sections through the nitrocellulose bridge (I) and associated tissue of the hemispheric midline of acallosal mice. The sections in **a**, **b**, and **c** are from animals implanted at "critical" stages; implantations were performed on P2 (**a**) and P8 (**b** & **c**); all implants were examined 48 hr after implantation. Compare **a**, **b**, and **c** to the sections in **d** and **e**, which were taken from animals implanted at "postcritical" stages. These implantations were performed 14 (**d**) and 21 (**e**) days after birth, and both implants were sacrificed 7 days later. In **a**, **b**, and **c**, the glia are more stellate, sending many cytoplasmic processes into the pores of the filter (I), whereas, in **c** and **d**, the cells near the implant appear flat, lacking extensive infiltration of processes. Directly above the infiltrated stellate glia of critical period implants are numerous axons (asterisks), but such axons were not apparent in postcritical stage implants. Original magnifications: **a** and **c**-**e**: ×400; **b**: ×125. The figure has been reduced to 65% of its original size. Reproduced from Smith *et al.*[57]

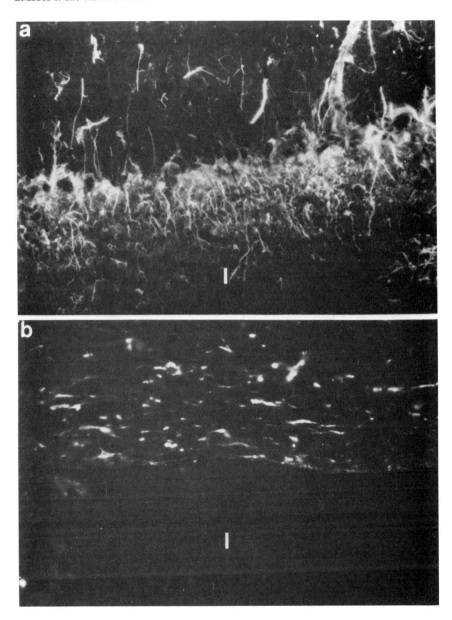

FIGURE 5. Coronal sections illustrating the staining pattern for antibodies against GFAP in animals implanted at critical and postcritical ages. (**a**) Acallosal neonates (P2) implanted with filters and examined after 5 days show extensive astrocytic processes within the implant (I) and within the cortex, retaining their stellate morphology. (**b**) The astrocytes in acallosal animals implanted at postcritical stages (P21) and examined after 1 week appear flat within the scar above the implant (I). Original magnification for **a** and **b**: ×300. The figure has been enlarged to 106% of its original size. Reproduced from Smith *et al.*[57]

lingering macrophages containing inclusions, however, as well as a few remaining islands of tissue debris. In contrast to P2 and P8 neonates, animals implanted on P14 and P21 showed only slight glial activity 48 hr after implantation. Filters examined at this stage were coated mainly with degenerating tissue and vascular elements (not shown). Thus, the reaction and migration of glia onto the filter in animals implanted on or later than P14 required a longer period of time, often taking a full week for cells to reach the vicinity of the filter. The reactive cells of older ages had a conspicuous change in shape from stellate (that is, inserted) to flat (compare FIGS. 4a-c with 4d,e; also 5a with 5b). Macrophages with inclusions, mesenchymal tissues, and large amounts of necrotic debris always persisted within these developing scars. Another significant variation of the host glial reaction in older animals was the relative inability of the mature form of reactive astrocyte to insert processes into the implant. Filters introduced intracerebrally at later stages (P21 and 8 months), and examined after 7 days, had limited penetration of glial processes into their pores (FIGS. 4d,e). Rather than inserting, the glia flattened on the surface of the filter and encapsulated the prosthesis by forming sheets several cell layers thick. Basal lamina was observed along the surface of many of these flattened astrocytes and may provide some impetus for their shape change since basal lamina is nonporous.

The anti-GFAP staining pattern at P21 showed sheets of flattened astrocytes having only a few short processes penetrating into the implant (FIG. 5b). These flattened astrocytes were often surrounded by nonstaining arachnoidal cells that constituted a larger proportion of the cell population encompassing the implant than at earlier stages.

Extracellular Matrices Associated with the Gliotic Response at Different Ages

The gliotic reaction that appeared 2 to 7 days after implantation in P2 neonates did not stimulate the production of collagen fibers or basal laminae within the parenchyma of the CNS. Only basal laminae that normally occur around capillaries and at the pial surface could be found. When animals implanted at P2 were examined for laminin (a major protein component of basal lamina), however, an unusual staining pattern was revealed. As expected, laminin appeared to be concentrated in the basal laminae of the blood vessels and the pia mater throughout the brain. Laminin was also found, however, within the pores of the filter in regions containing inserted glial processes, sites having no observable basal lamina (FIGS. 6a,b). Animals implanted at P2, P8, P14, P21, and 8 months, and compared as a group after 1 week of survival, showed gradual increases, correlated with age at implantation, in the observable amounts of basal lamina (compare FIGS. 6a,b with 6c,d), as well as in collagen associated with the glial scar. Ectopic basal laminae first appeared in small, isolated patches among cells surrounding the implant in some P8 individuals examined after 2 to 7 days. Interestingly, in P8 animals, axons were not observed juxtaposed to the ectopic basal lamina. Axons were observed clustered along the plasma membrane of astrocytes, however, less than 10 μm away from the basal lamina (FIGS. 2b-d). The antilaminin staining within the pores of the filter was greatly reduced or absent in brains implanted on or later than P14 (FIG. 6d). Collagen fibers were seen throughout the scar, occupying spaces between cells and cell layers. Transmission electron microscope (TEM) examination of the banding pattern for the fibers identified them as being composed of type I collagen (not shown, *cf.* Hay[31]).

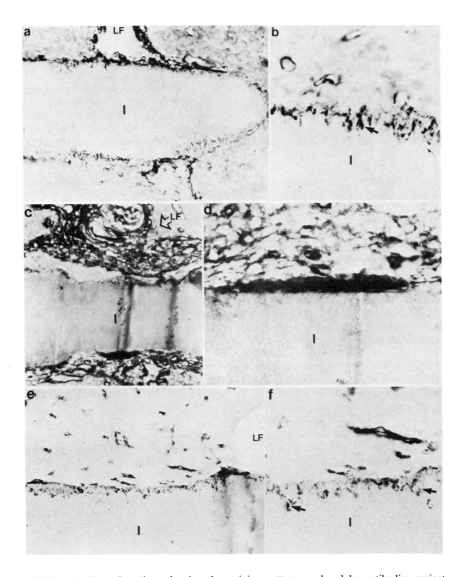

FIGURE 6. Coronal sections showing the staining pattern produced by antibodies against laminin protein. (a & b) In critically implanted P8 animals, laminin not only appears to be confined to the basal lamina of blood vessels and the pia, but is also along glial processes (arrow) within the filter (b). (c & d) When animals were implanted at postcritical stages (P21), anti-laminin stained the basal lamina in the scar that extends around the implant (I) and appears continuous with the longitudinal fissure (LF). The cells producing the laminin are flat (d). (e & f) Postcritical period animals (P17 and P34) implanted with glial-coated filters from P2 neonates show a laminin staining pattern identical to that in critical period animals given naked implants alone (compare to a & b). Original magnifications: a, c, and e: ×100; b, d, and f: ×250. The figure has been reduced to 63% of its original size. Reproduced from Smith *et al.*[57]

Transplantation of Glial-coated Implants from Neonatal to Postcritical Period Animals

Will glia that migrate onto an implant from P2-4 (critical stage) donors alter the gliotic reaction at the lesion site when transferred to an older (postcritical period) animal, and will such precoated implants (that is, transplants) promote callosal axon growth across the cerebral midline in postcritical period animals? In order to answer these questions, 2-day-old acallosal mice were implanted with nitrocellulose filters. After 48 hr, the glial-coated implants were removed and transferred into 17- or 34-day-old (postcritical period) acallosal mice. In most animals (14 out of 20 transplants), GFAP-positive glia survived the transplantation and were clearly demonstrable because of their inserted morphology (FIGS. 7c,d & 8b). [^{3}H]Thymidine injections into the donor neonate labeled cells before transplantation, and their presence in the host indicated that many of the inserted glia were, indeed, transferred (FIG. 8a). Silver grains were observed not only above glia attached to the filter but also above those along blood vessels away from the surface of the implant (FIG. 8).

The brains of transplanted animals displayed distinct changes in the glial reaction around the transplant, when compared with those of the same age receiving untreated implants. Implantation of naked filters into P14 or older animals consistently resulted in rampant tissue degeneration, followed by the formation of a dense, flat-cell form of glial scar associated with extensive basal laminae and collagen fibers (FIGS. 7a,b). In contrast, the majority of individuals given transplants of immature glia showed no scar formation, little basal lamina production, and negligible amounts of tissue necrosis and bleeding. In essence, the host gliotic response in transplanted animals became indistinguishable from animals implanted with naked implants during critical stages (FIGS. 7c,d). The transplanted animals also showed an antilaminin staining pattern identical to that seen in mice implanted on P2 (compare FIGS. 6a,b with 6e,f). Most transplants examined 3 to 6 days after insertion showed (in regions where donor glia were present) little or no cellular debris, and only a few macrophages at the donor-host interface (FIGS. 7c,d & 9). The astrocytes along the surface of the implant formed multiple branches that interdigitated with the injured cortex, appearing to "knit" the artificial material with the tissue of the living host. In such animals (lateral to the longitudinal fissure), apparently normal neuropil was present as close as one cell layer from the transplant (FIG. 9). In these successfully transplanted animals, there was minimal invasion of arachnoidal cells into the wound site. In a few instances, however, a dense collagenous scar with layers of basal lamina, fibroblasts, and flattened glia were located in discrete regions of tissue adjacent to areas of the transplant. This only occurred in those regions that lacked the penetrating, stellate form of astrocyte.

Induced Axon Growth over Glial Transplants

In 2 of the 20 postcritical period, transplanted animals examined after 4 to 11 days, several hundred "regenerating" or sprouting axons were present at the previously lesioned cerebral midline (directly below the longitudinal fissure) among the transplanted glia attached to the implant (FIGS. 7c,d & 10). The axons were all unmyelinated and bundled in small fascicles surrounded by glial processes (FIGS. 10b,c). Extensive examination of the implant indicated that no neurons and only nonneuronal cells, some capable of mitosis (FIG. 10d), and axons were present along the transplant surface itself.

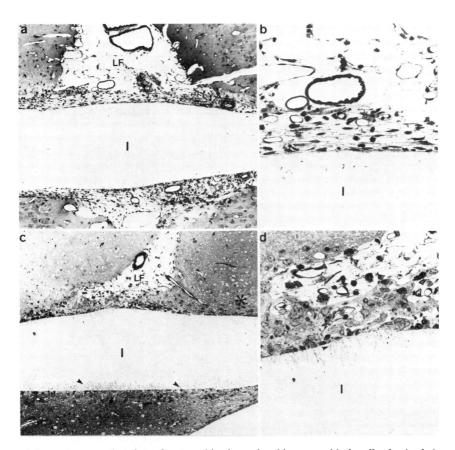

FIGURE 7. Coronal sections of untreated implants placed into postcritical acallosal animals (**a** & **b**), and transplanted filters precoated with glia harvested from neonates (**c** & **d**). Compare the difference in the gliotic reaction. The reacting cells along the untreated filter (**a** & **b**) are arranged in sheets and have a flattened morphology, with few processes extending into the implant. In contrast, the gliotic reaction produced in the postcritical brain by the transplant (**c** & **d**) resembles that in critical period implanted animals; numerous inserted processes (arrowheads) from stellate cells and minimal scar formation or necrosis are evident. Original magnifications: **a** and **c**: ×125; **b** and **d**: ×400. The figure has been reduced to 63% of its original size. Reproduced from Smith *et al.*[57]

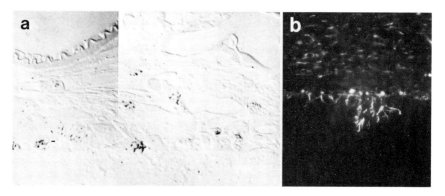

FIGURE 8. Coronal sections of P27 animals that received transplanted filters precoated with glia from neonates that were injected with [³H]thymidine (a). A majority of the glia attached to the filter are labeled with silver grains over the nuclei. Cells further removed from the implant surface and along blood vessels are also labeled by [³H]thymidine. Transplanted neonatal glia on Millipore placed into postcritical period animals (P34) retain their stellate morphology, as shown when stained with antibodies against GFAP (b). Original magnifications: **a**: ×450; **b**: ×300. The figure has been reduced to 67% of its original size. Reproduced from Smith *et al.*[57]

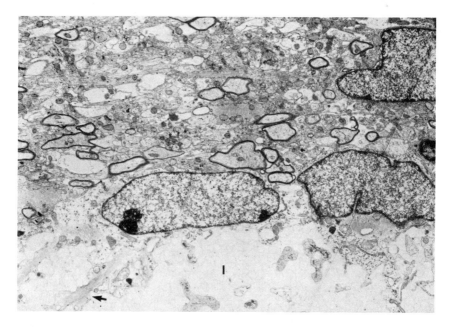

FIGURE 9. Transmission electron micrograph of the host-donor interface (far lateral to the midline) from a P17 acallosal animal that was given a precoated glial implant (transplant) and examined after 6 days. The astrocytes attached to the implant (I) retain their inserted processes, which are rich in intermediate filaments (arrow). The cortex above the attached glia shows little tissue degeneration and no scar formation. Original magnification: ×12 600; reduced to 63% of original size. Reproduced from Smith *et al.*[57]

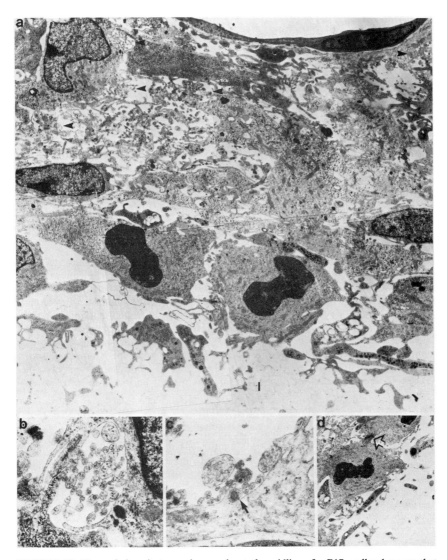

FIGURE 10. Transmission electron micrographs at the midline of a P17 acallosal mouse that received a preglial-coated implant from a 2-day-old neonate donor and was then examined 6 days after it had resided in the host. (**a**) The glia attached to the implant (**I**) have retained their stellate morphology and infiltrated cytoplasmic processes. Scarring and ectopic basal lamina are absent. Among the glia are many *de novo* formed axon bundles (arrowheads). Higher magnification shows loosely fasciculated unmyelinated axons (**b**) and others adjacent to astrocytic processes (**c**). Two daughter cells (**d**) above the implant (**a**) share a midbody (**d**). Thus, transplanted cells can divide. Original magnifications: **a**: ×10 000; **b** and **c**: ×20 000; **d**: ×3300. The figure has been reduced to 61% of its original size. Reproduced from Smith *et al.*[57]

DISCUSSION

In a previous study of surgically induced acallosal mice, it was shown that axons entrapped within Probst's neuromas in neonates retain the potential to regrow when presented with a properly aligned, glial-covered scaffold.[29] The present study demonstrates the existence of a critical period for such substrate-supported axon re-elongation. The *de novo* growth of commissural axons across the cerebral midline was observed in acallosal animals implanted with untreated prostheses on or before P8, but not later.

During critical stages, the migration of astrocytic glia onto the implant and the insertion of their processes are extremely rapid events occurring within 12 to 24 hr. During and after the initial glial invasion phase, the population of cells that moves onto the implant has the capacity to support the growth of axons, as well as vascular elements. The majority of these cells are GFAP-positive astrocytes, and, while in their youth, they not only have the ability to erect a three-dimensional scaffolding of processes pre-axonally (see Silver and Ogawa[29] and FIGS. 2c & 10b), but also appear to respond to the presence of growing axons by extending additional cytoplasmic processes around the fibers (see Navascués *et al.*[32]). In contrast, the reactive glial response in animals implanted 14 days or later after birth showed distinct differences from gliosis observed in neonates. The length of time it takes glial cells to reach the surface of the implant, the amount of bleeding from the implant site, the extent of secondary necrosis, the degree of basal lamina production, the degree of fibroblast contamination, and the density of tissue at and around the implant all increase with age (TABLE 1). The morphology of cells surrounding the implant also becomes altered, and, most importantly, these cells lose their ability to stimulate axon outgrowth. Thus, in contrast to adult "reactive" gliosis, we suggest that the gliotic response in neonatal mammals is an active rather than reactive phenomenon and, when controlled with a prosthesis, that it should be considered a beneficial and constructive process. We suggest the name "activated gliosis" when referring to the immature form of glial

TABLE 1. Induced Changes during and after the Gliotic Reaction[a]

	Critical[b]		Postcritical[b] (P14–Adult)	Transplant[c] (P2–P17,34)
	P2	P8		
Number of inserted GFAP⁺ cells	+++	++	−	++
Laminin along glial processes in filter	+	+	−	+
Axon outgrowth over filter	+++	++	−	+
Necrosis	−	+	+++	+
Blood surrounding filter	−	+	+++	+
Basal lamina	−	+	+++	+
Collagen	−	+	+++	+
Astrocyte shape	Stellate		Flat	Stellate
Inserted glial processes	+++	++	−	++
Time for glia to react to implant	24–48 hr		5–7 days	

[a] This table illustrates qualitatively the changes that occur during and after the gliotic reaction induced when acallosal mice are implanted with nitrocellulose filters at critical and postcritical stages, and when implants are transplanted from neonates to postcritical period animals. The +/− system represents an overall impression of the observable presence or absence of the described reactions.

[b] Untreated implants.

[c] Implants from P2 critical period mice.

response to injury. Phenomenologically similar "activated astrocytes" have been described in the developing[33] or regenerating optic nerve of *Xenopus laevis*[34–36] and along the regenerating olfactory nerve in adult rats,[37,38] suggesting that the adult CNS of amphibia and the peripheral olfactory system in mammals may retain the primitive "activated" form of glial cell. Consequently, there may be many features shared by the "activated" astrocyte in the mammalian neonatal CNS, one special part of the adult olfactory system, and in the adult CNS of amphibia.[37–40]

During development, the CNS is isolated from nonneural tissue by a basal lamina that forms at the endfeet of perivascular and pial astrocytes. In the developing optic[41–44] and central olfactory[8] pathways, as well as in the embryonic spinal cord[45,46] of most species of vertebrates (except teleosts[47]), growing axons tend to travel adjacent to the endfeet, but rarely touch the basal lamina. When penetrating injuries occur within the adult CNS, the resulting cellular disruption often stimulates reconstitution of glial-limiting membranes with connective tissue contaminants throughout the wound site.[23,48] In implanted acallosal neonates where axons were induced to extend across the midline, there was little extraneous basal lamina formation and growing axons were usually found directly adjacent to astrocytic processes, as they are in normal development.[42–44] In animals implanted with prostheses on P8 (a late critical stage when small patches of basal laminae sometimes developed), axons were rarely observed directly apposed to the basal laminae or connective tissue elements. Rather, they were usually positioned along membranes of stellate-shaped astrocytes, which sometimes appeared near the basal lamina. This observation suggests that when given a choice, callosal fibers prefer to associate directly with the plasma membrane of immature glia, rather than with basal lamina. Implantation of nitrocellulose prostheses after the critical period resulted in astrocytic scarring and the establishment of multiple layers of intracerebral basal laminae. Axons failed to regenerate across the midline through this terrain. During adult reactive gliosis, the dense encapsulation of the scar by limiting membranes has been considered to produce a barrier to regenerating axons.[17,49–51] Our observations support this hypothesis. We also suggest, however, that the basal lamina may not merely form a mechanical impediment to axons. Since the basal laminae that form within the scar cover the surfaces of many astrocytes, it may reduce the axon-astrocyte interaction that is apparently essential for the guidance and support of axons across the midline.[52,53]

Transplantation of Neonatal Glial-coated Implants into Postcritical Stage Animals

In comparison to postcritical period animals that received naked implants, older animals transplanted with bridges that were precoated with glia from P2 donor mice showed reduced amounts of tissue degeneration and glial-mesenchymal scarring. The lack of extensive tissue degeneration and bleeding in transplanted animals suggests that the transplant increases the survivability of cortical tissue near the site of injury. [³H]Thymidine labeling of donor glia before transplantation showed that many of the glia migrated away from the implant, and that some took up residence along blood vessels.

Nieto-Sampedro *et al.*[54] have shown that extracts containing injury-induced neurotrophic factors from lesioned animals increased the survival of transplants, when the tissue was transplanted with the extract. In adults, the production of injury-induced neurotrophic factors has a considerable lag time when compared with the neonatal counterpart.[55] We have shown that transplantation of "activated" astrocytes into postcritical period animals buffers the traumatic effect of the wound itself, perhaps by the production of a similar type of neurotrophic substance.[56] In turn, the increase in survivability of the cortical tissue near the lesion site and the reduction of gliosis in the host may further enhance the regeneration of axons onto the transplant.

Taken together with our earlier results,[26,28,29] the present findings suggest that immature astrocytes have the capability of attaching to a nitrocellulose sheet and functionally reproducing the "sling-like" structure that supports axon elongation between the hemispheres during normal development. The efficacy of astrocytes to recapitulate this structure postnatally and provide a properly aligned substratum for axon elongation is transitory, and diminishes quickly with age. When untreated filters are introduced into acallosal animals on or after P14, the resident astrocytes react to the wounding and implant by producing a dense glial-fibroblastic scar that lacks the ability to promote axon elongation. Finally, when activated astrocytes are removed from a neonate (retaining structural integrity) and transferred to a more mature or adult acallosal animal, the negative effects of reactive gliosis and scarring in the host are repressed, potentially reestablishing an environment conducive for axon regeneration. Our results are complementary to those of Kromer et al.,[16] who have shown that transplants of intact pieces of embryonic tissue placed into gaps between the septum and hippocampus can promote the long-distance regeneration of axons. Our study, however, suggests the possibility that it may be the immature glial environment within such embryonic grafts that supplies essential growth and guidance cues to the regrowing axons. Immature astrocytes appeared to aid the incorporation of the inanimate filter to the more mature cortex. These glia may also aid the fusion of embryonic grafts to the adult host.

ACKNOWLEDGMENTS

We wish to thank Catherine Doller for her technical assistance. We would also like to acknowledge and thank Dr. Irvine McQuarrie for suggesting the term "activated" astrocyte.

REFERENCES

1. GOLDMAN, P. S. & T. W. GALKIN. 1978. Prenatal removal of frontal association cortex in the fetal rhesus monkey: Anatomical and functional consequences in postnatal life. Brain Res. **152:** 451-485.
2. CARLSON, M. 1984. Development of tactile discrimination capacity in *Macaca mulatta.* III. Effects of total removal of primary somatic sensory cortex (SmI) in infants and juveniles. Dev. Brain Res. **16:** 103-117.
3. RAKIC, P. 1974. Intrinsic and extrinsic factors influencing the shape of neurons and their assembly into neuronal circuits. *In* Frontiers in Neurology and Neuroscience Research. P. Seeman & G. M. Brown, Eds.: 112-132. University of Toronto Press. Toronto.
4. DEVOR, M. 1975. Neuroplasticity in the sparing or deterioration of function after early olfactory tract lesions. Science **190:** 998-1000.
5. DEVOR, M. 1976. Neuroplasticity in the rearrangement of olfactory tract fibers after neonatal transection in hamsters. J. Comp. Neurol. **166:** 49-72.

6. KALIL, K. & T. REH. 1979. Regrowth of severed axons in the neonatal central nervous system: Establishment of normal connections. Science **205:** 1158-1161.
7. BREGMAN, B. S. & M. E. GOLDBERGER. 1982. Anatomical plasticity and sparing of function after spinal cord damage in neonatal cats. Science **217:** 553-555.
8. GRAFE, M. R. 1983. Developmental factors affecting regeneration in the central nervous system: Early but not late formed mitral cells reinnervate olfactory cortex after neonatal tract section. J. Neurosci. **3:** 617-630.
9. ARGIRO, V., M. B. BUNGE & M. I. JOHNSON. 1984. Correlation between growth form and movement and their dependence on neuronal age. J. Neurosci. **12:** 3051-3062.
10. SKENE, J. H. P. 1984. Growth-associated proteins and the curious dichotomies of nerve regeneration. Cell **37:** 697-700.
11. DAVID, S. & A. J. AGUAYO. 1981. Axonal elongation into peripheral nervous system "bridges" after central nervous system injury in adult rats. Science **214:** 931-933.
12. BENFEY, M. & A. J. AGUAYO. 1982. Extensive elongation of axons from rat brain into peripheral nerve grafts. Nature **296:** 150-153.
13. RICHARDSON, P. M., U. M. MCGUINNESS & A. J. AGUAYO. 1982. Peripheral nerve autografts to the rat spinal cord: Studies with axonal tracing methods. Brain Res. **237:** 147-162.
14. FRIEDMAN, B. & A. J. AGUAYO. 1985. Injured neurons in the olfactory bulb of the adult rat grow axons along grafts of peripheral nerve. J. Neurosci. **5:** 1616-1625.
15. KROMER, L. E. & C. J. CORNBROOKS. 1985. Transplantation of Schwann cell cultures promotes axonal regeneration in the adult mammalian brain. Proc. Natl. Acad. Sci. USA **82:** 6330-6334.
16. KROMER, L. E., A. BJÖRKLUND & U. STENEVI. 1981. Regeneration of the septohippocampal pathway in adult rats is promoted by utilizing embryonic hippocampal implants as bridges. Brain Res. **210:** 173-200.
17. RAMON Y CAJAL, S. 1928. Degeneration and Regeneration in the Nervous System. Hoffner. New York, NY.
18. BROWN, J. O. & G. P. MCCOUGH. 1947. Abortive regeneration of the transected spinal cord. J. Comp. Neurol. **87:** 131-137.
19. BERNSTEIN, J. J. & M. E. BERNSTEIN. 1971. Axonal regeneration and formation of synapses proximal to the site of lesion following hemisection of the rat spinal cord. Exp. Neurol. **30:** 336-351.
20. CLEMENTE, C. D. & W. F. WINDLE. 1954. Regeneration of the severed nerve fibers in the spinal cord of the adult cat. J. Comp. Neurol. **101:** 691-731.
21. CHAMBERS, W. W. 1955. Structural regeneration in the mammalian central nervous system in relation to age. *In* Regeneration in the Central Nervous System. W. F. Windle, Ed.: 135-146. Charles C. Thomas. Springfield, IL.
22. KIERNAN, J. A. 1979. Hypotheses concerned with axonal regeneration in the mammalian nervous system. Biol. Rev. **54:** 155-197.
23. REIER, P. J., L. J. STENSAAS & L. GUTH. 1983. The astrocytic scar as an impediment to regeneration in the central nervous system. *In* Spinal Cord Reconstruction. C. C. Kao, R. P. Bunge & P. J. Reier, Eds.: 163-195. Raven Press. New York, NY.
24. BERRY, M., W. L. MAXWELL, A. LOGAN, A. MATHEWSON, P. MCCONNELL, D. E. ASHHURST & G. H. THOMAS. 1983. Deposition of scar tissue in the central nervous system. Acta Neurochir. Suppl. **32:** 31-53.
25. PROBST, M. 1901. Uber den bau des balkenlosen grosshirns, sowie uber mikrogyrie und heterotopie der grauen substanz. Arch. Psychiatr. **34:** 709-786.
26. SILVER, J., S. E. LORENZ, D. WAHLSTEN & J. COUGHLIN. 1982. Axonal guidance during development of the great cerebral commissures: Descriptive and experimental studies, *in vivo,* on the role of preformed glial pathways. J. Comp. Neurol. **210:** 10-29.
27. LENT, R. 1983. Cortico-cortical connections reorganize in hamsters after neonatal transection of callosal bridge. Dev. Brain Res. **11:** 137-142.
28. HANKIN, M. H. & J. SILVER. 1984. Mechanisms of axonal guidance: The problem of intersecting fiber systems. *In* Developmental Biology: A Comprehensive Synthesis. L. Browder, Ed. Plenum. New York, NY.
29. SILVER, J. & M. Y. OGAWA. 1983. Postnatally induced formation of the corpus callosum in acallosal mice on glia-coated cellulose bridges. Science **220:** 1067-1069.

30. BOTTENSTEIN, J. E. & G. H. SATO. 1979. Growth of a rat neuroblastoma cell line in serum-free supplemented medium. Proc. Natl. Acad. Sci. USA **79:** 514-517.
31. HAY, E. D. 1981. Extracellular matrix. J. Cell Biol. **91:** 205-223.
32. NAVASCUÉS, J., L. RODRIGUEZ-GALLARDO, G. MARTIN-PARTIDO & I. S. ALVAREZ. 1985. Proliferation of glial precursors during the early development of the chick optic nerve. Anat. Embryol. **172:** 365-373.
33. SILVER, J. & J. SAPIRO. 1983. Axonal guidance during development of the optic nerve: The role of pigmented epithelia and other extrinsic factors. J. Comp. Neurol. **202:** 521-538.
34. REIER, P. J. & H. F. WEBSTER. 1974. Regeneration and remyelination of *Xenopus* tadpole optic nerve fibers following transection on crush. J. Neurocytol. **3:** 592-618.
35. BOHN, R. C., P. J. REIER & E. B. SOURBEER. 1982. Axonal interactions with connective tissue and glial substrata during optic nerve regeneration in *Xenopus* larvae and adults. Am. J. Anat. **165:** 397-419.
36. BOHN, R. C. & P. J. REIER. 1985. Retrograde degeneration of myelinated axons and reorganization in the optic nerves of adult frogs (*Xenopus laevis*) following nerve injury or tectal ablation. J. Neurocytol. **14:** 221-244.
37. LIESI, P. 1985. Laminin-immunoreactive glia distinguish regenerative adult CNS system from nonregenerative ones. EMBO J. **4:** 2505-2511.
38. RAISMAN, G. 1985. Specialized neuroglial arrangement may explain the capacity of vo-meronasal axons to reinnervate central neurons. Neuroscience **14:** 237-254.
39. ANDERS, J. J. & M. W. BRIGHTMAN. 1979. Assemblies of particles in the cell membranes of developing, mature and reactive astrocytes. J. Neurocytol. **8:** 777-795.
40. WUJEK, J. R. & P. J. REIER. 1984. Astrocytic membrane morphology: Differences between mammalian and amphibian astrocytes after axotomy. J. Comp. Neurol. **222:** 607-619.
41. SILVER, J. & R. M. ROBB. 1979. Studies on the development of the eye cup and optic nerve in normal mice and in mutants with congenital optic nerve aplasia. Dev. Biol. **68:** 175-190.
42. SILVER, J. & R. C. SIDMAN. 1980. A mechanism for the guidance and topographic patterning of retinal ganglion cell axons. J. Comp. Neurol. **189:** 101-111.
43. SILVER, J. 1984. Studies on the factors that govern directionality of axonal growth in the embryonic optic nerve and at the chiasm of mice. J. Comp. Neurol. **223:** 238-251.
44. SILVER, J. & U. RUTISHAUSER. 1984. Guidance of axons *in vivo* by a preformed adhesive pathway on neuroepithelial endfeet. Dev. Biol. **106:** 101-111.
45. NORDLANDER, R. H. & M. SINGER. 1982. Morphology and position of growth cones in the developing *Xenopus* spinal cord. Dev. Brain Res. **4:** 181-193.
46. SINGER, M., R. H. NORDLANDER & M. EGAR. 1979. Axonal guidance during embryogenesis and regeneration in the spinal cord of newt: The blueprint hypothesis of neuronal pathway patterning. J. Comp. Neurol. **185:** 1-22.
47. EASTER, S. S., B. BRATTON & S. S. SCHERER. 1984. Growth-related order of the retinal fiber layer in goldfish. J. Neurosci. **4:** 2173-2190.
48. GUTH, L., C. P. BARRETT, E. J. DONATI, F. D. ANDERSON, M. V. SMITH & M. LIFSON. 1985. Essentiality of a specific cellular terrain for growth of axons into a spinal cord lesion. Exp. Neurol. **88:** 1-12.
49. KAO, C. C., L. W. CHANG & J. M. B. BLOODWORTH. 1977. Axonal regeneration across transected mammalian cord: An electron microscopic study of delayed micronerve grafting. Exp. Neurol. **54:** 591-615.
50. PUCHALA, E. & W. F. WINDLE. 1977. The possibility of structural and functional restitution after spinal cord injury. Exp. Neurol. **55:** 1-42.
51. STENSAAS, L. J., P. R. BURGESS & K. W. HORSCH. 1979. Regenerating dorsal root axons are blocked by spinal cord astrocytes. Soc. Neurosci. Abstr. **5:** 684.
52. NOBLE, M., J. FOK-SEANG & J. COHEN. 1984. Glia are a unique substrate for the *in vitro* growth of central nervous system neurons. J. Neurosci. **4:** 1892-1903.
53. FALLON, J. 1985. Preferential outgrowth of central nervous system neurites on astrocytes and Schwann cells as compared with nonglial cells *in vitro*. J. Cell Biol. **100:** 198-207.
54. NIETO-SAMPEDRO, M., S. R. WHITTEMORE, D. L. NEEDELS, J. LARSON & C. W. COTMAN. 1984. The survival of brain transplants is enhanced by extracts from injured brain. Proc. Natl. Acad. Sci. USA **81:** 6250-6254.

55. NIETO-SAMPEDRO, M., M. MANTHORPE, G. BARBIN, S. VARON & C. W. COTMAN. 1983. Injury-induced neurotrophic activity in the adult rat brain: Correlation with survival of delayed implants in the wound cavity. J. Neurosci. **3:** 2219-2229.
56. RUDGE, J. S., M. MANTHORPE & S. VARON. 1985. The output of neurotrophic and neurite-promoting agents from rat brain astroglial cells: A microculture method for screening potential regulatory molecules. Dev. Brain Res. **19:** 161-172.
57. SMITH, G., R. MILLER & J. SILVER. 1986. Changing role of forebrain astrocytes during development, regenerative failure, and induced regeneration upon transplantation. J. Comp. Neurol. **251:** 23-43.

DISCUSSION OF THE PAPER

S. C. McLOON (*University of Minnesota, Minneapolis, MN*): It is interesting that the laminin is on the membrane side of the astrocytes, and, since we know that young astrocytes are moving, it might be interesting to pursue the idea of the laminin being produced by them being important for adhesion of the astrocytes themselves.

SILVER: Yes. If one coats the filters with laminin before putting them into the brain, we find that adhesions tend to increase. There seems to be more pronounced astrocyte reactions. It seems laminin could play an adhesive role. I recently spent 10 days in Dr. Lisi's lab learning her techniques. It is very clear that our staining pattern is probably the weakest we or a lot of people can produce. Dr. Lisi, however, uses special freezing techniques and very little washing. We can see laminin being produced in the cell bodies for the astrocytes on the surface of the filter. There is no doubt that laminin is being produced by astrocytes. What we do not know is if this laminin is being expressed on the surface. Right now, there is no good evidence to suggest that laminin is being touched by growth cones, but I am not willing to rule out this possibility yet. I think it is an important thing to study. Electron microscopy analysis could be done to see what growth cones touch, to see if growth cones contact laminin on the surface. It would be easy enough to do. We are certainly going to pursue it, and I am sure you will, too.

McLOON: I might just say that we have not been able to find a growth cone on laminin yet.

SILVER: It is not so easy to find growth cones, but laminin is not going to be the only player in this story. I discussed the production of N-CAM. Preliminary observations, which I did not discuss, showed that scars themselves make very little N-CAM. This may be because of all the mesodermal contaminants, which do not normally express N-CAM. Matrix molecules of the extracellular matrix that are produced in young brain may also be important. We always characterize glial scars as being dense. Why are they dense? Embryonic tissue is full of holes. We know now that there may be modulation of extracellular matrix substances. Astrocytes in young animals have the ability to move and make a beautiful three-dimensional structure. The brain is three dimensional, and astrocytes in young animals have fantastic abilities to respond to the presence of fibers by making ramifying processes. Old astrocytes are flat, slow, and sluggish, and they make a two-dimensional surface: that is just about it. It is going to be a very complicated story, but I think we can use similar paradigms to get at this question.

McLOON: Maybe I could ask a question.

SILVER: No. I do not want to answer that question of whether laminin is a magic molecule.

MCLOON: You showed N-CAM staining on the astrocytes that were on your substrate. Is that prior to the arrival of the axons? Or, if the axons have arrived, could that N-CAM be from the axons?

SILVER: There are not enough axons in the system: not all of the staining is axonal; the bulk of it is astrocyic. The axons take a different course. An important offshoot of this question would be whether axons could induce the presence of any of these molecules on these cells. Clearly, the glia nonneuronal elements might grow out first. They are the first characters on the scene, and they begin to express these molecules at least before or during the time course when axons and blood vessels are moving. It is almost simultaneous.

QUESTIONER: Is there a published study showing N-CAM staining on astrocytes alone?

SILVER: N-CAM on astrocytes alone in culture? I have not published such a study, but Martin Opel has. We have shown in the normal developing optic system of a variety of species, chicks and others, that astrocytes for the optic system produce N-CAM exactly, in the region near where growth cones grow. Where axons do not grow, you do not see it.

N. KALDERON (*Rockefeller University, New York, NY*): I have a comment about confirming the hypothesis you presented. You commented that the young astrocytes might make plasminogen activating factor. I found that developing astrocytes make plasminogen activating factor and that when they are mature it declines tremendously. So it has a nice correlation with the production of N-CAM. When in the differentiated state, they make a lot of it; when in the mature state, or when they are reactive, astrocytes probably do not make it.

SILVER: I think that is fantastic. I think James Turner also has a poster that shows that transplants in retina can actually dissolve the glial scar. An important question in terms of chronic paralysis would be whether cells such as this dissolve a basal lamina scar that has been present in the brain for long periods of time. It would be very important and exciting if it could happen. And it could be due to plasminogen activator.

KALDERONE: But they definitely make the young ones dissolve.

SILVER: That is very important.

F. H. GAGE (*University of California, La Jolla, CA*): You said you put laminin on the cell surface. What is the effect of laminin antibodies?

SILVER: Dr. Lisi and I tried antilaminin and we saw there was no change from the control; that is, it did not seem to inhibit migration.

GAGE: What is the antibody that you used?

SILVER: The antibodies are polyclonals against affinity-purified laminin. We have also used the Lisi's antibody. Our techniques show what most people show in terms of basal lamina staining in around the blood vessels. If we use Lisi's techniques, there is no doubt you can see more beautiful patterns of lamina staining. You can see the cytoplasmic localization of laminin in the cells that make it, and if it is being shipped to the basal lamina, blood vessels are invading this system. The scar is forming, and there is a lamina response by some kinds of cells. One of these is astrocytes: there is no doubt about it. But is it all being shipped to the basal lamina of the blood vessel and being inserted into the membrane? Lisi is convinced it is being inserted. We put stick filters in antilaminin and saw no effect. Maybe this is not a good blocking antibody, and maybe there are other players. Laminin may not be the whole story. But I do not think we can rule it out.

Identification of Trophic Factors and Transplanted Cellular Environments That Promote CNS Axonal Regeneration[a]

LAWRENCE F. KROMER[b] AND
CARSON J. CORNBROOKS[c]

[b]Department of Anatomy and Cell Biology
Georgetown University
Schools of Medicine and Dentistry
Washington, DC 20007

[c]Department of Anatomy and Neurobiology
University of Vermont
Given Medical Building
Burlington, Vermont 05045

INTRODUCTION

It has long been recognized that axons within the cellular environment of the adult mammalian peripheral nervous system (PNS) maintain their capacity to regenerate functional connections following peripheral nerve damage.[1,2] In contrast, most axons located within the cellular milieu of the mature mammalian central nervous system (CNS) appear to exhibit no spontaneous regeneration after a CNS lesion.[1,3–5] The classical observations of abortive regenerative responses within the CNS raise the question whether the failure of CNS axonal regeneration is due to the glial environment or intrinsic cellular properties of CNS neurons. Experimental evidence now indicates that there is considerable inherent plasticity within the adult mammalian CNS and that extensive synaptic reorganization and paraterminal sprouting from uninjured axons can occur within the CNS neuropil in response to injury.[4–7] Axonal regeneration through existing CNS fiber tracts or over long distances, however, rarely occurs, and retrograde neuronal degeneration often is observed following CNS injuries.[1,3–5,8] These observations indicate there are multiple cellular events that must be regulated in order to promote successful CNS axonal regeneration *in vivo*. In particular, neuronal viability must be enhanced following axotomy, axonal regrowth over long distances must be promoted, regenerating axons must be directed to their proper terminal regions, and synaptogenesis between the regenerating presynaptic elements and their appropriate postsynaptic targets must be insured. To accomplish this complex task, it is essential

[a]This work was supported by the March of Dimes Birth Defects Foundation and by Grants NS-23522 and NS-20189 from the National Institutes of Health.

207

to develop new experimental approaches that can be used to both identify and utilize selective cellular and/or molecular components that promote neuronal survival and the regeneration of appropriate and functional neuronal circuits following CNS injuries.

One promising experimental approach that has been developed to further explore what cellular components influence regeneration in the immature or adult mammalian CNS is the transplantation of adult PNS[9-15] or embryonic CNS[14-20] tissues. The rationale behind this experimental approach is to present injured CNS axons with an environment that is known to be conducive for axonal growth. For example, embryonic CNS tissue must contain a complex array of guidance cues that direct growing axons to their appropriate termination points. Possible mechanisms for this axonal guidance could combine the use of nonselective channels for axonal growth[21] with selective chemical substrates at specific locations that further direct the axons.[22,23] The mechanisms responsible for promoting regeneration in the PNS also appear to involve special "terrains" composed of cellular elements (Schwann cells and fibroblasts), extracellular matrix (basal lamina), and soluble trophic factors, that are necessary in order to facilitate PNS axonal regeneration.[2,24-28]

The precise cellular and extracellular factors that are responsible for the positive axonal growth observed in embryonic CNS tissue and in peripheral nerves have not been characterized. The use of *in vitro* cell preparations, however, where the cytology and molecular mechanisms of cell-cell interactions can be studied within the confines of restricted cell populations and chemically defined environments, has greatly facilitated the identification of substances that possess neurotrophic and neurotropic properties.[28-31] For example, neurotrophic factors, such as nerve growth factor (NGF), brain-derived neurotrophic factor, and ciliary neurotrophic factor, promote the survival, maintenance, and general metabolism of neurons. These neurotrophic factors appear to be soluble components that can be obtained from PNS and CNS tissue extracts or culture media conditioned by a variety of cells, including CNS glia.[31-41] Neurotropic factors or neurite growth-promoting factors are defined as molecules that are involved with the elongation and guidance of axonal processes.[28,42,43] These factors are released from cells into the culture media where they are associated with cell surfaces and extracellular matrices.[29,42,43] Thus far, two well-characterized extracellular matrix (ECM) components, laminin and fibronectin, which are synthesized by a variety of cell types including Schwann cells,[44] have been demonstrated to possess neurite-promoting properties but lack neurotrophic activity.[43,45-49] Only laminin, however, is reported to promote consistent neurite growth from CNS neurons in culture.[43,47-49] In addition to ECM components, molecules associated with the cell membrane of glial cells also appear to influence neurite growth *in vitro.*[50,51]

In the present review, we will describe some of the recent experimental results obtained in our laboratories that evaluate the roles of specific cell products and more complex cellular environments in promoting CNS axonal regeneration. The emphasis of this research, which utilizes the septohippocampal formation as a model system, is to 1) evaluate neurotrophic molecules, which have been identified in tissue culture, for their ability to promote neuronal survival *in vivo* and 2) identify selective cellular environments that enhance axonal regeneration following axotomy by providing a positive neurotropic effect *in vivo.* The septohippocampal lesion model system has been extensively described in previous experiments that have employed embryonic hippocampal transplants to promote the regeneration of lesioned septal cholinergic axons and the reinnervation of their terminal fields within the hippocampus.[18,19] The basic paradigm that we currently utilize is to perform complete bilateral aspiration lesions of all axons projecting in the dorsal septohippocampal pathways (composed of the supracallosal stria-cingulum bundle and the dorsal fornix and fimbria). This procedure results in severe retrograde degeneration of most cholinergic neurons within the medial septum as well as a persistent cholinergic denervation of the dorsal hippocampus.[19] This preparation also produces an extensive intracephalic cavity (approximately 4-6 mm long) that separates the lesioned surfaces of the septum and hippocampus (FIG. 1), thus providing an excellent site for the introduction of soluble cellular products or defined transplant materials that can be analyzed for their ability to inhibit retrograde neuronal death within the septum and promote cholinergic axonal regrowth over long distances.

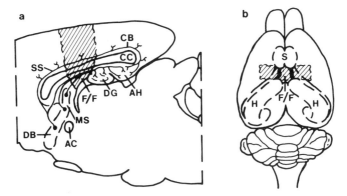

FIGURE 1. Schematic illustrations of the location and extent of the bilateral aspiration lesions (hatched areas) used to transect the dorsal septohippocampal pathways. (**a**) Sagittal drawing demonstrating the position of the lesion that extends through the cortex, corpus callosum (CC) and fornix-fimbria (F/F). This lesion, which transects all septal cholinergic axons that project through the fornix-fimbria, supracallosal stria (SS), and cingulum bundle (CB), produces a complete denervation of the dorsal dentate gyrus (DG) and Ammon's horn (AH). AC: anterior commissure; DB: diagonal band; MS: medial septum. (**b**) Dorsal view of a rat brain illustrating the lateral extent of the bilateral intracephalic lesion (hatched area) that completely severs the fornix-fimbria. Bilateral transplants (solid black strips) are positioned within the cavity so that they completely bridge the gap separating the injured surfaces of the septum (S) and hippocampal formation (H).

NEUROTROPHIC MOLECULES THAT PROMOTE CNS NEURONAL SURVIVAL

Since the discovery of NGF several decades ago,[52] extensive experimentation has demonstrated that target-derived macromolecules play an important role in regulating axonal growth, naturally occurring cell death during development, and neuronal maturation in the PNS.[28–30] The loss of specific target-derived trophic factors also may be involved in the process of retrograde cell degeneration that occurs following axotomy[3–5,8,28,53] and is observed in certain neuropathological diseases such as Alzheimer's dementia.[54] Conversely, it has been postulated that trophic substances may be instrumental in promoting regeneration in the PNS[25–27] and might influence cell survival in the CNS.[40] By utilizing *in vitro* assay procedures it has been possible to partially identify several putative neurotrophic factors of PNS[32–35,37] and CNS origin.[38–41] Moreover, some of these trophic factors, which are released in response to CNS injury, can support the survival of several types of neurons in culture[40,41,55] and enhance the survival of developing neurons within embryonic CNS and PNS transplants.[40,56]

Recent experimental studies strongly suggest that NGF is one of these endogenous CNS neurotrophic factors. For example, basal forebrain cholinergic neurons possess receptors for NGF[57] and exhibit selective uptake and retrograde transport of NGF following injections of exogenous NGF into their CNS target regions,[58,59] which also contain significant levels of endogenous NGF and its mRNA.[60,61] Moreover, the endogenous NGF levels within the hippocampus are elevated following septal deafferentation.[62] Both NGF and hippocampal extracts elevate cholinergic enzyme levels in basal forebrain neurons *in vitro*.[37,39] Chronic intraventricular injections of NGF also elevate levels of the biosynthetic enzyme for acetylcholine, choline acetyltransferase (ChAT), in the septum and hippocampus.[63,64] There is some ambiguity, however, concerning the ability of NGF to promote septal neuronal survival *in vitro*,[65] although recent evidence does suggest that it may influence neuronal viability *in vivo* following partial unilateral fornix-fimbria lesions.[66]

If NGF does act as a trophic molecule for forebrain cholinergic neurons, then it is important to determine whether the administration of exogenous NGF subsequent to CNS axonal injury can prevent neuronal degeneration that normally occurs within such regions as the medial septum.[19,67] To evaluate this possibility, three groups of adult rats were given complete bilateral transections of the dorsal septohippocampal cholinergic projections. In one group of animals, NGF (250 ng of 2.5s NGF/μl) was continuously infused for 2 weeks (total dose: 40 μg NGF) into the right lateral ventricle. A second group received cytochrome c under the same conditions as above, whereas the remaining operated animals received no treatment and constituted a lesioned, but nontreated group. Three groups of unlesioned control animals also were prepared: one group received no treatment and the remaining two received either NGF or cytochrome c. All animals were allowed to survive for 2 weeks before being prepared for Nissl staining and for ChAT immunocytochemistry to identify cholinergic neurons in the medial septum.

Results from these experiments[68] indicate that the number and distribution of ChAT-positive (ChAT$^+$) neurons within the medial septum and vertical limb of the diagonal band is similar in all nonlesioned animals (that is, NGF- and cytochrome c-treated and untreated controls). This suggests that the intraventricular infusion of NGF into normal unlesioned animals does not induce the expression of the cholinergic enzyme, ChAT, in septal neurons that normally do not contain this protein. Evaluation of animals that received complete bilateral lesions of the dorsal cholinergic septohippocampal pathways indicated that there is a significant loss of about 80% of cholinergic neurons within the medial septum (FIG. 2; TABLE 1) in all animals that were untreated or had received an intraventricular infusion of cytochrome c. In contrast, animals that received the NGF treatment after the lesion exhibit a remarkable and statistically significant increased survival of cholinergic neurons within the medial septum (approximately 85% survival both ipsilateral and contralateral to the site of NGF infusion). Observations based on Nissl-stained tissue sections also suggest that there is survival of noncholinergic septal neurons. If this NGF treatment is delayed for several days following the initial axonal transection, however, then neuronal survival is greatly diminished.[69] Thus, these results complement and extend the initial findings of Hefti[66] and clearly demonstrate that NGF is a neurotrophic molecule for certain classes of CNS neurons.

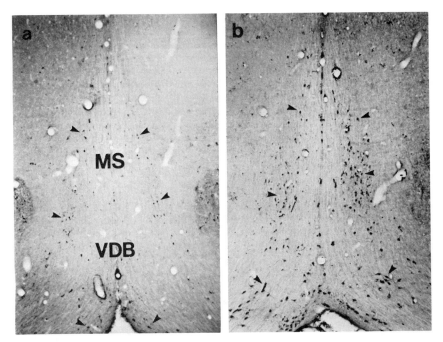

FIGURE 2. Coronal sections through the medial septum (MS) and vertical limbs of the diagonal band (VDB) illustrating the immunocytochemical localization of ChAT$^+$ neurons that have been stained with the peroxidase-antiperoxidase procedure. (a) Very few ChAT$^+$ neurons (arrows) are present in this specimen 2 weeks after receiving bilateral transections of the fornix-fimbria. (b) Numerous ChAT$^+$ cells can be identified in this specimen with bilateral fornix-fimbria lesions that received a continuous intraventricular infusion of NGF for 2 weeks after the lesion. From reference 68.

TABLE 1. Cholinergic Neuronal Survival in Medial Septum following Axotomy[a]

	Control	Lesioned		Lesioned + NGF	
	Number of Cells[b]	Number of Cells	Survival (%)	Number of Cells	Survival (%)
Right side	1300 ± 101	245 ± 47[c]	19	1104 ± 23[d]	85
Left side	1036 ± 77	190 ± 18[c]	18	868 ± 73[d]	84
Total	2336 ± 169	435 ± 64[c]	19	1971 ± 89[d]	85

[a] The control group indicates the number of ChAT$^+$ medial septal neurons present in the entire nucleus and its right and left counterparts. The lesioned group includes animals that received bilateral fornix-fimbria lesions. Approximately 80% of the ChAT$^+$ neurons within the medial septum undergo retrograde degeneration within 2 weeks following complete bilateral lesions of the dorsal septohippocampal pathways. In the lesioned + NGF group there is a highly significant survival of cholinergic neurons with only about a 15% loss in total cell number at 2 weeks after the lesion. Adapted from reference 68.

[b] Mean ± SEM.

[c] Significantly different from controls, $p < .001$

[d] Significantly different from animals with lesions alone, $p < .001$

CELLULAR COMPONENTS THAT INFLUENCE CNS AXONAL REGENERATION

Peripheral Nerves as Transplants

Several studies have demonstrated that PNS grafts can facilitate CNS axonal elongation[12,13]; however, few axons within the grafts appear to reenter the host CNS neuropil.[70] In particular, Wendt *et al.*[71] report that septal cholinergic axons within PNS transplants fail to reenter the denervated host hippocampus. In contrast, septal axons that are provided with embryonic CNS tissue as a substrate readily reinnervate the cholinergically denervated hippocampus.[19,71] Because of this discrepancy, we decided to reevaluate the ability of adult sciatic nerve grafts to function as a cellular bridge that could promote the cholinergic reinnervation of the hippocampus. During our investigation, we carefully evaluated whether the ability of septal cholinergic axons to regenerate through grafts of sciatic nerve was influenced by 1) the degree of fusion of the transplant to the host septum and hippocampus and 2) the extent of Wallerian degeneration within the nerve preparation. In these experiments either freshly axotomized sciatic nerve segments or sections from predegenerated sciatic nerves were used as transplants. The predegenerated sciatic nerves were prepared by completely transecting the right sciatic nerve at its exit from the spinal cord and ligating the cut distal end with surgical suture 10 days before taking the distal portion of the nerve for transplantation. Both freshly axotomized and predegenerated sciatic nerves were placed in sterile Leibovitz-15 medium, stripped of their epineurium, and cut into segments (approximately 5 mm long). These nerve segments were positioned in the cavity so that the cut ends were in direct apposition to the septum and hippocampus (FIG. 1b). Regenerative growth in these preparations was analyzed at 1, 3, 5, 8, 10, 14, and 28 days after transplantation.

The progress of CNS regeneration in this and in subsequent studies was monitored by neuroanatomical and immunohistochemical methods. Cholinergic neurons and their processes were visualized by the acetylcholinesterase (AChE) staining technique.[72] Neuronal processes, regardless of type, also were visualized with a monoclonal antibody directed against the phosphorylated subunits of the neurofilament protein (NFP). Laminin (LAM), a known component of basal laminae of peripheral nerves[73] and a molecule that appears in several brain areas following injury,[74-76] was visualized with polyclonal antibodies. Cells in the cavity were visualized using antibodies against glial fibrillary acidic protein (GFAP), a cytoskeletal protein in astrocytes[77] and mature nonmyelinating Schwann cells.[78] Schwann cells were visualized using a specific monoclonal antibody, "C4," which decorates the membranes of these peripheral glial cells when they are in contact with peripheral or central neurons.[79]

The results from this study (FIG. 3) suggest that there is a general sequence of events that occurs during the process of regeneration in this paradigm. Within 3 days thick GFAP$^+$ processes extend between the transplants and the host septum. At this time point AChE$^+$ fibers extend along these glial processes and begin to enter the grafts. Within 5 days after the lesion, numerous AChE$^+$ and NFP$^+$ fibers are within the grafts. There is considerable variation, however, in the amount of innervation present in the different transplants. Freshly axotomized nerve grafts with smaller diameters possess a moderately dense pattern of AChE$^+$ fibers, whereas grafts with larger diameters often contain necrotic centers. Predegenerated nerve grafts appear to possess a more extensive fiber ingrowth. The growth of cholinergic axons into both types of grafts, however, was greatly influenced by the degree of fusion between the

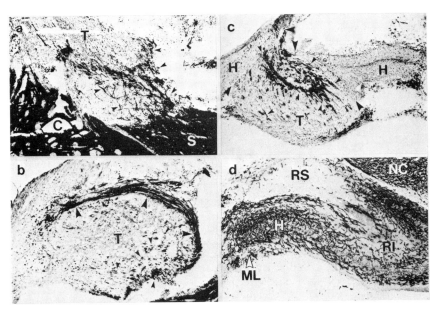

FIGURE 3. Coronal sections through specimens that received bilateral sciatic nerve grafts 6 days following bilateral fornix-fimbria lesions. All sections have been stained for AChE: **a-c** are of sciatic nerve grafts that were axotomized immediately before transplantation; **d** is from a specimen that received a predegenerated PNS graft. (**a**) Three days after transplantation, numerous AChE$^+$ fibers (arrows) traverse the cellular strands at the interface between the host septum (S) and the PNS transplant (T). Few cholinergic axons, however, have entered the graft at this survival time. C: caudate nucleus. (**b**) This PNS transplant does not possess a uniform distribution of AChE$^+$ fibers but contains fascicles of fibers along its periphery. Because of twisting of the nerve within the cavity, axons appear oriented both perpendicular (small arrows) and parallel (large arrows) to the plane of section. Posttransplant survival: 2 weeks. (**c**) Interface between the graft (T) and host hippocampus (H) demonstrating that there are several fascicles of AChE$^+$ fibers (small arrows) within this sciatic nerve graft that do not enter the host hippocampus although there is direct fusion (large arrows) between the transplant and host CNS. Posttransplant survival: 2 weeks. (**d**) Distribution of AChE$^+$ fibers within the host hippocampus of a specimen that received a predegenerated nerve graft 1 month previously. In this specimen there is extensive reinnervation of the dentate hilus (H) and molecular layer (ML), and regio inferior (RI) of Ammon's horn, with a sparse reinnervation of regio superior (RS). NC: adjacent neocortex that was not denervated by the lesion.

transplants and the host septum. Those specimens where the grafts were directly fused with the septum or were separated from the host CNS by short glial strands exhibited the greatest ingrowth of AChE$^+$ fibers. Axonal elongation within both types of grafts is rapid, but outgrowth into the host hippocampus is much slower. In this regard, reinnervation of the hippocampus via predegenerated nerve grafts appears more extensive than the limited outgrowth that occurred from freshly axotomized grafts. These experimental results are consistent with previous studies using freshly axotomized PNS nerve grafts[70,71] in that they also demonstrate relatively poor outgrowth of CNS axons from transplants of freshly axotomized sciatic nerve. Our results, however, suggest that there is better reinnervation of the host hippocampus when predegenerated nerves are used as transplants. The present results further indicate that there are at least two important parameters that influence the ability of septal cholinergic axons to utilize PNS nerve grafts as successful regeneration substrates. First, the growth of CNS axons into both predegenerated and freshly axotomized grafts is critically dependent on a very close approximation of the graft to the injured surfaces of the CNS (both septum and hippocampus). Second, the outgrowth of the cholinergic axons from the grafts into the host hippocampus is more extensive when predegenerated nerves are used as transplants.

Schwann Cell-ECM Cultures as Transplants

The ability of fresh or predegenerated peripheral nerve transplants to foster regeneration of the injured adult mammalian septohippocampal system has prompted us to initiate similar studies using cultured cells. The premise behind this approach was to take advantage of the technical advances in *in vitro* methodologies that allow the preparation of cultures containing discrete cell populations.[80] By systematically separating the cellular components of the peripheral nerve environment, which is favorable for CNS regeneration, we plan to identify the cells and eventually the molecules most germane to promoting axonal regrowth *in vivo*.

The initial studies with cultured cells as transplants utilized sections from mature Schwann cell-neuron cultures.[74] These explant cultures were derived from embryonic day 15 dorsal root ganglia (DRG) that were cultured on a collagen substratum using methods to eliminate any fibroblasts. The cultures were then maintained for 2 months in order to allow the explanted neurons to extend an extensive network of neuritic processes that were ensheathed or myelinated by differentiated Schwann cells and encased in robust basal laminae.[81,82] Transplants were prepared by removing all neuronal somata and sectioning the cultures into 1×5-mm strips such that the fascicles of neurites with their associated Schwann cells extended approximately parallel with the long axis of the transplant. Subsequently, the Schwann cell-ECM transplants were positioned in close proximity to the septum with the channels of matrix and peripheral glia spanning the lesioned area of the host CNS such that their posterior ends were in close apposition with the denervated hippocampus. This cellular transplant preparation thus provides a partially defined environment, containing degenerating neurites and myelin but viable Schwann cells within ECM channels, which can be evaluated for its ability to promote CNS axonal regeneration.

Controls for the cellular transplants consisted of three types. Some animals received lesions without transplants, whereas other recipients were given transplants of the collagen substratum incubated in medium identical to that used to grow the cultured cells. A third type of control was inherent to the Schwann cell-ECM transplants. Since the neurites and associated Schwann cells organize into fascicles on the collagen substratum *in vitro*, there are areas of the substrate that do not contain cells but are exposed to any secreted molecules synthesized by the Schwann cells. In the control experiments, axonal sprouts initially extend from the septal area within 3 days after the lesion; however, no regenerating axons are associated with the control collagen transplants or with the acellular regions of the Schwann cell-ECM transplants. Moreover, even 2 months after transplantation, no AChE$^+$ axons innervate the target hippocampus in the control specimens.

In the presence of transplants containing viable Schwann cells and extracellular matrix channels, axons from several areas of the injured adult mammalian CNS make contact with the cellular portions of the transplants. The majority of these axons

(AChE$^+$ and NFP$^+$) arise from the septum and caudate nuclei and reinnervate the hippocampus when given optimal conditions and adequate time (FIGS. 4a-c). As in the control experiments, axonal growth from the injured septum and caudate began as early as 3 days after transplantation. These growing fibers are associated with the GFAP$^+$ and/or LAM$^+$ tissue strands that are interposed for short distances between

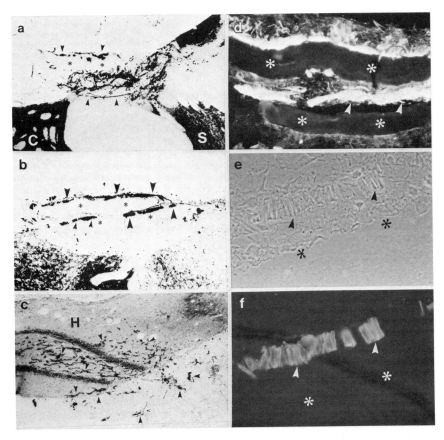

FIGURE 4. Coronal sections from specimens with bilateral Schwann cell-ECM transplants 2 weeks after transplantation. (a-c) This series of micrographs illustrates the location of AChE$^+$ fibers (arrows) that form the regenerated pathway from the septum to the hippocampus. From reference 74. (a) Numerous fascicles of AChE$^+$ fibers sprout from the host septum and travel along cellular strands to reach the Schwann cell-laden surface of the Schwann cell-ECM transplants (asterisks). (b) Dense bundles of AChE$^+$ axons (large and small arrows) are specifically associated with the discrete cellular areas along the dorsal surface of the collagen substratum (asterisks) throughout the length of each transplant. (c) A loose plexus of AChE$^+$ fibers is present in the rostral end of the host hippocampus (H). These axons reach the hippocampus by traveling along short tissue strands interconnecting the transplant and hippocampus. (d-f) These micrographs are from sections adjacent to the section illustrated in b. The arrows in d-f indicate the same AChE$^+$ cellular layer that is indicated by the small arrows in b. Asterisks localize the collagen substratum. (d) LAM immunoreactivity is localized to the cellular layer dorsal to the collagen. (e & f) These micrographs illustrate the same section under phase contrast (e) and fluorescence (d). The elongated cells above the arrows are positively identified as Schwann cells by their staining in f with the C4 antibody, which is specific for Schwann cells.

the intact CNS parenchyma and the cellular aspects of the transplants. Regenerating fibers are first seen on the transplants at 5 days after transplantation, where they are intimately associated with the cellular, and not the collagen, portion of the previously cultured tissue. These CNS fibers form fiber bundles associated with the LAM$^+$ matrix channels in the transplants (FIGS. 4b,d). This organization is analogous to that observed *in vitro* and in the PNS transplants discussed above. Further analysis also revealed that the Schwann cells express the antigen specifically recognized by the C4 antibody (FIGS. 4e-f). Thus AChE$^+$ areas associated with the transplants are also LAM$^+$, NFP$^+$, and C4$^+$. This shows that regenerating CNS axons are intimately associated with the Schwann cells and the LAM$^+$ extracellular matrix. Fibers so positioned on the transplant maintain direct contact with the bundles of cultured material, and, within 10 days after transplantation, they traverse the entire length of the transplant and are directed toward their correct target, the hippocampus. There are, however, many additional areas in the cavity that are LAM$^+$, presumably due to LAM expressed by injured CNS cells,[74,75] that do not contain AChE$^+$ or NFP$^+$ processes. At longer time points (for example, 14 days after transplantation), the AChE$^+$ fibers vacate the PNS terrain of the transplants, traverse the short GFAP$^+$ and/or LAM$^+$ cellular strands along the transplant-hippocampal interface and reinnervate the host hippocampus, which lacks LAM and C4. Within the hippocampus, the cholinergic fibers occupy terminal space in the dentate gyrus and regio inferior and superior of Ammon's horn. The extent of reinnervation of these areas varies depending on the location of the transplant-hippocampus interface. In some instances, when the transplant is directed toward but not in close proximity to the intact brain, the AChE$^+$ fibers remain associated with the transplant and do not traverse the longer tissue strands at the transplant-host interface. This is true at the septum-transplant as well as the transplant-hippocampus interfaces. In most experiments, however, when the transplant is correctly positioned adjacent to the lesioned surface of the hippocampus, the cholinergic fibers associated with the transplant provide a rich reinnervation of the host hippocampus that persists for the life of the animal.

Glial-derived ECM as Transplants

To continue our segregation of the peripheral nerve environment in order to characterize the source of factors that facilitate regeneration of CNS axons, we next examined the role of ECM channels.[83] Beginning with mature Schwann cell-ECM preparations, which were previously demonstrated to promote CNS axon elongation,[74] we prepared a cell-free substrate consisting of ECM channels synthesized by the differentiating Schwann cells. To obtain these ECM preparations, we removed the neuronal explant region from mature Schwann cell-DRG cultures, which were then osmotically shocked with water; successively treated with triton X-100, DNase, and deoxycholate; and extensively washed. Previous reports have demonstrated that this detergent treatment of the cultures preserves the major components of ECM reported in the peripheral nerve.[84-87] Furthermore, recent *in vitro* studies (reference 88 and Schinstine and Cornbrooks, unpublished observations) have shown that this preparation both supports and promotes neurite elongation from PNS neurons (sympathetic and DRG) as well as embryonic CNS neurons (spinal cord, neocortex, and septum). Matrix transplants were dissected and placed into bilateral cavities (two per side) so that the long axis of the ECM channels was parallel to the septal-hippocampal axis. The intracephalic cavities were prepared 6 days before transplantation, and the transplants were examined 1, 3, 5, and 10 days after transplantation. The results from these experiments (FIG. 5) indicate that the LAM immunoreactivity always remains

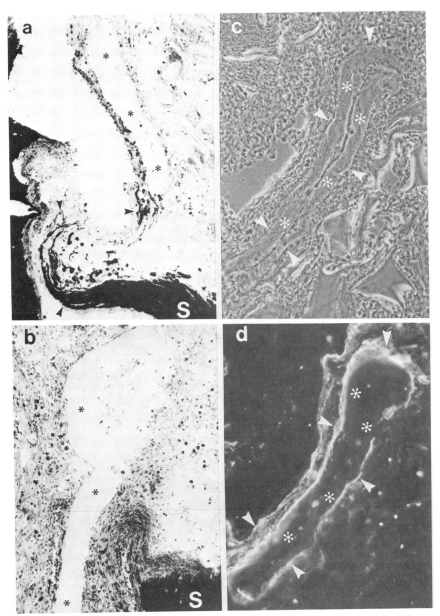

FIGURE 5. Coronal sections through ECM transplants that can be identified within the intra-cephalic cavity by the presence of the collagen substratum (asterisks). (a & b) AChE-stained sections illustrating the close proximity of the transplants to the host septum (S). (a) Although sprouting AChE⁺ fibers from the septum reach the transplant, they do not continue in association with the transplant. (b) This specimen is representative of many specimens in which there was no sprouting of AChE⁺ axons from the septum toward the transplant. (c & d) Adjacent sections to that illustrated in **a** viewed with phase contrast optics (c) and LAM immunofluorescence (d). This transplant has been folded so that the LAM⁺ ECM layer is present along the exterior surface of the folded collagen sublayer. Although LAM immunoreactivity is present in this transplant, it does not appear to attract or maintain the growth of AChE⁺ fibers.

associated with the matrix channels that are located on only one side of the transplants. At the septum-transplant interface there is a close approximation of the LAM$^+$ transplants both to the lesioned surface of the septum and to the numerous axonal sprouts emanating from the septum. Despite the continued presence of the LAM$^+$ matrix, however, no AChE$^+$ or NFP$^+$ axons are associated with the transplants during the times examined and no hippocampi are reinnervated.

DISCUSSION

Prevention of retrograde neuronal degeneration, which often occurs following injuries to the adult mammalian CNS, is one of the inherent problems that must be addressed in order to promote functional regeneration. One explanation for this phenomenon postulates that axotomy results in the loss of a specific retrogradely transported target-derived trophic molecule that is essential for neuronal survival.[3–5,8,28,53] Since it has been postulated that the survival of basal forebrain cholinergic neurons is dependent upon a continuous supply of the retrogradely transported neurotrophic factor, NGF,[54] we tested this hypothesis by infusing NGF into the lateral ventricle following complete bilateral lesions of the dorsal septohippocampal pathways, which contain all cholinergic axons projecting to the dorsal hippocampus. This study clearly demonstrates that the exogenous administration of NGF can inhibit the death of cholinergic and noncholinergic neurons within the medial septum. Thus, these results confirm and extend the initial findings of Hefti,[66] in which NGF was administered in conjunction with only a partial unilateral lesion of the fornix-fimbria. Since it is uncertain whether NGF receptors are present only on cholinergic septal neurons,[57] it is not possible at present to state whether the survival of the noncholinergic neurons is a secondary transneuronal effect due to the NGF-induced survival of the cholinergic cells or whether there is a direct effect of NGF on these neurons. Moreover, although the above studies have begun to address some questions concerning the role of NGF in promoting CNS neuronal survival, it remains to be determined whether the rescued septal cholinergic neurons will degenerate if the NGF treatment is withdrawn. It also is not known whether NGF treatments alone can prolong the life of these axotomized cholinergic neurons indefinitely or whether the combined use of NGF with an embryonic neural transplant is necessary for the continued survival of these septal neurons. Further investigations are currently being conducted to address these questions.

A second major obstacle to CNS axonal regeneration is the apparent lack of a favorable CNS terrain for axonal growth in the adult. Thus, an important use for the transplantation methodology is to identify what cellular environments are necessary for facilitating axonal regeneration in vivo. Our initial studies using cultured cells have demonstrated the feasibility of bridging a CNS lesion with characterized cellular fractions previously maintained in long-term culture.[74] By taking advantage of tissue culture methodologies that allow the separation of defined cell populations, we have initiated experiments that can examine the cellular source and eventually identify the individual molecules that influence CNS regeneration in a trophic and/or tropic manner. In using Schwann cell-ECM cultures devoid of fibroblasts, we are able to demonstrate that of the numerous peripheral nerve constituents, fibroblasts are not necessary for CNS regeneration. Moreover, experiments that utilize transplants of glial-derived ECM alone reveal that axonal regrowth is not facilitated when this acellular material is used to bridge the cavity between the septum and hippocampus. When comparing these results to the prolific outgrowth obtained when Schwann cells are transplanted in conjunction with the ECM, there is a clear indication that viable Schwann cells contribute factors that promote the successful reinnervation of the host hippocampus by injured septal neurons.

How do Schwann cells influence CNS regeneration? It is obvious from the control experiments that some septal neurons are capable of sprouting after injury without the influence of PNS tissue. Although these sprouts are initiated, they are not capable of extensive elongation and are not directed to the correct target areas except in the cases where transplants containing Schwann cells are present. Furthermore, there is more extensive axonal sprouting from the injured CNS in association with transplants of viable Schwann cells. These peripheral glial cells are known to synthesize and secrete a number of molecules[84-86,88] that may exert at least two types of influence on injured CNS axons. The first type of influence might be termed a chemotactic or chemotropic influence. This would require that sprouting axons recognize and be attracted to a soluble or substrate-bound gradient extending from the transplant.

The ability of putative Schwann cell-synthesized molecules to influence regenerating CNS neurons in a chemotropic manner is most likely related to the number of Schwann cells and their distance from the axonal sprouts. Although CNS axonal sprouts are capable of traversing short distances between the intact brain and the Schwann cell-laden transplants, longer interface distances are associated with a virtual absence of fibers on the transplants. This paucity of axonal growth could be due either to the loss of a continuous mechanical pathway if endogenous CNS glia and Schwann cells do not form a continuous cellular bridge at the host-transplant interface, or to the failure of the Schwann cells to establish a chemotactic gradient over long distances replete with astrocytic processes. Whether the putative chemotactic factor is not produced in adequate quantities or cannot attach to the astrocytic strands at the host-transplant interface to form a continuous pathway conducive to axonal growth remains to be determined.

There are several good candidates for Schwann cell-secreted factors that may attract growing CNS axons. LAM is a molecule secreted by Schwann cells[44] that has repeatedly been demonstrated to promote axon growth.[43,45,47-49,89-91] Although LAM is expressed for long periods of time by astrocytes in CNS regions that exhibit the potential for regeneration in the adult,[76] astrocytes in many other CNS areas also express transient LAM immunoreactivity in reaction to trauma.[74-76] Thus, caution should be exercised in suggesting that LAM alone can promote CNS axonal regeneration because our studies show that AChE$^+$ and NFP$^+$ fibers are not associated with many LAM$^+$ areas in the traumatized CNS. Moreover, LAM$^+$ extracellular matrix transplants, derived from peripheral glia and placed in very close apposition to the injured septum, do not promote CNS axonal elongation. This scenario creates a dichotomy in that LAM suitable for axonal elongation, as demonstrated in vitro with CNS and PNS axons,[43,45,47-49,89-93] also is present in the ECM-only transplants (reference 88 and Schinstine and Cornbrooks, personal observations), yet no axons extend on these matrix transplants. Although we can not assess whether the matrix channels in the ECM transplants are compromised by their CNS hosts, it is possible that the configuration of the molecule could have been altered in the CNS environment. Earlier descriptions of neurite-promoting factors containing LAM also describe the presence of a proteoglycan that is hypothesized to configure LAM such that the tropic aspect of the molecule is accessible to the neuronal plasmalemma.[89,91] Thus it is conceivable that the proteoglycans necessary for the precise stereochemical configuration required for the tropic activity of LAM may be absent from the endogenous CNS LAM produced by most reactive astrocytes and that the LAM present in the transplanted ECM preparations, which lack Schwann cells, may be altered by the CNS milieu of the host. In this context, it is important to note that Schwann cells maintain LAM, a known neurotropic factor, on their plasmalemmae[44,94] and that Schwann cell surfaces also may act as a suitable substrate for axonal growth *in vitro.*[50,51] Thus, the correct display of a tropic factor(s) on the glial plasmalemmae and/or in the ECM may require the metabolic participation of viable Schwann cells. In order for this to occur, Schwann cells would have to maintain the critical factors in a conformation suitable to influence the growing CNS axons. Schwann cells also may contribute to the structural stability of the ECM, and the matrix may, in turn, constrain the glia, thus establishing cell-matrix channels that mechanically and tropically guide regenerating axons.

A second type of factor potentially produced by Schwann cells that may affect CNS axons in a trophic manner is NGF. As we have indicated, there is consistent evidence that NGF can rescue axotomized septal cholinergic neurons from retrograde degeneration.[57,68,69] There also is preliminary evidence that Schwann cells, orphaned from a partnership with neurons, produce or accumulate NGF.[57,95] A recent study hypothesizes that the up regulation of NGF receptors on Schwann cells in the traumatized peripheral nerve may correlate with the establishment of a gradient of NGF molecules attached to the receptors.[96] If Schwann cells secrete NGF (or other trophic molecules), this may result in the rescue of neurons in addition to those that normally survive after fornix-fimbria transection. Furthermore, since NGF increases neuronal metabolism and process formation, one would predict an increased number of axons on transplants with denser Schwann cell populations. Indeed, although this is difficult to quantitate, our general impression is that there is a direct correlation between the number of AChE$^+$ or NFP$^+$ fibers and the number of Schwann cells in the transplants. Thus, NGF may act as both a trophic and tropic factor in the present paradigm by promoting the survival of septal cholinergic neurons and providing an excellent substrate, in addition to or in combination with LAM, for the elongation of septal axons.

SUMMARY

As indicated in this review, we have begun to elucidate cellular environments and trophic factors that promote the regeneration of adult mammalian CNS neurons. In the present paradigm, bilateral aspiration lesions of the fornix-fimbria are used to axotomize septal neurons and transect the septal cholinergic projection to the dorsal hippocampus in order to evaluate 1) the influence of trophic factors, such as NGF, on neuronal survival and 2) the ability of cellular transplants of PNS tissue to promote axonal regeneration *in vivo.* Initial results demonstrate that NGF is a potent trophic molecule that prevents retrograde degeneration of septal cholinergic neurons. Observations from transplantation studies demonstrate that viable Schwann cells obtained from PNS nerve grafts or Schwann cell-ECM cultures provide a favorable cellular milieu for CNS regeneration. These cellular transplants induce a remarkable sprouting response from septal cholinergic neurons and promote the rapid elongation of septal axons that reinnervate the denervated hippocampus. In stark contrast to the Schwann cell-laden transplants, transplants including only ECM channels synthesized by cultured Schwann cells do not promote axonal regeneration within the time periods that we have examined.

Therefore, we hypothesize that viable Schwann cells are crucial for the process of regeneration because they contribute both trophic and tropic factors to the injured CNS neurons. The significant early sprouting phenomenon associated with transplants containing Schwann cells strongly suggests that soluble Schwann cell-synthesized factors induce axon elongation and possibly enhance the survival of injured septal neurons. The trophic factors probably function in a manner similar, if not identical, to the action of NGF on axotomized septal neurons. Moreover, Schwann cells appear to provide tropic signals, such as LAM or a LAM-NGF complex, that can act, when in the proper stereoconfiguration, to promote the elongation and orientation of regenerating axons. Thus, our current data indicate that in order to promote optimal axonal regeneration from injured CNS neurons, both trophic and tropic factors must be supplied from exogenous sources.

ACKNOWLEDGMENTS

The authors wish to thank Robin Kleiman, Tim Neuberger, and J. Scott McDonald for their valuable assistance in several of the experiments.

REFERENCES

1. RAMON Y CAJAL, S. 1982. Degeneration and Regeneration in the Nervous System. Vols. 1 & 2. Hafner. New York, NY.
2. GUTH, L. 1956. Physiol. Rev. 36: 441-478.
3. GUTH, L. 1975. Exp. Neurol. 48: 3-15.
4. PURCHALA, E. & W. F. WINDLE. 1977. Exp. Neurol. 55: 1-42.
5. VERAA, R. P. & B. GRAFSTEIN. 1981. Exp. Neurol. 71: 6-75.
6. RAISMAN, G. & P. M. FIELD. 1973. Brain Res. 50: 241-264.
7. COTMAN, C. W. & G. S. LYNCH. 1976. In Neuronal Recognition. S. H. Barondes, Ed.: 69-108. Chapman & Hall. London.
8. BARON, K. D. 1983. In Spinal Cord Reconstruction. C. C. Kao, R. P. Bunge & P. J. Reier, Eds.: 7-40. Raven Press. New York, NY.
9. JAKOBY, R. K., C. C. TURBES & L. W. FREEMAN. 1960. J. Neurosurg. 17: 385-393.
10. KAO, C. C. 1974. Exp. Neurol. 44: 424-439.
11. BJÖRKLUND, A. & U. STENEVI. 1979. Physiol. Rev. 59: 62-100.
12. RICHARDSON, P. M., U. M. McGUINNESS & A. J. AGUAYO. 1980. Nature 284: 264-265.
13. DAVID, S. & A. J. AGUAYO. 1981. Science 214: 931-933.
14. BJÖRKLUND, A., U. STENEVI & N. A. SVENDGAARD. 1976. Nature. 262: 787-790.
15. STENEVI, U., A. BJÖRKLUND & N. A. SVENDGAARD. 1976. Brain Res. 114: 1-20.
16. LUND, R. D. & S. D. HAUSCHKA. 1976. Science 193: 582-584.
17. KROMER, L. F., A. BJÖRKLUND & U. STENEVI. 1979. Science 204: 1117-1119.
18. KROMER, L. F., A. BJÖRKLUND & U. STENEVI. 1981. Brain Res. 210: 153-171.
19. KROMER, L. F., A. BJÖRKLUND & U. STENEVI. 1981. Brain Res. 210: 173-200.
20. LEWIS, E. R., J. C. MUELLER & C. W. COTMAN. 1980. Brain Res. Bull. 5: 217-221.
21. SINGER, M., R. H. NORDLANDER & M. EGAR. 1979. J. Comp. Neurol. 185: 1-22.
22. WEISS, P. 1955. In Analysis of Development. B. H. Willier, P. Weiss & V. Hamberger, Eds.: 346-401. Saunders. Philadelphia, PA.
23. SPERRY, R. W. 1963. Proc. Natl. Acad. Sci. USA 50: 703-710.
24. SATINSKY, D., F. A. PEPE & C. N. LIU. 1964. Exp. Neurol. 9: 441-451.
25. LUNDBORG, G., L. B. DAHLIN, N. DANIELSEN, R. H. GELBERMAN, F. M. LONGO, H. C. POWELL & S. VARON. 1982. Exp. Neurol. 76: 361-375.
26. POLITIS, M. J., K. EDERLE & P. S. SPENCER. 1982. Brain Res. 253: 1-12.
27. LONGO, F. M., S. D. SKAPER, M. MANTHORPE, L. R. WILLIAMS, G. LUNDBORG & S. VARON. 1983. Exp. Neurol. 81: 756-769.

28. VARON, S. & R. BUNGE. 1978. Annu. Rev. Neurosci. 1: 327-361.
29. VARON, S. & R. ADLER. 1980. Curr. Top. Dev. Biol. 16: 207-252.
30. THOENEN, H. & Y.-A. BARDE. 1980. Physiol. Rev. 60: 1284-1335.
31. PEREZ-POLO, J. R. 1985. In Cell Culture in the Neurosciences. J. E. Bottenstein & G. Sato, Eds.: 95-123. Plenum. New York, NY.
32. ADLER, R. & S. VARON. 1980. Brain Res. 188: 437-448.
33. EBENDAL, T., L. OLSON, A. SEIGER & K. O. HEDLUND. 1980. Nature 286: 25-28.
34. SCHONFELD, A. R., L. J. THAL, S. G. HOROWITZ & R. KATZMAN. 1981. Brain Res. 229: 541-546.
35. RIOPELLE, R. J., R. J. BOEGMAN & D. A. CAMERON. 1981. Neurosci. Lett. 25: 311-316.
36. MULLER, H. W. & W. SEIFERT. 1982. J. Neurosci. Res. 8: 195-204.
37. HONEGGER, P. & D. LENOIR. 1982. Dev. Brain Res. 3: 229-238.
38. BARDE, Y.-A., D. EGAR & H. THOENEN. 1982. EMBO J. 1: 549-553.
39. OJIKA, K. & S. H. APPEL. 1984. Proc. Natl. Acad. Sci. USA 81: 2567-2571.
40. COTMAN, C. W. & M. NIETO-SAMPEDRO. 1985. Ann. N. Y. Acad. Sci. 457: 83-104.
41. COLLINS, F. & K. A. CRUTCHER. 1985. J. Neurosci. 5: 2809-2814.
42. LETOURNEAU, P. C. 1979. Exp. Cell Res. 124: 127-134.
43. MANTHORPE, M., E. ENGVALL, E. RUOSLAHTI, F. M. LONGO, G. E. DAVIS & S. VARON. 1983. J. Cell Biol. 97: 1882-1890.
44. CORNBROOKS, C. J., D. J. CAREY, J. A. MCDONALD, R. TIMPL & R. P. BUNGE. 1983. Proc. Natl. Acad. Sci. USA 80: 3850-3854.
45. BARON VAN EVERCOOREN, A. B., H. K. KLEINMAN, S. OHNO, P. MARANGOS, J. P. SCHWARTZ & M. E. DUBOIS-DALCQ. 1982. J. Neurosci. Res. 8: 179-194.
46. CARBONETTO, S., M. M. GRUVER & D. C. TURNER. 1983. J. Neurosci. 3: 2324-2335.
47. ROGERS, S. L., P. C. LETOURNEAU, S. L. PALM, J. MCCARTHY & L. T. FURCHT. 1983. Dev. Biol. 98: 212-220.
48. ROGERS, S. L., J. B. MCCARTHY, S. L. PALM, L. T. FURCHT & P. C. LETOURNEAU. 1985. J. Neurosci. 5: 369-378.
49. SMALHEISER, N. R., S. M. CRAIN & L. M. REID. 1984. Dev. Brain Res. 12: 136-140.
50. NOBLE, M., J. FOK-SEANG & T. COHEN. 1984. J. Neurosci. 4: 1892-1903.
51. FALLON, J. R. 1985. J. Cell Biol. 100: 198-207.
52. LEVI-MONTALCINI, R. & V. HAMBURGER. 1951. J. Exp. Zool. 116: 321-361.
53. LANDMESSER, L. & G. POLAR. 1978. Fed. Proc. 37: 2016-2022.
54. HEFTI, F. 1983. Ann. Neurol. 13: 109-110.
55. YOSHIDA, K., S. KOHSAKA, T. IDEI, S. NII, M. OTANI, S. TOYA & Y. TSUKADA. 1986. Neurosci. Lett. 66: 181-186.
56. GAGE, F. H., A. BJÖRKLUND & U. STENEVI. 1984. Nature 308: 637-639.
57. TANIUCHI, M., J. B. SCHWEITZER & E. M. JOHNSON, JR. 1986. Proc. Natl. Acad. Sci. USA 83: 1950-1954.
58. SCHWAB, M. E., U. OTTEN, Y. AGID & H. THOENEN. 1979. Brain Res. 168: 473-483.
59. SEILER, M. & M. E. SCHWAB. 1984. Brain Res. 300: 33-39.
60. KORSCHING, S., G. AUBURGER, R. HEUMANN, J. SCOTT & H. THOENEN. 1985. EMBO J. 4: 1389-1393.
61. SHELTON, D. L. & L. F. REICHARDT. 1986. Proc. Natl. Acad. Sci. USA 83: 2714-2718.
62. KORSCHING, S., R. HEUMANN, H. THOENEN & F. HEFTI. 1986. Neurosci. Lett. 66: 175-180.
63. GNAHN, H., F. HEFTI, R. HEUMANN, M. E. SCHWAB & H. THOENEN. 1983. Dev. Brain Res. 9: 45-52.
64. HEFTI, F., A. DRAVID & J. HARTIKKA. 1984. Brain Res. 293: 305-311.
65. HEFTI, F., J. HARTIKKA, F. ECKENSTEIN, H. GNAHN, R. HEUMANN & M. SCHWAB. 1985. Neuroscience 14: 55-68.
66. HEFTI, F. 1985. Soc. Neurosci. Abstr. 11: 660.
67. DAITZ, H. M. & T. P. S. POWELL. 1954. J. Neurol. Neurosurg. Psychiatry 17: 75-82.
68. KROMER, L. F. 1987. Science 235: 214-216.
69. KROMER, L. F. 1986. Soc. Neurosci. Abstr. 12: 983.
70. RICHARDSON, P. M., U. M. MCGUINNESS & A. J. AGUAYO. 1982. Brain Res. 237: 147-162.
71. WENDT, J. S., G. E. FAGG & C. W. COTMAN. 1983. Exp. Neurol. 79: 452-461.
72. TSUJI, S. 1974. Histochemistry 42: 99-110.

73. TIMPL, R., H. ROHDE, P. GEHRON-ROBEY, S. I. RENNARD, J. M. FOIDART & G. R. MARTIN. 1979. J. Biol. Chem. **254**: 9933-9937.
74. KROMER, L. F. & C. J. CORNBROOKS. 1985. Proc. Natl. Acad. Sci. USA **82**: 6330-6334.
75. LIESI, P., S. KAAKKOLA, D. DAHL & A. VEHERI. 1984. EMBO J. **3**: 683-686.
76. LIESI, P. 1985. EMBO J. **4**: 2505-2511.
77. ENG, L. F. 1980. *In* Proteins of the Nervous System. R. A. Bradshaw & D. M. Schneider, Eds.: 85-117. Raven Press. New York, NY.
78. JESSEN, K. R. & R. MIRSKY. 1984. J. Neurocytol. **13**: 923-934.
79. CORNBROOKS, C. J. & R. P. BUNGE. 1982. Am. Soc. Neurochem. Abstr. **13**: 171.
80. WOOD, P. 1976. Brain Res. **115**: 361-375.
81. UITTO, J. & J. J. JEFFREY. 1980. J. Cell Biol. **84**: 184-202.
82. BUNGE, M. B., A. K. WILLIAMS & P. M. WOOD. 1982. Dev. Biol. **92**: 449-460.
83. CORNBROOKS, C. J. & L. F. KROMER. 1986. Soc. Neurosci. Abstr. **12**: 697.
84. CAREY, D. J., C. F. ELDRIDGE, C. J. CORNBROOKS, R. TIMPL & R. P. BUNGE. 1983. J. Cell Biol. **97**: 473-479.
85. CORNBROOKS, C. J. 1983. Soc. Neurosci. Abstr. **9**: 346.
86. ELDRIDGE, C. F., J. R. SANES, A. Y. CHIU, R. P. BUNGE & C. J. CORNBROOKS. 1986. J. Neurocytol. In press.
87. CORNBROOKS, C. J. 1985. Soc. Neurosci. Abstr. **11**: 175.
88. CAREY, D. J. & R. P. BUNGE. 1981. J. Cell Biol. **91**: 666-672.
89. LANDER, A. D., D. K. FUJII & L. F. REICHARDT. 1985. J. Cell Biol. **101**: 898-913.
90. ADLER, R., J. JERDAN & A. HEWITT. 1985. Dev. Biol. **112**: 100-114.
91. DAVIS, G. E., S. VARON, E. ENGVALL & M. MANTHORPE. 1985. Trends Neurosci. **8**: 528-532.
92. IDE, C., K. TOHYAMA, R. YOKOTA, T. NITATORI & S. ONODERA. 1983. Brain Res. **288**: 61-75.
93. SCHWAB, M. E. & H. THOENEN. 1985. J. Neurosci. **5**: 2415-2423.
94. BIGNAMI, A., N. H. CHI & D. DAHL. 1984. J. Neuropathol. Exp. Neurol. **43**: 94-103.
95. ASSOULINE, J., E. P. BOSCH, R. LIM, R. JENSEN & N. J. PANTAZIS. 1985. Soc. Neurosci. Abstr. **11**: 933.
96. TANIVCHI, M., H. B. CLARK & E. M. JOHNSON. 1986. Proc. Natl. Acad. Sci. USA **83**: 4094-4098.

DISCUSSION OF THE PAPER

F. H. GAGE (*University of California, La Jolla, CA*): How do you know you are really getting cell death and survival and not just enzyme suppression and subsequent increase in ChAT activity? I believe in your results, but you have not discussed the bilateral effect.

KROMER: They are bilateral lesions, so we can look at all the cells that survive in the septum. You can count the magnocellular neurons that are left, and this count would correlate very nicely with the number of ChAT$^+$ cells. So there is a survival of magnocellular neurons in the medial septum after NGF treatment, and these neurons would normally die without the NGF. So, regardless of determining what the transmitter is for these cells, just looking at the number of cells using Nissl stains indicates there is an increased number of magnocellular neurons in this region.

S. McLOON (*University of Minnesota, Minneapolis, MN*): Do your septal neurites grow on a collagen substrate in culture?

KROMER: They do.

McLOON: Does it not seem strange that they would not grow on a collagen substrate when transplanted?

KROMER: No, not to me anyway. I think that in culture cells quite often are sending out processes because there are no other competing cells. This *in vitro* situation results in extensive neurite growth on the collagen. When we transplant a collagen substrate, cells in the CNS of the recipient may bind any factors in the collagen that neurites may be able to meagerly cling to in culture and very slowly grow on. Neurite outgrowth in culture on collagen is not very exciting. With all these other CNS cells growing out on the collagen transplants *in vivo,* slowly regenerating axons may never get a chance to grow out on the collagen. The same is true for the ECM. There is a lot of cell migration from the host CNS around the ECM, and the axons may grow too slowly to reach it before the other cells have got there. The active sites for neurite binding, therefore, may be lost before the axons reach the ECM.

But with Schwann cells present in these ECM tubes that does not occur, and you get robust rapid growth of axons. It suggests to us that the Schwann cells are providing either a soluble factor such as NGF or some cell-surface-bound factor, or are preventing degradation or producing basal lamina components that the axons can then find. Indeed, there may be a slight decrease in the amount of laminin staining with long-term survival of these ECM transplants. And so there may be some degradation of laminin occurring by these other CNS cells that are migrating out on the substrates.

McLOON: Is the other still migrating in?

KROMER: We are beginning to use antibodies for staining the different cell types so that we can identify leptomeningeal cells. There are also many endothelial cells that are present around the transplants. And it is known that endothelial cells do break down basal lamina.

J. M. GORELL (*Henry Ford Hospital, Detroit, MI*): How much NGF do you need, and what is the time course for infusion? Is there a critical period of responsivity? Have you measured NGF in a situation in which Schwann cells are provided?

KROMER: At this stage, we do not know how soon we have to give NGF after the lesion. I should reemphasize that these cholinergic cells appear to have NGF receptors on them, so it is likely that not all cells are going to respond to NGF, just cells that normally have receptors to NGF.

GORELL: How much have you used to get this exuberant response you have shown?

KROMER: In these studies I have used Alzet minipumps with a 2-week delivery time. It delivers about 10 microliters of NGF per week, which is a heavy dose, at a constant infusion of about 0.4 microliters per hour. The concentration is 250 nanograms per microliter. The dose is very large just to see if there is any cell survival.

D. STEIN (*Clark University, Worcester, MA*): I just want to make a comment that supports some of your findings. Several years ago, Bruno Will and I injected intra-ventricularly about 125 BUs of NGF and found that if you test the animals after fornix-fimbria, hippocampal, or entorhinal cortex lesions, following a single injection of NGF you can get significant sparing of function on both spatial alternation tests as well as on radial maze performance. These results do basically support your anatomical data. At the time we did not have a specific notion of what cells are spared. Still, our behavioral work does correlate very nicely with your anatomical findings.

We also found that if you waited up to 4 hr after the lesions that you did not get any of the beneficial behavioral consequences. This might be something to take into consideration in your experiments.

Summary

S. M. CRAIN (*Albert Einstein School of Medicine, New York, NY*): I will not attempt a serious summary here, but I would like to emphasize the power of the methods that have been presented—particularly with respect to systematic attempts to coordinate transplantation techniques together with analytical tissue and cell culture techniques. These experimental methods have greatly stimulated and accelerated the development of brain transplantation studies.

During the previous decade, tissue culture prototypes were developed for many of the techniques that have now been applied so dramatically in transplantation studies within adult organisms. The neurons in tissue cultures of fetal spinal cord and brain explants survived, matured, and developed functional and structural integrity so successfully that the *in vitro* studies encouraged and, in some respects, guided the recent transplantion studies in animals. The work done by Dr. Levi-Montalcini, who demonstrated the importance of nerve growth factor, provides a good example. Her studies were carried out in tissue culture systems with chick embryo dorsal root ganglia and sympathetic ganglia. The development of those pioneering experiments in the 50s have now reached a dramatic climax in the recent plethora of demonstrations that the nerve growth factor is probably playing a crucial role in the development of many types of central nervous system neurons, as well as peripheral ganglion neurons.

The cross-fertilization between these two fields—brain transplantation *in vivo* and brain explantation *in vitro*—is becoming increasingly fruitful, and I think we will hear a lot more about this as the symposium continues.

Transplantation of Retina and Visual Cortex to Rat Brains of Different Ages

Maturation, Connection Patterns, and Immunological Consequences[a]

RAYMOND D. LUND,[b] KANCHAN RAO,[b]
MARK H. HANKIN,[b] HEINZ W. KUNZ,[c] AND
THOMAS J. GILL III[c]

[b]Department of Neurobiology, Anatomy, and Cell Science

and

[c]Department of Pathology
University of Pittsburgh School of Medicine
Pittsburgh, Pennsylvania 15261

INTRODUCTION

There are several fundamental questions that underlie any study of the developing visual system. These include the following: why optic axons normally grow to the right places in the brain; why, when they have reached their targets, they stop growing; why, at a particular stage of development, more than half of the ganglion cells die[1,2]; and why regeneration after injury is not a normal property of the mature optic axon.[3,4]

There are many ways to approach these questions, but one important technique we have used over the past 10 years has been to transplant regions of the developing visual system from rat or mouse embryos into different locations in host rats of a variety of ages.[5-7] The subsequent maturation of the transplants and the development of interconnections between transplant and host are then studied to see how these are affected by the new environment with which the transplanted cells are confronted.

In this review, we will focus on two sets of transplant studies. The first set will examine how retinae mature when placed in newborn rat brains at different distances from their normal target regions and how this maturation is affected by transplanting tissue to adult recipients. The second group of transplant studies examines the immunological consequences of placing embryonic mouse neural tissue in rat brains of different ages. While it was originally thought that the brain is an immunologically

[a]This work was supported by Grants EY05283, NS07817, and CA18659 from the National Institutes of Health and by a grant from the Samuel and Emma Winters Foundation.

227

privileged site that could accept allografts without rejection,[8-11] current literature suggests that this is not altogether correct.[12-14] There is, however, considerable ambiguity with regard to survival of both allografts[15,16] and xenografts.[17-22] Therefore, it is important to conduct a comprehensive series of experiments to examine the effects of transplant location and condition (dissociated or solid), host age, and immunogenetics of host and donor on transplant rejection. In this report, work involving xenografts of dissociated mouse cortical cells to rat cortex and of mouse retinae to the midbrain of neonatal rats will be discussed together with preliminary experiments involving allografts.

Retinal Transplants

The first part of this study is focused on how retinae taken largely from mouse embryos of gestational age E12 and E13 survive after transplantation into neonatal rats and how similar transplants placed in adult rats fare.

Transplants Placed in Neonatal Hosts

All transplants differentiated according to a timetable dictated by the donor age rather than that of the host. If the lens was transplanted with the retina, the eye cup formed relatively normally with considerable lengths of apparently normal retina, and only small areas of rosette formation. If the lens was removed, more of the retina generally became folded into rosettes (FIG. 1A).

Detailed examination of mature retinal transplants showed that all the normal cell and plexiform layers were present.[23] Outer segments were clearly differentiated, and, with the electron microscope, they were seen as poorly organized stacks of membrane. Cell types unique to each layer could be recognized, and it was apparent, at least for transplants placed close to the superior colliculus, that there was a diversity of ganglion cell types which compared with that seen normally.[24] In silver stains of such transplants, a distinct optic fiber layer containing bundles of ganglion cell axons was seen. In contrast to normal retina, these axons most often left the transplants in a series of axon bundles rather than in a single optic nerve. In cases in which a single nerve was encountered, we counted the number of axons in it and found slightly less than 10 000[25] compared with about 120 000 in the normal rat optic nerve.[26]

Transplants placed close to the superior colliculus innervated both the colliculus and the more rostrally located visual centers. If one eye was removed from the recipient at birth, the transplant innervation to the denervated tectum was heavier, invading the whole stratum griseum superficiale with a density of innervation comparable to that of the normal crossed optic pathway.[27] Projections could also be traced to pretectum, dorsal lateral geniculate nucleus, and nuclei of the accessory optic tract. Within the superior colliculus, the transplant axons formed synaptic patterns that closely resembled those of optic axons in the normal superior colliculus. Physiological studies showed not only that transplants responded to light, but that light-triggered units could be recorded in the superior colliculus.[28] The responses were quite specific, some units responding transiently to light "on" or "off" whereas others responded to illumination by a cessation of spontaneous activity. Attempts to label small focal areas

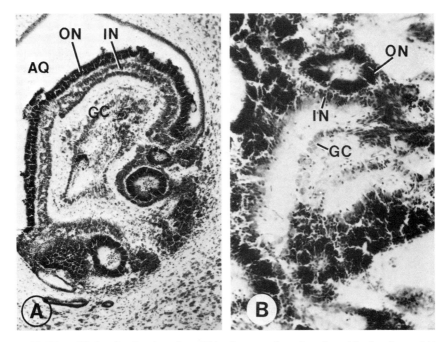

FIGURE 1. Nissl stain of retinae from E13 mice transplanted to the midbrain of rats. (A) Retina 1 month after transplantation to the aqueduct (AQ) of a newborn rat. (B) Retina 2 months after transplantation to the tectum of an adult rat with cyclosporin A treatment. The normal retinal laminae can be recognized. ON: outer nuclear layer; IN: inner nuclear layer; GC: ganglion cell layer. Magnifications for **A** and **B**: ×60 and ×149, respectively.

of ganglion cells in transplants by local injections of horseradish peroxidase or other labels in the tectum have failed (Rao and Lund, unpublished results), raising the possibility that, although many aspects of specificity of connections between retina and tectum were preserved after transplantation, topographic specificity may not be.

We were next interested in examining how retinae placed at a distance from the superior colliculus survived, and whether outgrowing axons would be directed toward the tectum. The first set of studies showed that retina placed over the inferior colliculus emitted axons that ran rostrally to enter the superior colliculus.[29] There was an indication that the earliest outgrowth was also directed.[30] Retinae placed over the cerebellum[7] or in the spinal cord[31] differentiated to form the normal laminae, but failed to maintain ganglion cells or optic fibers and did not sustain ingrowth into the adjacent host neuropil. Whether there was transient ingrowth that later disappeared was not investigated. This was studied in more detail for retinae transplanted from E12 mice to neonatal rat cortices (Perry and Lund, unpublished results). Such transplants differentiated by a normal timetable, including the timing of a sequence of cell death from the ganglion cell to the receptor layer. Somewhat surprisingly, ganglion cells survived for at least 4 weeks after transplantation, and there was evidence of an optic fiber layer within the retina. Using a series of antibodies specific to mouse neuronal cell surface proteins, however, there was no clear indication of axonal outgrowth into the host brain. A loss of ganglion cells was seen in similar studies in which E13 rat retinae were transplanted to neonatal rat cortex and allowed to survive for 2 months.[32]

In another study we transplanted mouse or rat retinae deeper in the midbrain adjacent to the aqueduct.[33] Using silver stains and, in the case of mouse transplants, species-specific labels, we found that at the earliest time they were identifiable, optic axons grew dorsally toward the tectum, which had been deprived of most of its optic input by unilateral eye removal at birth. There was no indication of transient ventral outgrowth from the transplant or of outgrowth on the surface of the aqueduct. Cortical transplants placed in the same location had a more broadly distributed outgrowth. It appears, therefore, that transplanted retinae placed in maturing brains have the capacity to direct axonal outgrowth toward an appropriate target region as long as the distance between transplant and target is not too great, or there are appropriate channels to permit such growth, or both. This will be discussed further.

Transplants Placed in Adult Rats

Retinae transplanted to adult hosts have been studied in somewhat less detail. In an earlier study involving transplantation between embryos and adults of a closed Sprague-Dawley colony, transplants placed over the tectum did not differentiate as well as transplants to neonatal hosts, and ingrowth into the adjacent host tectum was very limited even when the host eye innervating that tectum had been removed at the time of transplantation.[34] In more recent work, we have transplanted mouse retinae into the tectum of adult Sprague-Dawley rats and allowed them to survive for periods of 1-4 weeks. Cyclosporin A was administered daily (10 mg/kg body weight) from 1 day before transplantation to the time of sacrifice. The transplants were well integrated with the host brain, and although they tended to show more evidence of rosette formation than similar transplants to neonates, they developed a more robust laminar structure than in the previous study (FIG. 1B). In fiber preparations, a clearly defined optic fiber layer was seen, and, in some animals, there was a substantial ingrowth of axons to the host tectum (FIG. 2B). This differed from the ingrowth when using neonatal hosts in that the axons were grouped into small bundles, which appeared to run parallel to blood vessels coursing through the tectum from the surface. Mouse-specific antibody staining confirmed the identity of these axons as being of retinal origin (FIG. 2A). It has yet to be determined whether these axons make the same synaptic connections as are made from transplants placed in neonates. Thus, these studies on transplants to adults suggest that there is substantial ingrowth of retinal transplant axons into the host and that these transplant axons into hosts, as with transplants into neonates, exhibit a highly specific distribution.

Immunological Consequences of Cross-species Transplantation

The second issue raised in this paper is that of immunological incompatibility, which may lead to graft rejection or at least limitation in the degree of integration of graft and host tissues. The results reported here are centered around the development of immunological tolerance in the immature rat to embryonic mouse cerebral cortical cells that were dissociated and injected with minimal trauma into the occipital cortex

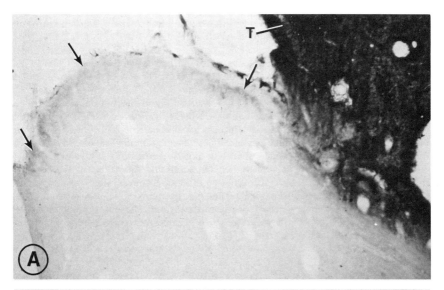

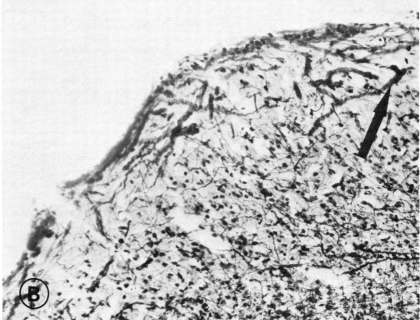

FIGURE 2. Mouse retina transplanted to the rostral part of the superior colliculus of an adult rat from which the host eye innervating that colliculus has been removed at the time of transplantation. (**A**) A mouse neuron-specific antibody, M6, demonstrating the transplant (T) and the projection from it to the host superior colliculus (arrows). This is a sagittal section, rostral to the right. (**B**) Detail of adjacent section stained for normal axons in the caudal part of the superior colliculus. Note the bundles of axons, one indicated by an arrow, which would not normally be present and are attributable to transplant ganglion cell outgrowth. Magnifications for **A** and **B**: ×67 and ×228, respectively.

of the recipients, and the stability of mouse retinal transplants placed in rat brains before the development of immunological competence.

Cortex was taken from embryonic mice of gestational age E14 and dissociated in Ca^{2+}- and Mg^{2+}-free medium. The cells were checked for density and viability and then concentrated to about 350 000-400 000 cells/ml. They were allowed to initiate aggregration, and then 0.5-1.0 μl of fluid was injected into the cortex of rats aged 0, 8, 12, 16, and 20 days and 8-12 weeks. Care was taken not to damage any major vessels on the surface of the cortex, and very little bleeding occurred as a result of the injection procedure. Despite these precautions, there must inevitably have been interruption of the blood-brain barrier. In addition, the surface of the brain was flushed with saline to remove cells that may have leaked from the injection site.

Survival of the graft cells was studied by examining the brains of the recipient rats at various ages 9-47 days after transplantation, using a variety of histological techniques. Transplants placed in rats at 0 and 8 days postnatal matured and integrated well with the host nervous system. At early survival times, the cell bodies were packed together, but, with longer survival times, they became more dispersed as a network of neural processes developed between them. In Nissl preparations, a diversity of cell shapes and sizes was seen (FIG. 3A), and, in silver stains, a rich axon plexus was noted, some of which appeared to be axons of host origin coursing through the transplant. Other axons were clearly of intrinsic origin and could, on rare occasions, be traced to large pyramidal neurons. Sections stained with a mouse-specific antibody to a neuronal cell surface glycoprotein, M6,[35] showed the transplants to be clearly differentiated from the adjacent host tissue with no evidence of cell mixing with host neurons.

For those transplants lying in and adjacent to the white matter, large axon bundles were seen entering the corpus callosum crossing to the opposite site of the brain (FIG. 3C), as well as running laterally into the internal capsule. Connections were more limited for transplants located superficially in the cortex, although these also differentiated to a stage where, in Nissl preparations, it was difficult to distinguish transplant and host cells without the aid of the species-specific antibody.

Transplants placed in 12-, 16-, and 20-day-old rats could be clearly identified 9 days later. They were, however, obviously infiltrated with macrophages and lymphocytes (FIG. 3B), the latter being clustered around blood vessels. The severity of the response varied among individuals, and there was quantitative variation in the response: smaller transplants showed significantly less lymphocytic infiltration than large ones. In silver-stained preparations, coarse fiber bundles were seen crossing the transplants, but the only fibers intrinsic to the transplants were extremely fine and appeared beaded in some cases. Antibody stains failed to show projections from these transplants. With longer survival, the transplants became totally infiltrated with lymphocytes and macrophages, and their internal organization became completely obscured.

Transplants placed in adults were invariably in an advanced state of rejection within a week of transplantation. If the animals were treated with cyclosporin A, however, transplants survived for months, as indicated for the retinal transplants, described in the previous section. Thus it appears that while xenografts from mouse to rat survive if placed in the brain during the first postnatal week, they elicit an immune response if transplanted when the host is 12 days of age or older. This is in contrast to allografts made between rat strains, where transplants to mature hosts can survive for long periods. We have found that embryonic cerebral cortex taken from donors of the inbred DA strain of rats and placed in the cerebral cortex of BN strain recipients as solid transplants will survive for at least 1 month without signs of rejection and without detection of a serum antibody response to DA major histocompatibility complex (MHC) antigens. These two strains differ in both MHC and non-MHC antigens. Similar survival was found using DA.BN donors and BN recipients, which

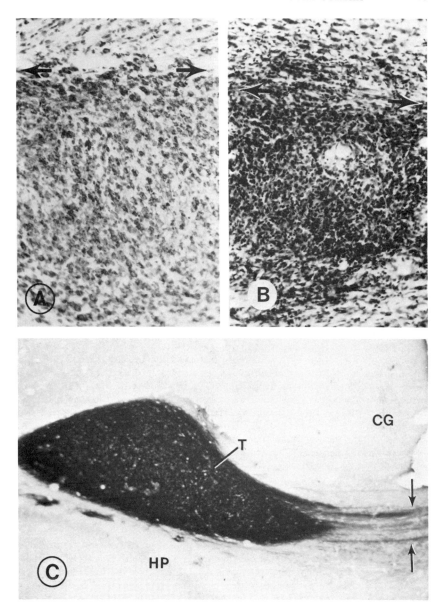

FIGURE 3. Dissociated cells from E14 mouse cortex injected into the fiber layer underlying the cortex of rats. (A) Nissl stain of transplant placed in 8-day-old rat and allowed to survive for 16 days. The arrows mark the dorsal border of the transplant. (B) Nissl stain of a similar-sized transplant injected into the rat at 16 days postnatal with 15 days survival. The dark appearance is the result of a massive invasion of lymphocytes. The arrows mark the dorsal boundary of the transplant. (C) Transplant placed in 8-day-old rat and allowed to survive for 31 days. The mouse-specific antibody staining shows axon bundles leaving the transplant to enter the corpus callosum (arrows). T: Transplant; CG: cingulate cortex; HP: hippocampus. Magnifications for **A** and **B** and for **C**: ×139 and ×67, respectively.

differ only in non-MHC antigens. Comparable transplants (from DA donor to BN recipients) placed through the atlanto-occipital membrane into the fourth ventricle showed signs of rejection within 3 weeks after transplantation, and elicited an antibody response to DA MHC antigens (average titer: 1:128). Since there was no bleeding associated with the introduction of the transplant and the positive pressure of cerebrospinal fluid would have limited invasion of mesodermal cells into the ventricle during the short period during which the membrane remained patent, it would seem unlikely that opening of the blood-brain barrier was the cause of the rejection reaction.

One critical question may be raised: Are the xenografts placed in neonatal rats stable? In our studies involving transplantation of mouse retina to the midbrain of neonatal rats, some grafts survived for as long as 1 year after transplantation. It is not practical to compare survival rates with previous rat-to-rat transplants because there are so many variables, including minor differences in technique attributable to different investigators. Still, although most of the transplants surviving for the longest times appeared perfectly normal and made appropriate connections with the host brain, one-fifth of the transplants showed indication of lymphocyte infiltration, with occasional ones showing an advanced immune rejection response as long as 18 weeks after transplantation. Similar destruction was extremely rare, and immune rejection was not seen in comparable transplants of rat retinae placed in rat brains. Since such destruction was relatively uncommon, we proposed that it results from events external to the transplantation process. For example, extraneously introduced antigens may have provoked a rejection reaction of the donor tissue. This hypothesis was tested by deliberately placing a provoking tissue—mouse skin—on the abdomen of mature rats that at birth had received retinal transplants in the brain. The skin graft showed signs of rejection 3 days after being placed on the host. After a further 3 days, the animals were sacrificed and their brains examined histologically. In each case studied, there was a profound rejection reaction in progress, and only the general outline of the retina was visible (FIG. 4A). Large numbers of lymphocytes were evident in the transplants and in the adjacent host brain, with notable concentrations around blood vessels (FIG. 4B). At this survival time, the transplants still retained a projection to the host superior colliculus (FIG. 4C). Thus, it appears that the neonatal rat was not sensitized by the mouse retinal transplant and that the effector arm of the immune response was not activated. The skin transplant in adult life did that.

DISCUSSION

The studies described here show that retina transplanted from fetal rat or mouse to the midbrain of neonatal rats survives and matures on a relatively normal timetable. Many of the features of normal retina, including gross potential responses to light flashes, are found in these transplanted retinae. The projections from the transplants to the host brain are limited to regions that normally receive optic input, and these projections are capable of transmitting precise functional information. This degree of specificity is achieved even though the transplant axons enter the host by a route quite different from that followed by normal optic axons and even though the donor and host are not age matched. Retinae placed on the dorsal surface of the midbrain send axons across the surface of the brainstem to enter the superior colliculus, in contrast to either cortical[36] or tectal[7] transplants, whose axons grow deep into the midbrain tegmentum. Since normal developing optic axons also grow on the surface of the brain,[37-41] an essential property of these axons may be that their growth follows substrates present on the surface of the brain such as the basal lamina or the glial

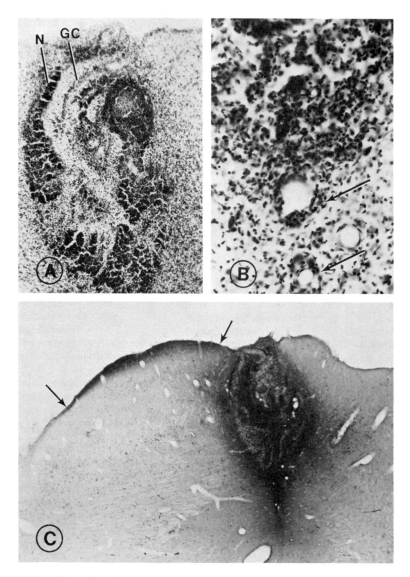

FIGURE 4. Coronal sections of mouse retinal transplant in the superior colliculus of 5-week-old rat. The E13 retina was placed in the colliculus on postnatal day 1. After a survival of 1 month, a mouse skin graft was placed on the abdomen. The animal was fixed 6 days later. (**A**) Nissl stain of retina. Note massive infiltration of lymphocytes into transplant. This infiltration largely obscures normal lamination. Control tissue would appear as in **A**. GC: ganglion cell layer; N: nuclear layers. (**B**) Detail of a ventral region of the transplant shown in FIGURE 1 to show cellular infiltration and the concentration of these cells around blood vessels (arrows). (**C**) Low-power view of section adjacent to that shown in **A**, stained for a mouse-specific antibody M4. Although there is nonspecific staining by secondary antibody around the transplant, there is also specific staining showing a projection from the transplant to the superior colliculus between the arrows on the left, but not on the right of the transplant. Magnifications for **A**, **B**, and **C**: ×53, ×203, and ×32, respectively.

end feet.[40] Indeed, many of these studies of early development suggest that optic axon growth is a passive process that follows a relatively nonspecific channel and is not obviously target directed, and this is followed by secondary process of error elimination by which axons that have failed to reach the right place are removed.[42,43] Thus, once axons enter the optic stalk, they are to some extent confined by the cells in the stalk, and this may be important for their subsequent distribution. At the optic chiasm, although many axons enter the appropriate optic tract, some grow into the opposite optic nerve[39-44] whereas others enter the wrong side of the brain.[39,45] Some axons enter the wrong brain region,[39,46] and some of those forming terminal arbors in the appropriate region may, nevertheless, project to the inappropriate part of the topographic representation of the retina on the brain region.[47] In rats and mice, there is an ordered sequence of cell death in the retina, during which time the anomalous projections are lost.[43,48,49]

The studies in which retinae were placed deep in the midbrain[33] suggest first that optic axons can grow on substrates other than those present on the surface of the brain and second that their growth may be directed specifically toward an appropriate target region, rather than passively following particular substrates to a target, where they then ramify a terminal arbor.

At the time that axons grow out from the transplants, radial glia are still present in the midbrain, and it is possible that these cells and the glial band occurring at the midline provide the necessary substrate for growth. It is known that tectal tissue contains factors that prolong the survival of retinal ganglion cells in vitro,[50,51] and it is possible that, like nerve growth factor (NGF),[52] these could also have a neurotropic role. One point of possible significance is that in previous studies, in which eyes of immature rats were injected with horseradish peroxidase, the enzyme was detected not only in the terminal regions of optic axons but in cell bodies lining the aqueduct below those regions.[39] Thus radial glia may be capable of transporting a variety of extracellular molecules from the surface of the tectum toward the aqueduct. If a retinal ganglion cell-sustaining factor is among these, it is possible that axons of retinal transplants are responding to a concentration gradient of such a substance, much as axons of the peripheral nervous system grow along an NGF concentration gradient in vitro,[52,53] and that such a factor directs their growth to the tectal surface.

A second point emerges from the experiments in which retina was placed in cortex. The sequence of cell death from ganglion cells to receptor cells occurred on a normal timetable indicating that it is an intrinsic property of the retinal cells and not the result of a global event such as an endocrine change in the animal and that it is not initiated by interactions between ganglion cells and their terminals. Somewhat surprisingly, unlike in vitro studies of similar design,[51] cell death in the ganglion cell layer in the absence of axonal growth into an appropriate target was protracted. One significant difference between the present studies and the in vitro experiments is that the axons of the ganglion cells in our studies have yet to grow out at the time of transplantation, whereas the ganglion cells studied in vitro were more mature and had already innervated terminal regions. It is possible that by having formed terminals, the cells become more dependent on sustaining factors produced by the target region.

Since the present work has shown that retinal transplant axons in neonatal rats are capable of considerable adaptive growth in order to establish relatively normal connections, it is important to know whether the substrates present in more mature brains are capable of supporting similar directed growth. The results reported here indicate that substantial specific ingrowth is possible from embryonic retinal transplants embedded in adult tecta. The much more restricted projection that occurs when retinae are connected by a stalk with the tectum suggests that when such transplants are distant from an adult host target region, alternate strategies, such as the use of peripheral nerve grafts, may be necessary to substitute for the loss of substrates for growth that are present only during development.

The second part of this study shows that the immunological consequences of transplantation, especially when using xenografts, are profound. There is a substantial literature showing that a variety of tissues, including embryonic neural tissue,[54] skin,[9,13-15] and tumor cells,[55,56] may be used as allografts into the adult central nervous system. Several authors, however, have shown that skin placed in the brain can be rejected,[13,14] as can neural tissue placed in brains of rats of different strains that vary in both major and minor MHC antigens.[12] One possible criticism of these studies is that in introducing the transplant, the blood-brain barrier may have been opened enough to expose the transplant to antigen-presenting cells not normally given access to the central nervous system. The results reported here using allografts into the brain or into the fourth ventricle suggest that other factors may be more significant. Transplants placed in the ventricular system are exposed to an environment that may contain antigen-presenting dendritic cells normally excluded from the brain parenchyma.[15] Furthermore, studies examining the expression of MHC antigens in the brain have shown them to be restricted under normal circumstances to the cells lining blood vessels.[57] Since solid transplants already have blood vessels that persist and connect with host vessels,[58] host lymphocytes will be directly exposed to the transplant vascular lining with which they may be immunologically incompatible. Destruction of the vascular system supplying the transplant would then lead to transplant destruction. This raises the possibility that solid grafts may be more vulnerable to rejection than dissociated cells, which would depend for their viability on ingrowth of recipient vessels.

These findings suggest that there may be a number of significant variables in neural transplants: the immunogenicity of the donor tissue, the disruption of the blood-brain barrier, the transplant location, the vascularization of the transplant, and the relative immunogenetic differences between the recipient and donor tissues. Other problems include the size of the transplant and whether the tissue is introduced as a solid tissue or as dissociated cells. Given this level of complexity, the current differences in the reported success of allogeneic and xenogeneic graft survival in the brain is not at all surprising.

Our studies show that xenografts placed in neonatal hosts generally survive for as long as 1 year without evidence of rejection. This is in marked contrast to mouse skin grafted onto the flank of newborn rats, which survive 8-13 days.[59] We found that mouse neural transplants placed in rat brains 13 days or older were rejected. Although neural transplants placed in neonatal hosts do not usually themselves elicit an immune response, they are rejected if mouse skin is later transplanted onto the flank of the recipient rats. Thus, they are not accessible to surveillance by the immune system, unlike xenografts placed outside the brain. It is important to know whether other foreign cells protected within the brain might be rejected following peripheral immunization. Most important among such cells may be those transformed by events such as viral infections, which may lie unrecognized in the brain unless an extrinsic immune stimulus is applied. The immune model described in this paper may be particularly valuable for studying pathogenesis and treatment of a variety of "autoimmune" diseases afflicting the central nervous system. An attractive feature of this system over a comparable experimental paradigm involving allografts into adult brains[12] is that the pathology associated with introducing the transplant has already disappeared by the time immunocompetence has developed in the hosts, and that the transplanted cells have already integrated substantially with host neurons.

ACKNOWLEDGMENTS

We acknowledge the valuable technical help of Mary Houston, Fran Shagas, Bob Reinhart, Peggy Bierer, Eric Huczko, and Tracy Sailer, as well as the secretarial assistance of Sharon Wesolowski.

REFERENCES

1. LAM, K., A. SEFTON & M. R. BENNETT. 1982. Loss of axons from the optic nerve of the rat during postnatal development. Dev. Brain Res. **3:** 487-491.
2. CRESPO, D., D. D. M. O'LEARY & W. M. COWAN. 1985. Changes in the numbers of optic nerve fibers during late prenatal and postnatal development in the albino rat. Dev. Brain Res. **19:** 129-134.
3. RAMON Y CAJAL, S. 1928. Degeneration and Regeneration of the Nervous System. Transl.: R. M. May. Oxford Press. London.
4. RICHARDSON, P. M., V. M. K. ISSA & S. SHEMIE. 1982. Regeneration and retrograde degeneration of axons in the rat optic nerve. J. Neurocytol. **11:** 949-966.
5. LUND, R. D. & S. D. HAUSCHKA. 1976. Transplanted neural tissue develops connections with host rat brain. Science **193:** 582-584.
6. LUND, R. D., A. R. HARVEY, C. B. JAEGER & S. C. MCLOON. 1982. Transplantation of embryonic neural tissue to the tectal region of newborn rats. *In* Changing Concepts of the Nervous System. A. R. Morrison & P. L. Strick, Eds.: 361-375. Academic Press. New York, NY.
7. MCLOON, L. K., S. C. MCLOON, F.-L. F. CHANG, J. G. STEEDMAN & R. D. LUND. 1985. Visual system transplanted to the brain of rats. *In* Neural Grafting in the Mammalian CNS. A. Björklund & U. Stenevi, Eds.: 267-283. Elsevier. Amsterdam.
8. WILLIS, R. A. 1935. Experiments on the intracerebral implantation of embryo tissues in rats. Proc. Roy. Soc. London Ser. B **117:** 400-412.
9. MEDAWAR, P. B. 1948. Immunity to homologous grafted skin. II. The fate of skin homografts transplanted to the brain, to subcutaneous tissue, and to the anterior chamber of the eye. Br. J. Exp. Pathol. **29:** 58-69.
10. BARKER, C. F. & R. E. BILLINGHAM. 1977. Immunologically privileged sites. Adv. Immunol. **23:** 1-54.
11. HEAD, J. R. & R. E. BILLINGHAM. 1985. Immunologically privileged sites in transplantation immunology and oncology. Perspect. Biol. Med. **29:** 115-131.
12. FREED, W. J. 1983. Functional brain tissue transplantation: Reversal of lesion-induced rotation by intraventricular substantia nigra and adrenal medulla grafts, with a note on intracranial retinal grafts. Biol. Psychiatry **18:** 1205-1267.
13. GEYER, S. J. & T. J. GILL III. 1979. Immunogenetic aspects of intracerebral skin transplantation in inbred rats. Am. J. Pathol. **94:** 569-580.
14. RAJU, S. & J. B. GROGAN. 1977. Immunologic study of the brain as a privileged site. Transplant. Proc. **9:** 1187-1191.
15. HEAD, J. R. & W. S. T. GRIFFIN. 1985. Functional capacity of solid tissue transplants in the brain: Evidence for immunological privilege. Proc. Roy. Soc. London Ser. B **224:** 375-387.
16. SCHEINBERG, L. C., D. G. KOTSILIMBAS, R. KARPF & N. MAYER. 1966. Is the brain "an immunologically privileged site?" III. Studies based on homologous skin grafts to the brain and subcutaneous tissues. Arch. Neurol. **15:** 62-67.
17. ALBRINK, W. S. & H. S. N. GREENE. 1953. The transplantation of tissues between zoological classes. Cancer Res. **13:** 64-68.
18. CLEMENTS, L. G. & P. S. STEWART. 1985. Lack of immunological privilege in chick brain as a transplantation site. Can. J. Zool. **63:** 223-227.

19. VINOGRADOVA, O. S., A. G. BRAGIN & V. F. KITCHIGINA. 1985. Spontaneous and evoked activity of neurons in intrabrain allo- and xenografts of the hippocampus and septum. *In* Neural Grafting in the Mammalian CNS. A. Björklund & U. Stenevi, Eds.: 409-419. Elsevier. Amsterdam.

20. DANILOFF, J. K., J. WELLS & J. ELLIS. 1984. Cross-species septal transplants: Recovery of choline acetyltransferase activity. Brain 324: 151-154.

21. LOW, W., C. J. K. DANILOFF, R. R. BODONY & J. WELLS. 1985. Cross-species transplants of cholinergic neurons and the recovery of function. *In* Neural Grafting in the Mammalian CNS. A. Björklund & U. Stenevi, Eds.: 575-584. Elsevier. New York, NY.

22. INOUE, H., S. KOHSAKA, K. YOSHIDA, M. OHTANI, S. TOYA & Y. TSUKADA. 1985. Cyclosporin A enhances the survivability of mouse cerebral cortex grafted into the third ventricle of rat brain. Neurosci. Lett. 54: 85-90.

23. LUND, R. D. & S. C. McLOON. 1983. Transplantation of brain tissue: Retinal transplants. R. B. Wallace & G. D. Das, Eds. Plenum. New York, NY.

24. PERRY, V. H., R. D. LUND & S. C. McLOON. 1985. Ganglion cells in retinae transplanted to newborn rats. J. Comp. Neurol. 231: 353-365.

25. LUND, R. D. & D. J. SIMONS. 1985. Retinal transplants: Structural and functional inter-relations with the host brain. *In* Neural Grafting in the Mammalian CNS. A. Björklund & U. Stenevi, Eds.: 345-354. Elsevier. Amsterdam.

26. FORRESTER, J. & A. PETERS. 1967. Nerve fibers in optic nerve of rat. Science 214: 245-247.

27. McLOON, S. C. & R. D. LUND. 1980. Specific projections of retina transplanted to rat brain. Exp. Brain Res. 40: 273-282.

28. SIMONS, D. J. & R. D. LUND. 1985. Fetal retinae transplanted over tecta of neonatal rats respond to light and evoke patterned neuronal discharges in the host superior colliculus. Dev. Brain Res. 21: 156-159.

29. McLOON, L. K. & R. D. LUND. 1982. Embryonic retinae transplanted to the inferior colliculus of newborn rats. Soc. Neurosci. Abstr. 8: 452.

30. McLOON, S. C. & L. K. McLOON. 1985. Factors mediating the pattern of axonal branches from retinal transplants into the host brain. *In* Neural Grafting in the Mammalian CNS. A. Björklund & U. Stenevi, Eds.: 355-362. Elsevier. Amsterdam.

31. McLOON, L. K., M. A. SHARKEY & R. D. LUND. 1983. Embryonic neural retina transplanted to spinal cord. Soc. Neurosci. Abstr. 9: 373.

32. McLOON, S. C. & R. D. LUND. 1984. Loss of ganglion cells in fetal retina transplanted to rat cortex. Dev. Brain Res. 12: 131-135.

33. HANKIN, M. H. & R. D. LUND. 1985. Development of retinotectal projections from retinae transplanted to the cerebral aqueduct. Soc. Neurosci. Abstr. 11: 223.

34. McLOON, S. C. & R. D. LUND. 1983. Development of fetal retina, tectum, and cortex transplanted to the superior colliculus of adult rats. J. Comp. Neurol. 217: 376-389.

35. LUND, R. D., F.-L. F. CHANG, M. H. HANKIN & C. F. LAGENAUR. 1985. Use of a species-specific antibody for demonstrating mouse neurons transplanted to rat brains. Neurosci. Lett. 61: 221-226.

36. JAEGER, C. B. & R. D. LUND. 1980. Transplantation of embryonic occipital cortex to the tectal region of newborn rats: A light microscopic study of organization and connectivity of the transplants. J. Comp. Neurol. 194: 571-597.

37. LUND, R. D. & A. H. BUNT. 1976. Prenatal development of central optic pathways in albino rats. J. Comp. Neurol. 165: 247-262.

38. SILVER, J. & J. SAPIRO. 1981. Axonal guidance during development of the optic nerve: The role of pigmented epithelia and other extrinsic factors. J. Comp. Neurol. 202: 521-538.

39. BUNT, S. M., R. D. LUND & P. W. LAND. 1983. Prenatal development of the optic projections in albino and hooded rats. Dev. Brain Res. 6: 149-168.

40. SILVER, J. & U. RUTISHAUSER. 1984. Guidance of optic axons *in vivo* by a preformed adhesive pathway on neuroepithelial end feet. Dev. Biol. 106: 485-499.

41. HORSBURGH, G. M. & A. J. SEFTON. 1986. The early development of the optic nerve and chiasm in embryonic rat. J. Comp. Neurol. 243: 547-560.

42. COWAN, W. M., J. W. FAWCETT, D. D. M. O'LEARY & B. B. STANFIELD. 1984. Regressive events in neurogenesis. Science 225: 1258-1265.

43. LUND, R. D. & F.-L. F. CHANG. 1983. The normal and abnormal development of the mammalian visual system. *In* Developmental Neuropsychobiology. W. T. Greenough & J. M. Juraska, Eds.: 95-118. Academic Press. New York, NY.

44. BUNT, S. M. & R. D. LUND. 1981. Development of a transient retino-retinal pathway in hooded and albino rats. Brain Res. **211:** 399-404.

45. McLOON, S. C. & R. D. LUND. 1982. Transient retinofugal pathways in the developing chick. Exp. Brain Res. **45:** 277-284.

46. FROST, D. O. 1982. Anomalous connections to somatosensory and auditory systems following brain lesions in early life. Dev. Brain Res. **3:** 627-635.

47. McLOON, S. C. 1982. Alterations in precision of the crossed retinotectal projection during chick development. Science **215:** 1418-1420.

48. POTTS, R. A., B. DREHER & M. R. BENNETT. 1982. The loss of ganglion cells in the developing retina of the rat. Dev. Brain Res. **3:** 481-486.

49. SEFTON, A. J., G. M. HORSBURGH & K. LAM. 1985. The development of the optic nerve in rodents. Aust. N. Z. J. Opthalmol. **13:** 135-145.

50. NURCOMBE, V. & M. R. BENNETT. 1981. Embryonic chick retinal ganglion cells identified *in vitro:* Their survival is dependent on a factor from the optic tectum. Exp. Brain Res. **44:** 249-258.

51. McCAFFERY, C. A., M. R. BENNETT & B. DREHER. 1982. The survival of neonatal rat retinal ganglion cells *in vitro* is enhanced in the presence of appropriate parts of the brain. Exp. Brain Res. **48:** 377-386.

52. GUNDERSON, R. W. & J. N. BARRETT. 1979. Neuronal chemotaxis: Chick dorsal-root axons turn toward high concentrations of nerve growth factors. Science **206:** 1079-1080.

53. LETOURNEAU, P. C. 1973. Chemotactic response of nerve fiber elongation to nerve growth factor. Dev. Biol. **66:** 183-196.

54. BJÖRKLUND, A. & U. STENEVI, EDS. 1985. Neural Grafting in the Mammalian CNS. Elsevier. Amsterdam

55. CIRCOLO, A., R. BIANCHI, B. NARDELLI, P. RIVOSECCHI-MERLETTI & E. BONMASSAR. 1982. Mouse brain: An immunologically privileged site for natural resistance against lymphoma cells. J. Immunol. **128:** 556-562.

56. GREENE, H. S. N. & H. ARNOLD. 1945. The homologous and heterologous transplantation of brain and brain tumors. J. Neurosurg. **2:** 315-331.

57. WHELAN, J. P. & L. A. LAMPSON. 1985. Expression of MHC Class I molecules in normal brain, area postrema, and olfactory epithelium. Soc. Neurosci. Abstr. **11**(2): 1105.

58. KRUM, J. M. & J. M. ROSENSTEIN. 1985. Temporal sequence of angiogenesis in neural transplant models. Soc. Neurosci. Abstr. **11:** 1149.

59. STEINMULLER, D. 1961. Transplantation immunity in the newborn rat. I. The response at birth and maturation of response capacity. J. Exp. Zool. **147:** 233-258.

DISCUSSION OF THE PAPER

M. PERLOW (*University of Illinois, Chicago, IL*): I think what is interesting about the transplants is that what may often be considered a problem with them may be made into an advantage. If your transplants are not working properly or seem to be deleterious to the animal, then one could conceivably cause these transplants to be rejected. If one were to transplant something, in the way shown in your work, into a human being, and were to find the transplant did not work, one could not very well go back and dig it out. But one might be able to cause the transplant to be rejected. At least a patient might not be worse off as a result of a failed transplant. Transplanting across species or between unrelated species might in fact be a useful way to approach the problem.

L. F. KROMER (*Georgetown University, Washington, DC*): You indicated that you thought that in the transplants into the cerebral acqueduct of neonates that the axons from the transplants are coursing along radial glia. Have you looked at electron micrographs to see if you can actually see whether the axons are following the radial glia?

LUND: We feel the radial glial cells are the most likely candidates. Some of our transplants are very carefully confined to the acqueduct, and the radial glial cells are the only elements that run all the way from the acqueduct to the surface. There is no fiber bundle that would run that way, and even the blood vessels could be stopped at the edge of the central gray. We should do electron microscopy studies on it, but it might be a little bit like looking for needles in hay stacks.

Cerebellar Transplantations in Adult Mice with Heredo-degenerative Ataxia[a]

C. SOTELO [b] AND R. M. ALVARADO-MALLART

Institut National de la Santé
et de la Recherche Médical Unité 106
Centre Medio-Chirurgical Foch
92150 Suresnes, France

INTRODUCTION

The high degree of differentiation achieved by the neurons in the mammalian brain is offset by a total lack of proliferative ability. Once the period of ontogenesis is finished, there is no known intrinsic possibility of neuronal increase. On the contrary, either a progressive and inevitable loss due to the physiological process of aging[1] or a faster, more selective loss resulting from various pathological processes[2] can occur. Neuronal loss causes partial deafferentation of surviving neurons and their subsequent adaptation to new conditions to compensate the loss. Despite the adaptive behavior of adult neurons,[3] functional recovery of impaired systems is always incomplete.

One of the primary concerns of current research in neuroscience is to find a way to manipulate the adaptive capability of the brain in order to allow a functional recovery as complete as possible. At present, experimental neurotransplantation is one of the most popular and promising techniques directed toward realizing this goal. Its lack of lymphatic drainage and, therefore, of dendritic cells[4] renders the central nervous system (CNS) immunologically privileged, since allogeneic grafts can survive in this system without immunosuppression for prolonged periods of time, potentially throughout a life span. A growing number of recent publications has been devoted to this subject[5]; these studies conclusively demonstrate that embryonic mammalian brain pieces, taken from donors syngeneic to the hosts, can survive without rejection when grafted to the adult CNS.

Most studies on embryonic neuron transplantation into adult animal brain have dealt with "global" systems. In these, a few nerve cells of the same type innervate very extensive terminal domains, composed of hundreds of thousands of neurons of very different categories (monoaminergic systems or cholinergic cortical systems). Despite the strict topographical arrangement of the projections in global systems, they probably function not only by specific synaptic contacts but also in a paracrine fashion. The neurotransmitter thus released can diffuse over long distances and affect numerous

[a] This work was supported by Grant 84 C 1314 from the Ministère de la Recherche et de la Technologie (Action Concertée: Neurosciences).

[b] Present address: INSERM U106, Hôpital de la Salpêtrière, 75651 Paris Cedex 13, France.

neurons equipped with adequate receptors. This seems to be the case in the noradrenergic innervation of the rat frontal cortex[6] and in the serotonergic innervation of the rat facial nucleus.[7] Because of the presumptive paracrine role of neurons in global systems, it is possible, in principle, to replace missing neurons of this kind by transplanting homologous embryonic neurons to their terminal domains. Functional recovery from this type of graft does not imply the formation of either specific afferent inputs or specific synaptic contacts with target neurons. The survival of the embryonic neurons and their morphological and biochemical differentiation, involving the development of release sites and the synthesis of appropriate neurotransmitters, would theoretically be enough to permit recovery. A number of investigators dealing with the nigrostriatal dopaminergic system,[8–12] with the ceruleohippocampal noradrenergic system,[13] and with the septohippocampal cholinergic system,[14–16] have corroborated these theoretical considerations with experimental results.

The conditions necessary for functional recovery from transplantations in "point-to-point" systems are much more definite and difficult to obtain. Point-to-point systems are those in which each nerve cell contacts no more than a few target neurons, as in most sensory and motor systems. Neurons in these systems do not act by a paracrine release of neurotransmitters but through a precise balance in input-output interactions involving a high specificity of the afferent and efferent synaptic contacts. It can be postulated that functional recovery would depend on the reestablishment of these synaptic interactions. Therefore, in order to restore function in point-to-point systems, grafted neurons would need to replace missing neurons in a very precise manner by reconstituting an equivalent synaptic circuitry. This implies three morphological prerequisites. The grafted neurons must 1) leave the graft and migrate to the exact location of the missing neurons; 2) provoke the sprouting of host axon terminals, which would lead to the formation of specific afferent synapses; and 3) grow axons that could synaptically contact proper targets in the host.

A few years ago, we started a series of experimental neurotransplantations[17,18] aimed at testing the possibilities of neuronal replacements in point-to-point systems. The biological material used in these experiments was the cerebellum of small rodents (rat and mouse). We first analyzed the behavior of Purkinje cells (PCs), grafted heterotopically in pieces of cerebellar primordia to the cerebral cortex or to the hippocampus. Under these conditions, the grafted embryonic neurons survive but remain confined to the graft, where they differentiate anomalous dendritic trees. An important reactive gliosis develops around the grafts, but, in spite of this gliosis, a few PC axons manage to leave the graft, although they do not establish synaptic contacts with nearby host neurons and eventually degenerate. On the contrary, serotonergic axons (global system) from the adult host brain can penetrate the implants, providing them with a serotonergic innervation that mimics that of the normal cerebellum. These studies indicate that although grafted PCs can grow axons within the host parenchyma, they preserve their input-output specificity; this, in turn, indicates that these neurons conserve the molecular mechanisms that subserve synaptogenesis during normal development and are necessary for the synaptic integration of PCs into a defective cerebellar circuitry.

New experiments,[19,20] which are summarized in this paper, were carried out to see whether the three morphological prerequisites for neuronal graft replacement can occur when embryonic PCs are implanted to cerebella with heredo-degenerative ataxia. "Purkinje cell degeneration" (pcd) mutant mice were selected for these experiments (pcd is an autosomal recessive mutation, mapped on chromosome 13, that arose spontaneously in the C57BR/cdJ strain and causes the death of virtually all PCs 15-45 days postnatally[21]). In pcd mice aged between 3 and 4 months, the number of residual PCs is about 0.05% of control value.[19] In spite of the lack of PCs at this age, a large proportion of the synaptic inputs to these neurons remains intact in the molecular layer; they are covered by thin astrocytic processes or are clustered in small groups, as in the hemispheres of adult "nervous" cerebellum,[22] another mutation affecting PCs in the mouse. Granule cells and inferior olivary neurons, the most important sources of PC afferents, begin to follow a slow process of transneuronal retrograde degeneration, but they are still numerous. Both neuronal populations almost completely disappear in older pcd mice, that is, in mice about 6 to 12 months old (see reference 23 for granule cells; Sotelo, unpublished results, for inferior olivary neurons). The adult pcd cerebellum (3 to 4 months old) thus offers an optimal situation for testing and analyzing the capabilities of neural grafts for substituting missing PCs.[19,20]

MATERIALS AND METHODS

Transplantation Procedures

In all experiments to be described in this paper, donor tissue was obtained from the cerebellar primordia of 12-day-old C57BL embryos. The fetuses were removed from the uterus and dissected at room temperature in phosphate-buffered saline (pH 7). Two different grafting procedures were performed: either the cerebellar primordia were mechanically dissociated in tissue culture medium[24] (and the cell suspensions used for grafting) or they were sliced into small pieces (and the individual pieces used in solid graft transplantation).

The hosts were pcd mutant mice that were 3 to 4 months old. They were anesthetized with chloral hydrate and fixed in a stereotaxic frame. Two small symmetrical craniotomies were made in the occipital bone to expose the posterior surface of the cerebellum at the border between vermis and hemisphere. Both types of graft were injected at variable depths with a 10-μl Hamilton syringe fitted with a glass pipette, so that each hemicerebellum contained one implant.

Morphological Procedures for the Analysis of Grafted Cerebella

Two to 3 months after transplantation, the mice were anesthetized with chloral hydrate and perfused through the heart with aldehyde fixatives for routine electron microscopy and immunocytochemistry.

Sagittal and frontal 25-μm-thick sections of the cerebellum were processed freely floating according to the peroxidase-antiperoxidase method.[25] Two primary antisera were used to identify PC somata, dendrites, and axons: one against cyclic GMP-dependent protein kinase (cGK),[26,27] which was donated by Professor P. Greengard; and the other against vitamin D-dependent binding protein or choleocalcin (CaBP),[28] which was donated by Dr. M. Thomasset. Two nontransplanted pcd mice, aged about 4 months, and two normal C57BL mice, about 6 months old, were also fixed for routine electron microscopy. The cerebellum was sliced in the sagittal plane and the blocks embedded in Araldite after osmification.

Morphometric Analysis

The percentage of the volume of cerebellar molecular layer occupied by grafted PCs was calculated stereologically with the point counting method.[29] The number of synaptic contacts between parallel fibers and PC dendritic spines per unit area of molecular layer was calculated from five sets of photomontages, which covered large areas (8350 μm^2) of molecular layer in two cerebella grafted with cell suspensions. Control density was obtained in a similar manner from the cerebella of two nongrafted C57BL mice that were about 6 months old.[19]

RESULTS

Our results will be grouped to correspond to three main questions. These questions will address the issue of whether the morphological prerequisites for functional restoration in point-to-point systems can occur.

Do Embryonic PCs Move out of the Grafts and Replace Missing Neurons of the pcd Mutant Cerebellum?

Cerebella Grafted with Cell Suspensions

All transplanted cell suspensions succeed in providing PCs to the mutant cerebellum. The distribution of the grafted cells follows a similar pattern: although a variable number of PCs remains in the zone occupied by the pipette track at the injection site, the vast majority move out and spread on both sides of the track to the nearby molecular layer parenchyma (FIG. 1A). Thus, molecular layer regions of different sizes and belonging to diverse folia, having in common only their proximity to the injection site, contain most of the grafted PCs. In the largest transplants, the diameter of the spread is about 1300 μm, suggesting that PCs migrate within an adult cerebellar parenchyma for distances over 600 μm. The immunohistochemical material, in which only PCs were stained, showed that these neurons (with the exception of those remaining in the pipette track) are selectively attracted to the molecular layer (FIG. 1A), since they are never encountered outside this layer. To see whether other neurons from the grafted cell suspensions are able to migrate and to invade the molecular layer of the mutant, 1-μm-thick sections were examined. Large ectopic PC perikarya are distributed over the superficial two-thirds of the molecular layer, the area in which grafted PCs migrate. Stellate and basket cells did not increase in density, and ectopic granule cells were not encountered; it can thus be concluded that only PCs are able to leave the graft and to migrate to the molecular layer.

Since the anti-cGK and anti-CaBP antibodies immunostain PC somata and dendrites in a Golgi-like fashion, they permit a close examination of the tridimensional arrangement of grafted PCs. The somata are distributed at random in a 3- to 5-cell-deep zone within the upper two-thirds of the molecular layer. The dendrites spread

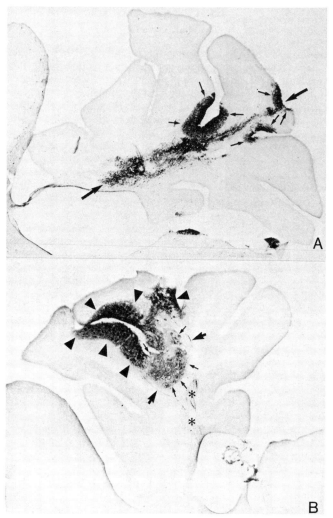

FIGURE 1. Distribution of grafted PCs 3 months after transplantation to the cerebellum of pcd mutant mice. The PCs were identified immunohistochemically. (**A**) This micrograph illustrates an example of the fate of grafted cell suspensions. Even in this region, which corresponds to the center of the injection, most PCs have moved out of the graft to precise areas of the cortical molecular layer (small arrows). Some neurons remain within the pipette track, which is clearly visible (large arrows). Note the closeness of the pipette track to areas of the molecular layer filled with grafted PCs. Immunostaining with anti-CaBP. (**B**) Fate of a grafted solid implant. As in **A,** most PCs have moved out of the graft and occupy molecular layer regions (arrowheads). A small remnant of the solid implant can still be seen in the white matter and adjacent cortex (small arrows). This remnant is composed of a few PCs and many PC axons, converging on a zone of immunonegative neurons corresponding to the deep nuclei. The large arrows point to two fine bundles of PC axons that leave the cortical areas and reach the deep nuclei of the host (asterisks) through the white matter (see FIG. 9A for a higher magnification of this nuclear area). Immunostaining with anti-cGK. Original magnification for **A** and **B**: ×40; figure reduced to 77% of original size.

throughout this layer but stop abruptly at the granular layer interface (FIG. 2B). Most PCs are monopolar, although bi- and multipolar forms do exist. The dendritic trees are composed of proximal thick branches and distal spiny branchlets, as in normal PCs. Those PCs with somata located under the subpial surface commonly have inverted dendritic trees that can span the whole molecular layer. Despite these abnormalities, the basic dendritic organization is maintained: in sagittal sections the dendrites display a maximal extension, whereas in transverse sections this extension is minimal. Therefore, they are confined to a single plane perpendicular to the direction of the folia and flattened in the transverse plane, indicating their disposition orthogonal to the bundles of parallel fibers preexisting in the molecular layer of the mutant cerebellum.

Cerebella Grafted with Solid Grafts

As with cell suspensions, the survival of implanted solid grafts is 100%. Instead of the unique behavior of grafted cell suspensions, solid grafts evolve in various ways, which can be divided into three main groups. In all of them, large areas of the host molecular layer are occupied by grafted PCs, which have succeeded in leaving the implants and in migrating within the parenchyma of the adult cerebellum.

1. In some instances, small remnants of the grafts are found in an extracerebellar location, between two folia. These remnants contain a few PCs intermingled with granule cells and, occasionally, other interneurons (FIG. 2A). Most PCs are located in the molecular layer of the host, where they are distributed in the same fashion as the grafted cell suspensions described above. Their dendritic trees are confined to the plane perpendicular to the bundles of parallel fibers and never penetrate the granular layer (FIG. 3A). Close examination of 1-μm-thick plastic sections also reveals the absence of ectopic granule cells and the unchanged density of molecular layer interneurons (FIG. 2A).

2. Most often, a more or less important remnant of the solid graft remains at the white matter of the cerebellum, close to the cortex or partially replacing it. These remnants are neither lobulated nor laminated (FIG. 1B). In immunostained material, they contain numerous bundles of immunopositive PC axons, in addition to some disarranged PCs. The axons form bouton-shaped varicosities that terminate around immunonegative neurons, clustered in certain areas of the graft. This arrangement clearly indicates that deep cerebellar nuclear neurons from the grafts are still present 3 months after transplantation and have succeeded in attracting the vast majority of axons from the grafted PCs (FIG. 1B). The presence of these remnants does not impede the migration of most of the transplanted PCs, since they occupy large regions of the host molecular layer, sometimes almost filling up to two folia. PCs in the host molecular layer have dendritic trees with features identical to those of PCs from the grafted cell suspensions (FIG. 3B).

3. In a few cases in which the pipette was inserted in a posteroanterior direction across the entire cerebellum, the implant was positioned extraparenchymatously in the space between the inferior colliculus and the anterior surface of the cerebellum (FIG. 4A). These implants develop lobulated structures that become integrated with the mutant cerebellum through a rather extensive interface. The lobulated structures consist of a trilaminated peripheral zone with PCs separating a molecular layer from a granular layer, and a central region, the equivalent of the deep nuclei (FIG. 4B). This contains numerous immunonegative cells through which the immunopositive

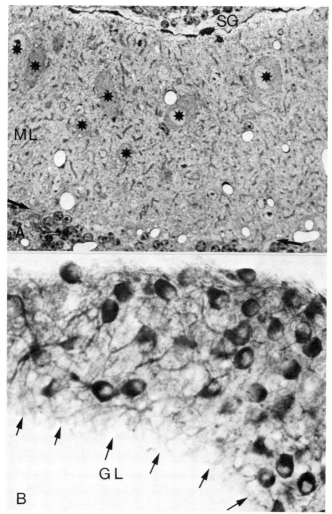

FIGURE 2. Light micrographs illustrating grafted PCs in the molecular layer of the host cerebellum. (**A**) Semithin plastic section stained with toluidine blue. The upper central part of the photograph shows a small remnant of a solid graft (SG) extruded between two folia in which a few granule cells are present. The molecular layer (ML) of the host cerebellum contains large perikarya in its superficial two-thirds, which belong to grafted PCs (asterisks). Dark, sinuous thin processes, corresponding to PC dendrites, spread throughout the molecular layer. Note the absence of granule cells outside the granular layer, the absence of PCs at the interface between the molecular layer and the granular layer (GL) (arrows), and the normal density of molecular layer interneurons. (**B**) The molecular layer (delimited by arrows) of a pcd cerebellum implanted with cell suspensions. It contains numerous PCs immunostained with anti-cGK. The perikarya are mostly within the superficial two-thirds of the molecular layer, where they are randomly arranged in a three- to five-cell-deep zone. The dendrites exhibit a maximal extension in this sagittal section. Note that they do not invade the granular layer but stop precisely at the interface between the molecular and granular layers. Original magnifications for **A** and **B**: ×600 and ×400, respectively; figure reduced to 77% of original size.

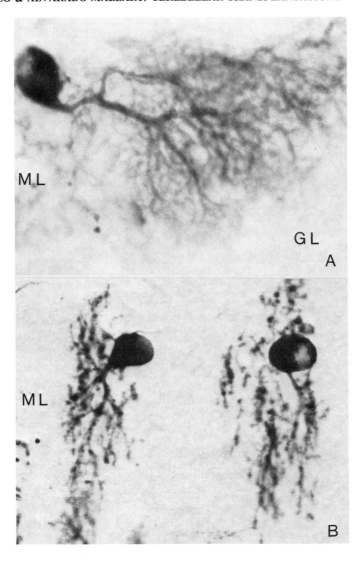

FIGURE 3. Monoplanar organization of the PC dendritic trees in cerebella transplanted with solid implants and observed at the most distant extension of the molecular layer invasion (transplant border). (**A**) Sagittal section (anti-cGK). The soma of the PC is located in the upper region of the molecular layer (ML) and gives rise to a single-stemmed primary dendrite oriented parallel to the cerebellar surface. The dendrite branches profusely and invades for some distance the neuropil of the molecular layer devoid of PCs. This dendritic tree exhibits a maximal extension, and, despite its orientation, resembles that of a normal PC, in which proximal and distal compartments have developed. Note that the dendrites do not enter the granular layer (GL). (**B**) Transverse section (anti-CaBP). Two distal PCs are illustrated in this micrograph. Note that their perikarya are in the upper third of the molecular layer and that their dendritic trees exhibit a minimal extension. Original magnifications for **A** and **B**: ×950 and ×600, respectively; figure reduced to 80% of original size.

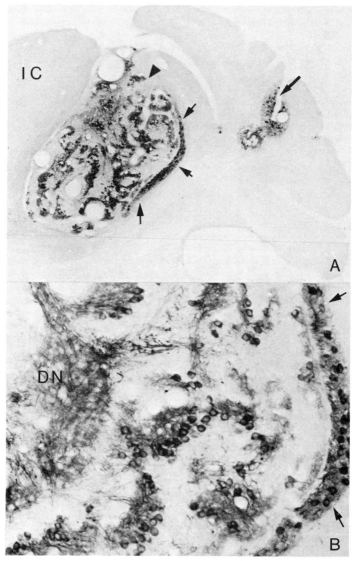

FIGURE 4. Extraparenchymal development and organization of a transplanted solid graft into a minicerebellum. Immunohistochemical staining of PCs with anti-cGK. (**A**) At the anterior surface of the cerebellum, behind the inferior colliculus (IC), a solid graft has formed a lobulated minicerebellum, which remains attached to the mutant cerebellum (arrowhead). Note that PCs are also present in near (small arrows) and far (large arrows) areas of the host molecular layer. (**B**) The minicerebellum is formed by a lobulated peripheral region, corresponding to the cerebellar cortex with PC perikarya at the interface between molecular and granular layers, and by a central deep nuclear region (DN). The latter contains immunonegative neurons surrounded by numerous immunoreactive PC axons. The arrows point to the PCs, which have succeeded in invading the host molecular layer. Original magnifications for **A** and **B**: ×40 and ×125, respectively; figure reduced to 83% of original size.

axons of the cortical PCs converge. Minicerebella of this sort always develop when solid grafts are transplanted in an extraparenchymatous location, both when they are isolated from the host brain[17] and when they are partially integrated into it.[18] Even in these extreme cases, PCs leave the graft and occupy extensive zones of the host molecular layer close to the interface between the implant and the mutant cerebellum or in folia far from it but affected by the pipette track during transplantation (FIG. 4). As expected, the dendritic trees of the PCs within the host molecular layer are organized according to the same rules as in the preceding cases.

Do Grafted PCs Provoke a Reactive Synaptogenesis with Proper Presynaptic Axons of the Host Cerebellar Cortex?

Regardless of the transplantation technique, all grafted PCs showed a similar synaptic investment. Therefore, the results from grafted cell suspensions and solid implants will be pooled.

Although an important study exists concerning young pcd mice during the critical period of PC death,[21] a complete analysis of the molecular layer of nontransplanted pcd cerebellum in 3- to 4-month-old mutant mice has never been undertaken. Since an analysis of this type is necessary for understanding the reactive synaptogenesis leading to synaptic investment of the grafted PCs, we shall begin with a brief description of these cerebella.

Ultrastructural Analysis of the Molecular Layer of Nontransplanted pcd Mice, 3 to 4 Months Old

The main feature of the pcd molecular layer at this age is the complete lack of normal PC elements. Neither thick dendrites nor distal branchlets and spines can be encountered. Some remnants of these neurons persist, however, and appear as distorted dendritic profiles with a very dense cytoplasmic matrix containing dying mitochondria and small clear vacuoles. These profiles are surrounded by a ring of healthy axon terminals. More often, only necrotic debris corresponding to the PCs remains, appearing as sinuously contoured dark bands to which healthy presynaptic terminals are attached (FIG. 5A).

Although molecular layer interneurons and the ascending branches of Golgi cell dendrites are normally innervated, the disappearance of PCs has deprived most presynaptic elements of their postsynaptic target. Thus, the vast majority of axon terminals are either associated to necrotic debris (FIGS. 5A & 5B) or, more often, concentrated in clusters of 2 to 10 bouton-shaped varicosities directly apposed to one another and partially covered with thin astrocytic processes. As in the cerebellar hemispheres of nervous mutant mice,[22] these clusters correspond mainly to presynaptic varicosities of parallel fibers formerly in synaptic contact with a spiny branchlet. In addition, a few isolated axon terminals exhibiting either the features of inhibitory terminals or of climbing fiber varicosities (FIG. 5C) are spread throughout the molecular layer. Occasionally, degenerating parallel fiber varicosities are observed in older animals (FIG. 5A), indicating that a slow transneuronal retrograde degeneration started shortly

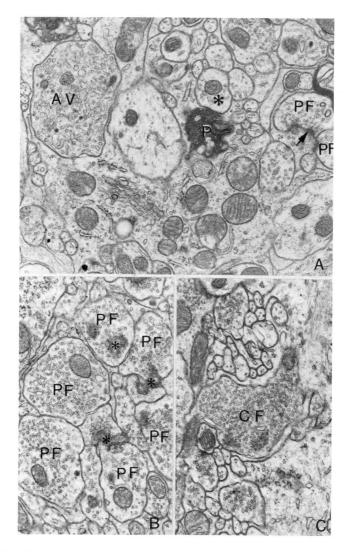

FIGURE 5. Electron micrographs of the molecular layer of a 3- to 4-month-old pcd cerebella. (**A**) In addition to the absence of PC elements in the molecular layer, this micrograph shows three features that characterize a nontransplanted pcd cerebellum: 1) an enlarged axonal varicosity (AV) containing abundant smooth endoplasmic reticulum and large granular vesicles; 2) a degenerating parallel fiber varicosity (P), still maintaining a synaptic relationship with an interneuron dendrite (asterisk); and 3) small, dark, necrotic debris (arrow), representing the remnant of a PC dendrite still attached to healthy axon terminals belonging to parallel fibers (PF). (**B**) A cluster of parallel fiber varicosities devoid of their postsynaptic elements, the distal spines of PC dendrites. Note the presence of necrotic remnants (asterisks) still associated to some of the parallel fiber axon terminals. (**C**) A climbing fiber varicosity (CF), characterized by the clustering of synaptic vesicles, the electron density of the axoplasmic matrix and the presence of a large granular vesicle. This varicosity lacks a postsynaptic element and is partially covered by thin astrocytic processes. Original magnifications for **A**, **B**, and **C**: ×21 000, ×22 000, and ×18 000, respectively; figure reduced to 76% of original size.

after the PCs disappeared. In addition, a few abnormal axonal varicosities of variable size, but always larger than normal, can be observed. They contain large numbers of tubular profiles of smooth endoplasmic reticulum, dense and multivesicular bodies, and large granular vesicles (FIG. 5A). These varicosities are always partially surrounded by thin astrocytic processes. They probably represent axon terminals that are devoid of their targets and are either at the beginning of retrograde degeneration or in a reactive stage of transient growth.

Interestingly enough, at the interface between the molecular and granular layers, there is an almost continuous zone containing numerous "empty baskets," which, like those of the nervous cerebellum,[22] maintain the cytological features of basket axons and even their organization into pinceau formations. An important difference, however, is the lack of an initial PC axon segment at the center of the empty pinceau formations.

Synaptic Investment of Grafted PCs

Electron microscopic immunocytochemical study confirms that only profiles belonging to PCs contain immunoprecipitate (FIG. 6A). This immunoprecipitate which spreads over somata, proximal and distal dendrites, spines, and even axons. Since these profiles are absent in nontransplanted pcd cerebellum, they must belong solely to grafted PCs. Moreover, this study shows that grafted PCs develop all of their intrinsic cytological features and, therefore, that it is possible to identify these neurons with cytological criteria in material prepared for routine electron microscopy, considerably facilitating a thorough ultrastructural analysis.

Although PC somata are located ectopically in the superficial two-thirds of the molecular layer, from a qualitative viewpoint they are synaptically invested like normal PCs with, however, one important difference: basket fiber-pinceau formations are absent around the initial segment of the PC axon (FIG. 8A). Axon terminals of stellate cells and basket axon ascending collaterals synapse on the perikaryal surface (FIG. 6B) and, occasionally, on the surface of the initial segments. Thus, the grafted PCs receive an adequate contingent of inhibitory inputs on their perikarya and their initial axon segment. Since the density of molecular layer interneurons is not increased, it is not possible that the inhibitory inputs originate from implanted neurons.

PC dendritic inputs also mimic normality. Almost all primary thick dendritic branches receive climbing fiber varicosities, which synapse on the stubby spines (FIG. 7A). Furthermore, the smooth membrane of these thick dendritic branches receives axon terminals from basket and stellate cells (FIG. 8B). The distal dendritic compartment is composed of typical spiny branchlets, studded with long-necked spines. These spines are contacted by axonal varicosities of the parallel fibers (FIG. 7B). Despite the high degree of normality in the synaptic investment of grafted PCs, indicating that these neurons almost succeed in correctly segregating their synaptic inputs, some minor abnormalities exist. Often, a few distal-like spines stem ectopically from thick proximal dendrites and receive synapses from axon terminals of parallel fibers (FIG. 8B). Occasionally, thin distal branchlets also receive inhibitory synapses on their smooth segment.

One of the characteristics of pcd parallel fibers is that, as reported above, they remain attached to necrotic debris of PC dendrites for long periods of time. In molecular layer areas containing grafted PCs, the relationship between host parallel fibers and host degenerative debris persists. Since it was important to know the fate of parallel fibers after grafting, we paid particular attention to these fibers when they

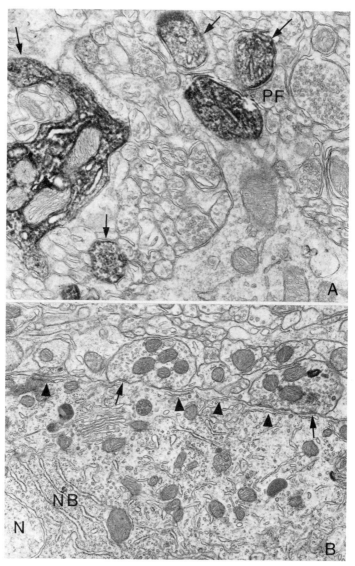

FIGURE 6. Ultrastructural features of transplanted PCs. (**A**) Immunocytochemical identification of PC elements with anti-CaBP. The only elements labeled are dendritic profiles of various sizes belonging to the grafted PCs. At the left of the micrograph the stem of a distal dendritic branch giving off long-necked spines (arrows) can be seen. One of the spines is synaptically contacted by a parallel fiber (PF) varicosity. Solid implant. (**B**) Electron micrograph of the perikaryon of a grafted PC. Note the presence of the hypolemmal cistern (arrowheads) and the typical cytology of this perikaryon with a small Nissl body (NB) in a perinuclear location (N: nucleus). Two axon terminals containing a pleomorphic population of synaptic vesicles and establishing type II synaptic contacts (arrows) belong to the molecular layer interneurons, most probably to stellate cells. Grafted cell suspension. Original magnifications for **A** and **B**: ×30 000 and ×19 000, respectively; figure reduced to 82% of original size.

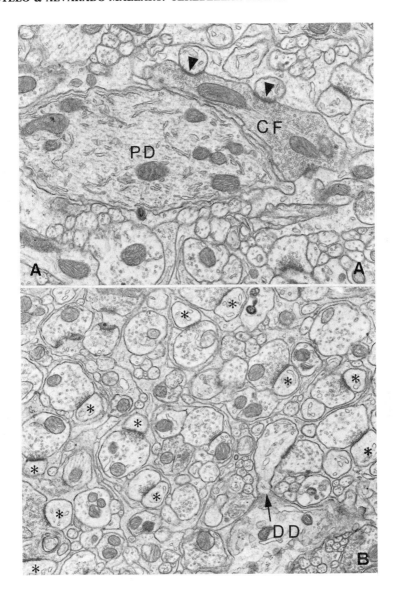

FIGURE 7. Synaptic investment of proximal and distal PC dendritic compartments. (**A**) Electron micrograph of a proximal dendrite (PD) of a grafted PC. Note the close relationship with an axonal varicosity belonging to a climbing fiber (CF) and synapsing on two small stubby spines (arrowheads). Solid graft. (**B**) Electron micrograph of a distal dendrite (DD) of a grafted PC. The arrow points to the emergence of a distal spine, synaptically contacted by a parallel fiber varicosity. Numerous axon terminals belonging to parallel fibers synapse on distal spines (asterisks) of a grafted PC dendrite. Solid graft. Original magnifications for **A** and **B**: ×21 000 and ×17 000, respectively; figure reduced to 85% of original size.

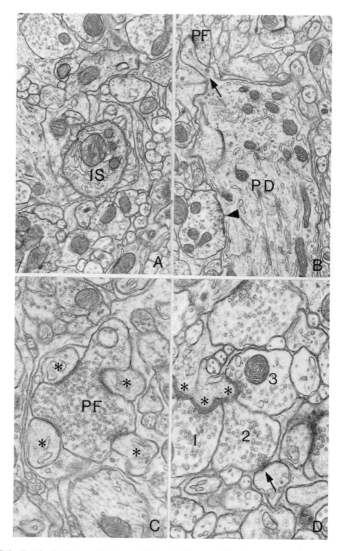

FIGURE 8. Particularities and abnormalities of the synaptic investment of grafted PCs. (**A**) Electron micrograph illustrating the initial segment (IS) of a PC axon within the molecular layer. Note its glial envelopment and, especially, the lack of a pinceau formation. Solid implant. (**B**) Electron micrograph of a proximal dendritic segment of a grafted PC (PD) receiving an axon terminal on its smooth surface (arrowhead). The terminal, which has pleomorphic vesicles and a type II synaptic contact, belongs to a stellate cell axon. The arrow points to an ectopic long-necked distal spine synaptically contacted by a parallel fiber (PF) varicosity. Grafted cell suspensions. (**C**) Enlarged axon terminal belonging to a parallel fiber and establishing synaptic contacts with four spines (asterisks) of distal PC dendrites. Grafted cell suspensions. (**D**) Necrotic debris (asterisks) remains attached to three parallel fiber varicosities (1-3), one of which has developed a new synaptic contact with the dendritic spine (arrow) of a grafted PC. Solid implants. Original magnifications for **A, B, C,** and **D**: ×18 000, ×19 000, ×29 000, and ×25 000, respectively; figure reduced to 77% of original size.

TABLE 1. Volumetric Proportion of Graft versus Cerebellum

| Case Number | Type of Graft | Volumetric Proportion[a] (%) | | |
		ML/Cerebellum	Graft/Cerebellum	Graft in ML/ML
85-5	Grafted cell suspension	30	0.8	3
85-10	Grafted cell suspension	26	1.3	5
85-11	Solid graft	27	2	12
85-91	Solid graft	21	6	17

[a] Percentage of the molecular layer (ML) volume occupied by the graft versus the total ML volume.

were located in the vicinity of grafted PCs. Some of them enlarge and attain a distal dendritic spine. At the sites where both membranes are directly apposed, a synaptic junction is formed (FIG. 8D). The new, active zone is located opposite the varicosal region still attached to the necrotic remnant. Their presence indicates that even host parallel fiber varicosities engaged in residual contacts with remnants of necrotic PCs are able to participate in the general process of reactive synaptogenesis provoked by the arrival of new PCs from the implants. Another feature of parallel fiber varicosities is that some of them are much larger than normal; they establish multiple synaptic contacts mainly on PC dendritic spines (FIG. 8C).

Morphometric Studies

Two types of morphometric analysis were performed to evaluate two different parameters.
Transplantation Yield. Stereology was used to determine the percentage of the total molecular layer volume per hemicerebellum occupied by grafted PCs. As indicated in TABLE 1, this study concerned two grafted cell suspensions and two solid implants. The yield is much greater with solid implants, since it reaches a high of 17%, as compared to the 5% maximum obtained with cell suspensions.
Ratio of Parallel Fiber Inputs to Grafted PCs. This was established by determining the surface density of synapses between parallel fiber varicosities and distal dendritic spines. TABLE 2 summarizes the results concerning grafted PCs originating from cell suspensions. The density obtained is only 52.6% of control values. Despite this important reduction, parallel fibers of the host react favorably to the presence of grafted PCs, and synaptogenesis is massive.

TABLE 2. Density of Parallel Fiber-PC Synapses

Material	Area of ML Surface (μm^2)	Number of Spines Contacted by Parallel Fibers	Number of Parallel Fiber-PC Synapses per 100 μm^2
Control	3950	766	19 (100%)
Grafted pcd/pcd	8350	840	10 (52.6%)

Do Grafted PCs Grow Axonal Projections That Synapse with Proper Target Neurons in the Deep Cerebellar Nuclei of the Host?

Immunocytochemistry with two PC markers (anti-cGK and anti-CaBP) was extremely valuable in answering this question. Both antibodies immunostain the entire PC axon, allowing the delineation of its course and terminal trees. In many, but not all, grafted cerebella, immunoreactive axons emerging from molecular layer PCs form thin bundles, which reach the deep nuclei through the white matter. The axons follow a rather rectilinear path and give off neither varicosities nor collateral branches. Once these axons reach their terminal domain at the most dorsal end of the deep nuclei, they branch profusely into thinner axonic segments, which become varicose from multiple enlargements, similar to bouton-shaped varicosities "en passant," and invade the deep nuclear parenchyma in variable numbers (FIG. 9A). These terminal plexuses can sometimes form intricate nests covering the perikarya of immunonegative nuclear neurons, but, more often, immunopositive axons border unreactive dendrites. The electron microscopic study of two cerebella immunostained with the antiserum against CaBP, one grafted with a cell suspension, the other with a solid implant, permitted the assessment of the synaptic contacts established between host nuclear neurons and grafted PCs. Although infrequent, immunoreactive axon terminals are present within the deep cerebellar nuclei. Often, they appear grouped in clusters, like the terminal axon branches observed with light microscopy, and resemble small bunches of grapes. Despite the immunoprecipitate, which obscures some of the cytological features of the reactive terminals, the axon terminals appear as large, ovoid varicosities filled with densely packed flattened synaptic vesicles and occasional mitochondria (FIG. 9B). These bouton-shaped varicosities establish gray type II synaptic junctions with perikarya or dendrites of large and small deep cerebellar neurons or both.

As mentioned above, the integration of grafted PCs to the circuitry of the cerebellar cortex is always achieved, both in grafted cell suspensions and in solid implants. However, corticonuclear interactions—which suppose the formation of correct PC projections—are not systematically produced, since in many of the grafted cerebella, PC axons do not leave the cortical region. Another important observation is that the distance between transplanted PCs and host deep nuclei is determinant for the development of appropriate PC axon projections. When grafted PCs, present in the host molecular layer or ectopic in the white matter, are less than 500 μm from the mutant deep nuclei, they are able to project to these nuclei, even if the remnant of a solid graft containing its own deep nuclei is nearby. On the contrary, in cases of very superficial transplantation (when the graft is deposited on the posterior or anterior cerebellar surface), axons from the grafted PCs do not succeed in reaching the distant deep cerebellar nuclei of the host. Therefore, the presence within the grafts of regions equivalent to the deep nuclei and an overly long distance between grafted PCs and host deep nuclei will prevent corticonuclear interactions from occurring, thus explaining the variability of the experiments reported in this study.

DISCUSSION

The results reported in this study demonstrate that regardless of the transplantation technique used, grafts obtained from genetically normal cerebellar primordia are able to survive in the cerebellum of adult pcd mutant mice. PCs identified with immu-

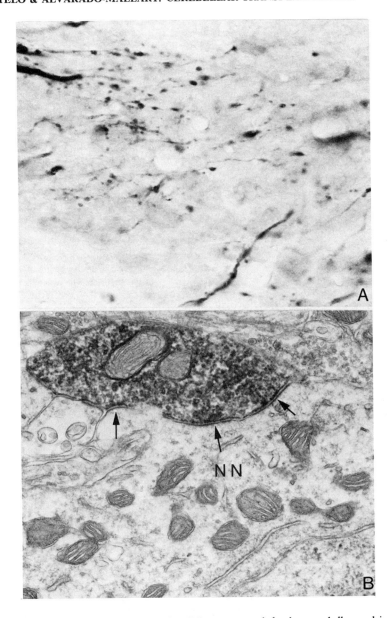

FIGURE 9. Efferent projections of grafted PC axons toward the deep cerebellar nuclei of the host. (**A**) Light micrograph of the dorsal region of the medial nucleus of the same cerebellum as that in FIGURE 1B, illustrating the terminal arborization of the PC axons. Note the low density of this projection and the varicose appearance of the PC axons. PCs identified with anti-cGK. (**B**) Electron micrograph of a PC axon terminal, immunolabeled with peroxidase precipitate. The axon terminal establishes type II synaptic contacts (arrows) with the perikaryon of a large nuclear neuron (NN). PCs immunostained with anti-CaBP. Original magnifications for **A** and **B**: ×600 and ×38 000, respectively; reduced to 85% of original size.

nohistochemical and electron microscopical methods were systematically encountered in all grafted cerebella. The long-term survival of this neuronal population within the mutant cerebellum indirectly corroborates previous results obtained by Mullen[30] from tetraparental animals (experimental chimeras containing mixtures of homozygous pcd and genetically normal cells), which showed the intrinsic action of the pcd genetic locus within the PCs. The long survival of the genetically normal grafted PCs (up to 12 weeks; in the mutant, they die between 3 and 8 weeks) is therefore an indication that the degeneration of this neuronal category in the mutant does not arise from either an abnormal cellular milieu or from a primary lesion to a different type of cell.

Cellular Composition of the Embryonic Grafts

In order to discuss the fate of the grafted PCs in the adult pcd cerebellum, it is necessary first to describe briefly the maturational state of the donor cerebellum. In the mouse, the cerebellar primordium appears on the 10th to the 12th day of gestation as a thickening of the primitive neuroepithelium, evaginated in the anterior region of the roof of the fourth ventricle. At E12, the date of our transplantations, this thickening contains an overlying mantle zone in addition to the primitive neuroepithelium. This mantle is composed of differentiating postmitotic neurons, corresponding to most of the deep nuclear neurons and PCs. Using [³H]thymidine, Miale and Sidman[31] reported that these two neuronal populations are formed between E11 and E13. At the moment of transplantation, the secondary neuroepithelium of the external granular layer is still absent, since it appears only in E13 embryos. Therefore, both the cell suspensions and the solid implants used in our experiments are composed of stem cells derived from the primitive neuroepithelium, deep nuclear neurons, and PCs. They do not contain interneurons, although some of their specific precursors are present in the transplanted material.

The main goal of the present experiments was to answer the following question: Is neuronal transplantation a good way to replace synaptically the missing neurons in a point-to-point system? In the following discussion, we shall evaluate the chances that grafted embryonic neurons have of fulfilling the three morphological requirements essential for neuronal replacement.

PC Migration

The results obtained from the long-term survivals do not allow the migratory pathways of the grafted PCs to be studied, but they do show that these neurons, in both types of transplantation, are indeed able to move out of the implants and migrate into the parenchyma of the adult mutant cerebellum because they are able to invade the molecular layer and settle within it. In another series of experiments aimed at analyzing the developmental sequence of grafted PCs (Sotelo and Alvarado-Mallart, unpublished results), we showed that these neurons leave the graft and migrate into the host molecular layer within the first 5 days after transplantation, when PCs are still very immature, before they reach a real age of E17. Therefore, they lose their positional relationships with other grafted neurons before the onset of proliferation of the stem cells of the external granular layer, which in the mouse occurs during the first 2 postnatal weeks.[31]

The early migration of PCs is of theoretical importance for the fate of the transplanted granule cell precursors. Data obtained from the study of the staggerer[32] and the reeler[33] mutant mice indicate that PCs could play a regulatory role in the proliferative activity of granule cell precursors. From the beginning of its formation, the external granular layer is lined on its lower surface with the apical processes of immature PCs. The intimate relationship between PC dendrites and precursor cells is enhanced during the period of bulk formation of granule cells, since in 10-day-old rats apical segments of certain PC dendrites penetrate into the external granular layer (Wassef, unpublished results). In the reeler and staggerer mutants, this relationship is much less important quantitatively, and a common feature of both cerebella is the notable reduction in granule cell numbers. Mallet *et al.*[32] and Mariani *et al.*[33] proposed a tentative explanation for this atrophy by suggesting that the reduction in the number of PCs in close association with the external granular layer could provoke granule cell hypoplasia. Therefore, if a reduction in the mitotic rate of granule cell precursors results from a lack of PCs in close topographical proximity, the early departure from the implant of these neurons might provoke an important slowdown in the production of transplanted granule cells. This hypothetical mechanism would explain why in the remnants of solid implants, either outside or inside the cerebellum, the number of granule cells is so low, whereas in the implants organized in minicerebella they are much more numerous.

For the purposes of this study, the most interesting result is that the neuronal invasion of the host molecular layer seems to be a very selective process: only PCs are able to penetrate this layer. The defective molecular layer of the adult pcd cerebellum appears to exert a positive neurotropism, in the sense used by Cajal,[34] to attract embryonic cells homologous to the missing neurons. We have deliberately chosen the classic terminology of Cajal because we still know nothing about the nature (chemical action, electrical influences) of the mechanisms used by the defective molecular layer to orient embryonic PCs during migration. The present observations, however, indicate that an adult central neuropil deprived of its main neuronal population seems to be as efficient in attracting neuronal replacements as a peripheral terminal domain is in orienting the growth of axons during morphogenesis or regeneration.

Analysis of PC distribution within the host molecular layer in the long-term survivals shows that these neurons can migrate for only a limited distance. The zone of tissue covered by the PCs in migrating is a rough sphere whose center is the pipette track and whose diameter never exceeds 1.5 mm. Therefore, the first prerequisite for neuronal replacement in transplantations dealing with point-to-point systems is only partially fulfilled, since the neurotropic effect of the defective molecular layer is limited to a distance of about 750 μm.

Integration of Grafted PCs in the Cerebellar Cortex Circuitry

Grafted PCs penetrate the host molecular layer when still very immature, before the final formation of the dendritic trees (Sotelo and Alvarado-Mallart, unpublished results). When these dendritic trees attain an adult morphology, as in the PCs analyzed in long-term transplants, they differ from those of control animals but nonetheless show two characteristic features: 1) a monoplanar disposition and 2) an almost complete segregation of synaptic inputs into proximal and distal compartments. During normal development, the acquisition of these two morphological features has been considered to be the result of an interplay between genetic factors and cellular interactions (namely synaptic) taking place during dendritic growth.[35] The formation of dendritic trees by the grafted PCs must also result from a similar interplay. This implies that the adult, postsynaptically deprived axons of the host molecular layer will start synaptogenesis immediately after the arrival of the still-immature neurons and that synaptogenesis will proceed normally. Therefore, the adult axonal field seems to influence PC differentiation by means of a mechanism very closely related to that operating during normal cerebellar morphogenesis.

Synaptic investment of the grafted PCs probably reflects the synaptic interactions presumed to occur between host axon terminals and grafted neurons. The main dendrites are contacted by climbing fibers and axons emerging from molecular layer interneurons, whereas the distal spiny branchlets receive inputs almost solely from parallel fibers. Although parallel fiber-PC synapse density is reduced by as much as 48%, it is unlikely that synapses are established between grafted granule cells and grafted PCs: 1) as discussed in the preceding section, the number of granule cells outside the granular cell layer is very low, suggesting that most of the grafted granule cell precursors have failed to proliferate; 2) some of the parallel fibers synapsing on PC spines remain attached to dark debris from mutant PCs, indicating that they belong to the host cerebellum; and 3) the number of these synapses is too high to account for the possibility that they arise only from grafted granule cells that could have succeeded in migrating to the host granular layer.

The 48% reduction in the number of parallel fiber-PC synapses per unit area could be explained by the progressive transneuronal process of degeneration, which affects granule cells after the death of mutant PCs. Indeed, in 3- to 4-month-old pcd mice (our recipient animals), numerous granule cells have already degenerated.[23] Therefore, the number of remaining parallel fibers at the time of transplantation is reduced, and, despite an effort at adaptation, they cannot produce enough presynaptic elements to reestablish a normal density of parallel fiber-PC synapses. The most obvious signs of adaption of parallel fibers are as follows: 1) the many enlarged varicosities provided with multiple synaptic contacts, always occurring in situations where the proportion of parallel fibers to distal spines of PC dendrites is unbalanced; and 2) the less frequently observed varicosities, still attached to necrotic debris but establishing new synaptic contacts on spines of grafted PCs. In both instances, the preexisting varicosities of parallel fibers adapt to their new situation through a well-known process, which we have previously described as "terminal sprouting."[36]

These considerations lead to the conclusion that the vast majority, if not all, of the abundant synaptic inputs established on grafted PCs are the result of early inter-actions between the host brain and the transplanted neurons. Furthermore, these interactions appear to maintain a specificity like that of normal ontogenesis. Therefore, the second prerequisite for neuronal replacement seems to be met, since in view of the synaptic investment of PCs in long-term survivals, it can be inferred that the presence of embryonic, nonafferented PCs must provoke terminal sprouting of target-deprived axon terminals in the host molecular layer. The end result of this process is the synaptic integration of grafted neurons into the cortical circuitry of the mutant cerebellum.

To what degree is this integration successful? Despite the qualitative normalcy of the synaptic investment of the grafted PCs, it is not identical to that of control PCs. The most obvious difference is the lack of baskets and pinceau formations around grafted PCs; this absence could stem from the abnormal location of the PC somata within the upper two-thirds of the molecular layer, and from the behavior of basket cell axons in PC-deprived cerebella. These axons remain clustered in "empty baskets," which persist for long periods, even for as long as the animal lives,[22] and prevent the occurrence of terminal spouting. Nonetheless, inhibitory inputs from host molecular layer interneurons establish abundant synaptic contacts on the soma and primary dendrites of grafted PCs. From a physiological viewpoint, however, these inhibitory inputs cannot totally restore the powerful inhibition normally provided by the pericellular baskets and the pinceau formations.

Another important result of the synaptic integration of grafted PCs is their role in preventing neuronal retrograde cell death. The presence of numerous synapses between climbing fibers and PCs, parallel fibers and PCs, and molecular layer interneurons and PCs, indicates that the grafted neurons provide trophic factors to stabilize their presynaptic partners. In nontransplanted pcd mice 6 months old, granule cells and inferior olivary neurons show a massive retrograde cell death. Although a quantitative analysis has not yet been made in the transplanted pcd mice, degenerating olivary neurons and granule cells are much less evident than in nontransplanted mutants. These observations indicate that at least some of the presynaptic neurons contacting PCs are spared from the transsynaptic retrograde death occurring in adult pcd mutants.

PC Projections: Cortico-Nuclear Interactions

The only output of the cerebellar cortex is PC axonal projection. Thus, the restorative value of neuronal grafting is dependent on the ability of the grafted PCs to grow axons that could, by projecting to normal terminal domains, establish appropriate synaptic connections with target neurons. Despite some important restrictions, grafted PCs seem to be able to send projections to the deep nuclei of the host cerebellum. As in cases of neural transplantation dealing with global systems, the axonal growth of the transplanted neurons is specifically regulated by interactions with the surrounding tissue. Thus, dopaminergic neurons are capable of extensive axonal outgrowth only when grafted into their corresponding terminal domains, for instance, within the neostriatum.[37] Similarly, the ingrowth of grafted PC axons is specifically oriented toward a target tissue, either the deep nuclear neurons grafted with the implants or the deep cerebellar nuclei of the host. In both cases, the denervated target cells give rise to a positive neurotropism that attracts the proper afferent fibers. Although the nature of this attraction remains unknown, it is most probable that the target cells exert a growth-stimulating effect similar to that exerted by peripheral denervated targets.[cf.38] As mentioned concerning the attraction of migrating PCs to the host molecular layer, the distance between the attractive forces (the nuclear neurons of the host) and the origin of the afferent projection (the grafted PCs) is also a limiting factor for the successful development of corticonuclear interactions: only those PCs less than 0.5 mm from the deep nuclei of the host can potentially provide innervation to the nuclear neurons. These results point to the existence of neurotrophic factors that could, when released by deafferented deep nuclear neurons, create chemical gradients to regulate specifically the ingrowth of the grafted PC axons. A similar mechanism has been suggested for axonal ingrowth in transplantations dealing with global systems.[39]

The third prerequisite for neuronal replacement in point-to-point systems seems to be at least partially satisfied, even though it is the most restrictive of the three. Thus, neuronal grafting can succeed, to a certain extent, in replacing the missing elements of the pcd cerebellum.

CONCLUSION

From a series of long-term survival cerebellar transplantations into the cerebellum of adult pcd mutant mice, we have evaluated the chances for embryonic PCs of replacing the missing neurons in the mutant cerebellar circuitry. The results, obtained either with grafted cell suspensions or with solid implants, point to the possibility of fulfilling most of the conditions necessary for functional recovery from transplantation in point-to-point systems such as the cerebellar circuitry. First, the defective molecular layer of the host cerebellum selectively attracts grafted embryonic PCs, causing them to leave the grafts and migrate to the location of the missing neurons. Once there, the embryonic PCs provoke the axon terminal sprouting of host fibers, resulting in the synaptic integration of the grafted neurons into the cortical circuitry of the host cerebellum. Finally, the grafted PCs grow axons that are able to reach their appropriate targets in the deep cerebellar nuclei of the host, where they establish synaptic connections on large and small neurons.

Therefore, in mice with heredo-degenerative ataxia, the missing PCs can be partially replaced by grafted embryonic neurons of the same category. This replacement preserves the synaptic specificity of afferent and efferent inputs. The present results provide a solid morphological basis in favor of a functional restoration by neuronal transplantations in systems in which neurons are connected in a point-to-point manner.

ACKNOWLEDGMENTS

We are grateful to Professor P. Greengard and to Dr. M. Thomasset for their generous gifts of anti-cGK antibody and anti-CaBP antibody and to Dr. J. L. Guénet for his supply of pcd mutant mice. We would also like to thank D. Le Cren for photographic work; J. P. Rio, J. Simons, and B. Cholley for technical help; and B. Alvarado for secretarial work and for reviewing the English.

REFERENCES

1. TOMLINSON, B. E. & G. HENDERSON. 1976. Some quantitative cerebral findings in normal and demented old people. *In* Neurobiology of Aging. R. Terry & S. Gershon, Eds.: 183-204. Raven Press. New York, NY.
2. BLACKWOOD, W. & J. A. N. CORSELLIS, EDS. 1976. Greenfield's Neuropathology. 3rd edit. Edward Arnold. Edinburgh.
3. COTMAN, C. W., M. NIETO-SAMPEDRO & E. W. HARRIS. 1981. Synapse replacement in the nervous system of adult vertebrates. Physiol. Rev. **61**: 684-761.
4. MASON, D. W., H. M. CHARLTON, A. JONES, D. M. PARRY & S. J. SIMMONDS. 1985. Immunology of allograft rejection in mammals. *In* Neural Grafting in the Mammalian CNS. A. Björklund & U. Stenevi, Eds.: 91-98. Elsevier. Amsterdam.
5. DUNNETT, S. B. & A. BJÖRKLUND. 1985. Intracerebral, intraspinal and intraocular transplantation in mammals: A bibliography. *In* Neural Grafting in the Mammalian CNS. A. Björklund & U. Stenevi, Eds.: 673-700. Elsevier. Amsterdam.
6. MOBLEY, P. & P. GREENGARD. 1985. Evidence for widespread effect of noradrenaline on axon terminals in the rat frontal cortex. Proc. Natl. Acad. Sci. USA **82**: 945-947.

7. DOLPHIN, A. C. & P. GREENGARD. 1981. Serotonin stimulates phosphorylation of protein I in the facial motor nucleus of rat brain. Nature. **289:** 76-79.

8. BJÖRKLUND, A. & U. STENEVI. 1979. Reconstruction of the nigrostriatal dopamine pathway by intracerebral nigral transplants. Brain Res. **177:** 555-560.

9. BJÖRKLUND, A., S. B. DUNNETT, U. STENEVI, M. E. LEWIS & S. D. IVERSEN. 1980. Reinnervation of the denervated striatum by substantia nigra transplants: Functional considerations as revealed by pharmacological and sensorimotor testing. Brain Res. **199:** 307-333.

10. DUNNETT, S. B., A. BJÖRKLUND, U. STENEVI & S. D. IVERSEN. 1982. CNS transplantation: Structural and functional recovery from brain damage. Prog. Brain Res. **55:** 431-444.

11. FREED, W. J., M. J. PERLOW, F. KAROUM, A. SEIGER, L. OLSON, B. J. HOFFER & R. J. WYATT. 1980. Restoration of dopaminergic function by grafting of fetal rat substantia nigra to the caudate nucleus: Long-term behavioral, biochemical and histochemical studies. Ann. Neurol. **8:** 510-519.

12. PERLOW, M. J., W. J. FREED, B. J. HOFFER, A. SEIGER, L. OLSON & R. J. WYATT. 1979. Brain grafts reduce motor abnormalities produced by destruction of nigrostriatal dopamine system. Science **204:** 643-647.

13. BJÖRKLUND, A., M. SEGAL & U. STENEVI. 1979. Functional reinnervation of rat hippocampus by locus coeruleus implants. Brain Res. **170:** 409-426.

14. DUNNETT, S. B., W. C. LOW, S. D. IVERSEN, U. STENEVI & A. BJÖRKLUND. 1982. Septal transplants restore maze learning in rats with fornix-fimbria lesions. Brain Res. **251:** 335-348.

15. BJÖRKLUND, A. & U. STENEVI. 1977. Reformation of the severed septohippocampal cholinergic pathway in the adult rat by transplanted septal neurons. Cell Tissue Res. **185:** 289-302.

16. LOW, W. C., P. R. LEWIS, S. T. BUNCH, S. B. DUNNETT, S. R. THOMAS, S. D. IVERSEN, A. BJÖRKLUND & U. STENEVI. 1982. Functional recovery following neural transplantation of embryonic septal nuclei in adult rats with septohippocampal lesions. Nature **306:** 260-262.

17. ALVARADO-MALLART, R. M. & C. SOTELO. 1982. Differentiation of cerebellar anlage heterotopically transplanted to adult rat brain: A light and electron microscopic study. J. Comp. Neurol. **212:** 247-267.

18. SOTELO, C. & R. M. ALVARADO-MALLART. 1985. Cerebellar transplants: Immunocytochemical study of the specificity of Purkinje cell inputs and outputs. *In* Neural Grafting in the Mammalian CNS. A. Björklund & U. Stenevi, Eds.: 205-215. Elsevier. Amsterdam.

19. SOTELO, C. & R. M. ALVARADO-MALLART. 1986. Growth and differentiation of cerebellar suspensions transplanted into the adult cerebellum of mice with heredo-degenerative ataxia. Proc. Natl. Acad. Sci. USA **83:** 1135-1139.

20. SOTELO, C. & R. M. ALVARADO-MALLART. 1987. Reconstruction of the defective cerebellar circuitry in adult pcd mutant mice by Purkinje cell replacement through transplantation of solid embryonic implants. Neuroscience **20:** 1-22.

21. LANDIS, S. C. & R. J. MULLEN. 1978. The development and degeneration of Purkinje cells in pcd mutant mice. J. Comp. Neurol. **177:** 125-143.

22. SOTELO, C. & A. TRILLER. 1979. Fate of presynaptic afferents to Purkinje cells in the adult nervous mutant mouse: A model to study presynaptic stabilization. Brain Res. **175:** 11-36.

23. TRIARHOU, L. C., J. NORTON, C. ALYEA & B. GHETTI. 1985. A quantitative study of the granule cells in the Purkinje cell degeneration mutant. Ann. Neurol. **18:** 146.

24. PROCHIANTZ, A., U. D. PORZIO, A. KATO, B. BERGER & J. GLOWINSKI. 1979. *In vitro* maturation of mesencephalic dopaminergic neurons from mouse embryos is enhanced in presence of their striatal target cells. Proc. Natl. Acad. Sci. USA **76:** 5387-5391.

25. STERNBERGER, L. A., P. H. HARDY, JR., J. J. CUCULIS & H. G. MEYER. 1970. The unlabeled antibody method of immunohistochemistry: Preparation and properties of soluble antigen complex and its use in identification of spirochetes. J. Histochem. Cytochem. **18:** 315-333.

26. WALTER, U., P. MILLER, F. WILSON, D. MENKES & P. GREENGARD. 1980. Immunological distinction between guanosine 3',5'-monophosphate-dependent protein kinases. J. Biol. Chem. **255:** 3757-3762.

27. DE CAMILLI, P., P. MILLER, P. LEVITT, U. WALTER & P. GREENGARD. 1984. Anatomy of cerebellar Purkinje cells in the rat determined by a specific immunohistochemical marker. Neuroscience 11: 761-817.
28. THOMASSET, M., C. O. PARKES & P. CUISINIER-GLEIZES. 1982. Rat calcium-binding proteins: Distribution, ontogeny and vitamin D dependence. Am. J. Physiol. 243: E483-E488.
29. WEIBEL, E. R. 1979. Stereological Methods: Practical Methods for Biological Morphometry. Vol. 1. Academic Press. London.
30. MULLEN, R. J. 1977. Site of pcd gene action and Purkinje cell mosaicism in cerebella of chimaeric mice. Nature 270: 245-247.
31. MIALE, I. L. & R. L. SIDMAN. 1961. An autoradiographic analysis of histogenesis in the mouse cerebellum. Exp. Neurol. 4: 277-296.
32. MALLET, J., M. HUCHET, R. POUGEOIS & J. P. CHANGEUX. 1976. Anatomical, physiological and biochemical studies on the cerebellum from mutant mice. III. Protein differences associated with the weaver, staggerer and nervous mutations. Brain Res. 103: 291-312.
33. MARIANI, J., F. CREPEL, K. MIKOSHIBA, J. P. CHANGEUX & C. SOTELO. 1977. Anatomical, physiological and biochemical studies of the cerebellum from reeler mutant mouse. Philos. Trans. R. Soc. London Ser. B. 281: 1-28.
34. RAMON Y CAJAL, S. 1910. Algunas observaciones favorables a la hipótesis neurotrópica. Trab. Lab. Inv. Biol. Univ. Madrid. 8: 63-135.
35. SOTELO, C. 1978. Purkinje cell ontogeny: Formation and maintenance of spines. Prog. Brain Res. 48: 149-170.
36. SOTELO, C. 1975. Synaptic remodeling in mutants and experimental animals. In Aspects of Neural Plasticity. F. Vital-Durand & M. Jeannerod, Eds.: 167-190. INSERM. Paris.
37. BJÖRKLUND, A., U. STENEVI, R. H. SCHMIDT, S. B. DUNNETT & F. H. GAGE. 1983. Intracerebral grafting of neuronal cell suspensions. II. Survival and growth of nigral cells implanted in different brain sites. Acta Physiol. Scand. Suppl. 522: 11-22.
38. HENDERSON, C. E. 1986. Activity and the regulation of neuronal growth factor metabolism. In The Neural and Molecular Bases of Learning. Dahlem Konferenzen. J. P. Changeux & M. Koniski, Eds. In press. Springer-Verlag. Berlin.
39. BJÖRKLUND, A. & U. STENEVI. 1984. Intracerebral neural implants: Neuronal replacement and reconstruction of damaged circuitries. Annu. Rev. Neurosci. 7: 279-308.

DISCUSSION OF THE PAPER

M. SEGAL (*Weizmann Institute, Rehovot*): I wonder if you have any behavioral recovery in this biological material?

SOTELO: For the moment, as a neuroanatomist, I am concentrating on the anatomy of this system. The problem of functional recovery is difficult because the motor behavior of the mutants varies very much from one animal to another. Since we still do not have a test for motor behavior to determine individual variability, we have not tried to investigate whether there is improvement in the mutant mice with grafted cerebellum.

SEGAL: There is no apparent improvement?

SOTELO: It is very difficult to say if there is apparent improvement. The problem is that some of the mice behave better than others. You cannot, just by looking at the colony, say whether a particular animal has an implant.

R. LINDSAY (*Sandoz Institute for Medical Research, London*): I think this biological material provides a very interesting paradigm. Could you explain the specificity? Have you, for example, transplanted it at later stages, when Purkinje cells are more developed, and do granular cells then migrate? Have you transplanted, for example, hippocampus, and do any of these cells migrate?

SOTELO: Your paradigm has been fitted with our biological material already. We have tried most of the experiments suggested in your question. We have injected hippocampal and septal nuclei neurons, as cell suspensions, into the pcd mutant cerebellum. The result is that the grafted cells do not migrate but stay inside the transplants.

Similarly, if you transplant cerebellum to hippocampus in which a lesion has been made with kainic acid (so that we know that neurons are missing in the hippocampus), again the transplant stays as a mass, and Purkinje cells do not invade the deficient hippocampus. Therefore, there is a very specific type of attraction of a cerebellar molecular layer devoid of Purkinje cells for transplanted neurons of the same category.

C. B. JAEGER (*New York University Medical Center, New York, NY*): I would like to ask two questions. First, in the migration of your Purkinje cells, do you ever see moving astroglia accompanied or followed by Purkinje cells? Second, do you see aberrant collaterals coming onto the Purkinje cells as an input? That is, does the axon come back to the cell bodies?

SOTELO: Yes for the first question. We have been doing double-labeling studies, using vimentin to identify immature glia and calcium-binding protein to recognized grafted Purkinje cells. Unfortunately, I did not know then that in the mouse, vimentin also stains adult astrocytes, and that there is as much vimentin as GFAP in an adult mouse astrocyte. From these double-labeling experiments, it appears that the glia of the host invades the transplant, but I do not know whether the glia of the transplants invades the host. Purkinje cells first migrate tangentially, migration which seems to be free of glia, followed by a perpendicular migration along the glial axis.

So a corridor is made at the surface of the cerebellum, between the glial and the basal membranes. There, the embryonic Purkinje cells move tangentially. Then, when they reach a certain distance they begin to move inward. In double-labeling experiments, radially migrating Purkinje cells appear parallel and in close proximity to the glial axes, formed by the Bergmann fibers. But do not forget, these Purkinje cells are moving in a direction opposite to that they normally follow during development.

The answer to the second question is yes. Some of the axons of grafted Purkinje cells, mainly in those cases where they cannot reach their target (the deep nuclei of the host), project either to deep nuclear cells present within the implant remnant, or contact other grafted Purkinje cells.

S. McLOON (*University of Minnesota, Minneapolis, MN*): Do you see any evidence of topography in the connection between the Purkinje cells?

SOTELO: The cerebellum is organized in sagitally functional compartments. What is important is not only the cell-to-cell recognition—which we have now proved and which is at the base of what we call synaptic specificity (indeed, climbing fibers contact grafted Purkinje cells whereas mossy fibers do not)—but the topographic organization of inputs and outputs for Purkinje cells. The cerebellar function is based on the fact that a limited column of cells in the inferior olive will project to very specific bands in the cortex, and we have no idea whether this topography is achieved with the grafted Purkinje cells. I suppose that it will be very difficult to imagine that the grafted Purkinje cells are moving to predetermined locations in the molecular layer, and have the positional information to go to places where they are supposed to go. I think what happens is that we are creating a new type of topography with the cannula track, since the cells move to the closest molecular layer and send projections to the closest deep nucleus of the host. I doubt that functional topography could be reconstructed at present with cerebellar transplants.

Synaptogenesis of Grafted Cholinergic Neurons

D. J. CLARKE,[a] F. H. GAGE,[b] S. B. DUNNETT,[c]
O. G. NILSSON,[d] AND A. BJÖRKLUND[d]

[a] Department of Pharmacology
Oxford University
Oxford, England

[b] Department of Neurosciences
University of California at San Diego
La Jolla, California

[c] Department of Experimental Psychology
Cambridge University
Cambridge, England

[d] Department of Histology
University of Lund
Lund, Sweden

INTRODUCTION

Over recent years, a wealth of morphological and electrophysiological evidence has emerged to suggest that grafts of fetal neurons form functional connections with the host central nervous system in a variety of anatomically distinct or chemically specific neuronal systems (for example, dopamine systems,[1,2] serotonin systems,[3,4] acetylcholine (ACh) systems,[5-8] noradrenaline systems,[9] retinal grafts,[10,11] cerebellar grafts,[12] and hippocampal grafts[13]). The cholinergic system has aroused much interest as a result of its implication in neurological disorders of learning and memory[14,15] and in the pathology of Alzheimer's Disease.[16] Grafts of cholinergic neurons from the fetal septal-diagonal band or basal forebrain areas have been demonstrated to be behaviorally and electrophysiologically active, in either young rats with prior denervation of the intrinsic cholinergic systems[8,17-21] or in behaviorally impaired aged animals.[22,23] Thus cholinergic-rich grafts are able to ameliorate impairments in learning and memory and to form electrically competent connections between graft and host. In view of these observations, the aims of the studies described here were to address the question of whether cholinergic grafts exert their effects by forming new, functional synaptic connections with host neuronal elements, and the extent to which these novel contacts resemble those normally found in control animals.

NORMAL CONNECTIVITY OF THE CHOLINERGIC SYSTEM IN HIPPOCAMPUS AND NEOCORTEX

It is now well established that cholinergic neurons in the basal forebrain send extensive projections to neocortex and hippocampus.[24–27] Until recently, however, with the advent of specific and sensitive antisera to choline acetyltransferase (ChAT), the synthetic enzyme for ACh, it was not possible to study the pattern of cholinergic termination and synaptic connectivity within cortical regions.

Hippocampus

Early studies of cholinergic termination using acetylcholinesterase (AChE) histochemical staining within the hippocampal formation revealed a laminar distribution of fiber staining.[28–30] Dense bands of fiber staining were observed adjacent to the pyramidal cell layers and the granule cell layer of the dentate gyrus.[28,31] The bulk of this cholinergic innervation originates in the medial septum and the nucleus of the diagonal band, and the pattern of septal termination as revealed by anterograde tracing techniques closely resembles the pattern seen with AChE staining.[32–35] Immunocytochemistry using monoclonal ChAT antibodies in the hippocampal formation support these earlier studies, in that a dense supragranular and suprapyramidal band was also visualized (FIG. 1A).[36,37] The ChAT-positive fibers are fine caliber with numerous large varicosities. Few fibers were found within the cell layers themselves; they seemed predominantly associated with the basal and apical dendrites of pyramidal neurons and primary dendrites of the granule cells.[36]

The hilar region of the dentate gyrus contained both cholinergic fibers and several ChAT-immunoreactive perikarya.[36,37] Cholinergic interneurons were also located in the stratum oriens, as well as in the stratum moleculare of both the dentate gyrus and the hippocampus itself (unpublished observation).

At the ultrastructural level, ChAT-immunoreactive boutons were identified by the dark, electron-dense coating of the immunoreaction product around the synaptic vesicles, giving the immunostained terminal an overall dark appearance (FIGS. 1B, 1C, 1E & 1F). Boutons were small (0.4-0.7 μm diameter) and had relatively large vesicles. Synaptic specializations were generally of the symmetrical type (Gray type II), though some contacts onto dendritic spine heads were asymmetrical.[36,37] The predominant postsynaptic target of the ChAT-immunoreactive boutons was dendritic shafts (65%) (TABLE 1 and FIGS. 1B & 1C), and only a small percentage of the identified synaptic terminals (5%) contacted neuronal perikarya.

These results are in agreement with other ultrastructural studies of cholinergic boutons in rat brain.[37–39]

Neocortex

Unlike the cholinergic innervation of the hippocampus, that of the neocortex originates from the magnocellular neurons of the basal forebrain. The innervation of neocortex is more diffuse than that of hippocampus, although some studies using

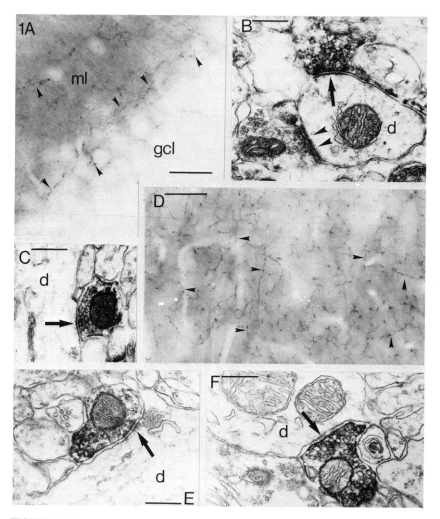

FIGURE 1. (A) Low-power light micrograph of ChAT fiber staining in control rat dentate gyrus. A dense band of ChAT-immunoreactive fibers (some of which are indicated by arrowheads) is found adjacent to the granule cell layer (gcl), at the base of the molecular layer (ml). Fibers are also apparent in the upper parts of the molecular layer. (B & C) Examples of ChAT-immunoreactive boutons forming symmetrical synaptic connections (arrows) with dendritic shafts (d). In **B**, a nonimmunoreactive bouton also forms an asymmetrical contact (arrowheads) onto the same dendritic shaft (d). (**D**) Light micrograph of layer IV of control frontoparietal cortex. ChAT-immunoreactive fibers (some of which are indicated by arrowheads) have a random distribution throughout the neuropil. (**E & F**) Electron micrographs of ChAT-immunoreactive boutons forming symmetrical membrane specializations (arrows) with dendritic shafts (d). Scale bars: **A**: 30 μm; **B, C, E & F**: 0.25 μm; **D**: 25 μm.

AChE histochemistry report bands of increased fiber density in layers II and III.[40,41] ChAT immunostaining, however, has revealed the presence of small, bipolar cholinergic interneurons. These interneurons were especially concentrated in layers II and III[5,38,42,43] but were not apparent in neocortex processed for AChE histochemistry.

Fine-caliber cholinergic fibers ramify throughout all cortical layers. Their orientation, however, varies according to their layer position: in layers I and VI fibers course parallel to the pia and white matter whereas in layers II-V the fibers have a more random distribution (FIG. 1D).

The appearance of these cholinergic boutons in the electron microscope was essentially similar to that previously described for the hippocampus.[5,38] Material from each layer of frontal neocortex was examined, and, in all layers, the predominant postsynaptic target of the symmetrical synapses from ChAT-positive boutons was dendritic shafts. It was often possible to identify the dendritic shafts as the apical

TABLE 1. Percentage Distribution of Postsynaptic Targets of ChAT-positive Boutons in Control, Young Grafted, and Aged Grafted Hippocampus

Postsynaptic Target	Control		Young Grafted		Aged Grafted	
	N	%	N	%	N	%
Dendritic shafts	51	64.6	31	23.7	85	64.9
Dendritic spines	17	21.5	12	9.1	28	21.4
Small dendrites or spines	5	6.3	—	—	11	8.4
Perikarya	4	5.1	88	67.2	7	5.3
Nonidentified	2	2.5	—	—	—	—
Total	79	100.0	131	100.0	131	100.0

dendrites of pyramidal neurons (TABLE 2 and FIGS. 1D & 1E). As in hippocampus, a small percentage of the boutons contacted neuronal perikarya (in this case, nonpyramidal neurons in layers II and IV). Synaptic specializations were generally symmetrical (Gray type II), though many axospinous specializations often displayed a greater density of postsynaptic thickening and may thus be classified as asymmetrical.[5,38,39]

CHOLINERGIC GRAFTS TO THE HIPPOCAMPAL FORMATION

In these experiments, suspension grafts prepared from the septal-diagonal band area of E14-16 rat fetuses (crown-to-rump length: 12-16 mm) were prepared according to the procedure of Björklund et al.[44] and injected directly into two sites within the hippocampal formation.[6,22]

Two groups of rats were studied using ChAT immunocytochemistry: a group of young rats, which received a denervating lesion of the fimbria-fornix at the time of transplantation (referred to later as the young, denervated group), and a group of aged rats, which were defined as being behaviorally impaired on the basis of their ability to learn a spatial navigation task in the Morris water maze[22] and which received

TABLE 2. Postsynaptic Targets of ChAT-immunoreactive Boutons in Control and Grafted Frontal Neocortex

Postsynaptic Target	I Control N	I Control %	II Control N	II Control %	III Control N	III Control %	IV Control N	IV Control %	IV Grafted N	IV Grafted %	V Control N	V Control %	V Grafted N	V Grafted %	VI Control N	VI Control %	VI Grafted N	VI Grafted %	Total[a] Control N	Total[a] Control %	Total[a] Grafted N	Total[a] Grafted %
Dendritic shafts	17	68	18	64	15	65	22	65	18	58	28	67	34	56	11	61	17	68	111	65	69	58
Dendritic spines	5	20	5	18	5	22	6	18	5	16	9	22	8	13	4	22	5	20	34	20	18	15
Small shafts or spines	3	12	4	14	3	13	4	12	2	6	5	12	3	5	3	17	3	12	22	13	8	7
Perikarya	—	—	1	4	—	—	2	6	6	20	—	—	16	26	—	—	—	—	3	2	22	19
Total	25	100	28	100	23	100	34	100	31	100	42	100	61	100	18	100	25	100	170	100	117	100

[a] All layers taken together.

a similar fimbria-fornix lesion just prior to sacrifice, but not at the time of grafting. The pattern of reinnervation in the hippocampus of these two groups of rats has previously been studied using AChE histochemistry[22,45]; the aims of the present studies were to examine the pattern of connectivity of graft-derived cholinergic fibers within the host hippocampal formation at both the light and electron microscopical levels using more specific and sensitive immunocytochemical methods as a marker for the cholinergic system. Septal grafts have been shown to be functionally active with respect to amelioration of behavioral impairments in both groups of animals.[22,46] Therefore, it is necessary to consider whether the functional recovery is mediated by new synapse formation in both groups and, if it is, whether the patterns of innervation for the two groups and for the group of young control rats are similar.

Twelve to 15 weeks after transplantation, suspension grafts were located in the host hippocampal formation (FIG. 2A) at the light microscopical level and appeared essentially similar in both young, denervated rats and in the aged animals, though the size and position of the grafts varied between individual animals in both groups. In some cases, grafts were large and occupied a large proportion of the host hippocampus whereas, at the other extreme, small grafts appeared confined to the choroidal fissure. Numerous intensely ChAT-immunoreactive neurons could be visualized within the graft, many of which appeared to be distributed along the border between the graft and the host tissue (FIG. 2A).

Within the graft neuropil, fine ChAT-positive fibers appeared intermingled with perikarya, and, on several occasions, fibers could be traced from the graft into the host hippocampal formation. The pattern of termination of these graft-derived fibers was carefully analyzed and compared to that seen in the control animals. In both grafted groups, the intrinsic cholinergic innervation had been removed by a fimbria-fornix lesion either acutely, as in the aged rats, or chronically, in the young, denervated group. Since this lesion is known to remove all extrinsic cholinergic innervation to the dorsal hippocampus, the ChAT fibers in the grafted hippocampus were predominantly of graft origin. The cholinergic interneurons may, however, account for some of the innervation, but, as a control, a few animals with fimbria-fornix transection but no grafts were examined in parallel. In the aged, impaired group, the cholinergic fibers appeared to terminate in the appropriate laminae, as compared to the control animals, but in the young, denervated group, an anomalous fiber pattern was observed.

Young, Denervated Grafted Animals

In these animals, where the fimbria-fornix was aspiration-lesioned at the time of grafting, the cholinergic fibers from the graft appeared to terminate predominantly within the granule cell layer (FIG. 2B) and the pyramidal cell layer of CA1 and did not form a dense band of staining adjacent to the cell layer at the base of the dendrites, as was seen in the control animals. In the lesion-only group, there was an almost complete absence of fiber staining in the cell body layers, though cholinergic interneurons were still visible.

This anomalous ChAT terminal distribution was also apparent at the ultrastructural level, where the predominant postsynaptic target of ChAT-immunoreactive boutons was neuronal perikarya (TABLE 1 and FIG. 2D), many of which could be identified as granule or pyramidal cells by their ultrastructural morphology.

Synaptic specializations were, again, generally of the symmetrical type, though a greater percentage of cholinergic, graft-derived boutons formed asymmetrical (Gray

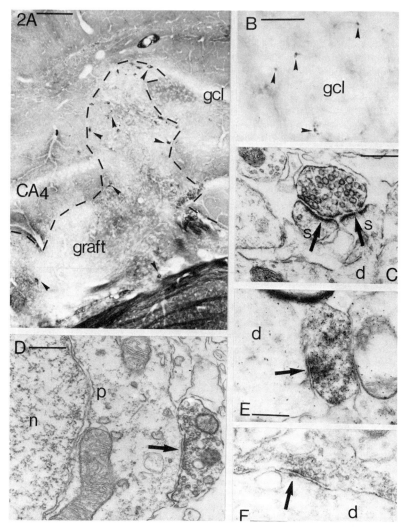

FIGURE 2. (A) Low-power light micrograph of a typical septal-diagonal band suspension graft within host hippocampus. The approximate boundary of the graft is shown by the dashed lines. The host granule cell layer (gcl) and pyramidal cell layer of CA4 remain virtually undisturbed by the presence of the graft. Numerous intensely ChAT-immunoreactive perikarya are visible within the graft (arrowheads), many of which are found adjacent to the graft-host interface. (B) In the young, denervated grafted rats, the majority of ChAT-immunoreactive fibers and varicosities (arrowheads) were found within the granule cell layer (gcl) itself and did not form a distinct supragranular band (see FIG. 1A). (C) Electron micrograph of a ChAT-immunoreactive bouton in a young, denervated grafted rat. The bouton forms two asymmetrical synaptic contacts (arrows) with two spine heads (s). One spine can be seen to emerge from a dendrite (d). (D) In the young, denervated grafted rats, the predominant postsynaptic target of the graft-derived ChAT-immunoreactive boutons was neuronal perikarya. In this electron micrograph a ChAT bouton forms a symmetrical membrane contact (arrow) with the perikaryon (p) of a probable granule cell (n: nucleus). (E & F) Electron micrograph of graft-derived ChAT-immunoreactive boutons in aged rats, both of which form symmetrical synapses (arrow) with dendritic shafts (d). The shaft in F could, in serial section, be traced to the perikaryon of a granule cell. Scale bars: A: 200 μm; B: 15 μm; C-F: 0.25 μm.

type I) synapses onto spines (FIG. 2C), dendritic shafts, and, occasionally, neuronal cell bodies. Thus, in the young, denervated groups of grafted animals, the graft-derived cholinergic fibers formed new synaptic specializations with host neuronal elements, but their pattern of termination and their postsynaptic targets were anomalous, in that a hyperinnervation of neuronal perikarya occurred.

These findings may reflect an ontogenetic effect. In immature animals, in other cortical regions, a greater number of synaptic boutons are found, especially in contact with cell bodies[47] that may be lost during development.[48] Thus, although information on the cholinergic innervation of hippocampus in immature animals is lacking, it seems possible that the innervation of the host hippocampus from graft-derived cholinergic fibers may reflect the situation in immature animals. Alternatively, a second hypothesis is that the ingrowing axons may fill spaces around the neuronal cell bodies normally occupied by noncholinergic septohippocampal terminals[49–51] or by hippocampal afferent terminals of different origin[52] that are removed as a result of the extensive fimbria-fornix lesion. The graft fibers may thus be guided toward the vacant synaptic sites.

Aged, Impaired Grafted Animals

In these animals, the intrinsic cholinergic input to the hippocampus was removed 5-7 days before sacrifice to ensure that any ChAT-immunoreactive fibers examined in the host tissue were probably of graft origin. A group of behaviorally impaired aged rats received similar acute unilateral fimbria-fornix lesions, but no grafts, to control for the efficacy of the lesion. In these animals, the contralateral side of the brain to the lesion provided a control for the staining procedure.

At the light microscopical level, numerous graft-derived cholinergic fibers were seen to cross the graft-host interface and ramify in the region adjacent to the granule cell layer of the dentate gyrus at the base of the molecular layer. In this study, only the dentate gyrus was examined. Thus, the cholinergic innervation from the graft, of the host dentate, appeared to form a distinct supragranular band of fiber staining, which was similar to that seen in young control animals. The innervation was never as complete as that seen in the young control group, however, in that fewer fibers and varicosities were visible. In the group that only received lesions, very few cholinergic fibers were seen in the dentate gyrus, though several ChAT-immunoreactive interneurons were apparent in the hilar region. On the contralateral side of the brain to the denervation, however, there also appeared to be a decreased level of fiber staining as compared to animals of the same age that were not behaviorally impaired (unpublished results).

At the electron microscopical level, many ChAT-immunoreactive terminals were studied, and, as with the young control group, the predominant postsynaptic target was dendritic shafts (TABLE 1 and FIGS. 2E & 2F). Occasionally, it was possible to identify the dendritic shaft as being of granule cell origin. In the host dentate gyrus in both the grafted animals and the animals that only received lesions, numerous dark, degenerating terminals were found. This degeneration resulted from the acute fimbria-fornix lesion. All degenerating terminals studied formed asymmetrical synaptic contacts with dendritic shafts or spines in the dentate molecular layer, and, in the grafted animals, although degenerating terminals appeared close to ChAT-immunoreactive boutons, the two bouton types were easily distinguishable.[7]

Thus the percentage distribution of postsynaptic targets in these aged grafted rats was essentially the same as that seen in the young, control rats but considerably different from that in the young, denervated grafted rats. This may suggest, therefore, that the graft reinnervation of host hippocampal formation in these aged, behaviorally impaired rats more closely resembles the "normal" situation than that obtained in rats with a prior denervating lesion. It appears that the fiber ingrowth from the graft occurs on top of the intrinsic cholinergic innervation, which suggests that the aging process may result in a partial denervation of the dentate gyrus, thus removing synaptic sites that the ingrowing cholinergic axons can occupy. It is, thus, plausible to speculate that the synaptogenesis in the host hippocampus in these intact aged animals may be functionally more appropriate than those partly anomalous connections formed in the young, grafted rats with prior denervation in the fimbria-fornix.

GRAFTS TO THE FRONTOPARIETAL NEOCORTEX

In this study, rats received unilateral ibotenic acid lesions of nucleus basalis (NBM), the region of origin of the cholinergic innervation of the neocortex. The rats were then subjected to a battery of sensorimotor tests as described in detail elsewhere.[18,53] One week after receiving a lesion, most animals received a suspension graft of fetal ventral forebrain area from rat embryos (crown-to-rump length: 16 mm) injected directly into two sites in host dorsolateral frontoparietal neocortex[5]; the remaining rats received only lesions and served as controls. Three to 4 months after receiving transplants, the rats were again behaviorally tested on the same sensorimotor tests and then processed for ChAT immunocytochemistry.

The suspension grafts located within neocortex were generally fairly small and often found in deeper layers of the cortex just above the corpus callosum. A typical graft is illustrated in FIGURE 3A. Clusters of ChAT-immunoreactive neurons were readily visible within the grafts and several were distributed along the graft-host interface. Fine-caliber ChAT-positive fibers were numerous within the graft and could often be traced into the surrounding deep cortical layers. Fibers extended 1-2 mm from the graft into, predominantly, layers IV-VI of neocortex, though, occasionally, also into layer III. The graft-derived fibers often appeared in close apposition to neuronal perikarya, especially in layers IV and V (FIG. 3B), although the graft-derived innervation of host neocortex was significantly less dense than that of the contralateral neocortex, which had received neither lesions nor grafts, and of neocortex from intact, control rats (FIG. 1D). In the animals that received only lesions, very little ChAT fiber staining was visible in layers IV-VI, though several cholinergic interneurons were seen in layers II and III and some fiber staining was seen in layers I and II. This fiber staining may represent fibers spared following the NBM lesion, fibers from the interneurons, or, alternatively, fibers from another source of cholinergic innervation such as the brainstem[54] or tegmentum.[51]

Specimens from layers IV-VI were taken for electron microscopical analysis, to determine whether new synaptic connections are formed between graft and host similar as they are in the hippocampus. Synaptic specializations were observed between ChAT-immunoreactive boutons of presumed graft origin in layers IV-VI and various neuronal elements in host neocortex. The predominant postsynaptic target was, as in the normal control animals, dendritic shafts (FIG. 3C), although a greater percentage of the contacts in layers IV and V contacted neuronal perikarya, especially layer V pyramidal neurons (TABLE 2 and FIG. 3D).

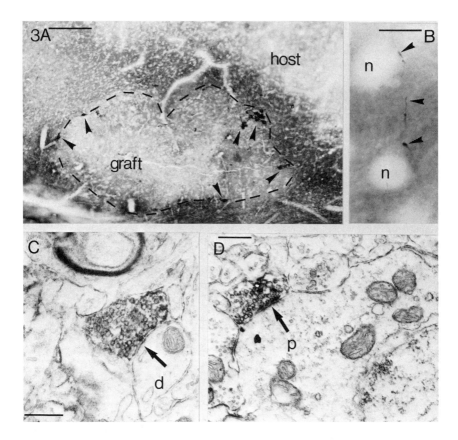

FIGURE 3. (A) Light micrograph of a ventral forebrain suspension graft in deep layers of frontoparietal cortex. Many ChAT-positive neurons are apparent, some of which are indicated by arrowheads, lying adjacent to the boundary of the graft, as shown by the dashed lines. **(B)** Fibers from the graft were seen in layers IV-VI of frontal cortex. In this light micrograph, a graft-derived ChAT-positive fiber (arrowheads) is in close apposition to two neuronal perikarya (n) in layer IV. **(C)** Electron micrograph of a ChAT-immunoreactive bouton forming a symmetrical synapse (arrow) with a dendritic shaft (d). **(D)** In the grafted animals, ChAT-immunoreactive boutons were found in symmetrical synaptic contact (arrow) with neuronal perikarya (p), many of which could be identified by their ultrastructural characteristics as pyramidal cells. Scale bars: **A**: 200 μm; **B**: 12 μm; **C** & **D**: 0.35 μm.

Bouton morphology was essentially the same as in both normal cortex and hippocampus, as well as in other brain areas,[6,36–39] and synaptic specializations were generally symmetrical, although many of the axospinous contacts were probably asymmetrical.

The differences in postsynaptic targets were not as great as those seen in the young, denervated hippocampal group, although an obvious perikaryal hyperinnervation of pyramidal neurons was demonstrated in layer V. The reasons for this hyperinnervation are not known, although more axosomatic contacts are established in early development that are either relocated or lost completely during development.[47,48,55] Thus the ingrowing fibers from embryonic graft tissue may become arrested upon establishment of an immature pattern of innervation. The cholinergic axons may exert a similar, or more powerful, physiological effect by directly contacting the cell body rather than more distal portions of the dendrites of the same neurons.

DISCUSSION

Until recently, synaptogenesis was considered an ontogenetic occurrence, one which ceased to be apparent in the fully mature central nervous system. More recent evidence, however, suggests that the brain remains plastic until senescence and retains the ability to incorporate new neuronal elements into a functional circuit of connectivity, presumably by the formation of new, active synaptic specializations. One line of evidence for such a phenomenon comes from studies of sprouting of afferent pathways following lesions of other primary inputs, a feature seen widely in the hippocampal formation.[56-60]

This phenomenon, often referred to as reactive synaptogenesis, has been clearly demonstrated in many such studies[56,58,61,62] where, following an extensive lesion of the entorhinal cortex, septal and commisural afferents to the dentate gyrus expand their fields of termination to occupy laminae normally occupied by perforant path connections to the granule cells. The time course of such synaptogenesis has been well documented.[56] The ability of the brain to accept and integrate new circuitry may also be seen following transplantation, as is demonstrated by the results presented here. Previous studies have suggested that the functional recovery following grafting may occur as a result of the formation of new synaptic connections in the host animal from ingrowing graft axons. Conversely, host elements themselves have also demonstrated an ability to form new synaptic contacts with neuronal elements in the graft.[13,63-65]

The results presented in this paper are consistent with previous electrophysiological studies on septal grafts in the hippocampal formation[29] and show that although functional synaptic connections are established between graft and host elements, their pattern of termination may be anomalous in animals that have undergone prior denervation of the intrinsic input. A similar study where dopaminergic mesencephalic tissue has been grafted to neostriatum[1] reports a similar erroneous termination upon large neuronal perikarya within host neostriatum. In these cases, the synaptogenesis observed may reflect a reinnervation of the initially denervated heterologous sites by the graft fibers.

In senescence, there is an overall decrease in neuronal elements within cortex and hippocampus. In the hippocampal formation, a notable feature of aging appears to be the loss or atrophy of dendritic spines and small branches.[66,67] Concomitant with this, several authors report a decrease in the number and density of synapses, especially in the dentate gyrus,[61,68,69] of up to 35%. This may reflect a partial denervation of the hippocampus as a result of an age-dependent degeneration process or, alternatively, a reduction in synaptic contacts as a result of the loss of postsynaptic elements. Despite such degenerative changes of the dentate gyrus during aging, however, it still retains the ability to incorporate the ingrowing graft axons and establish new synaptic contacts. In these cases, it is conceivable that the graft axons may be filling synaptic sites vacated by degenerating afferent pathways and thus be reinnervating a partially denervated target (as in the young, denervated group) or the fiber ingrowth may be formed on top of the intrinsic cholinergic input.

The former theory seems most plausible, however, in the light of other studies showing sprouting of cholinergic axons in the dentate gyrus after deafferentation in aged rats,[61] since a fairly "normal" pattern of termination was found in the present aged grafted animals, a pattern that could occur as a result of the reinnervation of specific cholinergic terminal sites, vacated by an age-dependent deafferentation of the hippocampal cholinergic input.

In conclusion, the results presented in this chapter provide unequivocal evidence that synaptogenesis from ingrowing, graft-derived cholinergic fibers occurs extensively within the host hippocampus and neocortex, irrespective of the age of the host animal. The formation of the new cholinergic synapses may, in part, be responsible for the ability of such cholinergic grafts to ameliorate functional impairments.

REFERENCES

1. FREUND, T., J. P. BOLAM, A. BJÖRKLUND, U. STENEVI, S. B. DUNNETT, J. F. POWELL & A. D. SMITH. 1985. Efferent synaptic connections of grafted dopaminergic neurons reinnervating the host neostriatum: A tyrosine hydroxylase immunocytochemical study. J. Neurosci. 5: 603-616.

2. MAHALIK, T. J., T. E. FINGER, I. STRÖMBERG & L. OLSON. 1985. Substantia nigra transplants into denervated striatum of the rat: Ultrastructure of graft and host interconnections. J. Comp. Neurol. 240: 60-70.

3. BEEBE, B. K., A. MOLLGÅRD, A. BJÖRKLUND & U. STENEVI. 1979. Ultrastructural evidence of synaptogenesis in the adult rat dentate gyrus from brainstem implants. Brain Res. 167: 391-395.

4. SEGAL, M. 1987. Interactions between grafted serotin neurons and adult host rat hippocampus. Ann. N.Y. Acad. Sci. This volume.

5. CLARKE, D. J. & S. B. DUNNETT. 1986. Ultrastructural organization of choline acetyltransferase-immunoreactive fibers innervating the neocortex from embryonic ventral forebrain grafts. J. Comp. Neurol. 250: 192-205.

6. CLARKE, D. J., F. H. GAGE & A. BJÖRKLUND. 1986. Formation of cholinergic synapses by intrahippocampal septal grafts as revealed by choline acetyltransferase immunocytochemistry. Brain Res. 369: 151-162.

7. CLARKE, D. J., F. H. GAGE, O. G. NILSSON & A. BJÖRKLUND. 1986. Formation of cholinergic synapses in the dentate gyrus of behaviorally impaired aged rats by grafted septal neurons. J. Comp. Neurol. 252: 483-492.

8. SEGAL, M., A. BJÖRKLUND & F. H. GAGE. 1985. Intracellular analysis of cholinergic synapses between grafted septal nucleus and host hippocampal pyramidal neurons. In Neural Grafting in the Mammalian CNS. A. Björklund & U. Stenevi, Eds.: 389-399. Elsevier. Amsterdam.

9. BJÖRKLUND, A. & U. STENEVI. 1979. Regeneration of monoaminergic and cholinergic neurons in the mammalian central nervous system. Physiol. Rev. 59: 62-100.

10. LUND, R. D. & D. J. SIMONS. 1985. Retinal transplants: Structural and functional interrelations with the host brain. In Neural Grafting in the Mammalian CNS. A. Björklund & U. Stenevi, Eds.: 345-354. Elsevier. Amsterdam.

11. McLOON, L. K., R. D. LUND & S. C. McLOON. 1982. Transplantation of reaggregates of embryonic neural retinae to neonatal rat brain: Differentiation and formation of connections. J. Comp. Neurol. 205: 179-189.

12. ALVARADO-MALLART, R. M. & C. SOTELO. 1982. Differentiation of cerebellar anlage heterotopically transplanted to adult rat brain: A light and electron microscopic study. J. Comp. Neurol. 212: 247-267.

13. RAISMAN, G. & F. F. EBNER. 1983. Mossy fiber projections into and out of hippocampal transplants. Neuroscience 9: 783-801.

14. BARTUS, R. T., R. L. DEAN, B. BEER & A. S. LIPPA. 1982. The cholinergic hypothesis of geriatric memory disfunction. Science 217: 408-417.

15. DEUTSCH, J. A. 1971. The cholinergic synapse and the site of memory. Science 174: 788-794.
16. COYLE, J. T., D. L. PRICE & M. R. DELONG. 1983. Alzheimer's disease: A disorder of cortical cholinergic innervation. Science 219: 1184-1190.
17. BUZSÁKI, G., F. H. GAGE, J. CZOPF & A. BJÖRKLUND. 1986. Restoration of rhythmic slow activity (theta) in the subcortically denervated hippocampus by fetal CNS transplants. Brain Res. Submitted for publication.
18. DUNNETT, S. B., G. TONIOLO, A. FINE, C. N. RYAN, A. BJÖRKLUND & S. D. IVERSEN. 1985. Transplantation of embryonic ventral forebrain neurons to the neocortex of rats with lesions of nucleus basalis mannocellularis. II. Sensorimotor and learning impairments. Neuroscience 16: 787-798.
19. FINE, A., S. B. DUNNETT, A. BJÖRKLUND, D. J. CLARKE & S. D. IVERSEN. 1985. Transplantation of embryonic ventral forebrain neurons to the neocortex of rats with lesions of nucleus basalis magnocellularis. I. Biochemical and anatomical and biochemical observations. Neuroscience 16: 769-786.
20. GAGE, F. H., A. BJÖRKLUND, U. STENEVI, S. B. DUNNETT & P. A. T. KELLY. 1984. Intrahippocampal septal grafts ameliorate learning impairments in aged rats. Science 225: 533-536.
21. LOW, W. C., P. R. LEWIS, S. T. BUNCH, S. B. DUNNETT, S. R. THOMAS, S. D. IVERSEN, A. BJÖRKLUND & U. STENEVI. 1982. Functional recovery following transplantation of embryonic septal nuclei into adult rats with septohippocampal lesions: The recovery of function. Nature (London) 300: 260-262.
22. GAGE, F. H. & A. BJÖRKLUND. 1986. Cholinergic septal grafts into the hippocampal formation improve spatial learning and memory in aged rats by an atropine-sensitive mechanism. J. Neurosci. 17: 89-98.
23. GAGE, F. H., S. B. DUNNETT, U. STENEVI & A. BJÖRKLUND. 1983. Intracerebral grafting of neuronal cell suspensions. VIII. Survival and growth of implants of nigral and septal cell suspensions in intact brain of aged rats. Acta Physiol. Scand. Suppl. 522: 67-75.
24. BAKST, I. & D. G. AMARAL. 1984. The distribution of acetylcholinesterase in the hippocampal formation of the monkey. J. Comp. Neurol. 225: 334-371.
25. INGHAM, C. A., J. P. BOLAM, B. H. WAINER & A. D. SMITH. 1985. A correlated light and electron microscopical study of cholinergic neurons that project from the basal forebrain to frontal cortex in the rat. J. Comp. Neurol. 239: 176-192.
26. MESULAM, M.-M., E. J. MUFSON, B. H. WAINER & A. I. LEVEY. 1983. Central cholinergic pathways in the rat: An overview based on alternative nomenclature. Neuroscience 4: 1185-1201.
27. WOOLF, N. J., F. ECKENSTEIN & L. L. BUTCHER. 1983. Cholinergic projections from the basal forebrain to the frontal cortex: A combined fluorescent tracer and immunohistochemical analysis. Neurosci. Lett. 40: 93-98.
28. FONNUM, F. 1970. Topographical and subcellular localization of choline acetyltransferase in rat hippocampal formation. J. Neurochem. 17: 1029-1037.
29. SHUTE, C. C. D. & P. R. LEWIS. 1966. Electron microscopy of cholinergic terminals and acetylcholinesterase-containing neurons in the hippocampal formation of the rat. Z. Zellforsch. Mikrosk. Anat. 69: 334-343.
30. STORM-MATHISEN, J. & T. W. BLACKSTAD. 1964. Cholinesterase in the hippocampal region: Distribution and relation to architectonics and afferent systems. Acta Anat. 56: 216-253.
31. GENESER-JENSEN, F. A. 1972. Distribution of acetylcholinesterase in the hippocampal region of the guinea pig. III. The dentate area. Z. Zellforsch. Mikrosk. Anat. 131: 481-495.
32. CHANDLER, J. P. & K. A. CRUTCHER. 1983. The septohippocampal projection in the rat: An electron microscopic horseradish peroxidase study. Neuroscience 10: 685-696.
33. CRUTCHER, K. A., R. MADISON & J. N. DAVIS. 1981. A study of the rat septohippocampal pathway using anterograde transport of horseradish peroxidase. Neuroscience 10: 1961-1973.
34. MEIBACH, R. C. & A. SIEGAL. 1977. Efferent connections of the septal area in the rat: An analysis utilizing retrograde and anterograde transport methods. Brain Res. 119: 1-20.
35. ROSE, A. M., T. HATTORI & H. C. FIBIGER. 1976. Analysis of the septohippocampal pathway by light and electron microscope autoradiography. Brain Res. 108: 170-174.

36. CLARKE, D. J. 1985. Cholinergic innervation of the rat dentate gyrus: A light and electron microscopical study using a monoclonal antibody to choline acetyltransferase. Brain Res. **360:** 349-354.
37. FROTSCHER, M. & C. LÉRANTH. 1985. Cholinergic innervation of the rat hippocampus as revealed by choline acetyltransferase immunocytochemistry: A combined light and electron microscopic study. J. Comp. Neurol. **239:** 237-246.
38. HOUSER, C. R., G. D. CRAWFORD, P. M. SALVATERRA & J. E. VAUGHN. 1985. Immunocytochemical localization of choline acetyltransferase in rat cerebral cortex: A study of cholinergic neurons and synapses. J. Comp. Neurol. **234:** 17-34.
39. WAINER, B. H., J. P. BOLAM, T. F. FREUND, Z. HENDERSON, S. TOTTERDELL & A. D. SMITH. 1984. Cholinergic synapses in the rat brain: A correlated light and electron microscopic immunohistochemical study employing a monoclonal antibody against choline acetyltransferase. Brain Res. **308:** 69-76.
40. HEDREEN, J. C., G. R. UHL, S. J. BACON, D. M. FARMBROUGH & D. L. PRICE. 1984. Acetylcholinesterase-immunoreactive axonal network in monkey visual cortex. J. Comp. Neurol. **226:** 246-254.
41. MESULAM, M.-M., A. D. ROSEN & E. J. MUFSON. 1984. Regional variations in cortical cholinergic innervation: Chemoarchitectonics of acetylcholinesterase-containing fibres in the macaque brain. Brain Res. **311:** 245-258.
42. ECKENSTEIN, F. & H. THOENEN. 1983. Cholinergic neurons in the rat cerebral cortex demonstrated by immunohistochemical localization of choline acetyltransferase. Neurosci. Lett. **36:** 211-215.
43. PARNAVELAS, J. G., W. KELLY & F. ECKENSTEIN. 1985. Cholinergic neurons and fibers in the rat visual cortex. Neurosci. Lett. Suppl. **21:** 510.
44. BJÖRKLUND, A., F. H. GAGE, U. STENEVI & S. B. DUNNETT. 1983. Intracerebral grafting of neuronal cell suspensions. VI. Survival and growth of intrahippocampal implants of septal cell suspensions. Acta Physiol. Scand. Suppl. **552:** 49-58.
45. BJÖRKLUND, A., F. H. GAGE, R. H. SCHMIDT, U. STENEVI & S. B. DUNNETT. 1983. Intracerebal grafting of neuronal cell suspensions. VII. Recovery of choline acetyltransferase activity and acetylcholine synthesis in the denervated hippocampus reinnervated by septal suspension implants. Acta Physiol. Scand. Suppl. **552:** 59-66.
46. DUNNETT, S. B., F. H. GAGE, A. BJÖRKLUND, U. STENEVI, W. C. LOW & S. D. IVERSEN. 1982. Hippocampal deafferentation: Transplant-derived reinnervation and functional recovery. Scand. J. Psychol. Suppl. **1:** 104-111.
47. MATES, S. L. & J. LUND. 1983. Developmental changes in the relationship between type 2 synapses of spiny neurons in the monkey visual cortex. J. Comp. Neurol. **221:** 98-105.
48. PURVES, D. & J. W. LICHTMAN. 1980. Elimination of synapses in the developing nervous system. Science **210:** 153-157.
49. BAISDEN, R. H., M. L. WOOFRUFF & D. B. HOOVER. 1984. Cholinergic and noncholinergic septohippocampal projections: A double-label horseradish peroxidase-acetylcholinesterase study in the rabbit. Brain Res. **290:** 146-151.
50. VINCENT, S. R. & E. G. MCGEER. 1981. A substance P projection to the hippocampus. Brain Res. **215:** 349-351.
51. VINCENT, S. R., K. SATOH, D. M. ARMSTRONG & H. C. FIBIGER. 1983. Substance P in the ascending cholinergic reticular system. Nature **306:** 688-691.
52. DENT, J. A., N. J. CALVIN, B. B. STANFIELD & W. M. CONWAN. 1983. The mode of termination of the hypothalamic projection to the dentate gyrus: An EM autoradiographic study. Brain Res. **258:** 1-11.
53. DUNNETT, S. B. 1987. Anatomical and behavioral consequences of cholinergic-rich grafts to the neocortex of rats with lesions of the nucleus basalis magnocellularis. Ann. N.Y. Acad. Sci. This volume.
54. MUFSON, E. J., A. LEVEY, B. WAINER & M.-M. MESULAM. 1982. Cholinergic projections from the mesencephalic tegmentum to neocortex in rhesus monkey. Soc. Neurosci. Abstr. **8:** 135.
55. BLUE, M. E. & J. G. PARNAVELAS. 1983. The formation and maturation of synapses in the visual cortex of the rat. I. Qualitative analysis. J. Neurocytol. **12:** 599-616.
56. COTMAN, C. W. & J. V. NADLER. 1978. Reactive synaptogenesis in the hippocampus. *In* Neuronal Plasticity. C. W. Cotman, Ed.: 227-271. Raven Press. New York, NY.

57. GAGE, F. H., A. BJÖRKLUND & U. STENEVI. 1983. Reinnervation of the partially deafferented hippocampus by compensatory collateral sprouting from spared cholinergic and nonadrenergic afferents. Brain Res. **268:** 27-37.
58. LEE, K. S., E. J. STANFORD, C. W. COTMAN & G. S. LYNCH. 1977. Ultrastructural evidence for bouton proliferation in the partially denervated dentate gyrus of the adult rat. Exp. Brain Res. **29:** 475-485.
59. MCWILLIAMS, R. & G. S. LYNCH. 1978. Terminal proliferation and synaptogenesis following partial deafferentation: The reinnervation of the inner molecular layers of the dentate gyrus following removal of its commissural afferents. J. Comp. Neurol. **180:** 581-616.
60. ZIMMER, J. 1973. Extended commissural and ipsilateral projection in postnatally deentorhinated hippocampus and fascia dentata demonstrated in rats by silver impregnation. Brain Res. **64:** 293-311.
61. HOFF, S. F., S. W. SCHEFF, L. S. BENARDO & C. W. COTMAN. 1982. Lesion-induced synaptogenesis in the dentate gyrus of aged rats. I. Loss and reacquisition of normal synaptic density. J. Comp. Neurol. **205:** 246-252.
62. MATTHEWS, D. A., C. COTMAN & G. LYNCH. 1976. An electron microscopic study of lesion-induced synaptogenesis in the dentate gyrus of the adult rat. II. Reappearance of morphologically normal synaptic contacts. Brain Res. **115:** 23-41.
63. ALBERT, E. N. & C. D. DAS. 1984. Neocortical transplants in the rat brain: An ultrastructural study. Experientia **40:** 294-298.
64. MATSUMOTO, A., S. MURAKAMI, Y. ARAI & M. OSANAI. 1985. Synaptogenesis in the neonatal preoptic area grafted into the aged brain. Brain Res. **347:** 363-367.
65. SCOTT, D. E. & M. SHERMAN. 1984. Neuronal and neurovascular integration following transplantation of the fetal hypothalamus into the third cerebral ventricle of adult Brattleboro rats. Brain Res. Suppl. **12:** 453-467.
66. GEINISMAN, Y., W. BONDAREFF & J. T. DODGE. 1978. Dendritic atrophy in the dentate gyrus of the senescent rat. Am. J. Anat. **152:** 321-330.
67. PARNAVELAS, J. G., G. LYNCH, N. BRECHA, C. W. COTMAN & A. GLOBUS. 1974. Spine loss and regrowth in hippocampus following deafferentation. Nature **248:** 71-73.
68. BONDAREFF, W. 1980. Changes in synaptic structure affecting neural transmissions in the senescent brain. *In* Proceedings of the Naito International Symposium of Aging. K. Oota & M. Makinodan, Eds. Raven Press. New York, NY.
69. GEINISMAN, Y., W. BONDAREFF & J. T. DODGE. 1977. Partial deafferentation of neurons in the dentate gyrus of the senescent rat. Brain Res. **134:** 541-545.

DISCUSSION OF THE PAPER

C. SOTELO (*INSERM U106, CMC Foch, Suresnes*): What is the pattern of distribution of your ChAT axons in adult aged brain? This was missing in the figure you presented.

CLARKE: This relates to a study I am doing at present in which I am comparing adult aged rats that have particular behavior impairments to aged rats that have no behavior impairments. I am also comparing aged rats to young rats.

SOTELO: It has not been proven that all aging rats have lost their ChAT innervation. Are you sure that in these aged animals that 5 days after transection of the fimbria-fornix is enough time for the total disappearance of the septal input into the hippocampus?

CLARKE: Yes, I am pretty sure. We saw many denervated terminals within the host hippocampal formation, but all of those that I looked at were forming asymmetric contacts. All of those degenerated terminals that were the result of the acute lesion were asymmetric contacts. I looked at 5 days and 10 days, and there appeared to be no difference in either the ChAT staining or the degeneration.

SOTELO: I would like to comment on the identification of the postsynaptic target neurons. In your distribution, you say 5.1% of the axons go to the soma, some go to the shaft, and some go to the spines, but you do not have features that allow you to say if these are dendrites. These dendrites could come from the GABA-ergic neurons or interneurons or wherever. So you still have a problem that you need to identify with Golgi staining on electron microscopy the postsynaptic neuron. Without the postsynaptic neuron, the distribution does not mean much.

CLARKE: With the cell bodies, in many cases, the neuron type is clearly obvious, and Golgi staining is in progress to allow one to definitely identify these targets, especially dendrites.

M. SHAPIRO (*Johns Hopkins University, Baltimore, MD*): Did the aged rats you examined show recovery on the task after the grafts?

CLARKE: Yes. I did not mention the behavior—it is not my field—but I suspect Prof. Björklund is going to give a more complete presentation about this group of animals.

SHAPIRO: Did you ever look at animals that did not show recovery of behavior?

CLARKE: No.

D. M. GASH (*University of Rochester, Rochester, NY*): Perhaps I missed the point you may have made, but, in the aged rats, did you also do lesions before you did the transplants? Is there any way that you can distinguish between recovery of the endogenous systems that might be important in the aged rats because of the transplant being there, and recovery because of the cholinergic neurons from the transplants providing innervation?

CLARKE: The rats were lesioned 4 to 5 days before perfusion, not before transplantation. I do not think there was enough time for a large reenervation from the intrinsic cholinergic system, that is, in the 4 to 5 days after it was lesioned.

SEGAL: Could the changing proportion that you see in the young rats be due to hyperinnervation of the soma? Could you count the total number of shaft synapses and look at the proportion of cholinergic synapses there, and then be able to say whether this is normal and whether the rest is just extra?

CLARKE: I have not actually done that, but it certainly appears that the cell bodies are receiving a far greater percentage. I have not looked at the shafts and the non-cholinergic and cholinergic synapses.

A. LINDOW (*Massachusetts General Hospital, Boston, MA*): Did you ever try doing the fibria-fornix lesions in the old animals to see whether you could get the distribution that you see in the young animals?

CLARKE: No.

Interactions between Grafted Serotonin Neurons and Adult Host Rat Hippocampus[a]

MENAHEM SEGAL

Center for Neurosciences
The Weizmann Institute of Science
Rehovot, Israel

INTRODUCTION

The past few years have witnessed a rapid expansion of research on plastic properties of transplanted CNS neurons. Two major developments contributed to this expansion. First was the demonstrated ability to identify chemically specific transplanted neurons in a host brain and follow their growth using standard histochemical methodologies.[1,2] Second was the suggestion that grafted neurons may substitute for damaged ones in providing the brain with specific chemicals needed for its normal operation.[3] The prospects of using brain grafts for the treatment of neurodegenerative diseases of the central nervous system have ignited the imagination of physicians and scientists alike. Current usage of brain grafting methods is motivated by different research goals: 1) An analysis of the factors underlying developmental specificity of neural connections; Will the grafted neurons form connections in a new brain akin to those formed by the native neurons, and if so, under what conditions would such connections be made?[4,5] 2) Analysis of the functions of a neuron group. Certain behavioral deficits can result from specific neuronal lesions. A most direct way of relating a function to a specific neuron group is the illustration that grafting of these neurons into a deficient brain can restore the deficient function.[6,7] 3) Reconstruction of neuronal connections for the simplification of their physiological analysis. Such is the case with long axon pathways that cannot be studied otherwise in an *in vitro* slice preparation.[8] 4) Clinical applications of graft methodology for treatment of degenerative diseases such as parkinsonism.[9]

Although the morphological analysis of graft-host interaction has been conducted quite extensively for several neuronal pathways and a functional recovery has been demonstrated elegantly for some neuroendocrine, motor, and, perhaps, some aspects of cognitive functions,[3,6,7,10] the physiological analysis of graft-host interaction lags behind, and only a few studies have been reported.[8,11] Three classes of questions have to be examined before we can assume that the grafted neurons integrate into the host brain. First, the grafted tissue has to receive afferents comparable to its normal counterpart such that stimulation of these afferents produces the same postsynaptic responses of the grafted neurons as seen normally. Second, the grafted neurons have

[a]This work was supported by the United States-Israel Binational Science Foundation.

284

to develop (or retain) physiological properties akin to those of their normal counterparts. Morphologically distinct neuronal types are known to possess characteristic ionic conductances, properties which determine their reactivity to incoming afferents and to drugs and pathological conditions. These might or might not develop in new and distinctly different conditions inherent in a graft-host relationship. Third, we need to know if the grafted neurons produce the same postsynaptic effects on their efferent targets as the normal cells do. Once an equivalence is established at the three levels between the grafted and the homotypic neurons, one can then assume that the grafted neurons had indeed replaced the lost ones, and proceed with a functional analysis of graft-host interactions.

PROPERTIES OF RAPHE NEURONS

We have begun a physiological analysis of graft-host interaction using the serotonin neurons grafted in the rat hippocampus. The hippocampus is a major target area of serotonin-containing fibers of midbrain raphe origin.[12] It has already been shown that raphe neurons containing serotonin at a relatively young embryonic age (E15) can be transplanted into the hippocampus, where they will innervate the host in a pattern similar to that of the normal innervation pattern of serotonin neurons originating from the raphe.[4] In the initial series of experiments, we investigated the properties of normal serotonin neurons recorded in a slice taken from the midbrain raphe. These neurons possess unique physiological properties that distinguish them from adjacent midbrain neurons and from hippocampal neurons recorded in a slice.[13] Some of these properties have been described elsewhere.[14,15] These cells have a relatively high input resistance (100-300 MΩ), higher than that of most central neurons. The high input resistance cannot be explained as being simply a function of the size of these neurons. It probably represents a genuine difference in membrane composition between raphe and other neurons. Passage of depolarizing or hyperpolarizing current pulses across the recorded membrane can uncover voltage-dependent membrane currents that govern the behavior of the cell at this membrane potential range. Most neurons exhibit inward rectification in response to large (> 25 mV) hyperpolarizing current pulses.[16] This is assumed to result from the hyperpolarization-induced opening of cationic channels that cause current to flow into the cell. This property is conspicuously absent in serotonin neurons. In response to depolarizing current pulses (or, when the cell is depolarized by a DC current, in response to hyperpolarizing current pulses), DR cells exhibit non-inactivating outward rectification. Action potentials can discharge spontaneously or in response to brief depolarizing current pulses. They are broad and contain a distinct Ca^{2+} component. The spikes discharged by serotonergic neurons are followed by a large afterhyperpolarization, which is associated with an increase in conductance and appears to consist of a fast component and a slow component. This large afterhyperpolarization is caused by activation of a Ca^{2+}-dependent K^+ current,[17,18] which brings the membrane close to K^+ equilibrium potential. The lack of inward rectification allows the membrane to reach such a polarized potential. During the hyperpolarization, a new species of K^+ current becomes activatable: the transient outward current (TOC),[19] which is activated by depolarization and prevents the membrane from reaching firing threshold (FIG. 1B). In fact, activation of this current clamps the membrane at a potential slightly below firing threshold for up to several hundreds of msec.[13] The presence of a potent TOC is unique to serotonin neurons and is not

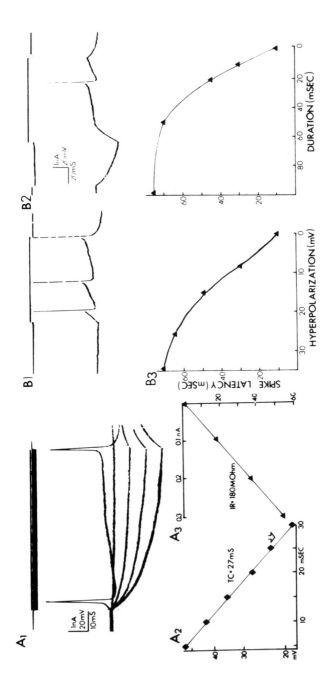

FIGURE 1. (A) Electrical properties of a dorsal raphe neuron. (A1) An intracellular recording was made from a putative serotonin-containing dorsal raphe neuron in a brainstem slice. Hyperpolarizing and depolarizing current pulses were applied to the neuron using a bridge circuit. (A2) An analysis of the hyperpolarizing charging curve indicated the presence of a single exponential curve with a time constant of 27 msec. (A3) The current-voltage curve of a family of pulses illustrated in A1 is linear down to 60 mV below resting potential (-65 mV) and indicates an input resistance of 180 MΩ. No sag in the voltage response can be seen at any of the potentials. (From reference 21.) (B) Properties of transient rectifications in a dorsal raphe neuron. (B1) A 100 msec depolarizing current pulse evokes a train of action potentials. (B2) A 50-msec priming hyperpolarization delays the action potential by 70 msec. Note the slow rise in membrane potential until it reaches firing level. (B3) A summary figure of the latency of the first spike as a function of the magnitude of hyperpolarization (left) or its duration (right). The duration at left was 50 msec. (From reference 8.)

present as such in most central neurons. The TOC restricts the number of spikes discharged by a serotonergic neuron under normal conditions. The coexistance of fast Na^+ and Ca^{2+} currents, which are followed by fast outward K^+ currents and the lack of inward rectification, produces a unique pattern of electrical activity that characterizes serotonergic neurons. One cell type that possesses nearly identical properties to those of serotonin neurons is the noradrenergic neuron of the nucleus locus ceruleus (LC).[20] Several of the properties, however, including the presence of hyperpolarizing rectification, distinguishes the latter from the former neuron type (Segal, unpublished results).

GRAFTED NEURONS

Two questions related to grafting of central neurons are pertinent: 1) Do these cells already possess the unique physiological characteristics by the time they are taken out of an embryo and grafted into the host brain? 2) Do they develop (or maintain) these properties when they grow in a host brain?

We have recorded the activity of neurons from the raphe in slices taken from brains of day 15-19 embryos. At the day of grafting (E15), the recorded cells did not exhibit any of the characteristics of the adult serotonergic neurons, with the exception, perhaps, of the lack of inward rectification (FIG. 2). Only within 2 additional days, that is, by E17, do cells in this region begin to express some of the identifying properties of serotonin neurons. Some cells begin to have adult physiological properties already by E18. It thus appears that on day of grafting (E15) the serotonin neurons still do not have any clear physiological properties. At this age, however, they do produce serotonin and appear to project serotonin fibers into terminal regions in the cortex. It is evident that if they possess adult physiological properties in a host brain they must have developed them in the host brain after grafting. Recording was made from regions in the hippocampal slice taken from a brain that was previously treated with a drug that destroys serotonin fibers (5,7-dihydroxytryptamine (5,7-DHT)) and was subsequently implanted with serotonin-rich E15 mesencephalic neurons.[21] We impaled neurons in the graft that possessed properties identical to those of adult midbrain serotonin-containing neurons. These properties include high input resistance, slow membrane time constant, lack of inward rectification, broad spikes, large afterhyperpolarization, presence of a large transient outward rectification, and lack of accommodation (FIG. 3). Furthermore, preliminary experiments suggest that these neurons have the same pharmacological properties seen in normal cells; that is, they respond to topical application of serotonin, acetylcholine, and noradrenaline in the same way normal cells do. These adult properties were recorded from 2 weeks to 6 months after grafting. These experiments indicate that neurons of the raphe nuclei that contain serotonin can be transplanted into the adult hippocampus where they will develop physiological properties similar to those seen in their natural location in the brain. These observations have important implications for the putative roles of growth conditions, afferent innervation, juvenile hormones, and environmental factors in the development of properties of serotonin neurons. Although the present studies do not rule out such factors, they indicate that these properties can be expressed without the presence of a juvenile environment.

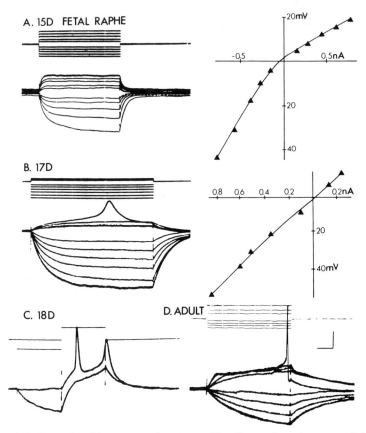

FIGURE 2. Properties of immature raphe neurons. Slices from embryonic mesencephalon were placed in the recording chamber, and intracellular recordings were made from putative raphe neurons. Series of hyper- and depolarizing current pulses were applied through the recording electrode. (**A**) In a neuron recorded at E15, there was no evidence for regenerative Na^+ or Ca^{2+} spikes, but there was a clear presence of outward rectification when the cell was depolarized. This is evident in the current-voltage plot (right) of the same cell. (**B**) Recording from a cell at E17. A small regenerative spike is evoked by depolarization. The lack of inward rectification is clear. (**C**) Recording from a E18 raphe cell exhibiting adult neuronal properties. These include high input resistance, broad spike, and a strong transient outward rectification. (**D**) Adult neuron. The typical raphe serotonergic properties are evident. Depolarizing current pulses evoke a transient outward rectification that delays the spike firing. Calibration for **A**-**D**: 10 msec, 20 mV, 0.5 nA.

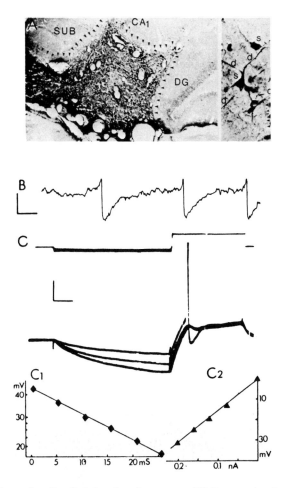

FIGURE 3. Properties of grafted dorsal raphe neurons. (A) Immunochemical staining of serotonin-containing neurons implanted into the hippocampus. Left: low-power view of the graft (DG: dentate gyrus; SUB: subiculum); right: high-power view of grafted neuronal somata (s) and dendrites (d) stained with serotonin-immunoreactive material. Calibration for the left and right sides: 100 μm and 10 μm, respectively. (B) Spontaneous activity of grafted neurons, recorded intracellularly. The action potentials are truncated by the recorder, but a large, slow afterhyperpolarization follows each spike. Calibration: 10 mV, 0.5 sec; resting membrane potential: -65 mV. (C) A series of hyperpolarizing current pulses applied to the grafted neuron results in downward voltage deflections. The hyperpolarization is followed by a depolarizing current pulse. (C1) The membrane time constant (24 msec) is derived from an exponential decay of the voltage. (C2) The current-voltage relation is linear and indicates an input resistance of 150 MΩ. Calibration: 10 msec, 20 mV, 1.0 μA. (From reference 21.)

GRAFT-HOST INTERACTIONS

The grafted neurons project serotonin-containing fibers into the host hippocampus. These fibers reach the same zones originally innervated by serotonin fibers of raphe origin. When these areas (for example, the dentate gyrus) are stimulated electrically, an antidromic spike can be recorded from grafted neurons present in the same slice at some distance away (FIG. 4). The properties of grafted central serotonin-containing fibers can thus be studied *in vitro*. These axons have slow conduction velocity and refractoriness. The antidromicity can be confirmed using a collision test: the spike traveling from the axon to the soma can be shown to collide with a spike evoked in the soma by a depolarizing current pulse. The conduction velocity (< 1 m/sec) indicates that the activated axons are unmyelinated. Stimulation at high frequencies can cause a dissociation between a soma-dendritic spike and an axon spike, which can follow higher frequencies of stimulation. This observation indicates that the soma is under a strong inhibitory control that can block invasion of axon spikes. The graft is selectively innervated by host fibers; stimulation of region CA3 of the host slice did produce an excitatory postsynaptic potential (EPSP) in some grafted cells positioned in the dentate gyrus (FIG. 4). No such response could be detected when the dentate gyrus or CA1 region was stimulated using the same stimulation parameters. The connections between the graft and host were not reciprocal as we could not find an antidromic response in grafted neurons even when stimulating the CA3 region with much higher currents.

The presence of functional connections between the raphe graft and the host hippocampus was assessed by electrical stimulation of the graft and recording intracellular activity in cells of the host hippocampus. It has been shown that topically applied serotonin hyperpolarizes hippocampal neurons.[22] This response is due to an

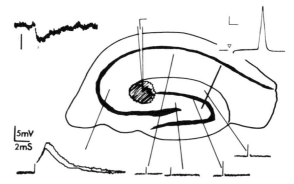

FIGURE 4. The raphe graft interacts with the host tissue. Three different experiments are depicted on a schematic diagram of a hippocampal slice containing a graft (hatched area). Top left: spontaneous EPSPs recorded in some grafted neurons. The recording was made with a KCl-containing pipette, and the hyperpolarizing PSP indicates that it is probably mediated by an increase in K^+ conductance. Top right: an antidromic response in a grafted neuron to stimulation of the dentate hilus. The antidromic response has a constant 6 msec latency and can collide with an orthodromic spike (not seen). Calibration: 2 msec, 10 mV. Bottom: traces showing orthodromic EPSPs evoked in grafted neurons. The traces on the left show responses to stimulation of region CA3 but not CA1 or the dentate gyrus. The larger EPSP is recorded after a tetanic stimulation (100 Hz for 100 msec).

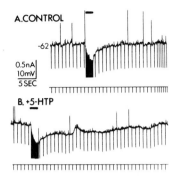

FIGURE 5. Postsynaptic effect of stimulation of a raphe graft on activity of a hippocampal neuron. (**A**) In normal medium, stimulation of the graft (10 Hz for 2 sec) produces a slow 1-3 mV hyperpolarization. (**B**) After addition of 5-HTP to the slice (a drop of 0.1 mM 5-HTP applied 2 min before stimulation), the same stimulation produces a much larger hyperpolarizing response.

increase in postsynaptic K^+ conductance. The possibility that graft stimulation will hyperpolarize hippocampal neurons was therefore tested. A distinct, long-lasting hyperpolarization was detected in hippocampal neurons located some 2-3 mm away from the stimulated graft. This hyperpolarization could be enhanced by loading the slice with a serotonin precursor, 5-hydroxytryptophane (5-HTP) (FIG. 5). The effect is distinctly different from that seen in response to stimulation of a graft taken from the septal region, where a pronounced and long-lasting depolarization is evident, and from that seen in response to stimulation of an LC graft (Segal, unpublished results).

FUNCTIONAL ANALYSIS

Once the normal properties of grafted serotonin neurons have been established, one can proceed and investigate functional aspects of these neurons. The serotonin innervation of the hippocampus has been implicated in the regulation of reactivity of the hippocampus to afferent stimulation. Reactivity of the hippocampus to stimulation of the perforant path, arising in the entorhinal cortex, exhibits a marked sleep-wakefulness variation; it is largest when the rat is in slow-wave sleep and smallest during wakefulness.[23] A similar variation exists in the commissural connection.[24] Srebro et al.[25] ascribed this variation to the serotonin innervation of the hippocampus. If indeed serotonin neurons emit an inhibitory action on postsynaptic neurons and they are silent during slow-wave sleep, one can expect evoked potentials to be largest then, and this is indeed the case. Srebro et al. found that 5,7-DHT treatment eliminates the sleep-wakefulness variation.[25] We confirmed this observation and have since proceeded to examine the possible restoration of the sleep-wakefulness variation after grafting of serotonergic neurons into the hippocampus. Preliminary observations indicate that, at least in some grafted rats, this variation does exist and is much larger than in 5,7-DHT-treated, ungrafted control rats (FIG. 6).

The present results suggest that a raphe graft can make specific functional connections with the host hippocampus. One major question related to the functional restoration of raphe-hippocampal connections is what controls raphe firing. Raphe neurons *in situ* fire spontaneously at different rates in relation to sleep-wakefulness cycles.[26] It is unlikely that grafted raphe neurons receive the same afferents as their normal counterparts do. One of the afferents that is likely to act in the new location is a noradrenergic input arising from the LC that innervates the host hippocampus.

The hippocampus itself might contribute to the regulation of activity of grafted raphe neurons, and, of course, the humoral factors that might be associated with sleep can still affect displaced raphe neurons.

Although the present and related studies indicate that grafting can, under certain conditions, restore functional connections with the host, it is quite clear that this property is shared with only a few brain nuclei. Most neuronal systems, where precision of afferent location and timing is crucial for information transfer, are not likely to be restored by grafting. This method, however, can be very useful for the analysis of the rules governing the developmental specificity of these structures.[27] The common denominator for the successful grafting of some nuclei is a diffuse and relatively slow efferent system. This is the case for some monoamines and acetylcholine nuclei in the brain. This is perhaps also the case for several peptide-containing nuclei in the hypothalamus. It is interesting to note that neurological and psychiatric disorders are associated with these nuclei, and thus the pursuit of grafting methods for these can eventually be of considerable help in understanding their mechanisms of action.

FIGURE 6. Hippocampal evoked responses to perforant path stimulation vary with sleep-wakefulness cycle. (**A**) Traces illustrating, on a slow time base, the shift from wakefulness to sleep in a 5,7-DHT-treated rat. Top: hippocampal electroencephalogram; bottom: trace made by a movement detector. Upward deflections are responses to perforant path stimulation applied once every 4 sec. The rat was monitored continuously, and the periods of sleep were marked. A small reduction in the responses is seen when the animal moves vigorously, but the responses are not much larger when he stops moving. (**B-E**) Averaged evoked responses during slow-wave sleep and quiet wakefulness. Each record is an average of eight consecutive responses. (**B**) Normal control rat. (**C**) Same rat with same stimulation parameters, 36 hr after an intraperitoneal injection of pharachlorophenylalanine (300 mg/kg). Note the disappearance of the sleep-wakefulness variation. (**D**) Averaged responses of a rat pretreated with intrahippocampal injection of 5,7-DHT. (**E**) A similar rat, but this one was grafted with serotonergic neurons of the MR. The sleep-wakefulness variation is evident.

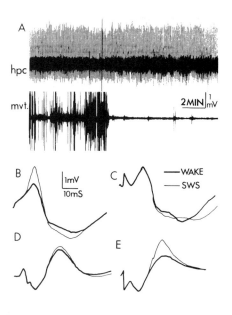

SUMMARY

We have followed the development of physiological and functional properties of serotonin-containing raphe neurons grafted into an adult host hippocampus as a model system for graft-host interactions. These raphe cells have no clear identifying properties on the day of grafting: they develop them while growing in the host. Raphe neurons, recorded 1 month after grafting, possess adult normal physiological properties. These include high input resistance, slow membrane time constant, lack of inward rectification, a transient outward rectification, broad spikes having a Ca^{2+} component, lack of accommodation, and a large afterhyperpolarization. The graft is first innervated by host fibers and later projects to the host tissue. When stimulated, postsynaptic hyperpolarized responses are recorded in hippocampal neurons. In the freely moving rat, raphe grafts can restore sleep-wakefulness variations in an evoked population response of the hippocampus to afferent stimulation, which is eliminated by depletion of serotonin. These studies illustrate that grafted serotonin neurons develop functional relations with a host brain.

ACKNOWLEDGMENTS

I would like to thank Dr. E. C. Azmitia for his collaboration in some of these experiments.

REFERENCES

1. BJÖRKLUND, A., M. SEGAL & U. STENEVI. 1979. Functional reinnervation of rat hippocampus by locus coeruleus implants. Brain Res. 170: 409-426.
2. BJÖRKLUND, A., U. STENEVI, R. H. SCHMIDT, S. B. DUNNETT & F. H. GAGE. 1983. Introduction and general methods of preparation. Acta Physiol. Scand. Suppl. 522: 1-7.
3. GASH, D., J. R. SLADEK & S. D. SLADEK. 1980. Functional development of grafted vasopressin neurons. Science 210: 1267-1369.
4. AZMITIA, E. C., M. J. PERLOW, M. J. BRENNAN & J. M. LAUDER. 1981. Fetal raphe and hippocampal transplants into adult and aged C57BL/GN mice: A preliminary immunocytochemical study. Brain Res. Bull. 7: 703-710.
5. BJÖRKLUND, A., F. H. GAGE, U. STENEVI & S. B. DUNNETT. 1983. Survival and growth of intrahippocampal implants of septal cell suspensions. Acta Physiol. Scand. Suppl. 522: 49-58.
6. DUNNETT, S. B., S. T. BUNCH, F. H. GAGE & A. BJÖRKLUND. 1984. Dopamine-rich transplants in rats with 6-OHDA lesions of the ventral tegmental area. I. Effects on spontaneous and drug-induced locomotor activity. Behav. Brain Res. 13: 71-82.
7. DRUCKER-COLIN, R., R. AGUILAR-ROBLERO, F. GARCIA HERNANDEZ, F. FERNANDEZ-CANCIN & F. BERMUDEZ RATTONI. 1984. Fetal suprachiasmatic nucleus transplants: Diurnal rhythm recovery of lesioned rats. Brain Res. 311: 353-357.
8. SEGAL, M., A. BJÖRKLUND, F. H. GAGE. 1985. Transplanted septal neurons make viable cholinergic synapses with a host hippocampus. Brain Res. 336: 308-312.
9. BACKLUND, E. O., P. O. GRANBERG, B. HAMBERGER, G. SEDVALL, A. SEIGER & L. OLSON. 1985. Transplantation of adrenal medullary tissue to striatum in parkinsonism. In Neural Grafting in the Mammalian CNS. A. Björklund & U. Stenevi, Eds.: 551-556. Elsevier. Amsterdam.
10. DUNNETT, S. B., W. C. LOW, S. D. IVERSON, U. STENEVI & A. BJÖRKLUND. 1982. Septal transplants restore maze learning in rats with fornix-fimbria lesions. Brain Res. 251: 335-348.
11. HAUNSGAARD, J. & Y. YAROM. 1985. Intrinsic control of electroresponsive properties of transplanted mammalian brain neurons. Brain Res. 335: 372-376.
12. AZMITIA, E. C. & M. SEGAL. 1978. The efferent connections of the dorsal and median raphe nuclei in the rat brain. J. Comp. Neurol. 179: 641-668.

13. SEGAL, M. 1985. A potent transient outward current regulates excitability of dorsal raphe neurons. Brain Res. **359:** 347-350.
14. AGHAJANIAN, C. K. & C. P. VANDERMAELEN. 1982. Intracellular recording from serotonergic dorsal raphe neurons: Pacemaker potentials and the effects of LSD. Brain Res. **238:** 463-469.
15. CRUNELLI, V., S. FORDA, P. A. BROOKS, K. C. P. WILSON, J. C. M. WISE & J. S. KELLY. 1983. Passive membrane properties of neurons in the dorsal raphe and periaqueductal gray recorded *in vitro.* Neurosci. Lett. **40:** 263-268.
16. PURPURA, D. P., S. PRELEVIC & M. SANTINI. 1968. Hyperpolarizing increase in membrane conductance in hippocampal neurons. Brain Res. **7:** 310-312.
17. BROWN, D. A. & W. H. GRIFFITH. 1983. Calcium-activated outward current in voltage-clamped hippocampal neurons of the guinea pig. J. Physiol. **337:** 287-301.
18. HOSTON, J. R. & D. A. PRINCE. 1980. A calcium-activated hyperpolarization follows repetitive firing in hippocampal neurons. J. Neurophysiol. **43:** 409-419.
19. SEGAL, M., M. A. ROGAWSKI & J. L. BARKER. 1984. A transient potassium conductance depresses the excitability of cultured hippocampal and spinal neurons. Neuroscience **4:** 604-609.
20. WILLIAMS, J. T., A. R. NORTH, S. A. SHELNER, S. NISHI & T. M. EGAN. 1984. Membrane properties of rat locus coeruleus neurons. Neuroscience **13:** 137-156.
21. SEGAL, M. & E. C. AZMITIA. 1986. Fetal raphe neurons grafted into the hippocampus develop normal adult physiological properties. Brain Res. **364:** 162-166.
22. SEGAL, M. 1980. The action of serotonin in the rat hippocampal slice preparation. J. Physiol. (London) **303:** 423-439.
23. WINSON, J. 1980. Influence of raphe nuclei on neuronal transmission from perforant pathway through dentate gyrus. J. Neurophysiol. **44:** 937-950.
24. SEGAL, M. 1978. A correlation of hippocampal responses to interhemispheric stimulation, hippocampal slow rhythmic activity and behavior. Electroenceph. Clin. Neurophysiol. **45:** 409-411.
25. SREBRO, B., E. C. AZMITIA & J. WINSON. 1982. Effect of 5-HT depletion of the hippocampus on neuronal transmission from perforant path through dentate gyrus. Brain Res. **235:** 142-147.
26. TRULSON, M. E. & B. L. JACOBS. 1979. Raphe unit activity in freely moving cats: Correlation with level of behavioral arousal. Brain Res. **163:** 135-150.
27. ZHOU, F. C., E. C. AZMITIA, S. AUERBACH & B. L. JACOBS. 1985. A specific serotonergic rowth factor from 5,7-DHT-lesioned hippocampus: *In vivo* evidence from fetal transplantation of raphe and locus coeruleus neurons. Soc. Neurosci. Abstr. **11:** 1084.

DISCUSSION OF THE PAPER

C. SOTELO (*INSERM U106, CMC Foch, Suresnes*): The cells you take from the raphe have their own inputs, and when you transplant them to the hippocampus they will have a totally different type of input. What about the spontaneous firing rate of these cells? Is it the same or very different?

SEGAL: I do not try to convince you that the normal innervation of the raphe is now coming from the hippocampus. It is puzzling that these cells still perform even though they do not see what they normally see coming from the habenula or any other place in the brain. A number of these cells to have spontaneous activity in the upper subiculum in the hippocampus, and they do perform. It has been shown by a number of people that these cells would normally have spontaneous firing with a very regular and slow rate, and that these cells also have this property in the hippocampus. I did not mention this as an identifying property of these neurons because there are quite a number of cells that under suitable conditions would produce this spontaneous firing activity. I do not know at the moment what regulates this activity.

SOTELO: You were talking about the maturation of membrane conductance. It was very nice to see that when you transplanted they remain immature and when they go to the hippocampus they mature. If you explant these cells into a tissue culture dish will membrane conductance show the same type of maturation?

SEGAL: I did not do it. I wish I could show that they do have the same properties in the dish, but I do not have this answer yet. Incidentally, these cells, when they are transplanted into the hippocampus, do get some of the input that they normally get. For example, the noradrenergic input coming to the raphe would be seeing them in the hippocampus. So it is not totally denervated with respect to the normal innervation.

GnRH Cell Brain Grafts

Correction of Hypogonadism in Mutant Mice [a]

MARIE J. GIBSON,[b] ANN-JUDITH SILVERMAN,[c]
GEORGE J. KOKORIS,[b] EARL A. ZIMMERMAN,[d]
MARK J. PERLOW,[e] AND HARRY M. CHARLTON[f]

[b]Department of Medicine
Mount Sinai School of Medicine
New York, New York 10029

[c]Department of Anatomy and Cell Biology
Columbia College of Physicians and Surgeons
New York, New York 10032

[d]Department of Neurology
Oregon Health Sciences Center School of Medicine
Portland, Oregon 97201

[e]Veterans Administration West Side Medical Center
Chicago, Illinois 60612

[f]Department of Human Anatomy
Oxford University
Oxford OX1 3QX, England

INTRODUCTION

In several models of induced or genetic neurochemical deficiency,[1-4] neuronal tissue grafts obtained from normal animals and containing the missing substance have been employed in attempts to correct the defects. The mutant hypogonadal mouse, lacking the neurohormone gonadotropin-releasing hormone (GnRH)[5] essential for maturation of the reproductive system, appeared spontaneously in a breeding colony at Harwell, England. Because the gonads of the animals do not develop after birth, adult animals are infertile and show no sexual behavior.

In the hypogonadal male, there is a juvenile scrotum, small penis, and short anogenital distance, accompanied by small undescended testes, an infantile reproductive tract, no spermatogenesis beyond the diplotene stage, and atrophic interstitial tissue. Pituitary and plasma gonadotropins and plasma testosterone concentrations are about 10% of the levels seen in normal mice of the same stock. The affected female mouse shows absent or delayed vaginal opening, tiny ovaries, little follicular development, and a thread-like uterus, as well as low gonadotropin levels.

[a]This work was supported by Grants NS20335 and HD19077 from the National Institutes of Health.

296

Several studies permit the conclusion that the primary defect in the hypogonadal mouse is the failure to produce GnRH. Electrical stimulation of the hypothalamus,[6] which stimulates luteinizing hormone (LH) release from the pituitary of normal mice, fails to do so in hypogonadal mice. But when exogenous GnRH is administered to these animals, the pituitary responds with increased LH and follicle-stimulating hormone (FSH) release.[7,8] If the ovaries or testes are transplanted to normal mice,[9] the ovaries are capable of ovulation and the testes of spermatogenesis.

In the normal rodent central nervous system (CNS), GnRH cells are found in small numbers throughout the rostral forebrain from the accessory olfactory bulb to the retrochiasmatic area of the basal hypothalamus,[10] and, in some reports, as far caudal as the arcuate nucleus.[11] Many GnRH cells are present in the septal-preoptic area, and major fiber projections are seen from rostral areas to the median eminence,[12] where GnRH has access to the pituitary portal plexus. We have not been able to detect any GnRH cells or fibers in adult hypogonadal untreated mice in any region from the olfactory bulb to the brainstem.

In the studies described here, we utilized brain grafts derived from the preoptic area of normal mouse fetuses, implanted into the third ventricle of adult hypogonadal mice, to determine whether GnRH cells in the grafts were capable of supporting the correction of any of the reproductive deficits. We have observed reproductive function and behavior in the treated mice, and have evidence of anatomical connectivity between graft and host brain.

METHODS

Hypogonadal and normal mice of the same stock (resulting from crossing the F1 hybrids between two inbred strains, C3H/HeH and 101/H) were used in these experiments. Animals were maintained in temperature and light-controlled quarters with food and water available *ad libitum*. In most experiments, tissue for each graft was dissected from the preoptic area of two fetal normal donor brains and pooled in a drop of sterile saline.[13] For certain studies, preoptic area tissue from neonatal or older normal mouse pups was utilized. Coronal cuts were made on the ventral surface of the donor brain. The rostral cut was made at the bifurcation of the anterior cerebral artery, and a second cut was made approximately 0.7 mm caudal to this. Lateral cuts were made 0.5 mm from the midline, and a final undercut 1.0 mm deep completed the preoptic area block. Host animals were anesthetized and received stereotaxic injections of graft material with a 20-ga needle into the anterior third ventricle of the brain.

Following survival periods determined by the experiment, animals were anesthetized with ether; blood was removed from the axillary artery and centrifuged; and the plasma was reserved at $-20°$ C for later radioimmunoassay of LH and FSH levels. In some cases, the mice were decapitated and the brains removed, fixed by immersion in Bouin's fixative before dehydration, and embedding in paraffin. Pituitaries from these animals were removed and frozen for subsequent radioimmunoassay of LH and FSH. Other animals were perfused intracardially with saline followed by Zamboni's fixative. The descending aorta in these animals was clamped before perfusion to spare the gonadal tissues for accurate weighing. Ovaries or testes were fixed in Bouin's for later histology. Brains were processed for immunocytochemical detection of GnRH cells and fibers as described in detail elsewhere,[14] using the antiserum LR-1, kindly supplied by Dr. R. Benoit.

RESULTS AND DISCUSSION

Physiological Recovery in the Hypogonadal Male

In the initial study, hypogonadal male mice aged 5 to 7 months received neural tissue grafts and were examined 2 months after implant surgery.[13] Of eight animals that received fetal preoptic area grafts, seven mice responded with testicular growth and seminal vesicle development (testes weight: 74.2 ± 15.0 mg), whereas none of the untreated hypogonadal mice (testes weight: 7.5 ± 1.0 mg) or those with control grafts obtained from cortical tissue (testes weight: 8.2 ± 0.8 mg) showed changes in reproductive measures. Despite the 10-fold increase in gonadal weights in the mice with preoptic area grafts, testes weights did not approach those seen in the normal males (207.7 ± 10.8 mg). This finding raised the possibility that the hypogonadal males could not respond with fully normal testicular development.

To test whether gonadal growth was related to the duration of time the graft was present, hypogonadal male mice aged 3 months received 16- to 18-day fetal preoptic area grafts and were studied at 10, 32, 60, 90, and 120 days after implantation.[15] Although no increase in testicular weight was evident at 10 days, within 30 days after implantation significant increases were seen, and a few individuals in the 60- and 90-day postimplantation groups had testes weights within the normal range. It appeared that the ability of the hypogonadal males to show reproductive organ development in response to the grafts was limited more by the orientation of GnRH cells within the grafts or of the graft within the ventricle or both than by any inability of the pituitary-gonadal axis of the hypogonadal mouse to respond to neurohormone. Steroid production of the testes was reflected in seminal vesicle growth, which is testosterone dependent, and scanning electron microscopy of the stimulated testes in the responding hosts showed full spermatogenesis. Within 2 months after implantation, pituitary LH and FSH levels in the treated hypogonadal mice were in the normal range, although plasma levels remained low at the time points studied.

Physiological Recovery in the Hypogonadal Female

Female hypogonadal mice responded to preoptic area grafts with vaginal opening (stimulated by estrogen secretion from the ovaries) and entered continual vaginal estrus, characterized by cornified cells in daily vaginal smears.[16] We did not, however, see evidence of the 4- to 6-day spontaneous ovulatory cycles normally present in the mouse. The ovarian and uterine weights of responsive females were in the normal range, as were the pituitary gonadotropins. Follicular development was evident in the ovaries examined histologically, but there were no corpora lutea present to indicate the occurrence of spontaneous ovulation.

In the next studies, we noted the sex of the fetal donors because we were concerned that the failure of the females to ovulate spontaneously could be related to some early sexual differentiation of the male brain. In addition, we were interested in determining whether the hypogonadal females with grafts would mate with normal males. Ten adult hypogonadal female mice aged 2 1/2 months received preoptic area tissue grafts from normal fetuses, with five mice receiving tissue derived from 17-day-old male fetuses, and five receiving tissue from 17-day-old female fetuses.[14]

At 3 months after surgery and at least 6 weeks after all females had entered continual vaginal estrus, each female was singly caged with a normal male for one night. Vaginal plugs, each formed from a male's ejaculate, were present in 9 of the 10 hypogonadal females, signifying successful copulation. The males were removed from the cages. Six of the hypogonadal females delivered litters of 4 to 6 pups each. All of the mothers nursed and retrieved their pups appropriately, and the pups thrived. A seventh female died on the 11th day of gestation, and three embryos were found at autopsy. Pituitary and plasma LH and FSH levels in these females were fully comparable to those found in normal females and were significantly higher than in the untreated hypogonadal mice.

The finding of ovulation in response to the male suggests that reflex ovulation occurred, an event described in seasonal breeders such as voles,[17] rabbits,[18] and cats,[19] as well as in rats that are in constant estrus as a result of being in a constant lighting regimen.[20] In this case, stimuli from the male trigger a reflexive ovulatory LH surge, presumably via hypothalamic GnRH. We were interested in evaluating LH release in relation to mating in hypogonadal mice that were in constant estrus as a result of preoptic area grafts.

When hypogonadal females were bled at 10 min after mating, plasma LH levels were significantly increased. Although plasma LH levels were not as high as the level seen at the time of the spontaneous LH surge in proestrus in normal female mice, they were sufficient to support ovulation in several of the mice.

In the previous study, of the seven females that became pregnant, four had received preoptic area tissue grafts that were derived from male fetuses, indicating that male fetal tissue is fully capable of sustaining ovarian development, reflex ovulation, and pregnancy.

Because the sex of the donor of fetal preoptic area tissue has not affected the outcome in our studies with male or female animals, we have attempted to use preoptic area tissue derived from older animals as a source of GnRH. Tissue obtained from 10- or 15-day-old pups has shown little success to date.[21] Although about 25% of male hypogonadal mice responded with testicular development when grafts were obtained from 5-day-old pups, we have not yet had any success in stimulating gonadal development in a smaller group of females with either male or female 5-day-old preoptic area tissue.

However, preoptic area tissue obtained from 1-day-old pups has been effective,[21] and, because testosterone levels are elevated in male mice in the perinatal period,[22,23] there may be some masculine differentiation of the neural tissue at this age.

Hypogonadal females with grafts of fetal or 1-day-old male or female preoptic area tissue were tested for sexual behavior with normal reproductively experienced male mice.[24] Comparisons were made with normal females that were in proestrus, the receptive stage of the ovulatory cycle. Graft recipients were as attractive as intact females in eliciting male mating behavior. In response to mounting by the males, the females showed lordotic responses that were similar to those shown by normal females in proestrus. Ovarian and uterine weights were similar whether the grafts were derived from fetuses or from neonatal males or females. Thus the sex of the fetal or neonatal donor does not affect the reproductive measures examined. It is not known at present why preoptic area tissue from fetal or neonatal female donors does not support normal spontaneous ovulation in the hypogonadal mouse. Whether gonadal steroid levels are not appropriate or whether necessary afferents to the grafted GnRH cell bodies or their fibers or both are lacking will be subjects of future study.

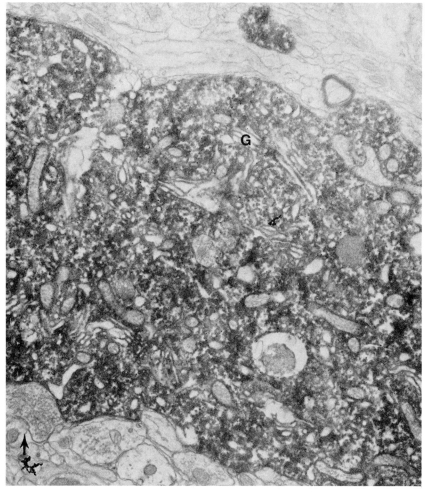

FIGURE 1. Electron micrograph of a portion of a GnRH cell body (note the Golgi apparatus (G)) in a transplant. There is a synapse (arrow) impinging on it. The presynaptic element has clear round vesicles. Original magnification: ×25 000; reduced to 62% of original size.

Anatomical Considerations

In a longitudinal study of GnRH fiber outgrowth from preoptic area grafts located in the third ventricle of the hosts, we were able to show that a small number of fibers had reached the median eminence within 10 days after implantation and that robust outgrowth was present within 30 to 60 days. This level of GnRH innervation of the host median eminence was maintained for the 120-day duration of the experiment.[15] Hence fiber outgrowth precedes statistically significant increases in testicular weight

(30 days) and detection of cornified vaginal smears (evidence of ovarian activation, seen as early as 12 days). We have concluded that GnRH fibers must arrive at and secrete into the primary portal plexus in order to drive pituitary gonadotropin release. This hypothesis has been further substantiated by our finding that transplants of preoptic area tissue that are placed in the lateral ventricle and contain viable GnRH neurons, but do not innervate the median eminence, are not capable of driving the pituitary-gonadal axis.[25] This rules out a ventricular delivery mechanism of the neurohormone.

The occurrence of reflex ovulations (vide supra) suggested that a high degree of integration had to occur between the host brain and cells in the transplant. We have begun, therefore, to explore the nature of the synaptic input to the transplant. We have shown that GnRH neurons are indeed innervated (FIG. 1),[26] though the degree of innervation (at least of the soma and dendrites within the transplant) seems to be very variable when compared to normal preoptic area GnRH neurons (Silverman *et al.*, unpublished results). In this instance we do not know if the synaptic input is derived from the host or is from neurons intrinsic to the graft.

It is clear that selected neuronal systems from the host do sprout axons into the transplanted tissue. Among those that we have studied, phenylethanolamine-N-methyltransferase (PNMT)-positive (adrenergic) fibers enter the transplant from the level of the arcuate and median eminence region and branch profusely in the graft (FIG. 2).

In our initial attempts to explore possible relationships between the restored reproductive physiology and behavior of our transplanted animals and the extrinsic innervation, we have studied neurotensin and neuropeptide Y networks. In female

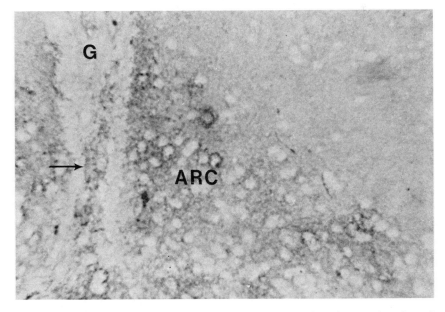

FIGURE 2. PNMT-positive fibers from the host arcuate nucleus (ARC) sprout into the graft (G). Original magnification: $\times 350$; reduced to 85% of original size.

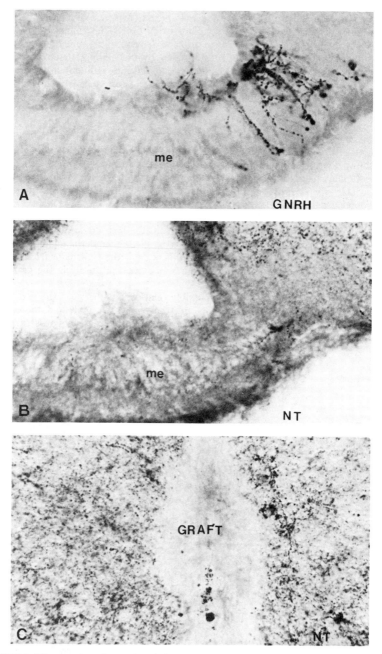

FIGURE 3. Three sections from a female hypogonadal mouse with a successful transplant. (A) GnRH fibers in their normal target, the lateral median eminence (me) of the host. (B) A serial section stained for neurotensin (NT). Note the lateral median eminence is essentially devoid of NT. (C) The graft at the level of the host paraventricular nucleus. No neurotensin fibers penetrate the graft in this area. Original magnification: ×350; reduced to 77% of original size.

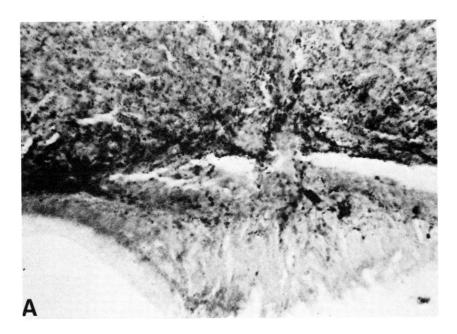

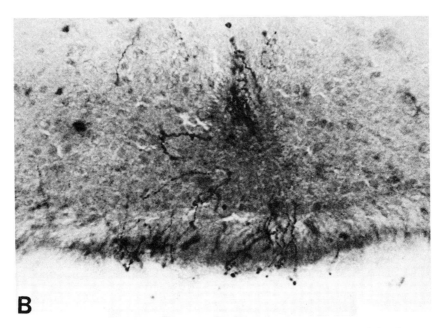

FIGURE 4. Two serial sections stained for neuropeptide Y (**A**) and GnRH (**B**). There are areas in graft and host where these two peptidergic systems overlap. Ultrastructural studies are necessary to determine if neuropeptide Y provides a synaptic input to GnRH cells or fibers. Original magnification: ×350; enlarged to 103% of original size.

hypogonadal mice displaying excellent gonadal recovery, intense patches of neurotensin fibers were found in the grafts of some, but not all, individuals. Similarly, the presence of neurotensin within the graft was apparently not essential for the display of lordosis in the presence of a normal male. In all animals, neurotensin fibers were present within the median eminence, but their distribution did not overlap with graft-derived GnRH fibers (FIG. 3). Hence, although neurotensin neurons may be among the population of preoptic area cells that concentrate estradiol (J. Morrell, personal communication), the input of this peptidergic system to the graft-GnRH neuron does not seem to be essential in mice to drive the reproductive axis.

In another group of females, also with excellent gonadal and behavioral recovery, we investigated the overlap of neuropeptide Y fibers and GnRH cells (graft) and fibers (host median eminence). Neuropeptide Y is colocalized with many dopamine-β-hydroxylase-positive and PNMT-positive neurons and fibers.[27,28] Although neuropeptide Y was present in all of these transplants, overlap with GnRH was most evident at the level of fibers in the median eminence (FIG. 4). It is not possible at this time to correlate the presence of this neuronal system and any aspect of reproductive recovery.

We are beginning light and electron microscopic studies of various putative modulators of GnRH function to see if these systems impinge on the GnRH neuron and, if so, to the same degree as that found in normal animals. Finally, the use of retrograde tracers placed into the transplant will permit an analysis of the afferent input to the grafts.

REFERENCES

1. BJÖRKLUND, A., U. STENEVI & N. A. SVENDGAARD. 1976. Nature 262: 787-790.
2. PERLOW, M. J., W. J. FREED, B. J. HOFFER, A. SEIGER, L. OLSON & R. J. WYATT. 1979. Science 204: 643-647.
3. GAGE, F. H., A. BJÖRKLUND, U. STENEVI, S. B. DUNNETT & P. A. T. KELLY. 1984. Science 225: 533-535.
4. GASH, D., J. R. SLADEK, JR. & C. D. SLADEK. 1980. Science 210: 1367-1369.
5. CATTANACH, B. M., C. A. IDDON, H. M. CHARLTON, S. A. CHIAPPA & G. FINK. 1977. Nature 269: 338-340.
6. IDDON, C. A., H. M. CHARLTON & G. FINK. 1980. J. Endocrinol. 85: 105-110.
7. FINK, G., W. J. SHEWARD & H. M. CHARLTON. 1982. J. Endocrinol. 94: 283-287.
8. CHARLTON, H. M., D. M. G. HALPIN, C. IDDON, R. ROSIE, G. LEVY, I. F. W. MCDOWELL, A. MEGSON, J. F. MORRIS, A. BRAMWELL, A. SPEIGHT, B. J. WARD, J. BROADHEAD, G. DAVEY-SMITH & G. FINK. 1983. Endocrinology 113: 535-544.
9. BAMBER, S., C. A. IDDON, H. M. CHARLTON & B. J. WARD. 1980. J. Reprod. Fertil. 58: 249-252.
10. WITKIN, J. W., C. M. PADEN & A.-J. SILVERMAN. 1982. Neuroendocrinology 35: 429-438.
11. SHIVERS, B. D., R. E. HARLAN, J. I. MORRELL & D. W. PFAFF. 1983. Neuroendocrinology 36: 1-12.
12. KING, J. C., S. A. TOBET, F. L. SNAVELY & A. A. ARIMURA. 1982. J. Comp. Neurol. 209: 287-300.
13. KRIEGER, D. T., M. J. PERLOW, M. J. GIBSON, T. F. DAVIES, E. A. ZIMMERMAN, M. FERIN & H. M. CHARLTON. 1982. Nature 298: 468-471.
14. GIBSON, M. J., D. T. KRIEGER, H. M. CHARLTON, E. A. ZIMMERMAN, A. J. SILVERMAN & M. J. PERLOW. 1984. Science 225: 949-951.
15. SILVERMAN, A. J., E. A. ZIMMERMAN, M. J. GIBSON, M. J. PERLOW, H. M. CHARLTON, G. J. KOKORIS & D. T. KRIEGER. 1985. Neuroscience 16: 69-84.
16. GIBSON, M. J., H. M. CHARLTON, M. J. PERLOW, E. A. ZIMMERMAN, T. F. DAVIES & D. T. KRIEGER. 1984. Endocrinology 114: 1938-1940.

17. CHARLTON, H. M., F. NAFTOLIN, M. C. SOOD & R. W. WORTH. 1975. J. Reprod. Fertil. **42:** 167-170.
18. HILLIARD, J., J. N. HAYWARD & C. H. SAWYER. 1964. Endocrinology **75:** 957-963.
19. CONCANNON, P., B. HODGSON & D. LEIN. 1980. Biol. Reprod. **23:** 111-117.
20. ZARROW, M. X. & J. H. CLARK. 1968. J. Endocrinol. **40:** 343-351.
21. CHARLTON, H. M., A. J. JONES, D. WHITWORTH, M. J. GIBSON, G. KOKORIS, E. A. ZIMMERMAN & A. J. SILVERMAN. 1987. Neuroscience. In press.
22. JEAN-FAUCHER, C., M. BERGER, M. DE TURCKHEIM, G. VEYSSIERE & C. JEAN. 1978. Acta Endocrinol. **89:** 780-788.
23. POINTIS, G., M.-T. LATREILLE & L. CEDARD. 1980. J. Endocrinol. **86:** 483-488.
24. GIBSON, M. J., H. C. MOSCOVITZ, G. J. KOKORIS & A. J. SILVERMAN. 1987. Horm. Behav. In press.
25. KOKORIS, G. J., A. J. SILVERMAN, E. A. ZIMMERMAN, M. J. PERLOW & M. J. GIBSON. 1987. J. Neurosci. In press.
26. SILVERMAN, A. J., E. A. ZIMMERMAN, G. J. KOKORIS & M. J. GIBSON. 1986. J. Neurosci. **6:** 2090-2096.
27. SAWCHENKO, P. E., L. W. SWANSON, R. GRZANNA, P. R. C. HOWE, S. R. BLOOM & J. M. POLAK. 1985. J. Comp. Neurol. **241:** 138-153.
28. EVERITT, B. J., T. HÖKFELT, L. TERENIUS, K. TATEMOTO, V. MUTT & M. GOLDSTEIN. 1984. Neuroscience **11:** 443-462.

DISCUSSION OF THE PAPER

D. M. GASH (*University of Rochester, Rochester, NY*): Our studies on vasopressin-deficient rats are very similar to yours, and we get results that very nicely parallel and complement the findings that you have. Furthermore, we also have to see very specific connections in the median eminence for function to return.

The issue I would like to raise concerns the small numbers of gonadotropin-releasing cells that you see. There are two possible explanations for this. The first is that these cells release so much of the peptide that they are producing that they are hard to see by immunocytochemistry. You might underestimate the number that are really there. The other possibility is that the receptors in the pituitary are supersensitive to the amount of peptides that might be released, or, conversely, that the receptors in the ovary may be more sensitive to lower levels of LH and FSH.

GIBSON: No, there is no evidence that these cells are supersensitive in the pituitary. The studies that have been done show that in an untreated hypogonadal mouse there is a lower number of receptors for GnRH in the pituitary, but that as GnRH is administered, either through injections or through a brain graft, that the numbers of receptors increase to normal levels. They are in the normal range in animals with a graft.

Morphological and Functional Correlates of Chromaffin Cell Transplants in CNS Pain Modulatory Regions[a]

JACQUELINE SAGEN AND GEORGE D. PAPPAS

Department of Anatomy
University of Illinois at Chicago
Chicago, Illinois 60612

INTRODUCTION

The ability to successfully transplant neural tissues into the adult central nervous system (CNS) has opened up the exciting possibility for repair of damaged neuronal circuitry. Although the survival of such transplants in the host CNS without appreciable immunological rejection is fairly well established, the ability of the transplanted tissue to function in the new environment and alter behavior in the host is a fairly recent discovery. In 1979, Perlow *et al.* first demonstrated that it is possible to reverse the motor abnormalities caused by unilateral dopamine deficiency in the striatum by transplanting fetal dopaminergic neurons.[1] Since then, these results have been reproduced and the techniques modified such that it is now fairly well established that grafting dopaminergic neurons into a deficient brain can reverse the motor abnormalities in these Parkinson's disease models.[2–6] Other studies have shown that it is possible to restore other functional deficits using grafting techniques. For example, the grafting of fetal serotonergic raphe neurons restores sexual behavior,[7] gonadotrophin-releasing hormone (GnRH)-containing preoptic area neuron grafts restore reproductive behavior and the ability to reproduce,[8,9] grafts of septal cholinergic neurons restore cognition,[10–13] and grafts of supraoptic/paraventricular vasopressin neurons restore the ability of rats to concentrate urine.[14] These studies are discussed in greater detail in other papers in this volume.

These results are promising and suggest a potentially clinically useful approach to the replacement and restoration of damaged neuronal tissue. In our own laboratory, we are interested in the modulation of pain sensitivity. Since pain is not necessarily the result of damaged neuronal tissue, it is essential to establish the function of neural transplants in intact, nonlesioned animals.

Adrenal medullary chromaffin cells are ideal candidates for these transplantation studies because they contain and release several neuroactive substances that modulate pain sensitivity in the CNS, including norepinephrine, epinephrine, Met- and Leu-

[a] This work was supported in part by National Research Service Award NS07630 and Research Grant GM37326 from the Department of Health and Human Services.

enkephalin, neurotensin, and other neuropeptides.[15–32] These studies suggest that some catecholamines and neuropeptides may be co-stored and co-released by chromaffin cells. Another advantage of using these cells for transplantation studies is that the rate of release of neuroactive substances from chromaffin cells can be readily modified by common pharmacological agents such as nicotine.

Chromaffin cells have been shown to survive for long periods of time when transplanted into the CNS, and have the ability to restore motor deficits in lesioned animals.[4,33–37] Recently, adrenal medullary homografts have been transplanted to the striatum of human Parkinson patients with encouraging results.[38]

Adrenal chromaffin cells apparently maintain a degree of plasticity, since they have been shown to change morphologically and biochemically in response to altered environmental conditions. For example, chromaffin cells in culture change their shape and form processes similar to those of the small granule cells in the sympathetic ganglia, particularly in the presence of nerve growth factor.[39–43] This is accompanied by a shift in the production of catecholamines from epinephrine to norepinephrine, most likely caused by the removal of the steroid-secreting adrenal cortex.[44,45] Denervation of the adrenal medulla in rats also produces a marked increase in the synthesis of opioid peptides.[46] Similarly, chromaffin cell transplants in the anterior eye chamber appear to differentiate into a more neuronal phenotype.[47,48] Moreover, these transplanted chromaffin cells receive synaptic contacts, possibly from the host,[49,50] and can innervate cortical tissue co-transplanted in the anterior eye chamber.[51] This may not be the case for chromaffin cell transplants into the CNS, since fiber outgrowth from the cells in lateral ventricle grafts are sparse and there is little evidence of host reinnervation by the grafts.[4] Rather, the appearance of a halo of catecholamine fluorescence surrounding the graft suggests that the behavioral effects observed are due to diffusion of catecholamines to host receptors.

Since the local injection of pharmacological agents into the brainstem and spinal cord produces profound alterations in pain sensitivity, a diffuse, nonsynaptic release of these substances from transplants may be sufficient to elicit these responses. The rationale for the following experiments was to transplant neural tissues capable of locally releasing neuroactive substances into brainstem and spinal cord pain-modulatory regions sensitive to these substances.

The classical model for pain modulation includes three major interconnecting links: the midbrain periaqueductal gray (PAG), the ventral medulla including the nucleus raphe magnus (NRM) and the adjacent nucleus reticularis paragigantocellularis (NRPG), and the dorsal horn of the spinal cord.[52–55] According to this model, neurons in the PAG activate neurons in the NRM and NRPG, which in turn inhibit pain transmission neurons in the spinal cord. Opioid peptides appear to play an important role at all levels of this modulatory system. The PAG contains a high density of opiate receptors[56] and enkephalin-containing neurons and terminals, particularly in the ventrolateral region.[57,58] Moreover, the microinjection of morphine into the PAG produces a more potent analgesia than anywhere else in the CNS.[59–61] The NRM and particularly the NRPG are also rich in opiate receptors and opioid peptides.[62–64] The microinjection of morphine in these regions produces analgesia.[65,66]

The final common pathway for these brainstem systems is the dorsal horn of the spinal cord where small-diameter primary afferent fibers carrying nociceptive information terminate.[67,68] Descending fibers originating from brainstem neurons in the NRM and NRPG inhibit these spinal cord pain transmission pathways.[54,55,69,70] Recent studies have also revealed a direct spinal projection from the PAG,[71] although the ventral medulla is still considered an important relay from the PAG to the spinal cord. Although the bulbo-spinal projection is mainly serotonergic, many peptide-containing neurons in these regions may also be involved in the modulation of nociception at the level of the spinal cord.[63,72] In addition to descending peptide influences, the dorsal horn contains enkephalinergic interneurons and high levels of opiate receptors.[57,73–75] The intrathecal injection of morphine elicits potent analgesia.[76]

In addition to the enkephalinergic components of this bulbo-spinal pain control system, catecholamine-containing neurons in the brainstem exert a significant influence on this system. Histochemical studies reveal a dense concentration of noradrenergic fibers concentrated in the superficial laminae of the dorsal horn of the spinal cord.[77,78] The intrathecal administration of norepinephrine into the lumbar subarachnoid space produces analgesia,[79–81] whereas the blockade of noradrenergic receptors in the spinal cord by antagonists[82,83] or the depletion of spinal cord norepinephrine by neurotoxins[84,85] produces increased sensitivity to noxious stimuli. Recent studies suggest that opioid peptides and catecholamines may act synergistically to produce their effects, and the maximum effect is dependent on the co-activation of both systems in the spinal cord.[86]

The ventral medulla also contains dense noradrenergic innervation,[87–90] but this input appears to exert the opposite effect on pain sensitivity, since the microinjection of noradrenergic antagonists into the NRM results in a potent, long-lasting analgesia.[91,92]

In addition to opioid peptides and catecholamines, the adrenal chromaffin cells also contain several other neuropeptides that may be important in the regulation of pain sensitivity in these brainstem regions. For example, vasoactive intestinal polypeptide (VIP) is produced by bovine chromaffin cells in culture, and is released by nicotine.[18,20] Immunoreactive VIP is also found in the PAG, where the microinjection of this peptide produces a potent analgesia not reversed by naloxone.[93] Another peptide, neurotensin, is localized to a subpopulation of norepinephrine-containing chromaffin cells.[28,94] It is thought that an important component of the PAG-medulla projection is neurotensinergic.[53,95,96] Finally, recent immunocytochemical studies suggest that substance P coexists with epinephrine in the rat adrenal medulla.[20] This peptide has been strongly implicated in pain transmission, since it is thought to be the major neurotransmitter in primary afferent fibers.[97–99] Substance P-containing neurons and terminals have also been identified in the PAG[100] and in the ventral medulla,[101,102] although their role in the modulation of nociception is unclear. It is thought that some of these neurons project to the spinal cord.

In summary, the purpose of the following studies was to assess the possibility of altering pain sensitivity following the transplantation of adrenal chromaffin cells into CNS regions involved in pain modulation, and to determine the underlying morphological mechanisms for such alterations.

TRANSPLANTS OF RAT ADRENAL MEDULLA INTO RAT SPINAL CORD

In all of the following studies, male and female Sprague-Dawley-derived rats weighing 300-350 g served as hosts. Pain sensitivity was measured in these animals using three standard analgesiometric tests sequentially: the tail flick test,[103] the paw pinch test, and the hot plate test.[104] To elicit the tail flick response, a focused beam of high-intensity light is applied to the dorsal surface of the rat's tail. The time interval between the onset of the stimulus and the tail flick response is measured at three regions of the tail, the average of which is defined as the "tail flick latency." To prevent tissue damage in the absence of a response, the stimulus is terminated at 14 sec and the tail flick latency assigned a value of 14. The paw pinch response is elicited by a commercially available apparatus (Ugo-Basile) that applies pressure at a constant rate of 64 g/sec. The force is applied to the ventral surface of both hind paws sequentially until the animal reacts by a withdrawal response. The hot plate response is determined by placing the rat on a 55° C copper plate enclosed in a plexiglass cylinder. The interval between placement on the hot plate and the response of either licking the hind paws or jumping off the plate is defined as the "hot plate latency." In the absence of a response, the animal is removed after 40 sec and assigned a hot plate latency of 40. Thus, both thermal and mechanical pain stimuli were employed, as well as both reflexive and integrated pain responses.

In all of the reported studies, baseline pain sensitivity and pain sensitivity following a low dose of nicotine (0.1 mg/kg, s.c.) were determined before surgery. For this group of studies, graft tissue consisted of dissected pieces of rat adrenal medulla obtained from the same group of adult rats as the host.[105,106] After cervical dislocation, adrenal glands were rapidly removed and placed in ice-cold Hanks' buffer. The medullary tissue was dissected from the cortical tissue, cut into small pieces (less than 0.5 mm³), and incubated in 2.5 S nerve growth factor (0.1 µg/ml) in Hanks' buffer for approximately 20 min. Tissue from one adrenal medulla was transplanted in each animal. Control animals received an equal volume of either heat-killed adrenal medullary tissue or sciatic nerve tissue.

Following a laminectomy to expose a 2-3-mm segment of the lumbar enlargement, a small incision was made in the dura and graft tissue was placed in the subarachnoid space. The skin was closed with wound clips, and the animals returned to their cages for observation. Animals exhibiting motor abnormalities after surgery were discarded from the study.

Pain sensitivity was determined at various time intervals after transplantation. Following the determination of baseline pain sensitivity, animals received an injection of nicotine (0.1 mg/kg) and pain sensitivity was again measured at 2, 10, 20, and 30 min after the injection. FIGURE 1 illustrates the pain responsiveness at 8 weeks after transplantation procedures. Initially, pain responsiveness in transplanted animals was similar to that of preimplanted animals (not shown) and control-implanted animals. Thus, the transplants do not alter baseline pain sensitivity. When animals are stimulated with a low dose of nicotine, however, potent analgesia is induced in the animals with adrenal medullary transplants in the spinal cord. This effect is not observed in the same animals before implantation (not shown) or in animals with control transplants. The analgesia observed was apparent for all three analgesiometric tests. It was most marked at 2 min after nicotine stimulation, and the pain threshold remained elevated for 10-20 min, tending toward baseline by 30 min.

Since the ability of nicotine to induce the release of chromaffin cell contents is well known, it is likely that these results are due to the local release of neuroactive substances into the subarachnoid space. The most likely candidates for eliciting the observed analgesia are the opioid peptides and the catecholamines, since these substances independently induce analgesia when injected intrathecally. To assess the contribution of opioid peptides, a second group of animals received identical transplants. Immediately after the induction of analgesia by nicotine, the animals received an injection of either opiate antagonist naloxone (2 mg/kg, s.c.) or saline vehicle. Results of this experiment are shown in FIGURE 2. The injection of naloxone immediately and dramatically reversed the induced analgesia. Pain threshold was reversed to baseline and remained there for the duration of testing. In contrast, pain threshold remained elevated in animals receiving saline injections.

To control for the tendency of the elevation in pain sensitivity to gradually decrease

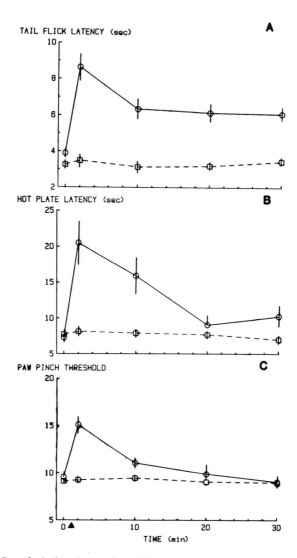

FIGURE 1. Effect of spinal cord adrenal medullary transplants on pain sensitivity. The ordinate is the threshold for response to noxious stimuli as assessed by the tail flick test (**A**), hot plate test (**B**), or paw pinch test (**C**). Each point represents the mean ± SEM. The abscissa is the time course of responses to noxious stimuli after nicotine stimulation. Time 0 indicates the preinjection values. The arrowhead indicates the point at which nicotine (0.1 mg/kg, s.c.) was injected. ○: animals with adrenal medullary transplants in the spinal cord ($N = 12$); □: animals with control transplants in the spinal cord. Comparisons between the two groups using two-way ANOVA indicated that the induction of analgesia was statistically significant for all three tests ($p < .01$, tail flick and hot plate tests; $p < .05$, paw pinch test). Taken from Sagen *et al.*[106]

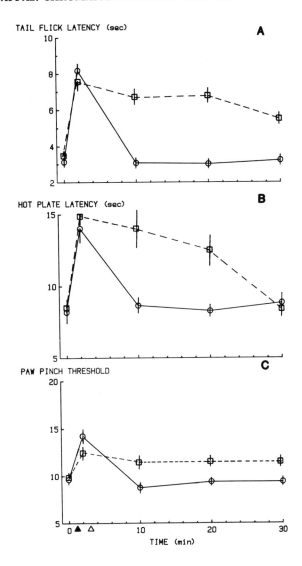

FIGURE 2. Effect of naloxone on the analgesia induced by spinal cord adrenal medullary transplants. The ordinate is the threshold for response to noxious stimuli as assessed by the tail flick test (**A**), hot plate test (**B**), or paw pinch test (**C**). Each point represents the mean ± SEM. The abscissa is the time course of responses to noxious stimuli after drug injections. Time 0 indicates the preinjection values. The closed arrowhead indicates the point at which nicotine (0.1 mg/kg, s.c.) was injected. After the induction of analgesia, animals received either naloxone (2 mg/kg, s.c.) or saline vehicle, indicated at the open arrowhead. ○: animals with spinal cord adrenal medullary transplants receiving naloxone after the induction of analgesia ($N = 9$); □: animals with spinal cord adrenal medullary transplants receiving saline after the induction of analgesia ($N = 9$). Comparisons between the two groups using two-way ANOVA indicated that the reversal of the analgesia by naloxone was statistically significant for all three tests ($p < .01$). Taken from Sagen et al.[106]

toward prenicotine baseline levels over time, some transplanted animals were pretreated with naloxone before nicotine injection. The induction of analgesia by nicotine was completely blocked in these animals.

These results suggest that changes in pain sensitivity can be brought about by the transplantation of adrenal medullary tissue in the spinal cord. The analgesia observed after stimulation by nicotine is most likely due to the local release of neuroactive substances, particularly opioid peptides into the spinal subarachnoid space. The contribution of catecholamines to this analgesia is not clear, but preliminary studies using the α-adrenergic antagonist phentolamine (10 mg/kg, s.c.) suggest that it is minimal. The important role of opioid peptides in the production of analgesia by rat adrenal medullary transplants is somewhat surprising considering the relatively low levels of opioid peptides in the rat adrenal.[30-46] These results suggest the possibility that the chromaffin cells differentiate in the new environment to produce more opioid peptides. This is supported by a study showing marked increases in the amounts of enkephalin and enkephalin-containing polypeptides after denervation of rat adrenal glands.[46]

BOVINE CHROMAFFIN CELL IMPLANTS IN RAT SPINAL CORD

One of the obvious disadvantages of transplanting solid tissue pieces of adrenal medulla is that the graft contains a heterogeneous cell population. The adrenal medulla contains several cell types besides chromaffin cells, including endothelial cells, fibroblasts, and ganglionic cells. To circumvent these variables, a homogeneous preparation of chromaffin cells can be used. Furthermore, since the survivability of the grafts most likely depends on its ability to obtain nutrients from the new host environment, it is likely that cell suspensions will be better able to survive the initial phases. Therefore, in the next group of studies, bovine chromaffin cells, which were generously provided by Dr. Harvey Pollard (National Institutes of Arthritis, Diabetes, and Digestive and Kidney Disease, National Institutes of Health, Bethesda, MD), were used as graft tissue. The cells were obtained from the adrenal glands of steers or cows as described by Pollard et al.[107] The resultant preparation from seven to nine glands contains 0.5-1.0×10^9 chromaffin cells and is essentially free of other cell types. A further advantage of this preparation is that bovine chromaffin cells contain much higher levels of opioid peptides than rat chromaffin cells.[32] The major disadvantage of this preparation is that the transplant is cross-species. Classical studies, however, suggest that the CNS is immunologically privileged to some extent; tissues with major histocompatibility differences transplanted to the CNS are rarely rejected.[108-112] Furthermore, Perlow et al.[113] have shown that dispersed, cultured bovine chromaffin cells survive at least 2 months without evidence of immunological rejection when transplanted to the cerebral ventricles of rats. In addition, these transplanted cells maintain the ability to synthesize and store catecholamines, as indicated by fluorescence histochemistry.

Suspensions of bovine chromaffin cells were shipped in air-tight culture media the day after preparation. They were concentrated by centrifugation and resuspended in small volumes of Hanks' buffer containing 0.1 μg/ml 2.5 S nerve growth factor and kept on ice until they were transplanted. The cells were injected via an intrathecal catheter following a modification of the technique of Yaksh and Rudy.[114] After a small incision was made in the dura overlying the atlanto-occipital junction, a catheter made of PE 10 tubing was threaded through the incision into the subarachnoid space and down the spinal cord to the level of the lumbar enlargement. Cell suspensions were injected through the catheter in 15-μl volumes over 20-30 sec and were followed by a 10-μl flush with Hanks' buffer. Each animal received approximately 100 000 cells. Cell viability was determined at the end of the surgical procedures to be approximately 85% by trypan blue exclusion. Control animals received equal volumes of either heat-killed cells or Hanks' buffer containing nerve growth factor.

Animals were tested for pain sensitivity and response to nicotine stimulation (0.1 mg/kg) at 1 day, 1 week, 2 weeks, 4 weeks, 8 weeks, and 16 weeks following bovine chromaffin cell or control implantation.[115,116] Statistical analysis was done using two-way analysis of variance and the Newman-Keuls test for multiple post hoc comparisons.[117] Typical results at 4 weeks are shown in FIGURE 3. The injection of nicotine induced potent analgesia in animals with chromaffin cell implants, but not in animals with control implants ($p < .01$ for all three analgesiometric tests). The peak increase in pain threshold was at 2 min after nicotine and gradually decreased toward baseline levels by 30 min.

The ability of nicotine to induce analgesia in implanted animals was tested at several intervals over a 16-week period. Results are summarized in FIGURE 4. Since this dose of nicotine did not significantly alter pain sensitivity at any time in control animals ($p > .05$), the data for these animals is omitted for clarity. Analgesia induced by nicotine stimulation could be observed as early as 1 day after cell injection, although the increases in both tail flick latencies and paw pinch thresholds above prenicotine baseline levels were smaller than at other time points. An explanation for this is that the baseline pain sensitivities were higher at 1 day after implantation than at other times during the study. Compared to the preimplantation pain sensitivities, tail flick latency was elevated from 3.2 $\pm$ 0.4 sec to 5.4 $\pm$ 0.6 sec and paw pinch threshold from 10.5 $\pm$ 0.5 to 13.1 $\pm$ 0.7. These differences were statistically significant ($p < .05$). The most likely explanation for this result is that the cells are initially releasing large amounts of their granular contents into the subarachnoid space after the trauma of manipulation during implantation. This also suggests the possibility that at longer time points after implantation there is either a minimal basal (nonstimulated) release of neuroactive substances from the chromaffin cells or that spinal cord receptors become tolerant to the level of catecholamines and neuropeptides that are spontaneously released by the chromaffin cells.

The ability to induce analgesia with nicotine in transplanted animals appears to be well maintained for at least up to 4 months. The differences between the pre- and postnicotine pain sensitivities were statistically significant at all the tested time points ($p < .01$). This supports the notion that the survival of chromaffin cells transplanted to the CNS from another species is quite good. There was a slight decrement in response toward the end of the study, however, suggesting that some of the implanted cells may ultimately die. One possible explanation for this may be an immunological rejection, since plasma cells are occasionally found infiltrating the transplants. In support of this possibility, a more recent group of transplanted animals receiving cyclosporin treatment (0.1 mg/kg daily for 3 weeks) appears to be more responsive to nicotine stimulation. Another possible explanation for the decrement in response may be an associated conditioning to the testing procedures over time, since the baseline levels also tend to be slightly decreased.

In order to determine the sensitivity of chromaffin cell implants to nicotine, another group of implanted animals received several doses of nicotine at weekly intervals on a rotating dose schedule. Results are illustrated in FIGURE 5. The lowest dose of nicotine, 0.05 mg/kg, produced a small but statistically significant ($p < .05$) elevation in tail flick latency and paw pinch threshold in animals with spinal cord bovine chromaffin cell implants. At the highest dose of nicotine (0.2 mg/kg), the elevations in all three tests are nearly maximal (91% maximum tail flick latency and 92%

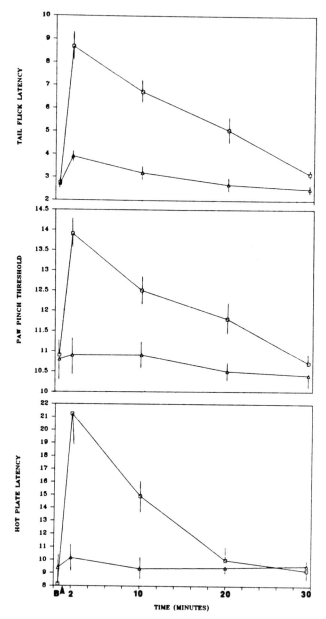

FIGURE 3. Effect of spinal cord bovine chromaffin cell implants on pain sensitivity. The ordinate is the threshold for response to noxious stimuli as measured by the tail flick test (sec) (**A**), paw pinch test (**B**), or hot plate test (sec) (**C**). Each point represents the mean ± SEM. The abscissa is the time course of responses (min) to noxious stimuli after nicotine stimulation. Time 0 indicates the preinjection values. The arrowhead indicates the point at which nicotine (0.1 mg/kg, s.c.) was injected. □: animals with bovine chromaffin cell implants in the spinal cord (N = 14); △: animals with control implants in the spinal cord (N = 10). Taken from Sagen *et al.*[116]

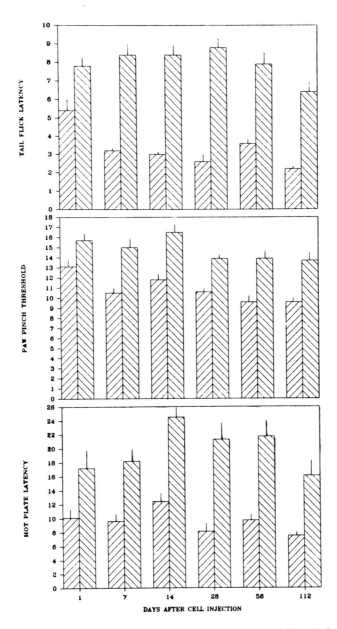

FIGURE 4. Long-term changes in pain responsiveness in animals with spinal cord bovine chromaffin cell implants. The ordinate is the threshold for response to noxious stimuli as determined by the tail flick test (sec) (**A**), paw pinch test (**B**), or hot plate test (sec) (**C**). The bars represent the mean ± SEM for each measurement ($N = 15$ animals). The ordinate is the time (days) after chromaffin cell implantation. Each set of bars represents the response latencies before (▨) and 2 min after (▧) nicotine injections (0.1 mg/kg, s.c.) in implanted animals. Since nicotine had no effect on pain sensitivity in animals with control implants at any of these times, these values are omitted for clarity. Taken from Sagen et al.[116]

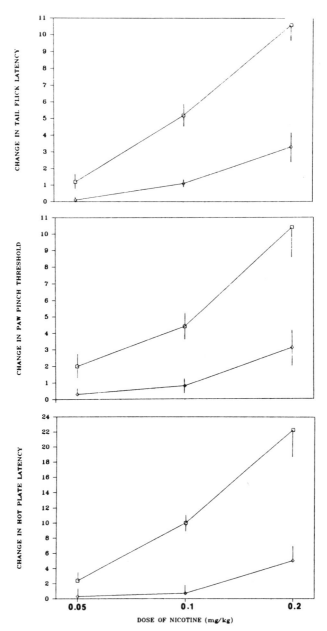

FIGURE 5. Dose-response relationships for the effect of nicotine on pain sensitivity in animals with spinal cord bovine chromaffin cell implants. The ordinate shows the changes in the nociceptive threshold for the tail flick test (sec) (**A**), paw pinch test (**B**), or hot plate test (sec) (**C**). Values were obtained by subtracting the prenicotine response latencies from the latencies determined 2 min after nicotine injections. Each point represents the mean ± SEM. The abscissa shows the nicotine doses (mg/kg) plotted on a log scale. □: animals with bovine chromaffin cell implants in the spinal cord ($N = 9$); ◇: animals with control implants in the spinal cord ($N = 8$). Taken from Sagen et al.[116]

maximum paw pinch threshold and hot plate latency). At this dose, however, there is also a slight elevation in pain threshold in control animals. This is not surprising, since nicotine in higher doses (0.5-2.0 mg/kg) has been shown to produce antinociception.[118,119] It does complicate the interpretation of the effect of transplants on pain sensitivity, however, since the relative contribution of nicotine itself to the analgesia must be considered. Therefore, the intermediate dose of 0.1 mg/kg was determined to be optimal for these studies, since it does not alter pain sensitivity in control animals.

In order to determine the contribution of catecholamines and opioid peptides to the analgesia induced by nicotine in implanted animals, a group of animals with spinal cord bovine chromaffin cell implants was pretreated with either opiate antagonist naloxone (2 mg/kg, s.c.), noradrenergic antagonist phentolamine (10 mg/kg, s.c.), or saline vehicle 10 min before nicotine injection. These doses were chosen since they do not produce any alterations in pain sensitivity.[120] Results are illustrated in FIGURE 6. Pretreatment with saline had no effect on the analgesia elicited by nicotine stimulation in implanted animals. Naloxone, however, severely attenuated this analgesia as assessed by all three analgesiometric tests ($p < .01$). Phentolamine completely blocked the elevation in hot plate latency ($p < .01$), and seemed to partially attenuate the elevation in tail flick latency and paw pinch threshold, but the latter were not statistically significant. These results again suggest that the release of opioid peptides from chromaffin cell transplants plays an important role in the induction of analgesia. The partial attenuation by phentolamine suggests that catecholamine release may also be involved. These results also underline the different mechanisms of pain control measured by the three analgesiometric tests. Since the hot plate test involves the integration with higher centers, changes in hot plate latency may be more dependent on multiple factors.

It is possible that the co-release of two or more pharmacologically active agents (such as norepinephrine and enkephalin) from implanted chromaffin cells would act synergistically to produce their effects. The synergistic action of opiates and catecholamines in the intrathecal induction of analgesia has been suggested by Yaksh.[86] This possibility is being explored further in our transplant studies.

The results of these studies demonstrate that it is possible to induce analgesia by implanting chromaffin cells into the spinal cord. This is potentially clinically useful, since it would provide a local and readily available source of opioid peptides and catecholamines for the relief of pain. One aspect that requires further study is the question of tolerance, both with respect to nicotine's ability to stimulate release of neuroactive substances from chromaffin cell granules, and with respect to spinal cord sensitivity to repeated release of opioid peptides and catecholamines from chromaffin cells. An interesting observation by Yaksh and Reddy[76] is that although there is significant tolerance to analgesic potency with repeated morphine injections intrathecally, the concurrent injection of lower doses of morphine and a noradrenergic agonist produces no decrement in analgesic potency. Since chromaffin cells have been shown to co-release catecholamines and opioid peptides,[22,30] they may provide an ideal combination for avoiding the development of tolerance. Furthermore, Eiden et al.[17] have shown that continued exposure of chromaffin cells to nicotine results in Met-enkephalin mRNA induction and increased Met-enkephalin synthesis, an effect that may offset a possible tolerance effect to repeated injections of nicotine. Preliminary work in our laboratory suggests that analgesia can be elicited by nicotine injections at daily intervals in animals with chromaffin cell implants. There does appear to be some tachyphylaxis, however, since potent analgesia cannot be induced 1 hr after the initial induction of analgesia.

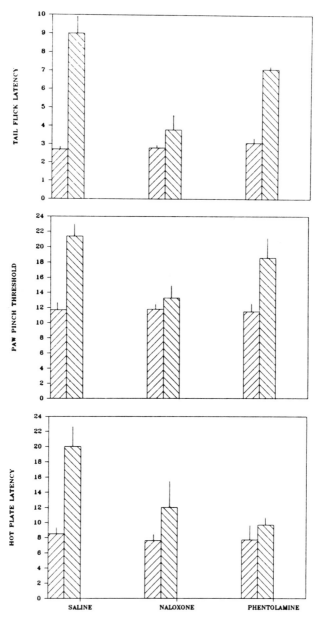

FIGURE 6. Effect of antagonists on the analgesia induced by nicotine in animals with spinal cord bovine chromaffin cell implants. The ordinate is the threshold for response to noxious stimuli as determined by the tail flick test (sec) (**A**), paw pinch test (**B**), or hot plate test (sec) (**C**). Each bar represents the mean ± SEM (N = 7). The first bar in each set (▨) is the pain threshold measured 10 min after the injection of either saline, naloxone (2 mg/kg, s.c.), or phentolamine (10 mg/kg, s.c.). The preinjection values are not shown since the antagonists did not alter these response latencies. The second bar in each set (▧) is the response to nicotine (0.1 mg/kg, s.c.), injected 10 min after the pretreatment with antagonists. Taken from Sagen *et al.*[116]

CHROMAFFIN CELL IMPLANTS IN THE PAG

As discussed above, the PAG is another important region in the control of no-ciception. We have conducted similar transplant studies in this region using both rat adrenal medullary tissue and bovine chromaffin cell suspensions as the graft tissue.[121] One important difference between the PAG implants and the spinal cord implants is that the PAG implants are intraparenchymal, whereas the spinal cord implants are in the subarachnoid space, such that there is no direct interference with CNS tissue. One advantage of intraparenchymal implantation is that there is greater potential for the development of host-graft interactions. However, this technique also produces more damage to the host CNS, and the opportunity for rapid delivery of nutrients to the graft tissue may be more limited.

Pieces of dissected rat adrenal medullae were stereotaxically introduced into the host PAG (A: 1.0 mm; L: 0.5 mm; H: 3.5 mm; incisor bar: -2.5 mm). Bovine chromaffin cells were injected in 0.5-μl volumes through a 27-gauge injection needle. Control animals received an equal volume of heat-killed cells, solid adrenal tissue, sciatic nerve tissue, or Hanks' buffer. Pain sensitivity was assessed using techniques identical to those described above.

Results of this study are illustrated in FIGURE 7. Eight weeks after the trans-plantation of rat adrenal medullary tissue into the PAG, analgesia was elicited by 0.1 mg/kg of nicotine ($p < .01$). This analgesia was less pronounced and of shorter duration than that induced by similar transplants in the spinal cord (see FIG. 1). Control transplants did not produce any alterations in pain sensitivity with nicotine stimulation ($p > .05$). In some cases, the adrenal transplants were found to be placed outside of the PAG region. Transplants in these areas failed to induce analgesia following nicotine injections ($p > .05$). Pretreatment of these animals with either opiate antagonist, naloxone, adrenergic antagonist, or phentolamine produces a partial attenuation of nicotine-induced analgesia (TABLE 1). Therefore, both opioid peptides and catecholamines released from the transplants may be partially responsible for the induced analgesia. It is possible that other neuropeptides released by chromaffin cells (for example, VIP, neurotensin, substance P) may contribute to this analgesia.

Bovine chromaffin cell implants in the PAG produced similar results to those of rat adrenal medullary tissue (FIG. 7). The induced analgesia, however, appears to be more potent. One possible explanation for this is that bovine chromaffin cells contain relatively greater amounts of opioid peptides than rat chromaffin cells.[32] Another possibility is that the survival of the bovine cell suspension is greater, since there is less interference with nutrient provision by the host in the initial stages. A third possibility is the tendency for the nonchromaffin cells in the solid tissue transplant to proliferate and produce a heavy collagen capsule (see FIG. 9), which may act as barrier to the diffusion of active substances to host receptors, or host-graft synaptic relationships.

ULTRASTRUCTURAL CORRELATES OF CHROMAFFIN CELL GRAFTS

In order to determine the underlying morphological changes responsible for the behavior that was observed, some animals were prepared for electron microscopy after the conclusion of testing procedures. Animals were perfused via the aorta with buffered

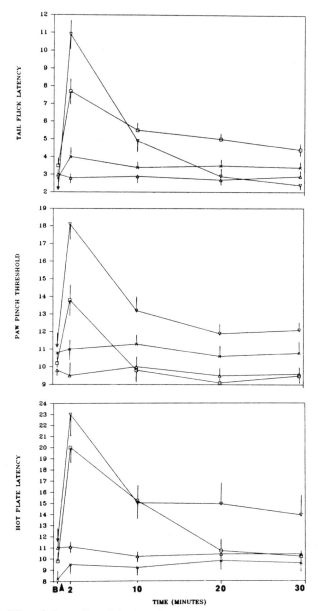

FIGURE 7. Effect of chromaffin cell implants in the PAG on pain sensitivity. The ordinate is the threshold for response to noxious stimuli as assessed by the tail flick test (sec) (**A**), paw pinch test (**B**), or hot plate test (sec) (**C**). Each point represents the mean ± SEM. The abscissa is the time course of responses to noxious stimuli after nicotine stimulation. Time 0 indicates the preinjection values. The arrowhead indicates the point at which nicotine (0.1 mg/kg, s.c.) was injected. △: animals with control implants in the PAG ($N = 7$); □: animals with rat adrenal medullary tissue implants in the PAG ($N = 9$); ▽: animals with bovine chromaffin cell implants in the PAG ($N = 8$); ✕: animals with rat adrenal medullary tissue or bovine chromaffin cells implanted outside of the PAG region ($N = 7$). Taken from Sagen *et al.*[121]

TABLE 1. Effect of Antagonists on Pain Sensitivity in PAG Bovine Chromaffin Cell Implants

	Tail Flick Latency (sec)			Paw Pinch Threshold			Hot Plate Latency (sec)		
	Saline	Naloxone	Phentolamine	Saline	Naloxone	Phentolamine	Saline	Naloxone	Phentolamine
Baseline	3.4 ± 0.2	3.4 ± 0.4	3.2 ± 0.2	9.9 ± 1.0	9.4 ± 0.5	9.5 ± 0.7	10.1 ± 0.6	9.8 ± 0.4	11.7 ± 0.5
After pretreatment	3.8 ± 0.9	3.7 ± 0.7	3.7 ± 0.2	9.8 ± 1.2	9.3 ± 0.4	9.4 ± 0.4	10.2 ± 0.5	10.8 ± 0.4	11.2 ± 0.6
After nicotine	7.7 ± 0.9	5.2 ± 0.4	5.3 ± 1.0	20.0 ± 2.2	14.2 ± 0.3	10.4 ± 0.6	13.8 ± 1.1	11.0 ± 0.3	11.1 ± 1.1

mixed aldehydes, and the brainstem or spinal cord regions containing the implants were dissected out and routinely processed for electron microscopy.[122,123] To assess the viability of the chromaffin cells in the transplants, catecholamine fluorescence histochemistry using the glyoxylic acid method[124] was also performed in some cases.

In general, the transplanted tissue was readily identifiable under a dissecting microscope, and both catecholamine fluorescence and toluidine blue-stained semithin sections revealed that the transplants were healthy and contained numerous chromaffin cells. Rat adrenal medullary tissue pieces implanted 8 weeks earlier in the subarachnoid space of the spinal cord were found to be tenuously attached to both the host spinal cord and the overlying dura mater (FIG. 8A). Ultrastructural studies revealed that the chromaffin cells in the graft contain numerous granules, primarily of the norepinephrine-containing type in that they are oval and have dense cores, in contrast to the epinephrine type found predominantly in the intact adrenal, which are round and have evenly dense cores (FIGS. 8B & 8D). This observation is supported by catecholamine assays that show an increased ratio of norepinephrine to epinephrine in the grafted adrenal medulla compared with the *in situ* case. Similar findings have been reported by other laboratories.[125]

The capillaries in the transplants are fenestrated (FIG. 8C), in contrast to those of the host nervous system, providing a potential for leakiness in the blood-brain barrier.[126,127] Occasionally, finger-like projections containing chromaffin granules can be seen protruding from chromaffin cells in the graft, suggesting the potential for the differentiation of the chromaffin cells into a more neuronal phenotype. In general, however, there does not appear to be an extensive integration between the graft tissue and the host CNS. Thus it does not appear that synaptic relationships between the host and graft are a necessary prerequisite for behavioral alterations. Rather, it is likely that the analgesia induced by these transplants is due to the humoral release of pharmacologically active substances into the subarachnoid space of the spinal cord.

In contrast, there is a much greater integration between host CNS and graft tissue when the transplants are placed in the CNS parenchyma, rather than the cerebrospinal fluid. FIGURE 9 shows a typical host-graft boundary 8 weeks after the transplantation of rat adrenal medullary tissue into the PAG. Astrocytic cell processes delineate the host parenchyma, whereas a thick collagenous layer identifies the adrenal medullary graft. Phagocytes are found both in the graft and host tissue in these border areas. These are most likely mobilized to eliminate host and graft hemorrhagic elements and other necrotic debris produced by local traumatic injury after the initial injection of the graft. These phagocytes apparently become permanent residents at the host-graft borders.

In order for the graft to initially survive transplantation, it must become vascularized by the host. The endothelial cells of the capillaries of the grafted tissue are attenuated and fenestrated, in contrast to those of the surrounding parenchymal tissue (FIG. 10). This has provided a leakiness in the blood-brain barrier, which can be demonstrated by the intravascular injection of the marker protein, horseradish peroxidase (FIG. 11). The horseradish peroxidase can be seen not only to penetrate the graft tissue containing the fenestrated capillaries, but also to penetrate the extracellular space of host parenchyma, where the capillaries are nonfenestrated. This observation has also been noted by Rosenstein and Brightman[128] after the transplantation of superior cervical ganglia. Thus, grafts of peripheral tissue may allow blood-borne substances normally excluded by the blood-brain barrier to reach CNS parenchyma.

Although there is clear delineation between the host and graft borders by glial processes and collagen deposits, this does not appear to act as an absolute barrier to graft-host interaction. Cellular elements, both glial and neuronal, may enter the graft, and chromaffin cells can be identified as "intruding" into the surrounding parenchymal

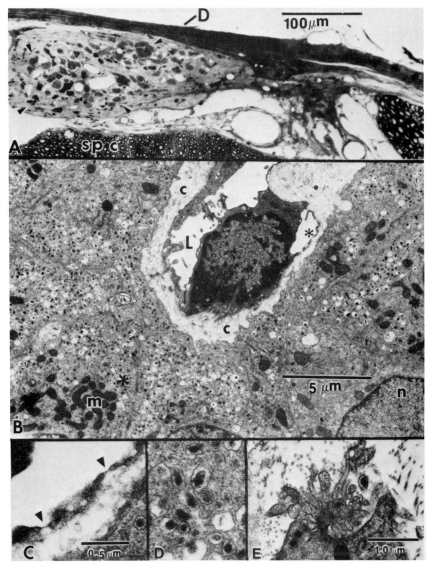

FIGURE 8. (A) Light micrograph of a section from a portion of the dorsal lumbar spinal cord. A piece of adrenal medullary transplant can be found in the subdural space. Dense chromaffin cells can be readily identified in the graft (arrowheads). D: dura; spc: spinal cord. (B) Electron micrograph of adrenal medullary tissue that was transplanted and left for 8 weeks in the spinal cord. The graft is made up primarily of compact granulated chromaffin cells. See D for an enlargement of the chromaffin granules (large asterisk). Note that portions of the blood vessel endothelial cells are attenuated and fenestrated. See C for an enlargement of the endothelial process (small asterisk). L: lumen of blood capillary; c: collagen; n: nucleus of chromaffin cell. (C) Diaphragms at arrowheads are seen in the fenestrae of the endothelial process. (D) The granules are of the norepinephrine type, in contrast to the predominant epinephrine type found in the rat adrenal medulla *in situ*. (E) Enlarged portion of a chromaffin cell in the subarachnoid space of the dorsal spinal cord where some short blunt processes are present 8 weeks after transplantation. Taken from Sagen *et al.*[123]

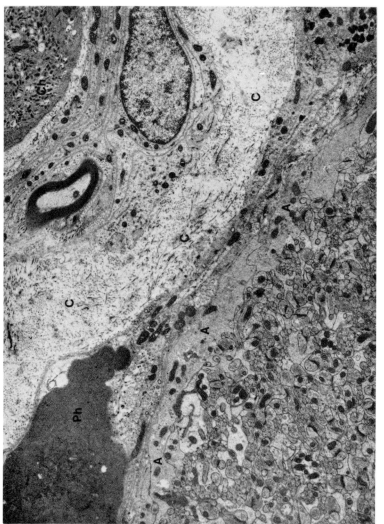

FIGURE 9. Electron micrograph of a section at the graft-host boundary. Note the astrocytic processes (A) delineating the neuropil of the PAG of the host tissue. The grafted adrenal medullary tissue has a thick collagen (C) border. Typically, phagocytes (Ph) and plasma cells can be found at the graft-host boundary. A myelinated fiber can be seen within the graft as well as a portion of a chromaffin cell (Ch). Original magnification: ×7000; reduced to 87% of original size. Taken from Sagen *et al.*[123]

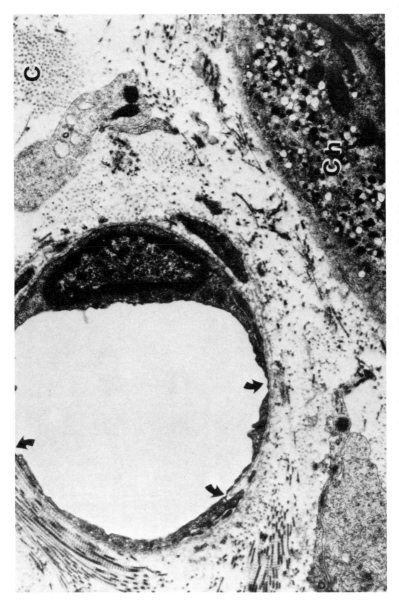

FIGURE 10. Electron micrograph of a section of grafted adrenal medulla tissue into the PAG. Note that the endothelium of the capillary is fenestrated (at arrows), unlike the surrounding host tissue where the endothelium is characterized as being continuous. A great deal of collagen (C) is present in this 8-week-old graft. Ch: chromaffin cell. Original magnification: ×12 400; reduced to 87% of original size. Taken from Sagen et al.[123]

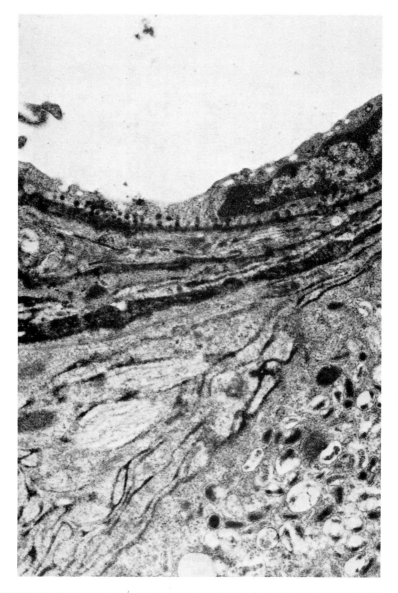

FIGURE 11. Electron micrograph of a section of adrenal medullary tissue grafted into the
PAG. The marker horseradish peroxidase (HRP) was intravascularly injected 20 min before
the rat was fixed with mixed aldehydes by intracardial perfusion. Note that virtually all of the
extracellular space contains HRP precipitate. the endothelial cell contains vesicles filled with
HRP on the basal lamina side and not on the luminal surface as this was washed away by the
saline rinse that preceded the perfusion fixation. The marker HRP can seep through the extracellular space from the graft into that of the host parenchyma. A portion of a chromaffin cell
is present in the lower right of the micrograph. Original magnification: ×20 000; reduced to
85% of original size.

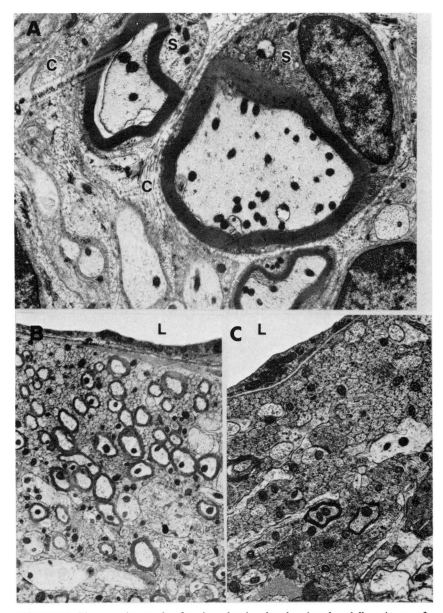

FIGURE 12. Electron micrographs of sections showing that the adrenal medullary tissue grafts into the PAG brings about a noticeable increased number of myelinated processes, both in the grafted adrenal medullary tissue (upper micrograph) and in the surrounding host tissue of the PAG. The graft contains abundant collagen (C), and the Schwann cells (S) can be readily identified. Compare the neuropil of the PAG that has grafts nearby (**B**) with a comparable section of normal neuropil (**C**). L: lumen of blood vessel. The original magnifications for **A** and for **B** and **C**: ×7400 and ×5200, respectively; the figure has been reduced to 97% of its original size. Taken from Sagen et al.[123]

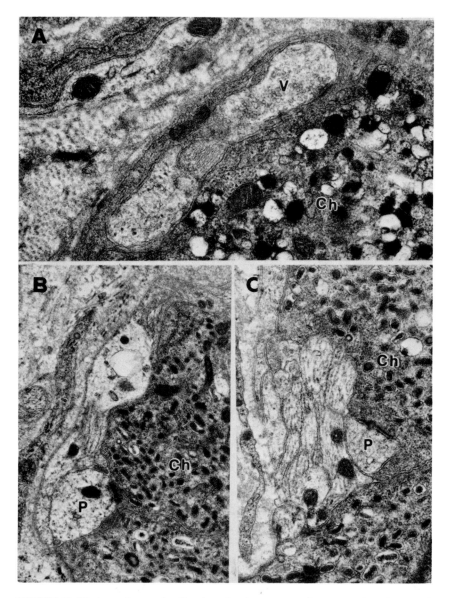

FIGURE 13. Electron micrographs of sections showing processes that apparently make synaptic contact with chromaffin cells (Ch) in 8-week-old transplants in the PAG. Some processes in **A** contain vesicles, indicating that they may be presynaptic; others (P) in the **B** and **C** can be interpreted morphologically to be postsynaptic processes. Original magnification: ×16 000; reduced to 97% of original size. Taken from Sagen *et al.*[123]

tissue. In addition, large numbers of myelinated axons can be found surrounded by Schwann cells throughout the transplant, in contrast to the intact adrenal medulla (FIG. 12). The origin of these large numbers of myelinated axons in the graft has yet to be determined. One possibility is the neuronal cell bodies normally present in the *in situ* adrenal. We have never found one of these in our grafts, however. Therefore, they may originate from the surrounding host parenchyma. It is possible that the placement of intraparenchymal grafts has activated not only an astroglial reaction, but an oligodendrocytic reaction as well. Areas near the transplant in the PAG host tissue also have an increased number of myelinated axons than in controls (FIG. 12). There are no Schwann cells in these areas, and the myelination appears to be of the CNS type, perhaps formed by "activated" oligodendrocytes.

Numerous neuronal processes forming synaptic contacts on the chromaffin cells can be observed (FIG. 13). These presynaptic endings have small clear vesicles, similar to the postganglionic cholinergic synapses found on the adrenal chromaffin cells in the intact medulla. Since neuronal cell bodies are not found in the grafts, however, it is likely that these presynaptic processes are from the host tissue. Occasionally, processes containing primarily microtubules and having junctional dense material can be seen in contact with chromaffin cells (FIG. 12). These may be postsynaptic processes to the chromaffin cells. Thus, chromaffin cells grafted into host CNS parenchyma may participate in both pre- and postsynaptic relationships with host tissue.

CONCLUDING REMARKS

Results of these studies indicate that adrenal chromaffin cells grafted into CNS pain-modulatory regions can reliably produce analgesia when stimulated by nicotine. This is most likely due to the stimulated release of neuroactive substances from chromaffin cell granules. Thus, these cells can provide a local supply of opioid peptides and catecholamines, readily available on demand. This technique may offer a new approach to therapy for intractable pain.

ACKNOWLEDGMENTS

We thank Dr. Mark Perlow for his valuable suggestions and his help for the formulation and initiation of this research endeavor. In addition, we also acknowledge the generous support and advice of Dr. Herbert K. Proudfit in lending us his analgesiometric equipment. We gratefully acknowledge the electron microscope facility of the Research Resources Center, University of Illinois at Chicago, for the use of their equipment.

REFERENCES

1. PERLOW, M. J., W. J. FREED, B. J. HOFFER, A. SEIGER, L. OLSON & R. WYATT, JR. 1979. Science **204:** 643-647.
2. BJÖRKLUND, A. & U. STENEVI. 1979. Brain Res. **177:** 555-560.
3. DUNNETT, S. B., A. BJÖRKLUND, U. STENEVI & S. D. IVERSEN. 1981. Brain Res. **229:** 209-217.
4. FREED, W. J., B. HOFFER, L. OLSON & R. J. WYATT. 1984. In Neuronal Transplants, Development and Function. J. Sladek & D. Gash, Eds.: 373-406. Plenum. New York, NY.
5. FREED, W. J., M. J. PERLOW, F. KAROUM, A. SEIGER, L. OLSON, B. J. HOFFER & R. J. WYATT. 1980. Ann. Neurol. **8:** 510-519.
6. OLSON, L., E.-O. BACKLUND, W. FREED, M. HERRERA-MARSCHITZ, B. HOFFER, A. SEIGER & I. STROMBERG. 1985. Ann. N.Y. Acad. Sci. **457:** 105-126.
7. LUINE, V. N., K. J. RENNER, M. FRANKFURT & E. AZMITIA. 1984. Science **226:** 1437-1439.
8. GIBSON, M. J., D. T. KRIEGER, H. M. CHARLTON, E. A. ZIMMERMAN, A. J. SILVERMAN & M. J. PERLOW. 1984. Science **225:** 949-941.
9. KREIGER, D. T., M. J. PERLOW, M. J. GIBSON, T. F. DAVIES, E. A. ZIMMERMAN, M. FERIN & H. M. CHARLTON. 1982. Nature **298:** 468-471.
10. BJÖRKLUND, A. & F. H. GAGE. 1985. Ann. N.Y. Acad. Sci. **457:** 53-81.
11. DUNNETT, S. B., W. C. LOW, S. D. IVERSON, U. STENEVI & A. BJÖRKLUND. 1982. Brain Res. **251:** 335-348.
12. GAGE, F. H., A. BJÖRKLUND, U. STENEVI, S. B. DUNNETT & P. A. T. KELLY. 1984. Science **225:** 533-536.
13. LOW, W. C., P. R. LEWIS, S. T. BUNCH, S. B. DUNNETT, S. R. THOMAS, S. D. IVERSON, A. BJÖRKLUND & W. STENEVI. 1982. Nature **300:** 260-262.
14. GASH, D., J. R. SLADEK, JR. & C. D. SLADEK. 1980. Science **210:** 1367-1369.
15. BOARDER, M. R., A. J. LOCKFELD & J. D. BARCHAS. 1982. J. Neurochem. **39:** 149-154.
16. CORCORAN, J. J., S. P. WILSON & N. KIRSHNER. 1984. J. Biol. Chem. **259:** 6208-6214.
17. EIDEN, L. E., P. GIRAUD, J. R. DAVE, A. J. HOTCHKISS & H.-U. AFFOLTER. 1984. Nature **312:** 661-663.
18. EIDEN, L. E., P. GIRAUD, A. HOTCHKISS & M. J. BROWNSTEIN. 1982. In Regulatory Peptides: From Molecular Biology to Function. E. Costa & M. Trabucchi, Eds.: 387-395. Raven Press. New York, NY.
19. HERVONEN, A., M. PELTO-HUIKKO & I. LINNOILA. 1980. Am. J. Anat. **157:** 445-448.
20. KONDO, H. 1985. Arch. Histol. Jpn. **48(5):** 453-481.
21. LEVINE, M., A. ASHER, H. POLLARD & O.ZINDER. 1983. J. Biol. Chem. **258:** 1311-1315.
22. LIVETT, B. G., D. M. DEAN, L. G. WHELAN, S. UDENFRIEND & J. ROSSIER. 1981. Nature **289:** 317-319.
23. MIZOBE, F., M. IWAMOTO & B. G. LIVETT. 1984. J. Neurochem. **42:** 1433-1438.
24. MIZOBE, F. & B. G. LIVETT. 1983. J. Neurosci. **3(4):** 871-876.
25. MUELLER, T. H. & K. UNSICKER. 1981. J. Neurosci. Methods **4:** 39-52.
26. STINE, S. M., H.-Y. T. YANG & E. COSTA. 1980. Neuropharmacology **19:** 683-685.
27. TAN, L. & P. H. YU. 1980. Biochem. Biophys. Res. Commun. **95:** 1901-1908.
28. TERENGHI, G., J. M. POLAK, I. M. VARNDELL, Y. C. LEE, J. WHARTON & S. R. BLOOM. 1983. Endocrinology **112:** 226-233.
29. VIVEROS, O. H., S. P. WILSON & K. J. CHANG. 1982. In Regulatory Peptides: From Molecular Biology to Function. E. Costa & M. Trabucchi, Eds.: 217-224. Raven Press. New York, NY.
30. WILSON, S. P., K.-J. CHANG & O. H. VIVEROS. 1982. J. Neurosci. **2(8):** 1150-1156.
31. WILSON, S. P. & O. H. VIVEROS. 1981. Exp. Cell Res. **133:** 159-169.
32. YANG, H.-T., T. HEXUM & E. COSTA. 1980. Life Sci. **27:** 1119-1125.
33. FREED, W. J., J. M. MORIHISA, E. SPOOR, B. HOFFER, L. OLSON, A. SEIGER & R. J. WYATT. 1981. Nature **292:** 351-352.
34. FREED, W. J., F. KAROUM, H. E. SPOOR, J. M. MORIHISA, L. OLSON & R. J. WYATT. 1983. Brain Res. **269:** 184-189.

35. KAMO, H., S. U. KIM, P. L. McGEER & D. H. SHIN. 1985. Neurosci. Lett. **57**: 43-48.
36. MORIHISA, J. M., R. K. NAKAMURA, W. J. FREED, M. MISHKIN & R. J. WYATT. 1984. Exp. Neurol. **84**: 643-653.
37. OLSON, L., E.-O. BACKLUND, G. SEDVALL, M. HERRERA-MARSCHITZ, U. UNGERSTEDT, I. STROMBERG, B. HOFFER & A. SEIGER. 1984. *In* Catecholamines. Part C. Neuropharmacology and Central Nervous System: Therapeutic Aspects. E. Usdin, A. Carlsson, A. Dahlstrom & J. Engel, Eds.: 195-201. Alan R. Liss. New York, NY.
38. BACKLUND, E.-O., P.-O. GRANBERG, B. HAMBERGER, E. KNUTSSON, A. MARTENNSSON, G. SEDVALL, A. SEIGER & L. OLSON. 1985. J. Neurosurg. **62**: 169-173.
39. ACHESON, A. L., K. NAUJOKS & H. THOENEN. 1984. J. Neurosci. **4**(7): 1771-1780.
40. TISCHLER, A. S., R. A. DELELLIS, B. BIALES, G. NUNNEMACHER, V. CARABBA & H. WOLFE. 1980. Lab. Invest. **43**(5): 399-409.
41. TISCHLER, A. S., R. L. PERLMAN, G. NUNNEMACHER, G. M. MORSE, R. A. DELELLIS, H. J. WOLFE & B. E. SHEARD. 1982. Cell Tissue Res. **225**: 525-542.
42. UNSICKER, K., B. KRISCH, U. OTTEN & H. THOENEN. 1978. Proc. Natl. Acad. Sci. USA **75**: 3498-3502.
43. UNSICKER, K., B. RIEFFERT & W. ZIEGLER. 1980. *In* Histochemistry and Cell Biology of Autonomic Neurons, SIF Cells, and Paraneurons. O. Eranko, S. Sonila & H. Paivarinta, Eds.: 51-59. Raven Press. New York, NY.
44. POHORECKY, L. A. & R. J. WURTMAN. 1971. Pharmacol. Rev. **23**: 1-35.
45. WURTMAN, R. J. & J. AXELROD. 1966. J. Biol. Chem **241**: 2301-2305.
46. LEWIS, R. V., A. S. STERN, D. L. KILPATRICK, L. D. GERBER, J. ROSSIER, S. STEIN & S. UDENFRIEND. 1981. J. Neurosci. **1**(1): 80-82.
47. OLSON, L. 1970. Histochemie **22**: 1-7.
48. UNSICKER, K., B. TSCHECHNE & D. TSCHECHNE. 1981. Cell Tissue Res. **215**: 341-367.
49. KONDO, H. 1978. J. Anat. **127**: 323-331.
50. UNSICKER, K., B. TSCHECHNE & D. TSCHECHNE. 1978. Brain Res. **152**: 334-340.
51. OLSON, L., A. SEIGER, R. FREEDMAN & B. HOFFER. 1980. Exp. Neurol. **70**: 414-426.
52. BASBAUM, A. I. & H. L. FIELDS. 1979. Ann. Neurol. **4**: 451-462.
53. BASBAUM, A. I. & H. L. FIELDS. 1984. Annu. Rev. Neurol. **7**: 309-338.
54. MAYER, D. J. & D. D. PRICE. 1976. Pain **2**: 379-404.
55. YAKSH, T. L. & T. A. RUDY. 1978. Pain **4**: 299-359.
56. ATWEH, S. F. & M. J. KUHAR. 1977. Brain Res. **129**: 1-12.
57. HÖKFELT, T., A. LJUNGDAHL, L. TERENIUS, R. ELDE & G. NILSSON. 1977. Proc. Natl. Acad. Sci. USA **74**: 3081-3085.
58. MOSS, M. S., E. J. GLAZER & A. I. BASBAUM. 1983. J. Neurosci. **3**: 603-616.
59. LEWIS, V. A. & G. F. GEBHART. 1977. Brain Res. **124**: 283-303.
60. MURFIN, R., J. BENNETT & D. J. MAYER. 1976. Neurosci. Abstr. **2**: 946.
61. YAKSH, T. L., J. C. YEUNG & T. A. RUDY. 1976. Brain Res. **114**: 83-103.
62. ATWEH, S. F. & M. J. KUHAR. 1977. Brain Res. **124**: 53-67.
63. HÖKFELT, T., T. TERENIUS, H. G. J. M. KUYPERS & O. DANN. 1979. Neurosci. Lett. **14**: 55-60.
64. UHL, G. R., R. R. GOODMAN, M. J. KUHAR, S. R. CHILDERS & S. H. SNYDER. 1979. Brain Res. **166**: 75-94.
65. AKAIKE, A., T. SHIBATA, M. SATOH & H. TAKAGI. 1978. Neuropharmacology **17**: 775-778.
66. TAKAGI, H. 1980. Trends Pharmacol. Sci. **1**: 182-184.
67. LIGHT, A. R. & E. R. PERL. 1979. J. Comp. Neurol. **186**: 151-172.
68. RALSTON, H. J. & D. D. RALSTON. 1979. J. Comp. Neurol. **184**: 643-684.
69. FIELDS, H. L. & A. I. BASBAUM. 1978. Annu. Rev. Physiol. **40**: 217-248.
70. LIEBESKIND, J. C., D. J. MAYER & H. AKIL. 1974. Adv. Neurol. **4**: 261-269.
71. MANTYH, P. W. & M. PESCHANSKI. 1982. Neuroscience **7**(11): 2769-2776.
72. BOWKER, R. M., H. W. M. STEINBUSCH & J. D. COULTER. 1981. Brain Res. **211**: 412-417.
73. ATWEH, S. F. & M. J. KUHAR. 1983. Br. Med. Bull. **39**: 47-52.
74. GLAZER, E. J. & A. I. BASBAUM. 1981. J. Comp. Neurol. **196**: 377-389.
75. LaMOTTE, C., C. B. PERT & S. H. SNYDER. 1976. Brain Res. **112**: 407-412.
76. YAKSH, T. L. & S. V. R. REDDY. 1981. Anesthesiology **54**: 451-467.
77. DAHLSTROM, A. & K. FUXE. 1965. Acta Physiol. Scand. Suppl. **247**: 1-36.

78. WESTLUND, K. N., R. M. BOWKER, M. G. ZIEGLER & J. D. COULTER. 1983. Brain Res. **263:** 15-31.
79. KURAISHI, Y., Y. HARADA & H. TAKAGI. 1979. Brain Res. **174:** 333-336.
80. REDDY, S. V. R., J. L. MADERDRUT & T. L. YAKSH. 1980. J. Pharmacol. Exp. Ther. **213:** 525-533.
81. REDDY, S. V. R. & T. L. YAKSH. 1980. J. Pharmacol. Exp. Ther. **213:** 525-533.
82. PROUDFIT, H. K. & D. L. HAMMOND. 1981. Brain Res. **218:** 393-399.
83. SAGEN, J. & H. K. PROUDFIT. 1984. Brain Res. **310:** 295-301.
84. PROUDFIT, H. K. & T. L. YAKSH. 1980. Soc. Neurosci. Abstr. **6:** 433.
85. SAGEN, J., M. A. WINKER & H. K. PROUDFIT. 1983. Pain **16:** 253-263.
86. YAKSH, T. L. 1985. Pharmacol. Biochem. Behav. **22:** 845-858.
87. FUXE, K. 1965. Acta Physiol. Scand. Suppl. **247:** 37-84.
88. LEVITT, P. & R. Y. MOORE. 1979. J. Comp. Neurol. **186:** 505-528.
89. SAAVEDRA, J. M., H. GROBECKER & J. ZINN. 1976. Brain Res. **114:** 339-345.
90. VERSTEEG, D. H., J. VAN DER GUGTEN, W. DE JONG & M. PALKOVITS. 1976. Brain Res. **113:** 563.
91. HAMMOND, D. L., R. A. LEVY & H. K. PROUDFIT. 1980. Pain **9:** 85-101.
92. SAGEN, J. & H. K. PROUDFIT. 1982. Brain Res. **223:** 391-396.
93. SULLIVAN, T. L. & A. PERT. 1981. Neurosci. Abstr. **7:** 504.
94. LUNDBERG, J. M., A. ROKAEUS, T. HÖKFELT, S. ROSELL, M. BROWN & M. GOLDSTEIN. 1982. Acta Physiol. Scand. **114:** 153-155.
95. BEITZ, A. J. 1982. Neuroscience **2:** 829-834.
96. KALIVAS, P. W., L. JENNES, C. B. NEMEROFF & A. J. PRANGE. 1982. J. Comp. Neurol. **210:** 255-238.
97. BARBER, R. P., J. E. VAUGHN, J. R. SLEMMON, P. M. SALVATERRA, E. ROBERTS & S. E. LEEMAN. 1979. J. Comp. Neurol. **184:** 331-352.
98. HÖKFELT, T., R. ELDE, O. JOHANSSON, R. LUFT, G. NILSSON & A. ARIMURA. 1976. Neuroscience **1:** 131-136.
99. RANDIC, M. & V. MILETIC. 1977. Brain Res. **111:** 197-203.
100. MOSS, M. S. & A. I. BASBAUM. 1983. J. Neurosci. **3:** 1437-1439.
101. HÖKFELT, T., A. LJUNGDAHL, H. STEINBUSCH, A. N. VERHOFSTAD, G. NILSSON, E. BRODIN, B. PERNOW & M. GOLDSTEIN. 1978. Neuroscience **3:** 517-538.
102. JOHANSSON, O., T. HÖKFELT, B. PERNOW, S. L. JEFFCOATE, N. WHITE, H. W. M. STEINBUSCH, A. A. J. VERHOFSTAD, P. C. EMSON & E. SPINDEL. 1981. Neuroscience **6:** 1857-1881.
103. D'AMOUR, F. E. & D. L. SMITH. 1941. J. Pharmacol. Exp. Ther. **72:** 74-79.
104. WOOLFE, G. & A. D. MACDONALD. 1944. J. Pharmacol. Exp. Ther. **80:** 300-307.
105. SAGEN, J., G. D. PAPPAS & M. J. PERLOW. 1986. Soc. Neurosci. Abstr. **11:** 615.
106. SAGEN, J., G. D. PAPPAS & M. J. PERLOW. 1986. Brain Res. **384:** 189-194.
107. POLLARD, H. B., J. PAZOLES, J. C. E. CREUTZ, J. H. SCOTT, O. ZINDER & A. HOTCHKISS. 1984. J. Biol. Chem. **259:** 1114-1121.
108. ALBRINK, W. S. & H. S. N. GREEN. 1953. Cancer Res. **13:** 64-68.
109. DAS, G. D., B. H. HALLAS & K. G. DAS. 1979. Experientia **35:** 143-153.
110. MEDAWAR, P. B. 1948. Br. J. Exp. Pathol. **29:** 58-69.
111. MURPHEY, J. E. & E. STURM. 1923. J. Exp. Med. **38:** 183-197.
112. PERLOW, M. J. 1981. Brain Res. Bull. **6:** 171-176.
113. PERLOW, M. J., K. KUMAKURA & A. GUIDOTTI. 1980. Proc. Natl. Acad. Sci. USA **77:** 5278-5281.
114. YAKSH, T. L. & T. A. RUDY. 1976. Physiol. Behav. **27:** 1031-1036.
115. SAGEN, J. & G. D. PAPPAS. 1986. Anat. Rec. **214(3):** 114A.
116. SAGEN, J., G. D. PAPPAS & H. B. POLLARD. 1986. Proc. Natl. Acad. Sci. USA. **83:** 7522-7526.
117. KEPPEL, G. 1973. Design and Analysis: A Researcher's Handbook. Prentice-Hall. Englewood Cliffs, NJ.
118. SAHLEY, T. L. & G. G. BERNTSON. 1979. Psychopharmacology **65:** 279-283.
119. TRIPATHI, H. L., B. R. MARTIN & M. D. ACETO. 1982. J. Pharmacol. Exp. Ther. **221:** 91-96.

120. JENSEN, T. S. & D. F. SMITH. 1983. Eur. J. Pharmacol. **86:** 65-70.
121. SAGEN, J., G. D. PAPPAS & M. J. PERLOW. 1987. Exp. Brain Res. In press.
122. PAPPAS, G. D., J. SAGEN & M. J. PERLOW. 1985. Soc. Neurosci. Abstr. **11:** 64.
123. SAGEN, J., G. D. PAPPAS & M. J. PERLOW. 1987. Exp. Brain Res. In press.
124. DE LA TORRE, J. C. & J. W. SURGEON. 1976. Histochemistry **49:** 81-93.
125. FREED, W. J., F. KAROUM, H. E. SPOOR, J. M. MORIHISA, L. OLSON & R. J. WYATT. 1983. Brain Res. **269:** 184-189.
126. PAPPAS, G. D. & J. SAGEN. 1986. Anat. Rec. **214**(3): 96A.
127. ROSENSTEIN, J. M. 1985. Soc. Neurosci. Abstr. **15:** 840.
128. ROSENSTEIN, J. M. & M. W. BRIGHTMAN. 1984. *In* Neural Transplants. J. R. Sladek & D. M. Gash, Eds.: 423-443. Plenum. New York, NY.

DISCUSSION OF THE PAPER

J. F. KORDOWER (*University of Rochester, Rochester, NY*): Did you give multiple injections of nicotine to the same animals to see whether you might be getting a tolerance to it?

SAGEN: This is something that we are looking at right now. The analgesia can be induced at daily intervals without evidence of tolerance, but we do get some tachyphylaxis to the nicotine itself in that the analgesia cannot be induced immediately after the initial induction.

L. OLSON (*Karolinska Institute, Stockholm, Sweden*): Did you try NGF in any of your studies? And did you not need cyclosporin A with the bovine cells?

SAGEN: Initially, we placed the tissue in NGF right before the transplantation. This treatment did not have any obvious effects on the transplants. Perhaps longer exposure to NGF would make a difference. As for cyclosporin A, it apparently was not necessary for the survival of some bovine cells for at least 4 months. However, you will notice there is a slight decrement over time in the response. I hope cyclosporin A will take care of that.

Morphological and Immunocytochemical Characteristics of PC12 Cell Grafts in Rat Brain[a]

C. B. JAEGER

Departments of Physiology and Pharmacology
New York University Medical Center
New York, New York 10016

INTRODUCTION

Several recent studies have suggested a beneficial influence of embryonic neural grafts on the recovery of function of animals with brain lesions [1–4] or endocrine deficiencies. [5,6] It is apparent from this work that such grafts can serve as biosynthetic prostheses to supply a vital transmitter or hormone. Other materials, such as trophic substances, which could aid the regeneration of the injured pathways, may also be released by such grafts. [7] Typical neural transplants, however, are composed of non-neuronal cell types, in addition to specific neurons, [1,8] making it difficult to pinpoint the source or target of various factors. Thus, homogeneous transplants consisting of only one cell type were chosen for this study so as to identify potential trophic effects and further clarify the direction and nature of cell interactions between neural transplants and the host brain.

PC12 cells were used because it is known from previous *in vitro* studies that such cells grow processes in the presence of nerve growth factor (NGF)[9–11] and other growth factors. [12–14] These factors drastically alter the morphology of PC12 cells, changing them from the initially round form into process-forming neuron mimics. The expression of processes in PC12 cells has been of particular value in the monitoring of "factors" different from NGF that were, for example, found in brain extracts, [13] cell line supernatants, [13] and other sources. [14] In the present work, PC12 cell aggregate grafts were placed into different brain regions of Sprague-Dawley rats for recognition of possible trophic interactions between the host brain and graft. Since PC12 cells synthesize catecholamines, [10] they contain the biosynthetic enzyme tyrosine hydroxylase (TH), which served as a probe in this work for immunocytochemical identification of the grafted PC12 cells.

Recent studies of grafted PC12 cells showed that they continue to grow in the brain of immature Sprague-Dawley rats. [15] The cells manufacture catecholamine transmitters, and the grafts become vascularized by host-brain-derived microvessels. Migration of astroglia from the host brain into the PC12 cell grafts takes place. Interestingly, it was found that the vascular-PC12 cell barrier that forms is leaky to

[a]This work was supported by Grant NS19699 from the U.S. Public Health Service and by the American Parkinson's Disease Association.

tracers introduced into the host circulation, indicating that the normally existing blood-brain barrier,[16] which structurally consists of endothelial cells and an astrocytic "glia limitans," was altered in the graft.[17] This raised the following question: What are the actual fine structural characteristics of the newly formed capillaries and their astrocyte associations in the PC12 cell grafts? This was studied further in the present work in addition to the identification of trophic interactions.

MATERIALS AND METHODS

Recipient animals were young rats of the Sprague-Dawley strain, of various sizes, of weights between 10 and 250 g, and of various postnatal ages (in days: P4, P10, P12, P14, P21, P30, and P40). Transplantation was carried out with either a 10- or 50-μl microsyringe, which was connected to a glass micropipette, which had a tip diameter of either 100 or 250 μm. PC12 cell aggregates were drawn into the pipette and were subsequently implanted stereotactically by injections of an estimated aggregate-fluid volume of approximately 2 to 5 μl. For each experiment, Dr. L. A. Greene generously provided the live PC12 cells that were grown and maintained in his laboratory on collagen-coated culture dishes.[9-11] The methods used for PC12 cell aggregate preparation and the histological and immunocytochemical procedures for grafts grown for variable time periods were similar to those described previously.[8,15]

RESULTS

Growth and Overall Morphology of Grafts

PC12 cell aggregate grafts survived in the brain of Sprague-Dawley rats as previously described.[15] Since transplant size increased substantially over time, it was necessary to sacrifice recipient animals within 2 months after implantation. The size of PC12 cell grafts at the time of sacrifice was proportional to the initial graft volume. It was estimated that over a period of 6 to 8 weeks the largest graft increase was approximately 60 to 100 times the original volume. This increase is less than the size increase that would be expected to accompany symmetrical cell divisions (all cells in the given volume) and less than the increase that would accompany cell doubling at a rate of twice per week.[9]

Similar growth of PC12 cell grafts occurred in different host brain regions, but modification of adjacent brain tissues varied. For example, the large PC12 cell graft illustrated in FIGURES 1a, 1b & 2a was situated within the dorsal mid- and hindbrain. It caused considerable distortion of the inferior colliculus and rostral regions of the cerebellum. Small grafts, on the other hand, like the PC12 cell graft situated ventrally within the hypothalamic third ventricle (FIGS. 1c & 1d), were not associated with obvious gross structural alterations of the surrounding host brain.

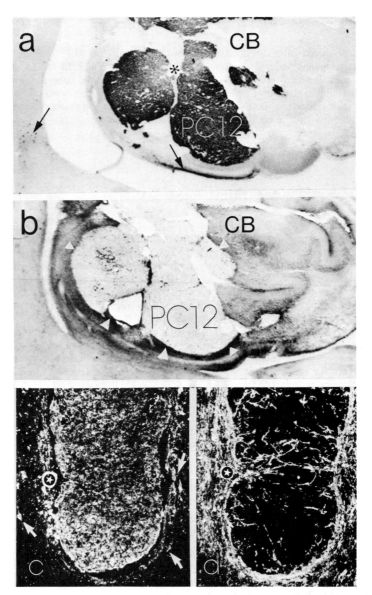

FIGURE 1. Low-power photomicrographs of PC12 cell aggregate grafts. Immunocytochemical localization of TH (**a** & **c**) and GFAP (**b** & **d**) using the peroxidase-antiperoxidase procedure. (**a**) The large graft (PC12, only partially shown here) occupied much of the dorsal tectum and rostral cerebellum. Note that the staining in the central portions of the graft (asterisk) is slightly less intense than that in the remaining areas, where TH levels are relatively high. Arrows point to host brain intrinsic catecholamine cells and fibers. (**b**) A section that was adjacent to that shown in **a** illustrating regions of astroglia reactive zones in the host brain abutting the graft (triangles). (**c** & **d**) Dark-field photomicrographs of a small graft situated ventrally in the third ventricle. The stars mark similar regions in the adjacent sections. Some periventricular TH-positive neurons of host are indicated by arrows in **c**. Host-derived astroglia extend long processes within the PC12 cell graft in **d**. Note the dense distribution of GFAP-positive material at the graft surface.

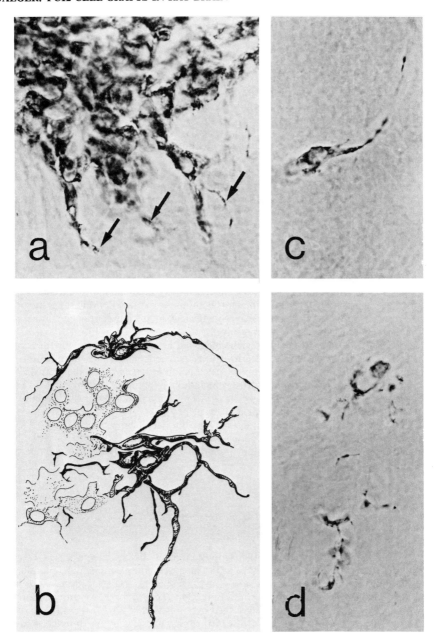

FIGURE 2. Process-forming PC12 cells stained with TH antisera. (**a**) Phase-contrast photomicrograph of a small TH-labeled PC12 cell cluster in the host hippocampus (unlabeled). Note processes (arrows) projecting into the interface region. (**b**) Camera lucida drawing of a region similar to that shown in (**a**). Processes of PC12 cells exhibit variable diameters. (**c** & **d**) Single-process-forming PC12 cells in the host's fimbria adjacent to the graft illustrated in **a**.

Immunocytochemistry

PC12 cells produce several enzymes necessary for biosynthesis of catecholamines.[10] Most notably, TH, which catalyzes conversion of tyrosine to L-dopamine (a catecholamine precursor), is consistently synthesized. Immunocytochemical visualization of TH results in intense and nearly uniform staining throughout the graft (FIGS. 1a & 1c). Since TH immunoreactivity is also distributed within the entire cytoplasmic compartment of PC12 cells, individual cells (which may have migrated) and small clusters of the grafted cells were readily identified by the immunohistological procedure.

Small and moderately grown grafts that were stained for TH between 3 and 5 weeks after transplantation exhibited relatively uniform enzyme activities throughout their depths (FIG. 1c). On the other hand, some very large grafts and grafts assayed at the longest survival times showed graded immunocytochemical staining of variable intensity in different PC12 cell clusters. Such grafts exhibited lower TH staining centrally in comparison to superficial areas (FIG. 1a). In addition to TH, two other catecholamine biosynthetic enzymes, namely aromatic amino acid decarboxylase and dopamine β-dehydroxylase, were detected in PC12 cell grafts. The PC12 cell aggregate grafts failed to stain with antisera directed against phenylamine N-methyl transferase (PNMT), the enzyme that catalyzes conversion of noradrenaline to adrenaline. On the other hand, adrenal medulla implants continue to express PNMT, suggesting that intracranial corticosteroid levels may be sufficient to sustain continued synthesis of this enzyme (Jaeger, unpublished results).

PC12 cells also synthesize acetylcholine,[13] but levels of histochemically detectable acetylcholinesterase (AChE), a degradative enzyme commonly present in cholinergic cells, were too low to precipitate any AChE reaction products within the grafted PC12 cells. This is in contrast to the intense staining obtained in the cell walls of invading microvasculature (see FIG. 4a), which is due to butyrylcholinesterase,[18] usually referred to as unspecific cholinesterase.

Immunocytochemical localization of glial fibrillary acidic protein (GFAP) was carried out in order to identify interactions at the interface between cells of the host brain and the PC12 cells of the grafts, and in order to identify possible migration of astroglia into the grafts.

Trophic Interactions

Several observations suggest that trophic interactions occur between PC12 cells and the surrounding host brain tissue at the interface. For example, differentiation of some PC12 cells, expressed by process growth, is seen in certain locations of the host brain (see below); furthermore, a graft-abutting zone (about 100 μm or more in width) of reactive astrocytes is established over a period of 2 to 4 weeks (FIG. 1b).[15] This graft-host brain interface region is further characterized by much reduced silver-staining capacity of the abutting neural tissue, suggesting a reduction of stainable tissue proteins. Other types of trophic signals may account for the migration of endothelial and astroglia cells from the host brain into grafts.

In some regions of the host brain, grafted PC12 cells that were located adjacent to the graft-host brain interface formed processes (FIG. 2). This occurred primarily in grafts apposed to deep areas of the cerebral cortex[15] or the hippocampus. Single

PC12 cells (FIGS. 2c & 2d) or small cell clusters consisting of a few PC12 cells were also observed to extend short processes when positioned in these host brain locations. A few grafts that were placed into the host hippocampus consisted of PC12 cells that had been treated with NGF for 2 weeks before implantation.[11] This NGF pretreatment resulted in some enhancement of process extension. Process formation by PC12 cells *in vitro* usually requires presence of growth factors, like NGF, neurite inducing factor (NIF),[14] or other growth factors.[12,13] It is likely that local release of growth factors from the host brain also triggers the process extension in the grafted PC12 cells.

Host-derived cells that were observed within the grafts were primarily the en- dothelial cells that formed an extensive graft vasculature, some associated pericytes, and astroglia. Two morphologically different types of astroglia were observed in the pial membranes that covered graft surfaces not directly apposed to host parenchyma. These GFAP-positive cells were either flat cells of epithelial-cell-like morphology or had long processes resembling fibrous astrocytes (FIG. 3b). Within the graft, predom- inantly fibrous astrocytes were recognized (FIG. 3c). This could be explained if certain environmental conditions, which may influence astrocyte shape, become relatively uniformly established within the PC12 cell grafts. Since endothelial cells were the first cell type to invade the PC12 cell grafts before large numbers of astroglia were de- tected,[15] it appears likely that endothelial cell migration into PC12 cell grafts is either independent of astrocyte migration or that additional requirements must be met for astroglial chemotaxis. One such possibility could be synthesis of extracellular matrix components by endothelium. Such a synthesis would allow astrocyte attachment and subsequent migration.

Transformation of Host-derived Endothelial Cells

An extensive microvasculature was established within PC12 cell aggregate grafts (FIG. 4a). Two weeks after grafting (earliest time studied), numerous AChE-reactive capillaries had invaded the grafts from the surrounding host brain and meninges. Very few astrocytes (see above) accompanied the capillaries in the young grafts. Subse- quently, in 3- and 4-week-old PC12 cell grafts, astrocytes were more numerous, and some GFAP-positive processes contacted the host-derived cerebral vasculature (FIG. 3c). A surprising observation was the formation of a leaky capillary system within the PC12 cell grafts.[15,17] This was demonstrated by the introduction of tracers, such as horseradish peroxidase,[16] into the peripheral circulatory system and the subsequent tracer localization within the grafts positioned in the central nervous system (FIG. 3a).

Ultrastructure of PC12 Cell Aggregate Grafts

PC12 cells within grafts were uniquely identified by their large dense core vesicles and their relatively high ribosome content within the cytoplasmic compartment (FIGS. 5a, 6 & 7).[9] PC12 cells were arranged in loose cord-like structures. The cells within them formed broad cytoplasmic contacts interposed by free surfaces from which numerous short processes and filopodia projected. Membrane specialization between

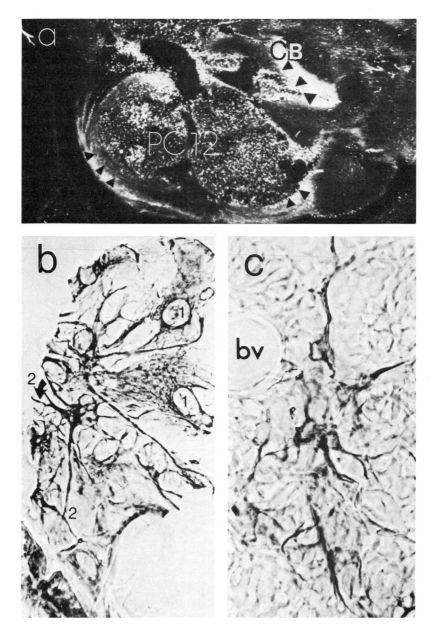

FIGURE 3. (a) Dark-field photomicrograph illustrating the distribution of horseradish per-oxidase (HRP) tracer within a PC12 cell aggregate graft (PC12) following injection of HRP peripherally into the tail vein. Note some leakage of HRP into host brain parenchyma abutting the graft (triangles). (b) Two types of GFAP-immunoreactive astroglia cells in graft pial mem-brane (1: flat cells of epithelial-cell-like morphology; 2: long processes resembling fibrous astro-cytes). (c) Host-derived GFAP-positive cells within the PC12 cell aggregate graft (bv: capillary).

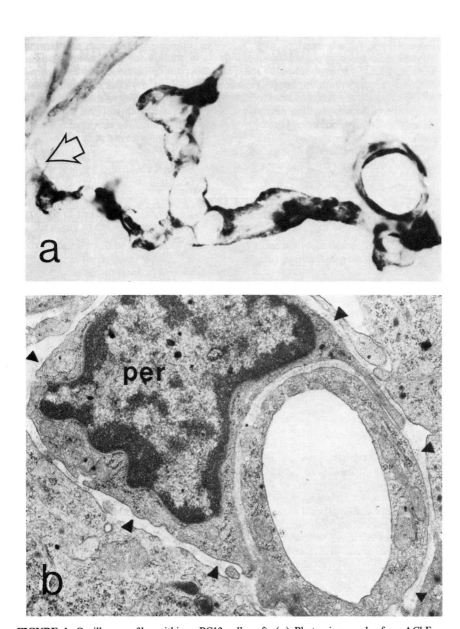

FIGURE 4. Capillary profiles within a PC12 cell graft. (**a**) Photomicrograph of an AChE-positive capillary. The open arrow marks the approximate position of a capillary branch point at the graft-brain interface. Note the convoluted course and variable vessel diameter. (**b**) Electron photomicrograph of constricted capillary lumen. Basal lamina between PC12 cells and endothelial cell and pericyte (per) are indicated by triangles.

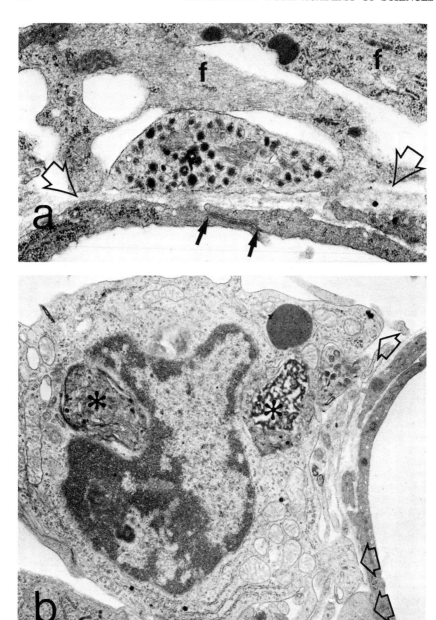

FIGURE 5. Electron micrographs of astrocyte soma and processes and their association to endothelium in a PC12 cell aggregate graft. The open arrows mark the endothelial cell contacts. (a) A PC12 cell process characterized by large electron dense vesicles surrounded by a filament (f)-containing glial process. Note the endothelial cell tight junction between the arrows. (b) Astroglia-like cell containing debris vacuoles (asterisk).

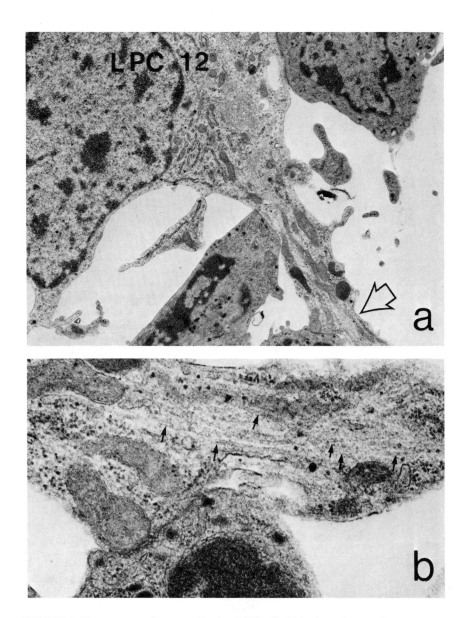

FIGURE 6. Fine structure of a process-bearing PC12 cell within the perimeter of an aggregate graft. (a) Low-power electron micrograph illustrating reduction of cytoplasmic density (LPC 12) in the process-bearing cell. The region of the process near the open arrow is shown in **b** at higher power. (b) Parallel microtubule arrays (arrows) packaged in a process of the PC12 cell.

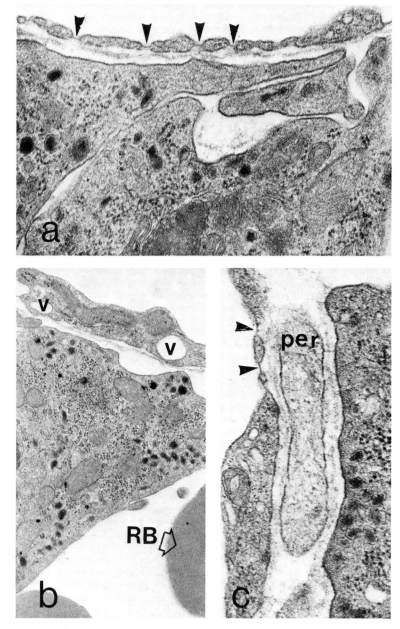

FIGURE 7. Electron micrographs of fenestrated endothelium in a PC12 cell graft. Note the "loose" appearance of endothelial basal lamina. Diaphragms within fenestra are indicated by arrowheads. (a) Endothelial wall exhibiting closely spaced diaphragms. (b) Large vacuoles (v) in endothelial cell cytoplasm and red blood cells (RB) in interstitial space of graft. (c) Portion of pericyte process (per) surrounded by "loose" basal lamina.

contacting cells was rarely seen, but obvious packaging of electron-dense vesicles into certain cytoplasmic compartments and flat processes (FIG. 5a) were apparent. Process-forming PC12 cells had cytoplasm of less density than that for round cells (FIG. 6a). PC12 cell processes contained characteristic microtubule assemblies (FIG. 6b).

Astroglia derived from the host brain were identified by the presence of filaments within cytoplasm and processes (FIG. 5a). Thin astrocytic processes made contacts with the basal lamina of endothelial cells. Typical astroglial endfoot structures[16] were lacking, however. Endothelial cell-astrocyte appositions were usually small, and PC12 cell processes contacted the basal lamina directly (FIG. 5a). At the graft-host interface, astrocytes formed thick stacks of thin membranous lamenae containing glycogen granules and filaments. Some astrocyte-like cells had large inclusion compartments, or "debris vacuoles," of degenerating organelles. An example is illustrated in FIGURE 5b. This cell had a nuclear profile very similar to that of a pericyte, but it lacked the surrounding basal lamina that usually distinguishes pericytes (FIG. 4b).

The fine structure of endothelial cell profiles was inhomogeneous within the PC12 cell grafts. Capillary profiles had lumina of variable size (FIG. 4b) and morphology. In thick light microscope sections, individual microvessels exhibited constrictions and expansion areas along their courses; FIGURE 4a shows a microvessel that is convoluted and multiply branched. Extended capillary walls usually coincided with the presence of fenestra in the endothelial cell cytoplasm (FIG. 7). Typically, formation of a glia limitans at endothelial basal lamina was incomplete in PC12 cell grafts (see above), and therefore PC12 cells were directly apposed to the basal lamina. Most notably, the basement lamina was loosely distributed (FIGS. 7a & 7c) and often multiply stacked.[17]

Commonly, large extracellular spaces occurred between endothelial cells and the contacting PC12 cells. Pericytes accompanying capillaries were scarce (FIG. 4b); in particular, the large extended capillary lumina appeared to lack pericytes entirely. Since some extravasated erythrocytes were found in interstitial spaces of localized graft regions (FIG. 7b), it is possible that open-ended capillaries or breaks within capillary walls existed in the graft microvasculature.

DISCUSSION

The results of this study provide further support for previous observations indicating survival and growth of PC12 cell aggregate grafts in the brain of allogeneic host rats. Furthermore, it was found that some regions of the brain, in particular, deep layers of the cerebral cortex, fimbria, and hippocampus, support process extension of grafted PC12 cells. Process formation by PC12 cells was restricted to peripheral areas of the graft, suggesting local release of trophic factors and limited diffusion of such materials into the graft. These observations show that PC12 cell grafts can be useful for *in vivo* detection of neuronotropic factors. Moreover, responses to hippocampal trophic factors were found to be enhanced in PC12 cells that were grown in suspension cultures and treated with NGF before implantation. Interestingly, recent mappings of NGF and its messenger ribonuclease in the rat brain indicated relatively high levels of these materials within the hippocampus and within cortical regions.[19] It is worth noting that for process formation to occur *in vitro* it is necessary to have both neuronotropic factors and a suitable substrate or matrix.[10,20] The experiments in this study suggest that these two conditions are satisfied *in vivo* in some brain regions.

Since PC12 cell grafts also persisted when they were placed into mature hosts, it appears unlikely that the *in vivo* growth of such grafts depends directly on the host's age. Similar conclusions were obtained from studies of intracerebral neural grafts of embryonic tissues.[1] Other observations, however, suggest that initial graft size, cell treatments, and, possibly, differences of transplantation procedures may account for conflicting observations obtained in different laboratories (see below).

The pheochromocytoma cell line, PC12, was originally isolated by Greene and Tischler[9] from an adrenal medullary tumor that had been found in rats of the New England Deaconess Hospital strain. The early studies had indicated that isografts of the tumor survive whereas grafts of tumor cells (that is, allografts) in a species different from this strain were rejected. Recent work,[15,17] however, has shown that allografts of PC12 cells to the brain of Sprague-Dawley rats survived and continued to grow into tumors. On the other hand, studies carried out in a different laboratory[21] showed that PC12 cell allografts failed to persist for periods longer than 2 weeks. At the present time, it is difficult to reconcile these differences in PC12 cell graft survival, but it appears that PC12 cell aggregates of a certain size persisted as grafts whereas small quantities of dissociated PC12 cells were not recovered. It is possible that dispersed PC12 cells are more vulnerable to drastic alterations of environmental conditions, and clustering may protect some of the cells during a "critical period" of metabolic adjustment. Alternatively, immunological adjustments may be required for PC12 cell survival in the brain.

Greene[22] and Scheineberg and co-workers,[23] who have used tumor iso- and homo-transplants to the brain of various mouse species, have concluded that the brain is only relatively immunologically privileged. This was based, in one case,[23] on observations that the growth and differentiation of homotransplants of an ependymoblastoma tumor that was generated within the brain of a C57BL/6J mouse were variable in other mouse species. The precise nature of species-related differences for the growth of a given transplant type in the brain remains to be resolved, although recently much progress has been made in identification of some of the candidates that may be involved in the cellular and molecular immune responses occurring in the relatively protected brain environment.[7,24] Cell types that present antigens to specific lymphocytes, macrophages, or other cells that in turn could subsequently transmit the initiation of molecular immune responses have been implicated; such cell types are astroglia and endothelial cells. In addition to their immune function, both endothelial cells and astroglia potentially encompass the regulation of the blood-brain barrier.[16] This study has found that both host-derived, GFAP-positive astroglia and endothelial cells migrate into PC12 grafts. The microvasculature that is formed in the graft, however, is morphologically totally altered from that of the host brain. Moreover, the fine structural relationships of astroglia to endothelial cells differed significantly from that seen within the host brain. PC12 cells may bring about structural changes of the endothelial cells directly or via mediation of an altered substrate environment.

The microvasculature of tumors is known to be variable.[25–27] Notably, the occurrence of fenestrated endothelium[28,29] characterized certain tumor capillaries. Recent *in vitro* studies have shown that endothelial cell morphology may also be affected by the surface structure or matrix composition upon which cell attachment takes place.[30] It is also known that many tumor cells secrete specific enzymes that have potentially the capacity to break down certain components of extracellular matrices.[31,32] This in turn could affect the endothelial cells that may be both attracted[25] and altered[29] by tumor cell secretion products.

Following an initial chemotactic event, cell interactions in PC12 grafts between astroglia and endothelial cells could be independently affected by PC12 cells or via signals derived from altered capillaries. Moreover, the existence of immunologically distinguishable astrocyte types within the brain[33] raises questions about whether the functional diversity (antigen presentation, metabolic hyperactivation as seen in "reactive" astroglia, barrier selection) associated with astroglia also defines astrocyte types. PC12 cell grafts may provide a unique model system, one that would allow answers to questions about the nature of the chemotactically sensitive astrocyte type that migrates into PC12 cell grafts, or would allow the identification of the particular enzymatic pathway followed in PC12 cells that direct structural information to endothelial cells. Further elucidation of such events will be useful for understanding immune functions, repair mechanisms of astrocytes, or blood-brain barrier control of the brain.

The third area of application of PC12 cell grafts that may be of some clinical importance involves their potential use as a bioimplant prostheses. It is known that PC12 cells synthesize high levels of dopamine and lesser quantities of norepinephrine.[10] Such materials are also synthesized in PC12 cell grafts.[15] Since implanted PC12 cells may affect behavioral paradigms,[21] this suggests that such materials are released from PC12 cell grafts. Implanted PC12 cell aggregate grafts, however, have the potential to form large tumors; therefore their utility for long-term studies is limited. A strategy of "mitosis inhibition" by X-ray irradiation has been recently employed, and preliminary findings show considerable growth reduction of PC12 aggregates transplanted to the forebrain of Sprague-Dawley rats (Jaeger et al., unpublished results) in paired grafting experiments with either treated or untreated cells. Moreover, experiments employing oncogen-transfected PC12 cells[34,35] indicate that the use of these probes may influence terminal differentiation in PC12 cells. It remains to be seen, however, whether complete inhibition of mitosis and longevity are compatible events in the PC12 cell system.

CONCLUSIONS

PC12 cell grafts provide an interesting alternative to convential embryonic neural grafts.[1–6,8] Transplantation of a homogeneous, "single-cell-type" bioimplant has the advantage of allowing more readily the recognition of graft-host brain interactions, such as trophic effects and cell migration between the two compartments. Such interactions were in fact identified using the PC12 cell aggregate grafts. Moreover, PC12 cell aggregate grafts synthesize transmitters that could appropriately serve as a dopamine replacement source; thus, PC12 cell grafts could have the potential to be used clinically. There is a major disadvantage that now excludes clinical application and sets a time limit on in vivo PC12 cell grafts. This is the continuation of mitosis of PC12 cells and the concurrent growth of such grafts at the expense of the host brain. For long-term studies and for the determination of an actual clinical usefulness of such single-cell-type grafts, it is therefore necessary to limit the growth of PC12 cells before transplantation or to insure a state of "permanent differentiation" within such transplants. Such studies are now being pursued.

ACKNOWLEDGMENTS

It is a pleasure to thank Dr. L. A. Greene for his generous and constant provision of PC12 cell cultures. Antisera to catecholamine biosynthetic enzymes were gifts of Drs. T. H. Joh and D. H. Park. Dr. R. Liem graciously provided antisera to GFAP.

REFERENCES

1. BJÖRKLUND, A. & U. STENEVI. 1984. Intracerebral neural implants: Neuronal replacement and reconstruction of damaged circuitries. Annu. Rev. Neurosci. **7:** 279-308.
2. DUNNETT, S. B., A. BJÖRKLUND & U. STENEVI. 1983. Dopamine-rich transplants in experimental parkinsonism. Trends Neurosci. **6:** 266-270.
3. FREED, W. J. 1983. Functional brain tissue transplantation: Reversal of lesion-induced rotation by intraventricular substantia nigra and adrenal medulla grafts, with a note on intracranial retinal grafts. Biol. Psychiatry **18:** 1205-1267.
4. FREED, W. J., J. M. MORIHISA, E. SPOOR, B. J. HOFFER, L. OLSON, A. SEIGER & R. J. WYATT. 1981. Transplanted adrenal chromaffin cells in rat brain reduce lesion-induced rotational behaviour. Nature **292:** 351-352.
5. GASH, D., J. R. SLADEK & C. D. SLADEK. 1980. Functional development of grafted vasopressin neurons. Science **210:** 1367-1369.
6. KRIEGER, D. T., M. J. PERLOW, M. J. GIBSON, T. F. DAVIES, E. A. ZIMMERMAN, M. FERIN & H. M. CHARLTON. 1982. Brain grafts reverse hypogonadism of gonadotropin-releasing hormone deficiency. Nature **298:** 468-471.
7. NIETO-SAMPEDRO, M., R. P. SANETO, J. DE VELLIS & C. W. COTMAN. 1985. The control of glial populations in brain: Changes in astrocyte mitogenic and morphogenic factors in response to injury. Brain Res. **343:** 320-328.
8. JAEGER, C. B. 1985. Cytoarchitectonics of substantia nigra grafts: A light and electron microscopic study of immunocytochemically identified dopaminergic neurons and fibrous astrocytes. J. Comp. Neurol. **213:** 121-135.
9. GREENE, L. A. & A. S. TISCHLER. 1976. Establishment of a noradrenergic clonal line of rat adrenal pheochromocytoma cells which respond to nerve growth factor. Proc. Natl. Acad. Sci. USA **73:** 2424-2428.
10. GREENE, L. A. & G. REIN. 1977. Release, storage and uptake of catecholamines by a clonal cell line of nerve growth factor (NGF)-responsive pheochromocytoma cells. Brain Res. **129:** 247-263.
11. RUCKENSTEIN, A. & L. A. GREENE. 1983. The quantitative bioassay of nerve growth factor: Use of frozen 'primed' PC12 peochromocytoma cells. Brain Res. **263:** 177-183.
12. BERG, D. K. 1984. New neuronal growth factors. Annu. Rev. Neurosci. **7:** 149-170.
13. EDGAR, D., Y.-A. BARDE & H. THOENEN. 1979. Induction of fiber outgrowth and choline acetyltransferase in PC12 pheochromocytoma cells by conditioned media from glial cells and organ extracts. Exp. Cell Res. **121:** 353-361.
14. WAGNER, J. A. 1986. NIF (neurite inducing factor): A novel peptide inducing neurite formation in PC12 cells. J. Neurosci. **6:** 61-67.
15. JAEGER, C. B. 1985. Immunocytochemical study of PC12 cells grafted to the brain of immature rats. Exp. Brain Res. **59:** 615-624.
16. ANDERS, J. J., K. DOROVINI-ZIS & M. W. BRIGHTMAN. 1979. Endothelial and astrocytic cell membranes in relation to the composition of cerebral extracellular fluid. Adv. Exp. Med. Biol. **131:** 193-209.
17. JAEGER, C. B. 1986. Fenestration of cerebral microvessels induced by PC12 cells grafted to the brain of rats. Ann. N.Y. Acad. Sci. **481:** 361-364.
18. FLUMERFELT, B. A., P. R. LEWIS & D. G. GWYN. 1973. Cholinesterase activity of capillaries in the rat brain: A light and electron microscopic study. Histochem. J. **5:** 67-77.
19. WHITTEMORE, S. R., T. EBENDAL, L. LARKFORS, L. OLSON, A. SEIGER, I. STROMBERG & H. PERSSON. 1986. Developmental and regional expression of nerve growth factor messenger RNA and protein in the rat central nervous system. Proc. Natl. Acad. Sci. USA **83:** 817-821.
20. VLODAVSKY, I., A. LEVI, I. LAX, Z. FUKS & J. SCHLESSINGER. 1982. Induction of cell attachment and morphological differentiation in a pheochromocytoma cell line and embryonal sensory cells by the extracellular matrix. Dev. Biol. **93:** 285-300.
21. HEFTI, F., J. HARTIKKA & M. SCHLUMPF. 1985. Implantation of PC12 cells into the corpus striatum of rats with lesions of the dopaminergic nigrostriatal neurons. Brain Res. **348:** 283-288.

22. GREENE, H. S. N. 1957. Heterotransplantation of tumors. Ann. N.Y. Acad. Sci. **69:** 818-829.
23. SCHEINBERG, L. C., F. L. EDELMAN & W. A. LEVY. 1964. Is the brain "an immunologically privileged site"? Arch. Neurol. **11:** 248-264.
24. FONTANA, A. & W. FIERZ. 1985. The endothelium-astrocyte immune control system of the brain. *In* Seminars in Immunopathology and Immunoneurology. P. A. Miescher & H. Muller-Eberhardt, Eds. Vol. **8:** 57-70. Springer. Berlin.
25. AUSPRUNK, D. H. & J. FOLKMAN. 1976. Vascular injury in transplanted tissues: Fine structural changes in tumor, adult and embryonic blood vessels. Virchows Arch. B. **21:** 31-44.
26. FARRELL, C. L., P. A. STEWART & R. F. DEL MAESTRO. 1984. Tumoral and peritumoral cerebral blood vessels in a rat glioma model. Soc. Neurosci. Abstr. **10:** 998.
27. VICK, N. A. 1980. Brain tumor microvasculature. *In* Brain Metastasis. L. Weiss, H. A. Gilbert & J. B. Posner, Eds.: 115-133. G. K. Hall. Boston, MA.
28. BEARER, E. L. & L. ORCI. 1985. Endothelial fenestral diaphragms: A quick-freeze, deep-etch study. J. Cell Biol. **100:** 418-428.
29. WOLFF, J. & H.-J. MERKER. 1966. Ultrastruktur und Bildung von Poren im Endothel von poroesen und geschlossenen Kapillaren. Zellforsch. **73:** 174-191.
30. MILICI, A. J., M. B. FURIE & W. W. CARLEY. 1985. The formation of fenestrations and channels by capillary endothelium *in vitro.* Proc. Natl. Acad. Sci. USA **82:** 6181-6185.
31. BERGMAN, B. L., R. W. SCOTT, A. BAJPAI, S. WATTS & J. B. BAKER. 1986. Inhibition of tumor-cell-mediated extracellular matrix destruction by a fibroblast proteinase inhibitor, protease nexin I. Proc. Natl. Acad. Sci. USA **83:** 996-1000.
32. JONES, P. A. & Y. A. DECLERCK. 1980. Destruction of extracellular matrices containing glycoproteins, elastin, and collagen by metastic human tumor cells. Cancer Res. **40:** 3222-3227.
33. RAFF, M. M., R. H. MILLER & M. NOBLE. 1983. A glial projenitor cell that develops *in vitro* into an astrocyte or an oligodendrocyte depending on culture medium. Nature **303:** 390-396.
34. ALEMA, S., P. CASALBORE, E. AGOSTINI & F. TATO. 1985. Differentiation of PC12 pheochromocytoma cells induced by *v-src* oncogene. Nature **316:** 557-559.
35. NODA, M., M. KO, A. OGURA, D. LIU, T. AMANO, T. TAKANO & Y. IKAWA. 1985. Sarcoma viruses carrying *ras* oncogenes induce differentiation-associated properties in a neuronal cell line. Nature **318:** 73-75.

DISCUSSION OF THE PAPER

G. D. PAPPAS: (*University of Illinois, Chicago, IL*): What I would like to ask you concerns your GFAP reaction. How soon can you see the reaction after injection? In some of the work that we have been doing on pain perception in the spinal cord, we inject PC12 cells in the subarachnoid space. Within 2 weeks, we have these invasive tumors that have caused paralysis in the lower limbs. At that time, we fix the rat and remove the tissue. We do not find any reactive astrocytes that we can identify. Are your astrocytes long term, or do you see reactive astrocytes within 2 weeks after injection?

JAEGER: At this stage, up to 2 weeks after injection, the area surrounding the graft does not contain the same level of reactive astrocytes as the one I showed you for grafts of about 1 month. I will not say there are no astrocytes because this technique is not absolutely perfect for detecting possibly reactive astrocytes. But just in comparison, I would say there is much less reaction at 2 weeks. Also, in the irradiated case, even after a month there was very little reactive material that could be related to more glia cells making more GFAP.

V. SINALI (*Institute of Neurology, Milan, Italy*): Do you have any biochemical evidence of plasticity of the cells in relation to a different region where they are grafted? Do they, for example, produce more acetylcholine?

JAEGER: I do not know.

M. F. D. NOTTER (*University of Rochester, Rochester, NY*): Does X-ray treatment of the PC12 cells *in vitro* or *in vivo* induce neurite extension?

JAEGER: Not that I have noticed in these experiments. Only a few experiments have been done in which PC12 cells have been looked at in tissue culture following X-ray treatment. These cells are still there. I do not see any neurites unless they are treated with something else.

Summary and Discussion

L. GREENE (*New York University, New York, NY*): I would like to thank the speakers for their excellent, lucid talks, the discussants for their excellent questions, and the audience for its attentiveness. I must say that I am quite impressed with the attentiveness of this large group.

I do not think it is worth, using Dr. Sotelo's terminology, my going over the papers "point to point." Let me just make a few general remarks.

I was impressed by the general use of markers. Although the topic of this session was specific cells, one was not, in every case, implanting a single type of cell. It was quite possible, however, for an experimentalist to follow a particular cell type by using a marker. More markers are becoming available, and they are surprisingly specific. I am quite impressed by this. The use of monoclonal antibodies and the employment of specific antibodies to detect particular enzymes was particularly powerful. From an outsider's point of view, these developments seem to be moving the field along very interestingly.

The other general point that interested me was that the transplants did not act as anticipated in every case. Although Dr. Segal mentioned that he did not think he would be here if his transplants had not worked as expected, I think the opposite was true in some cases. For example, Dr. Lund showed transplants that grew in the wrong direction if they were made too far away from the tectal region. Dr. Sotelo and Dr. Clarke also showed interesting cases in which there was a failure of axonal growth from transplants to reach the appropriate region. We can learn from these differences. There has been a lot of emphasis on saying, "Gee, things are working properly when we make the transplants." We can, however, learn as much when things do not work appropriately.

Let me now highlight a few general points from each paper. Dr. Lund made a very practical point: one has to be very careful to think about the role of the immunological system in transplants.

In Dr. Sotelo's paper, I was very taken by what I will call the Ulysses effect. In this effect, the appropriate neurons seem to be lured out of the transplants. This opens up the question of what it is that is luring or attracting these cells. I was also taken by the fact that there were distance limitations; that is, the Purkinje cells did not form the appropriate connections beyond 700 microns. I do not know what to make of the 700 micron figure. This number is something a mathematical biologist might find fascinating. It might correspond to the distance something can diffuse in gray matter.

In Dr. Clarke's paper, I was struck by the difference between the innervation for young animals and that for old animals. When Dr. Clarke used fairly young animals, she saw a hypo-effective innervation; when she used aged animals, the new connections seemed to be more or less normal. As she mentioned, it would be fascinating to correlate this difference with behavioral differences.

In Dr. Segal's paper, I was very taken by the way physiological markers were used. Dr. Segal's use of physiological properties to mark the particular cells he was interested in was very impressive.

I was also taken by the physiologic properties of the raphe cells he transplanted. The cells developed in a totally appropriate way, even in an inappropriate place. The acquisition and onset of certain characteristic physiologic properties seem to be built into these particular cells.

It would be particularly interesting to go back in the other direction. Dr. Segal did show that the cells may have lost a certain plasticity, but what about going back earlier? Is there a point at which one can make a transplantation of raphe cells in which they cannot show this appropriate type of formation of these physiologic markers? I was also impressed by Dr. Segal's assessment of behavioral responses in the experimental animals.

In Dr. Gibson's paper, I was very struck by the combination of techniques that were employed. We saw anatomy, we saw development, we saw behavior—a variety of impressive techniques. Obviously, a number of workers were involved, and they were able to coordinate their efforts and address a single question. And again, I was impressed by the use of appropriate markers.

Dr. Sagen and Dr. Jaeger each presented a paper using a simplification of cell type rather than using a piece of tissue containing different cell types. In each case, the attempt was to use a defined cell type. In both papers, the emphasis was not so much on formation of connections, but in using the implanted cells as vehicles to produce enzymes and thereby to produce particular biological products or, as discussed in these papers, catecholamines or opiates. So we have gone from the use of implants to form connections to their use as little factories to make particular biologically useful materials.

I was also struck by Dr. Sagen's point that there was a difference between spinal cord and CNS. In the spinal cord the cells did not seem to interact with the chromaffin cells, whereas in the CNS they did. I wondered why this might be and what could be responsible for this difference.

Dr. Jaeger's paper illustrated the point about markers and the point about using the cells as factories. I was also impressed by the effects on the vasculature. In transplantation research we generally consider the effects of connectivity or things being released, but clearly the implants that are made of various cell types are going to affect the vasculature. It is something that has come up here and there, but it is a very important area that one has to think about more: the blood supply to particular regions of the brain may in fact be directly affected by the implants that are put in.

Another point that Dr. Jaeger mentioned was the glia. One has to be very attentive to what's happening to glial cells that might be coming in to the explant. We know that neurons are not going to be moving long distances, but clearly glial cells are.

L. KROMER (*Georgetown University, Washington, DC*): I was particularly intrigued by Dr. Sotelo's discussion, and I have a question for him. Have you tried putting in grafts from normal cerebellar donors in time periods when you are getting the degeneration of the Purkinje cells in the mutant? If you have, have you looked to see whether the axons from the grafted Purkinje cells can follow the degenerating pathway that is being opened up by the degenerating Purkinje cells of the host? This might provide a better pathway for these axons in the grafted Purkinje cells to reach the deep nuclei.

C. SOTELO (*Inserm U106, CMC Foch, Suresnes*): That is a very nice question, but, as I emphasized in my paper, a competition for molecular layer territory is very important for the survival of these neurons. The degeneration of Purkinje cells in the mutant is fast, but slow compared to the speed of migration of the embryonic neurons from the graft to the molecular layer. We never did these types of experiments because I believe that you should transplant the Purkinje cells during the 2-4-week period in which the Purkinje cells are degenerating. If remnants of Purkinje cells and necrotic debris remain in the molecular layer, the new embryonic cells may not be able to migrate in. That is the only reason I did not try, but it is something that we are planning to do for a different reason.

The reason we want to do this is mainly neural. You know neural people like Richard Mullen have tried to do chimeric tetra-parental animals trying to see whether the nervous genetic loci act on the intrinsic Purkinje cells or not. Our results seem to indicate loci probably act intrinsically. When you have mirror images of these bands of Purkinje cells surviving, this is not the answer. Purkinje cells are dying, and the cells that are dying probably correspond to the supernumerary Purkinje cells in the cerebellum.

So, now we graft embryonic cells that have a normal genetic background. These cells survive very nicely for at least 3 or 4 months. Sure, when we put the cells in, the degeneration period is ended. If it is some cellular toxin effect or something, this can be transient.

QUESTIONER: I would like to ask Dr. Jaeger one or two questions. After X-irradiation of PC12 cells, have you looked at the biochemistry of the cells after a long period?

C. B. JAEGER (*New York University, New York, NY*): No, not the biochemistry.

QUESTIONER: About the time after transplantation, the longest time you mentioned was 1 month. Have you looked longer?

JAEGER: No. I showed you a cauliflower-shaped graft within the occipital cortex that was 7 weeks. I have them up to 2 months. I have usually tried to implant my grafts roughly into the forebrain, and if you implant large grafts there you will get neurological deficiencies developing in the animals. The cortical one not so much, obviously. Maybe the cortex is not so important for the animals. But a large graft may grow there quite effectively.

QUESTIONER: Cells are responsive to nerve growth factor after X-irradiation, I think.

JAEGER: That is possible. I have not done that.

G. D. PAPPAS (*University of Illinois, Chicago, IL*): This is just a general question that I have been wondering about. As Dr. Sagen showed, when one transplants into adult brain one talks about the gliotic reaction and the importance of the astrocytes. But what about oligodendrocytes? I do not know how prevalent myelination is in the periaqueductal brain that Dr. Sagen showed, but we see myelination where there should not be any. Does anybody care to comment about this? Could something be going on here with the oligodendrocytes?

A. W. DECKEL (*Johns Hopkins University School of Medicine, Bethesda, MD*): First, we recently reported that when you look at myelination with a few different sorts of stains, including neurofibrillary stains and stains of myelination itself, cortical transplants seem to have abnormal patterns of myelination.

Second, when using an old-fashioned silver stain in our striatal transplants, we found when we accidentally placed those transplants in the neocortex that we had an intense oligodendrocytic reaction. This corresponds with the abnormal sort of patch of myelination seen on the external perimeters of the striatal transplant. So, in two different systems, we have seen something very much like that.

SOTELO: I want to ask Dr. Pappas whether he has transplanted some solid piece of adrenal gland, and whether there are Schwann cells there or not.

PAPPAS: I believe there probably were a few. Yes.

SOTELO: These may be the cells responsible for the myelination.

PAPPAS: You really think so? If they do, the myelination that we see in the host is of the central or peripheral type.

D. M. GASH (*University of Rochester School of Medicine, Rochester, NY*): This is a question directed to Dr. Jaeger, and it goes back to using X-irradiation to inhibit mitosis of the cells. I wonder why you chose that? There are a number of chemical treatments that you can also use to induce differentiation and to inhibit mitosis. A number of these treatments will, for example, induce larger synthesis of dopamine. Studies that we have done with Dr. Notter have shown increases of 1000% in dopamine production after treatment with nerve growth factor and actinomycin C. Have you looked at various other treatments to see whether and how they would effect transplantation?

GREENE: Your studies refer to neuroblastoma cells, is that correct?

GASH: No, on PC12 cells. There we found that they do increase their production of dopamine as measured by HPLC.

JAEGER: To answer the first question of why X-irradiation was used: I tried various other chemical treatments, but I felt the chemical treatment might have been interfering with the experiments I was interested in. They were not very successful, so that is why in fact the X-irradiation was chosen.

QUESTIONER: I have two questions for Dr. Sotelo. What is the fate of the precursor of granular cells? What is the fate of the deep neurons in the suspensions after injection?

SOTELO: When I am transplanting a piece of cerebellum at E12, the only cells I am transplanting are stem cells, a few deep nuclei neurons, and Purkinje cells. The granular layers do not form. Whenever I transplant a cell suspension or solid implant, the stem cells will continue to proliferate. Theoretically, they are already committed.

What happens is that Purkinje cells move out of the transplants within 4 days after transplantation. Years ago, in a study with mutants, we speculated that there was a close correlation between the presence of normal Purkinje cells and the regulation of the proliferation rate of the standard granule layer. In the mutants we used, the absence of normal Purkinje cells suppressed the proliferation of the standard granular cells because these cells were few and the number of inert granular cells formed very low.

In the transplants, what happens is that the Purkinje cells leave the transplants very quickly before the beginning of proliferation of the standard granular layer. My guess is that the number of granular cells that are formed is very small. Dr. Lund uses markers that allow him to follow whole populations of cells he has implanted. A possibility is Thy-I and Thy-II. You have two different strains of mice: one is Thy-I positive and the other is Thy-I negative. We are planning to get the antibodies to follow the very short time—something like 2 weeks after transplantation—to see the fate of the older neurons in the cerebellum.

When we make a solid transplant the deep nuclear neurons normally remain at the cortical level. It is very easy with our Purkinje cell staining method to recognize these zones because you see the circumference of Thy-I-positive staining axons going on immunonegative cells. They have the same pattern as the deep nuclei in the normal animal. Deep nuclear cells do remain and are another limiting factor for the growth of the Purkinje cell axons toward the host nucleus because they have trapped a lot of axons.

QUESTIONER: Do you see migration of Purkinje cells from the graft into the host if you use donor tissue beyond E12, say, E14 or E16?

SOTELO: I do not know.

Neural Tissue Transplantation

Comments on Its Role in General Neuroscience and Its Potential as a Therapeutic Approach

RAYMOND T. BARTUS

Department of CNS Research
Medical Research Division
American Cyanamid Company
Pearl River, New York 10965
and
New York University Medical Center
New York, New York 10016

INTRODUCTION

By many standards, research involved with neural tissue transplantation represents one of the most exciting areas of basic neuroscience research; however, it also continues to be one of the most controversial. Although considerable evidence now indicates that transplanted brain tissue can indeed survive, differentiate, and innervate the host (thus forcing revision of many established neuroscience dogmas), many other important issues remain in dispute. Foremost among these are questions about the functional nature of the transplanted tissue and the therapeutic value the phenomenon and associated techniques may offer for treating certain neurological defects, such as Parkinson's disease and Alzheimer's disease.

The editors of this volume have asked me, as someone not directly involved with brain tissue transplant research, to discuss the work in this area, as it may impact the general neurosciences, as well as future therapeutic approaches for neurodegenerative problems. Although many independent purposes or objectives could be accomplished by brain tissue transplantation research, certain general goals seem to provide a particularly useful means of logically evaluating and discussing current progress and future prospects. These include 1) the impact this research has had on basic information about neural function; 2) the role it has played in opening new areas of scientific inquiry; and 3) the potential to facilitate functional recovery after brain damage.

Although the current contributions of brain tissue transplantation research seem most clear when the first two goals are considered, it is the third goal that has attracted the greatest excitement and promise, and also continues to generate the most controversy. It is hoped that by reviewing the work in this area from these perspectives, not only might it be easier to determine what has been accomplished to date, but, moreover, what remains to be done if work in this area is to evolve from one of basic query to one that offers promise of providing effective therapeutic relief for certain neurological defects.

355

CONTRIBUTIONS TO BASIC INFORMATION ON NEURAL
FUNCTION: REVISING OLD DOGMAS

One early contribution of the seminal work in this area involved the accumulation of basic information on developing and adult brain and the consequent reshaping of our perceptions and thinking about how the brain works. The very fact that it is now generally accepted that neural transplants survive and remain viable up to months after transplantation provides a prime example of how research in this area has contributed to a more general understanding of brain function. Although it was documented long ago that neonatal brain tissue could survive and then grow when transplanted into adult mammalian brain (see the excellent review by Gash et al.[1]), this early information was not generally accepted until recently. Consequently, the old dogma that claimed such a phenomenon was impossible continued to persist in the majority of neuroscience circles.

In the mid-1970s, renewed interest in this phenomenon was deservedly sparked by papers that carefully characterized some of the conditions that enhance survival of brain tissue grafts,[2] as well as by reports that new neural connections seemed to form between the graft and the host.[3] Over the last decade, tremendous progress has been made, with considerable attention devoted toward characterizing and quantifying the important physical and temporal parameters required for the successful transplantation of neural tissue into adult brain. Although a review of this careful and systematic work would be well beyond the scope of this paper, it is important to note that not only have numerous laboratories now successfully transplanted brain tissue, but that a reasonable degree of prediction and control of the phenomenon is now possible, including some of the variables important for the eventual establishment of physical contact between graft and host.[1,4]

Aside from the fundamental importance of these observations and the correction of many traditional views of the adult mammalian nervous system that they have forced upon us, research with brain tissue grafting continues to provide the opportunity for expanding our knowledge of brain function. Future research in this area is likely to continue to contribute to more accurate insight and principles regarding general nervous system development, as well as numerous specific issues, including neuron differentiation, neuron-to-neuron synaptic specificity, neuron-glial interactions, and peripheral versus central nervous system response to insult or injury. Moreover, when information from studies such as these is merged with knowledge gained from emerging disciplines in molecular neurobiology, great advances could be made in our understanding of the nervous system. Clearly, it can be expected that the role played by transplantation research will continue to have a significant impact on the development of thinking and research in the general neurosciences for a long time to come.

STIMULATION OF NEW AREAS OF SCIENTIFIC INQUIRY:
TROPIC FACTORS AND ASTROCYTE FUNCTION

Another general objective of neuroscience that has been served by neural tissue transplantation research involves the identification and empirical pursuit of new areas of scientific inquiry. In the course of characterizing the conditions under which the survival of the graft might be optimized, investigators have described two very different, but related, phenomena that deserve special attention: tropic factors and astrocyte function.

During the past several years considerable direct and circumstantial evidence has accumulated which suggests existence of so-called neurotropic factors, which, in addition to being present in (and passed along with) the transplanted tissue, are apparently released upon brain injury in the host. Many studies, including many of the papers in this volume, have demonstrated that some of these substances may be critical to the survival and differentiation of neurons in the central nervous system. Although evidence of the existence of such factors in the central nervous system developed independent of neuron transplantation research, the study of graft survival has helped confirm their presence in the brain and has, moreover, provided intriguing evidence of their multiplicity of type and function.

Recent evidence suggests that some factors apparently are primarily involved with promoting neuron survival, whereas others primarily promote neurite outgrowth.[5] Moreover, different putative factors seem to exhibit a degree of specificity for particular brain regions or neuron types, being ineffective when applied in brain regions foreign to their origin or purpose. Critical periods for optimal activity of the neurotropics are also being defined, so that time, as well as place, is relevant to their efficacy.[6] Finally, although efforts to purify and characterize the physical properties of these substances are in their early stages, several investigators have demonstrated that astrocytes represent at least one primary source for some of the factors.[6] Indeed, a number of neurofunctional improvements known to occur after brain tissue transplantation have also been effectively accomplished by increasing the local concentration of neurotropic factors derived from young astrocytes. These data indicate that some of the functional recovery reported to occur after neural tissue transplantation may be related to the presence of neurochemical factors within astrocytes, more so than to the transplantation of neurons per se.

The second phenomenon, briefly mentioned above, involves the study of astrocyte function. Investigators have demonstrated that, although the neurons that constitute a transplanted brain graft remain physically restricted to the site of transplantation, certain glial cells contained in the graft (especially astrocytes) migrate into the host, sometimes over relatively long distances (up to 2 mm).[7] Others have noted that the migrating astrocytes seem to induce vascularization of the host,[8] a process many believe to be crucial to proper transplant survival. Finally, it is suggested that the astrocytes are important for helping the graft to make physical contact with the host brain, possibly guiding development of new synaptic contacts between transplant and host.[8]

Although the study of neurotropic factors and astrocyte function will continue to enhance our understanding of why brain tissue transplantation is possible and how it might be more effectively performed, it is also clear that these two interrelated phenomena represent areas of study that clearly deserve attention in their own right. It may be said, with no intent of minimizing the excitement over, or interest in, the implications of neural tissue transplantation research (which is nevertheless a man-made aberration in the adult brain), that the therapeutic benefits derived from such research could be surpassed by those derived from the research on neurotropic factors and astrocyte function (presumably naturally occurring phenomena).

In conclusion, it seems reasonable to expect that a more complete understanding of neurotropic factors and astrocyte function should lead to a much broader understanding of general central nervous system function, the important variables involved with brain injury, and the various degenerative and regenerative processes involved with diseases of the nervous system. Furthermore, the search for an effective means of treating certain neurodegenerative problems might be facilitated by a more complete understanding of tropic factors and astrocyte function.

FUNCTIONAL RECOVERY: CURRENT STATUS AND THERAPEUTIC IMPLICATIONS

As mentioned earlier, of all the contemporary issues associated with brain tissue transplantation, those concerned with functional recovery and possible therapeutic applications are among the most interesting and controversial. In this regard, at least three general questions deserve special consideration: 1) Is the transplanted neural tissue truly or solely responsible for the behavioral recovery? 2) In those instances where one can conclude (or is willing to assume) that the transplant is responsible for recovery, what is the mechanism involved? An important corollary of this is as follows: What is the evidence that functional reinnervation of damaged brain has been achieved? 3) Finally, what is the evidence that neural tissue transplantation represents a viable approach for treating various neurodegenerative diseases? Two related questions are as follows: How valid or predictive are the animal models that are used to demonstrate functional recovery? How much more efficacious is tissue transplantation, relative to more conventional treatment approaches currently available in the clinic?

Is the Transplanted Tissue Responsible for the Behavioral Recovery?

Artificially induced brain lesions have been used for many decades by behavioral neuroscientists interested in defining the functional role of discrete brain regions and in studying the processes responsible for the gradual recovery that typically follows injury. When Perlow et al.[9] demonstrated that rats subjected to striatal lesions regained normal motor function after neural transplantation of fetal dopamine-containing neurons, interest in the use of brain lesions to study the functional consequences of brain tissue transplants quickly grew. The majority of this work, however, has been directed toward expanding the brain regions capable of inducing behavioral improvement and the types of behaviors that might be affected.

Although it now seems that many behavioral deficits can be reduced or reversed by neural tissue transplantation in both brain-damaged and aged rats, control groups are rarely included to conclusively demonstrate what factor(s) might be responsible. For example, many behavioral deficits that follow discrete brain lesions are known to recover spontaneously: sometimes it is difficult to be certain whether the observed functional recovery is simply, or even primarily, the result of innervating transplanted brain tissue. This may be a particularly serious problem with rodent lesion-models of Alzheimer's and Parkinson's disease, where long-term recovery of function following the lesion has been reported. One fairly simple control group, which is rarely employed in transplant studies, would involve relesioning the transplanted tissue following recovery to see if the deficit reappears. Additionally, the possibility that neurotrophic factors may be directly contributing to the functional recovery (independent of their beneficial effects on neuron graft survival) makes simple explanations even more difficult. Previously discussed studies demonstrating significant functional recovery after injections of tropic factors from astrocytes adds credence to this notion.

Has Functional Reinnervation Been Achieved?

Although not all studies clearly demonstrate that the transplanted brain tissue is responsible for the functional recovery, there are many studies which demonstrate that the grafted tissue most certainly plays an important role in the functional improvement. Even in these cases, however, it is difficult to determine the specific mechanism responsible, except, perhaps, in those instances where the graft is used as a bridge across a small lesion (usually done with spinal preparations).

Although many investigators attempt to interpret the observed recovery in terms of "functional reinnervation" by the graft (and this possibility continues to represent an important goal of this research), the probability that the transplant simply serves as a biological "chemical delivery system" that effectively replaces lost neurotransmitter or hormone cannot easily be dismissed.

Given that a primary function of living neural tissues is to secrete neurochemicals in accordance with changes in their homeostatic condition, and that the transplanted neurons continue to express this inherent, phenotypic response, it seems certain that one result of tissue transplantation involves the dumping of manufactured chemicals into the area surrounding the transplantation site. Thus, the major issue that remains is whether the transplanted tissue is doing more than merely acting as a biological chemical delivery system. Unfortunately, it is difficult to answer this question from the majority of the published studies. Many studies have used behavior as an end point, and although behavioral improvement is an important and often necessary condition for demonstrating functional recovery, it does not adequately define the nature of the recovery or the mechanism responsible. In this regard, it is noteworthy that some of the most impressive behavioral changes reported with neurotransplants have also been obtained, in other studies, with parenteral administration of drugs with appropriate mechanisms of action. Similarly, significant functional recovery has been reported after transplantation of tissue grafts void of neurons, but rich in chromaffin cells and astrocytes. Finally, in one of the more exceptionally controlled studies, similar degrees of recovery were achieved when Alza pumps were implanted and neurotransmitters thus infused directly into the ventricles (as compared with successfully transplanted brain tissue).[9] Collectively, those studies argue, in many instances, that the functional recovery observed with tissue transplantation may likely be unrelated to genuine functional reinnervation of damaged brain.

In many instances, it may be important to distinguish between *functional reinnervation* of the brain (which would represent partial repair of neural circuitry) and *synaptic innervation* between the graft and host (which would simply provide a source of replacement neurotransmitter). Of course, studies in which neural transplants are grafted directly onto the terminal field of the host could be expected to do little more than provide a renewed source of transmitter for the damaged brain, since the afferents that normally innervate the lesion site remain disconnected. Evidence of the formation of new synapses between the graft and host do little to diminish this functional limitation. The notable exceptions of examples where synapses also formed between the host and the terminal fields of the graft provide preliminary evidence of reinnervation, but many additional studies at the electrophysiological level or neurochemical level or both are required to establish that the reinnervation is complete and truly functional. This is not to imply that functional reinnervation may not be possible, although the conditions under which it might be expected to occur may be limited.[4] In the meantime, careful, multidisciplinary studies are required for any attempt to establish the extent to which functional reinnervation actually occurs and its role in the behavioral recovery seen after neural transplantation. Clearly, this question provides one of the foremost challenges for future research in this area.

Does the Transplant Represent a Viable Therapeutic Approach?

Although the available evidence for functional reinnervation may still be sparse, and the transplant may only be serving as a neural means of drug delivery to the brain, several arguments could be raised for why transplanted neural tissue may provide a superior therapeutic means of replacing diminished neurotransmitters or neurohormones in the brain. To begin, many chemical substances necessary for proper function in a region of the central nervous system are either quickly metabolized in the blood or do not readily cross the blood-brain barrier. Thus, viable neural tissue transplanted into the brain circumvents this problem. Additionally, by placing the tissue at the proper projection site, one can be more certain of achieving adequate concentrations at the area of need, while keeping levels in other areas to a minimum. Further, because the graft seems to achieve close physical contact (that is, form putative synapses) with the efferent neurons of the host, greater selectivity of effects might be expected. These variables collectively should be expected to maximize efficacy, while significantly reducing unwanted side effects of any transmitter released by the graft. Further, the possibility that the live biological chemical delivery system may retain some self-regulatory properties (for example, via presynaptic autoreceptors, sensitivity to the availability of precursors, or responsiveness to circadian rhythms) may provide a degree of functionally relevant fine tuning not easily obtained when more traditional means of replacing neurotransmitters are used. Finally, by transplanting brain tissue that is genetically programmed to innervate the host at that target site, it is possible that the normal phenotypic expression of the transplant will provide a number of essential transmitters or factors (some of which may still be unknown and may function synergistically). Thus, multiple neurotransmitters might be manufactured and delivered by the graft to the terminal field, possibly producing more complete replacement of deficient transmitters, resulting in more complete restoration of function.

Despite the conceptual reasons for believing that neural tissue transplantation represents a potentially superior means of replacing diminished neurotransmitters or hormones, two reservations must be expressed. First, like many current approaches to treating neurodegenerative diseases, brain tissue transplantation will not likely affect the pathogenesis of the disease, but can be expected to merely reduce a portion of the symptoms. In fact, given that the etiologic factor(s) is likely to still be present, a relapse might be considered the more likely probability. Second, although considerable optimism among investigators currently exists, relatively little direct empirical evidence of clear superiority of brain transplants has yet been established. Few studies have attempted to directly compare the effects of brain tissue transplantation with more conventional therapeutic approaches, such as parenteral drug injections or intrathecal infusions. For this reason, the recent evidence of significant reduction in parkinsonian symptoms in monkeys treated with 1-methyl-4-phenyl-1,2,3,6-tetrahydropyridine after receiving striatal transplants[11] should be tempered until careful and objective comparisons to currently available drug treatments are made, and long-term studies are completed, with appropriate control groups. Such comparisons are necessary if the relative value of the transplantation procedure is to be determined. Otherwise, there will be no way to distinguish those situations in which transplantation would offer clear advantages from those situations in which transplantation would introduce unjustifiable risk and expense. These types of comparisons are essential if this research in basic neuroscience is to develop logically into a field offering legitimate therapeutic relief.

ACKNOWLEDGMENTS

The author thanks Ms. Rochelle Gordon for assistance in preparing this manuscript, and Dr. Jeffrey Kordower for comments on an earlier draft.

REFERENCES

1. GASH, D. M., T. J. COLLIER & J. R. SLADEK, JR. 1985. Neural transplantation: A review of recent developments and potential applications to the aged brain. In Neurobiology of Aging. Vol. 6: 131-150. Ankho International.
2. STENEVI, U., A. BJÖRKLUND & N. A. SVENDGAARD. 1976. Transplantation of central and peripheral monoamine neurons to the adult rat brain: Techniques and conditions for survival. Brain Res. 114: 1-20.
3. LUND, R. D & S. D. HAUSCHKA. 1976. Transplanted neural tissue develops connections with host rat brain. Science 193: 582-584.
4. FISHMAN, P. S. 1986. Neural transplantation: Scientific gains and clinical perspectives. Neurology 36: 389-392.
5. AZMITIA, E. C. 1987. A serotonin-hippocampal model indicates adult neurons survive transplantation and aged target may be deficient in a soluble serotonergic growth factor. Ann. N.Y. Acad. Sci. This volume.
6. NIETO-SAMPEDRO, M., J. P. KESSLAK, R. GIBBS & C. W. COTMAN. 1987. Effects of conditioning lesions on transplant survival, connectivity, and function: Role of neurotrophic factors. Ann. N.Y. Acad. Sci. This volume.
7. LINDSAY, R. M., C. EMMETT, G. RAISMAN & P. J. SEELEY. 1987. Application of tissue culture and cell-marking techniques to the study of neural transplants. Ann. N.Y. Acad. Sci. This volume.
8. SMITH, G. M., R. H. MILLER & J. SILVER. 1987. Astrocyte transplantation induces callosal regeneration in postnatal acallosal mice. Ann. N.Y. Acad. Sci. This volume.
9. PERLOW, M. J. & W. J. FREED. 1979. Brain grafts reduce motor abnormalities produced by destruction of nigrostriatal dopamine system. Science 204: 643-647.
10. COLLIER, T. J., D. M. GASH & J. R. SLADEK, JR. 1987. Norepinephrine deficiency and behavioral senescence in aged rats: Transplanted locus ceruleus neurons as an experimental replacement therapy. Ann. N.Y. Acad. Sci. This volume.
11. SLADEK, J. R., JR., T. J. COLLIER, S. N. HABER, A. Y. DEUTCH, J. D. ELSWORTH, R. H. ROTH & D. E. REDMOND, JR. 1987. Reversal of parkinsonism by fetal nerve cell transplants in primate brain. Ann. N.Y. Acad. Sci. This volume.

A Serotonin-Hippocampal Model Indicates Adult Neurons Survive Transplantation and Aged Target May Be Deficient in a Soluble Serotonergic Growth Factor[a]

EFRAIN C. AZMITIA

Department of Biology
Washington Square Center for Neural Sciences
New York University
New York, New York 10003

INTRODUCTION

Neuronal transplantation offers the ability to observe the interactions of cells from different brain areas and of different ages. It has been observed that afferent neurons transplanted to their normal targets provide the best situation for subsequent survival, maturation, and function.[1-3] Likewise, fetal cells develop best when transplanted to neonatal host brain.[4,5] Thus, the conditions that most closely parallel the normal situation provide the most fertile environment for mixing neuronal cells from different animals.

The main theme of this paper is to establish the extreme conditions for success in neuronal transplantation. In order to examine the most appropriate model, we chose to transplant afferent cells into their normal target. Serotonergic neurons were selected as the afferent cells for several reasons: 1) The developmental history of these cells has been carefully described by a variety of laboratories. The cells complete their neurogenesis by day 14 of gestation in the rat[6] and immediately begin to extend neurites toward their target.[7-9] 2) These cells can be reliably visualized using available antibodies raised against serotonin.[10,11] 3) The neuroanatomy of this system has been clearly described in the adult[12-14] and in the fetal brain.[7,9] Thus, the fetal serotonergic cells that project to specific target areas can be isolated in fetal and adult tissue. Our question was as follows: "Can afferent (donor) cells of different ages develop after transplantation into the appropriate target area of an adult brain?"

The other side of this question deals with the age of the host target area. We have previously shown that fetal serotonergic cells survive for 1 month in an aged brain when transplanted into the hippocampus.[15] This observation should be considered in light of the evidence that endogenous afferent serotonergic neurons appear to be withdrawing from this same target area during aging.[16] This implies that the cause of the afferent neuronal decrease is a deficit in the afferent neuron itself rather than

[a] This work was supported by Grant BNS 86-07796 from the National Institutes of Health.

a decrease of a trophic factor in the aged target area. In fact, several authors have subsequently shown that transplanted fetal neurons can survive in the aged brain and may in fact reverse certain age-related abnormalities in these animals.[17-19]

Our strategy in studying the effects of age of the target area was to use *in vivo* and *in vitro* conditions. To examine the donor-host interactions *in vivo*, fetal serotonergic neurons were grown in adult and aged hippocampus for either a short (1-month) or long (3-month) period and the amount of high-affinity serotonergic uptake compared between these groups. *In vitro*, fetal serotonergic cells were grown in primary dissociated cultures, and the high-speed supernatant from adult and aged hippocampus was added to the cultures. The amount of high-affinity uptake by the cultured neurons was compared between these conditions. A description of our culture model and the effects of target tissue has been described.[20]

Previously, we have shown that the supernatant from adult hippocampus can stimulate serotonergic maturation in tissue culture.[21,22] The stimulation is most effective at dilutions of 1:1000 of the supernatant. Partial removal of serotonergic fibers from the adult hippocampus will induce homotypic collateral sprouting of the undamaged adult serotonergic neurons[23-26] and will cause an increase in the stimulation of the hippocampus supernatant factor at low (1:50) but not high (1:1000) dilutions. These results indicate that partial loss of the 5-hydroxytryptamine (5-HT) afferents to the adult hippocampus encourages the growth of adult serotonergic neurons *in vivo* and fetal serotonergic neurons *in vitro*. The fact that aged hippocampal tissue contains fewer serotonergic fibers could result in stimulated fetal serotonergic development if the normal production of target growth factors is functional. Therefore, our question was "Does aged target tissue support serotonergic neuronal maturation after transplantation and in tissue culture?"

METHODS

Adult (4-6-month-old) and aged (24-month-old) male C57B1/6N mice were used (Charles River Breeding Laboratories). Isogenetic pregnant mice (14-16 days of gestation) were killed by decapitation. The fetuses were removed with their placentae and placed in ice-cold oxygenated Ringer's buffer. A surgical approach was developed for removal of the fetal raphe 5-HT nuclei under the dissecting microscope, a mid-sagittal section of tissue between the mesencephalic and pontine flexures was cut out using a number 11 scalpel blade, the overlying tectum and meninges were removed, and a strip was cut 0.5 mm on each side of the midline. The strip was cut into small cubes (1 mm^3), which were then transferred to ice-cold sterile 1% glucose in minimal essential media (MEM) solution (GIBCO). The fetal hippocampus was removed from underneath the cortical tissue and also cut into small cubes.

Adult Cells and Co-transplantation

Adult serotonergic cells were removed from the dorsal raphe nucleus by making a cube (0.5 mm^3) from a coronal section at the level of the superior colliculus. The tissue was placed in ice-cold glucose-MEM solution until just before transplantation. In adult only transplantation, the adult tissue was placed on a sterile petri dish and cut into small pieces. In adult-fetal co-transplantation, fetal hippocampus and adult raphe cubes were minced together into smaller pieces.

The host mice were anesthetized with an intraperitoneal injection of Ketalar (ketamine HCl, 50 μg/g body weight, Parke-Davis) and followed 1 min later with an intramuscular injection of Rompun (xylazine, 20 μg/g body weight, Baynet). Blocks from a single embryo were aspirated into a glass micropipette and stereotaxically injected over 10 min in the hippocampus or lateral ventricle with a glucose-MEM solution (2 μl). The hippocampal coordinates were 2 mm caudal, 1.5-2.0 mm lateral, and 3.0 mm ventral to bregma. Postoperatively, the skull was sprayed with Neosporin aerosol (polymyxin B-bacitracin-neomycin powder, Burroughs Wellcome) and the closed incision was coated with an iodine solution.

Mice were singly housed in a quiet room on a 12/12 hr light/dark cycle with food and water *ad libitum*. One month following transplantation, the mice were perfused intracardially with 150 ml of a solution of 3.5% paraformaldehyde, 0.5% glutaraldehyde, and 0.05% magnesium sulfate in 0.1 M phosphate buffer (pH 7.4) chilled to 5° C. The brains were postfixed in the same fixative overnight before being washed in 0.9% saline in 0.1 M phosphate buffer and transferred to 0.9% saline in 0.1 M Tris buffer (TBS). Fifty-micron-thick sections were cut on a Vibratome (Oxford Sectioning System, Ted Pella) and stained immunocytochemically as described previously.[27] The primary antibody, rabbit anti-5-HT, was used at a 1:2000 dilution in 0.2% Triton and 1% normal sheep serum in TBS and incubated on sections for 17 hr at 5° C and 2-4 hr at room temperature. After the completion of the unlabeled antibody peroxidase-antiperoxidase procedure, selected sections were reacted with methyl green or cresyl violet. Specificity controls included preabsorption of anti-5-HT serum (1:2000) with 10^{-2} M 5-HT and use of NSS in place of the primary antibody.[15]

Isolation

The hippocampus and midbrain from adult mice were removed by blunt dissection and homogenized in 10 vol/weight (minimum volume was 1 ml) ice-cold 0.32 M sucrose with 10 strokes of a loosely fitted glass homogenizer (Thomas No. 04715) and a teflon pestle (No. 5952) using a Cole Palmer motor drive (model 442) set at 1000 rev/min. Synaptosomes were obtained by using a procedure modified from Jonec and Finch[28] that has already been described.[15] The homogenate was centrifuged (1000 g for 10 min) and the supernatant (S_1) carefully removed and saved. The pellet (P_1) was resuspended in 2 ml of 0.32 M sucrose and centrifuged again at low speed (1000 g for 10 min) to obtain another S_1. The S_1 supernatants were combined and centrifuged at 14 000 g for 10 min. The resulting P_2 pellet (crude synaptosomal preparation) was resuspended in 10 vol of original tissue weight of Krebs-bicarbonate buffer. The above centrifugations were performed at 2° C in the SM-24 rotor of a RC2-B Sorvall Centrifuge.

Reaction

Incubations were performed in triplicate or quadruplicate in tissue culture mul-tiwelled plates (Linbro-76002-04) with a total reaction volume of 300 μl, which contained 15 μl of the P_2 suspension. The incubation solution was raised to 37° C, and the reaction was started by the addition of 20 μl of [^{3}H]5-HT (5×10^{-8} M) prepared in Krebs-Ringer buffer. Nonspecific accumulation is determined by incubating as described with the addition of 10^{-5} M Fluoxetine (Fluoxetine was kindly provided by Lilly Research Laboratories, Eli Lilly and Company). The reaction was terminated after 3 min by filtering the incubation medium through GF-B Whatman filters and washing for 25 sec with 10 ml of ice-cold NaCl in 0.1 M phosphate buffer (pH 7.4), using an automatic Titertek cell harvester (Flow Laboratories). All chemicals were enzymatic or Sigma grade.

RESULTS

Fetal Raphe into Adult Host

The neuronal transplantation of fetal serotonergic cells into hippocampus of adult mice showed positive 5-HT-immunoreactive (IR) cells in all cases.[15] The donor fetal 5-HT-IR cells were found in dorsal hippocampus, lateral ventricle, and dorsal thalamus. The areas of the neuronal soma of 5-HT-IR cells were measured at various times after transplantation (5, 13, 20, and 26 days, as shown in TABLE 1). It can be seen that a large increase occurred between 13 and 20 days after transplantation (67% increase compared to day 13; $p < .05$) and remained relatively stable after this time (50% increase compared to day 13; $p < .01$).

The multipolar 5-HT-IR neurons could be clearly seen to extend processes out of the fetal tissue into the adult hippocampus. The fibers grew into their normal target areas in the hippocampus, the stratum lacunosum-moleculare, and the molecular and polymorphic areas of the dentate gyrus. The biochemical measure of high-affinity [^{3}H]5-HT uptake showed a small but significant increase 1 month after transplantation. There was a fairly large variation in that two animals showed a much larger increase than the others, probably due to placement of the cells (FIG. 1). Compare these results to those shown in the paper by Zhou, Auerbach, and Azmitia,[29] where the growth of serotonergic cells are shown in normal and 5,7-dihydroxytryptamine (5,7-DHT)-lesioned hippocampus. Examination of a group of mice 3 months after transplantation showed much better uptake than in the normal adult mice at 1 month (FIGS. 1 & 2).

Fetal Hippocampus into Adult Host

Fetal hippocampus could be successfully transplanted into the adult mouse brain. The fetal tissue grew much larger than the transplanted fetal raphe tissue, and the donor hippocampal tissue usually occupied a large area below the normal hippocampus; this area extended into the lateral ventricle. The fetal hippocampus was innervated quite effectively by adult 5-HT-IR fibers.[15]

Adult Raphe into Adult Host

Neuronal transplantation of adult raphe tissue into adult hippocampus showed that some 5-HT-IR cells were alive 1 week after transplantation. The size of the transplant was small, and the 5-HT-IR fibers formed dense swirls within the transplant. These fibers did not penetrate the adult hippocampus. One month after transplantation, no 5-HT-IR cells were visible, and all that remained of the transplanted tissue was a necrotic region filled with macrophages.

Co-transplantation of Fetal Hippocampus and Adult Raphe into Adult Host

In a number of adult animals, a co-transplantation of adult raphe cells and fetal hippocampal cells was made into the dorsal hippocampus. After 1 month, giant

TABLE 1. Area of 5-HT-IR Cells in Midsections of Raphe Transplants in Hippocampus

Days after Transplantation	Area (μ^2)	Number of cells
5	200 ± 16	11
13	213 ± 11	9
20	356 ± 67[a]	10
26	318 ± 19[b]	14

NOTE: The significance levels were determined with respect to the areas measured 13 days after transplantation using the Student t test.
[a] $p < .05$
[b] $p < .01$

surviving 5-HT-IR neurons could be found within the co-transplanted fetal hippocampus. These cells measured over 350 μm^2 in area (FIG. 3). These 5-HT-IR cells showed extensive branching around the soma, and somatic spines were apparent (FIGS. 4 & 5). This unusual morphology was never observed in the 5-HT-IR cells in the endogenous raphe nuclei of the midbrain or in the fetal neurons transplanted into the adult animal.

Supernatant Factor

We have previously shown that a high-speed supernatant fraction from adult rat hippocampus can stimulate the biochemical maturation of cultured fetal serotonergic cells.[21,22] This stimulation is most effective at dilutions around 1:1000 and can be destroyed either by heat or trypsin digestion. Supernatant fractions from cerebellum are not very effective in our culture preparation. We tested the ability for stimulating

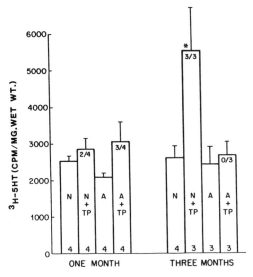

FIGURE 1. Each bar represents the average of the synaptasomal uptake of [³H]5-HT in mice 1 or 3 months after transplanting fetal serotonergic neurons into the hippocampus. The numbers at the bottom of the bars represent the number of transplanted mice; the numbers at the top of the bars represent the number of successful grafts. N: Normal adult hippocampus; A: aged hippocampus; TP: transplant. After 3 months, only the fetal raphe serotonergic cells transplanted into the adult hippocampus show a dramatic increase (>100% stimulation, $p < .05$).

maturation of fractions from the hippocampus and cerebellum of adult and aged mice on rat dissociated fetal serotonergic cells in tissue culture. Our results demonstrated that hippocampal supernatants at dilutions between 1:10 and 1:1000 were effective at stimulating serotonergic high-affinity uptake mechanisms in culture for 3 days (TABLE 2). There was no significant stimulation produced by hippocampal supernatant from an aged (26-month-old) male. Neither the young nor aged cerebellar tissue supernatant produced a significant stimulation in this study.

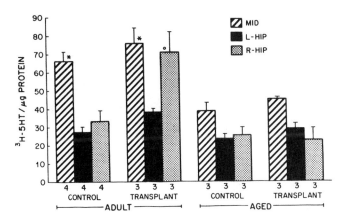

FIGURE 2. An analysis of the synaptosomal uptake of [³H]5-HT into adult and aged mice. The midbrain (MID), left hippocampus (L-HIP), and right hippocampus (R-HIP) were measured. The fetal mesencephalic cells were placed into the right hippocampus of adult and aged recipients. The adult midbrain showed greater uptake than the aged midbrain ($p < .01$). Transplanted fetal cells increased the hippocampal uptake only in the adult host ($p < .01$).

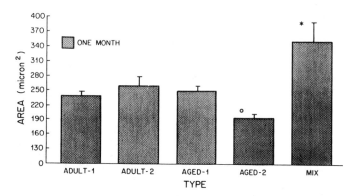

FIGURE 3. The averaged somal area of fetal 5-HT-IR cells transplanted into the hippocampus. Each of the first four bars shows an average value obtained from a different mouse; the areas of 10 cells were averaged for each bar. The size of the somal area is significantly reduced in the second aged mouse (fourth bar, $p < .05$). The last bar (MIX) indicates the average area of adult raphe cells co-transplanted with fetal hippocampus into three adult hosts. The area measurement of the soma is significantly increased over the adult groups combined ($p < .01$).

TABLE 2. Effects of Mouse Supernatant Fractions on the Biochemical Maturation of Fetal Rat Serotonergic Cells in Culture

Conditions	[³H]5-HT Uptake at Different Supernatant Dilutions				
	0	1:10	1:100	1:1000	1:10 000
Control	2930 ± 674 (3)				
Hippocampus					
Adult		5106 ± 435 C^a (4)	5718 ± 135 C^b (4)	6742 ± 1088 C^b (4)	4528 ± 632 (4)
Aged		5062 ± 562 C^a (4)	4270 ± 494 A^a (3)	4547 ± 1730 (4)	
Cerebellum					
Adult		4139 ± 871 (3)		4271 ± 125 (3)	
Aged		4271 ± 131 (3)		4392 ± 1016 (4)	

NOTE: Dissociated cultures of rat raphe of 14 days gestation were plated at 1.74×10^6 cells/cm^2 and grown for 3 days on poly-L-lysine substrate. Uptake of [³H]5-HT (5×10^{-8} M) was determined for 15 min at 37° C. The Student t test was used to determine significance. C: significance was determined with respect to the control values; A: significance was determined by comparing the adult and aged supernatant values.

$^a p < .05.$
$^b p < .01.$

In order to test whether the effect could be seen at an earlier time in culture, young and aged mouse hippocampal supernatants were tested for their effects the first day in culture. The results show that at a dilution of 1:50 the young hippocampus produced a significant increase, whereas the aged supernatant was not significantly changed from control levels (FIG. 6). These results strongly suggest that the poor growth seen after long-term fetal raphe transplants in aged brain may be a consequence of a decreased availability of a serotonergic growth factor that affects neurite outgrowth.

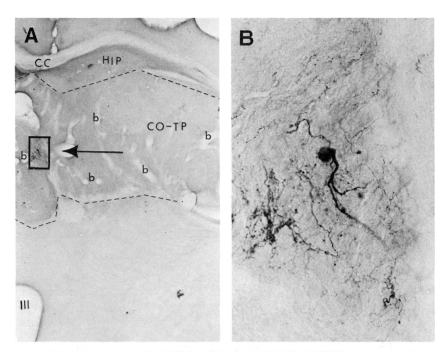

FIGURE 4. Photographs of a 5-HT-IR adult neuron. (A) The 5-HT-IR neuron was co-transplanted (CO-TP) with fetal hippocampus into the adult host hippocampus (HIP). The fetal hippocampus has expanded into the lateral ventricle. Many large blood vessels enter the graft (b). CC: corpus callosum; III: third ventricle. The area within the square marked by the arrow is shown in B. (B) High-power view of the neuron shown in A. The cell has a large soma and a single large process with many collaterals. Survival: 1 month.

DISCUSSION

Fetal Neuronal Transplants

Afferent neurons reach their target during normal development by a complicated series of steps, most of which may not be available in the adult brain. Yet, the target area itself has been shown to retain the crucial factors required for the induction of

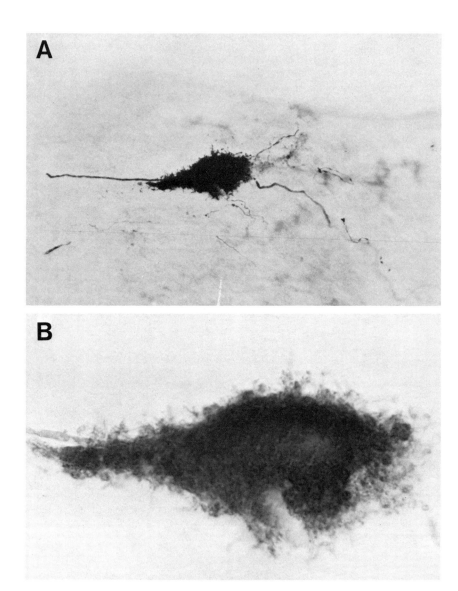

FIGURE 5. A high-power photograph of an adult dorsal raphe nuclei neuron co-transplanted with fetal hippocampus into adult brain. (**A**) The 5-HT-IR neuron has a thick single process exiting from one pole, which may be myelinated. Many processes exit from the other pole of the neuron. (**B**) Oil immersion photograph of the same cell to illustrate the many protrusions from the soma. These appear to be somatic spines. Survival: 1 month.

terminal branching of the afferent neurons.[30,31] Many studies, some of them described in this volume, have established that fetal neurons have more robust outgrowth when transplanted into their normal target area than into an area they do not innervate.

The serotonergic system has a very expansive innervation pattern in the adult brain.[12–14] These cells are located on the midline of the brainstem and densely project to hippocampus, cortex, olfactory bulb, thalamus, hypothalamus, and spinal cord. In these terminal areas, the 5-HT cells have specific cellular regions within the target area where the fiber branching is heaviest. They should not, therefore, be thought of as a "diffuse" or "nonspecific" afferent system. We and others have previously established that transplanted rodent fetal serotonergic cells can survive and innervate a variety of target areas. Mouse fetal raphe neurons can hyperinnervate the hippocampus of an adult mouse with the pattern of innervation being quite similar to that normally seen in the adult.[15] The same pattern of innervation occurs if the rat is used.[29,32]

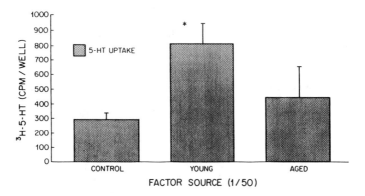

FIGURE 6. The uptake of [³H]5-HT by cultured raphe cells after 24 hr in culture is shown. Soluble factor at a dilution of 1:50 was obtained either from young (2-month-old) or aged (24-month-old) hippocampus. There was a significant stimulation after addition of factor from young but not aged tissue.

Fetal serotonergic neurons have also been transplanted into other areas. We have shown that these cells mature normally when transplanted into the lateral midbrain area.[33] These cells have also been transplanted to caudate-putamen, where they survive but show reduced outgrowth compared to those in the hippocampus.[34] Fetal serotonergic cells have also been transplanted into the spinal cord, the striatum,[35] and the fourth ventricle.[36] Finally, serotonergic fetal cells have been transplanted into the medial hypothalamic area after this region had been denervated with a prior injection of 5,7-DHT.[37] It is interesting to note that the serotonergic fetal neurons can "hyperinnervate"; that is, their innervation patterns exceed the pattern normally seen in the adult brain.

The transplanted serotonergic fetal cells in the hippocampus show morphological and physiological maturation similar to that normally seen in the adult. The cells increase in size (TABLE 1) and show a multipolar shape reminiscent of what is normally seen in the adult. Ultrastructural studies 1 month after transplantation show that the cellular organelles are as abundant in the transplanted fetal serotonergic cells as in the serotonergic cells of the adult dorsal raphe nucleus (Azmitia and Gannon, unpublished observation). The development of mature electrophysiological properties of transplanted serotonergic cells follows the same sequence as serotonergic neuronal development *in situ*.[38] This work is described elsewhere in this volume.[39] In addition, we have recorded from the transplanted cells *in situ* and noted that the cells have a rhythmic firing pattern that is sensitive to 5-methyltryptamine (Heym, Jacobs, and Azmitia, unpublished observation). Thus, it appears that most of the factors required for afferent cell maturation can be found within the normal target area of the adult hippocampus.

The function of these cells in the hippocampus has been studied behaviorally and biochemically. We have found that 5,7-DHT injections into the fornix-fimbria of rats results in a decrease in hippocampal 5-HT uptake and that this decrease is negatively correlated with nocturnal locomotor activity.[40] This same 5,7-DHT injection can induce homotypic collateral sprouting[23–26,30] and cause transplanted fetal serotonergic cells to greatly increase their innervation density in the adult brain.[29] This enhanced outgrowth produced a significant hypoactivity in nocturnal locomotor measures.[41] In addition, 5-HT turnover in transplanted adult hippocampus is accelerated compared to normal, suggesting that the synthesis and release mechanisms are functional.[42,43]

In the hypothalamus, we have shown that bilateral 5,7-DHT microinjections into the ventromedial hypothalamus of female rats results in decreased [^{3}H]5-HT uptake, decreased 5-HT and 5-HIAA levels, and fewer 5-HT-IR fibers.[44,45] The changes in the 5-HT system have been correlated with the rat's increased responsiveness to progesterone in inducing female sexual activity.[37] The bilateral transplantation of fetal serotonergic neurons into this area can restore the 5-HT innervation density, the 5-HT and 5-HIAA levels, and the normal response to progesterone.[46]

Adult Neuronal Transplantation

These studies confirm the ability of fetal serotonergic cells to survive after neuronal transplantation and to mature and function in adult brain. Adult serotonergic neurons survive for 1 week but then degenerate after transplantation into the adult hippocampus. The adult 5-HT cells produce a thick outgrowth of fibers, but these fibers do not penetrate the adult target areas. The fibers form extensive swirls near the borders with the host tissue and die within 1 month after transplantation. If fetal hippocampal tissue is mixed with the adult midbrain tissue during transplantation, however, a number of the adult 5-HT neurons do survive and mature. These cells have a very large somal area and show evidence of extensive somatic spines. It can be concluded, then, that fetal target tissue enables these adult neurons to survive and mature. Thus, if the proper conditions can be provided, adult neurons can be successfully transplanted.

The reason for this survival may be the decreased number of astroglial cells in the fetal tissue compared to the adult animals.[47] We have shown that transplantation into an adult brain results in an extensive astroglial scar.[33] This barrier, which would not form with a fetal target, may be deleterious to long-term survival.[48] It is interesting to note that we have recently observed the presence of a serotonergic inhibitory factor in primary astroglial cultures.[49]

Aged Hippocampal Host

In this report, we have confirmed our original observation that fetal serotonergic neurons transplanted to the aged hippocampus can survive and mature during the first month. It appears, however, that these cells do not maintain their viability in long-term studies. High-affinity uptake of serotonin in the aged animals returned to normal levels after 3 months, whereas 3-month survival and maturation in young adults was enhanced compared to the 1-month transplantation group. This study suggests that the target area environment in aged animals may not be as favorable as that seen in young adults. In previous work, we had observed that the endogenous serotonergic innervation of the aged hippocampus was reduced compared to young mice.[16] This observation raised the possibility that the target area may be responsible for the decreased 5-HT innervation. The hippocampus from aged rats shows a marked decline in the amount of reactive fiber sprouting after injury when compared to young adult rats.[50] This indicates that hippocampal aging affects many afferent systems. The cause for the decreased sprouting in this target area may be related to the increased density of glial cells seen in aged cortical regions.[51] Glial cells may be deleterious to new neuronal sprouts.[48]

A molecular explanation for the reduced innervation of endogenous aged and transplanted fetal serotonergic neurons is the decreased availability of growth factors. In the peripheral tissue, both nerve growth factor and EGF levels have been shown to significantly decline with age in the mouse.[52,53] In the rat hippocampus, injury-induced neuronotrophic factors concentrated by Gelfoam are not present in aged brains.[54] In order to test this hypothesis for the serotonergic system, adult and aged hippocampal supernatant fractions were compared in a tissue culture system of primary fetal serotonergic neurons. Our results indicate that aged tissue is deficient in the amount of a hippocampal supernatant fraction that is capable of stimulating serotonergic biochemical maturation in culture (TABLE 2 and FIG. 6). This fraction in adult animals is both heat and trypsin sensitive, suggesting that it is a protein molecule.[21] Furthermore, prior 5,7-DHT injections in the fornix-fimbria, which increases the homotypic collateral sprouting of endogenous serotonergic fibers, can increase the amount of this factor in the hippocampus.[22] Finally, the cerebellar supernatant fraction is without stimulatory effects in both adult and aged tissue. Current studies are directed at isolating this protein maturation factor and understanding its regulation in the brain.

REFERENCES

1. HARVEY, A. R. & R. D. LUND. 1984. Transplantation of tectal tissue in rats. IV. Maturation of transplants and development of host retinal projections. Dev. Brain Res. **12:** 27-37.
2. LUND, R. D. 1981. Cortical transplants: Model for the study of maturation of neuronal specificity. Neurosci. Res. Program, Bull. **20:** 513-520.
3. McLOON, S. C. & R. D. LUND. 1980. Specific projections of retina transplanted to rat brain. Exp. Brain Res. **40:** 273-282.
4. DAS, G. D., B. H. HALLAS & K. G. DAS. 1980. Transplantation of brain tissue in the brain of rat. I. Growth characteristics of neocortical transplants from embryos of different ages. Am. J. Anat. **158:** 135-145.
5. STENEVI, U., A. BJÖRKLUND & N. A. SVENDGAARD. 1976. Transplantation of central

and peripheral monoamine neurons in the adult rat brain: Techniques and conditions for survival. Brain Res. **114:** 1-20.

6. LAUDER, J. M. & F. E. BLOOM. 1974. Ontogeny of monoamine neurons in the locus coeruleus, raphe nuclei and substantia nigra of the rat. I. Cell differentiation. J. Comp. Neurol. **155:** 469-482.

7. LIDOV, H. G. W. & M. E. MOLLIVER. 1982. Immunocytochemical study of the development of serotonergic neurons in the rat CNS. Brain Res. Bull. **9:** 559-604.

8. OLSON, L. & A. SEIGER. 1972. Early prenatal ontogeny of central monoamine neurons in the rat: Fluorescence histochemical observations. Z. Anat. Entwicklungsgesch. **137:** 301-316.

9. WALLACE, J. A. & J. M. LAUDER. 1983. Development of the serotonergic system in the rat embryo: An immunocytochemical study. Brain Res. Bull. **10:** 459-479.

10. STEINBUSCH, H. W. M., J. DE VENTE & J. SCHIPPER. 1986. Immunohistochemistry of monoamines. *In* Neurochemistry: Modern Methods and Applications. P. Panula, H. Paivarinta & S. Soinila, Eds. Vol. **16:** 75-105. Alan R. Liss. New York, NY.

11. JACOBS, B., P. J. GANNON & E. C. AZMITIA. 1984. The serotonin nuclei of the cat brainstem: An immunocytochemical study. Brain Res. Bull. **13:** 1-31.

12. AZMITIA, E. C. & M. SEGAL. 1978. An autoradiographic analysis of the differential ascending projections of the dorsal and median raphe nuclei in the rat. J. Comp. Neurol. **179:** 641-667.

13. AZMITIA, E. C. & P. J. GANNON. 1986. The primate serotonergic system: A review of human and animal studies and a report on *Macaca musicularis.* Adv. Neurol. **43:** 407-468

14. STEINBUSCH, H. M. W. 1981. Distribution of serotonin immunoreactivity in the central nervous system of the rat: Cell bodies and terminals. Neuroscience **6:** 557-618.

15. AZMITIA, E. C., M. J. PERLOW, M. J. BRENNAN & J. M. LAUDER. 1981. Fetal raphe and hippocampal transplants in adult and aged C57BL/6N mice: An immunohistochemical study. Brain Res. Bull. **7:** 703-710.

16. AZMITIA, E. C., M. J. BRENNAN & D. QUARTERMAIN. 1983. Adult development of the hippocampal-serotonin system of C57BL/6N mice: Analysis of high-affinity uptake of [^{3}H]5-HT. Int. J. Neurochem. **5:** 39-44.

17. GAGE, F. H., S. B. DUNNETT, U. STENEVI & A. BJÖRKLUND. 1983. Aged rats: Recovery of motor impairments by intrastriatal nigral grafts. Science **221:** 966-969.

18. BJÖRKLUND, A. & F. H. GAGE. 1987. Grafts of fetal septal cholinergic neurons to the hippocampal formation in aged or fimbria-fornix-lesioned rats. Ann. N.Y. Acad. Sci. This volume.

19. COLLIER, T. J., D. M. GASH & J. R. SLADEK, JR. 1987. Norepinephrine and behavioral senescence in aged rats: Transplanted locus ceruleus neurons as an experimental replacement therapy. Ann. N.Y. Acad. Sci. This volume.

20. AZMITIA, E. C. & P. M. WHITAKER-AZMITIA. 1987. Target cell stimulation of dissociated serotonergic neurons in culture. Neuroscience **21**(1): 47-64.

21. AZMITIA, E. C. & F. C. ZHOU. 1985. A specific serotonergic growth factor from 5,7-DHT-lesioned hippocampus: *In vitro* evidence from dissociated cultures of raphe and locus coeruleus neurons. Soc. Neurosci. Abstr. **11:** 1085.

22. AZMITIA, E. C., M. I. DAVILA, P. J. LAMA, R. B. MURPHY, R. PELASEYED & P. M. WHITAKER-AZMITIA. 1986. Serotonergic growth factor from adult hippocampus supernatant stimulates the maturation of serotonergic neurons in dissociated mesencephalic cultures. Soc. Neurosci. Abstr. **12:** 159-162.

23. AZMITIA, E. C., A. M. BUCHAN & J. H. WILLIAMS. 1978. Structural and functional restoration by collateral sprouting of hippocampal 5-HT axons. Nature **274:** 374-377.

24. ZHOU, F. C. & E. C. AZMITIA. 1984. Homotypic collateral sprouting of hippocampal serotonergic fibers demonstrated by retrograde transport of horseradish peroxidase in the rat. Brain Res. **308:** 53-62.

25. ZHOU, F. C. & E. C. AZMITIA. 1985. The effects of adrenalectomy and corticosterone on homotypic collateral sprouting of serotonergic fibers in hippocampus. Neurosci. Lett. **54:** 111-116.

26. ZHOU, F. C. & E. C. AZMITIA. 1986. Induced homotypic sprouting of serotonergic fibers in hippocampus. II. An immunocytochemical study. Brain Res. **337:** 337-348.

27. AZMITIA, E. C. & P. J. GANNON. 1983. The ultrastructural localization of serotonin immunoreactivity in myelinated and unmyelinated axons within the medial forebrain bundle of rat and monkey. J. Neurosci. **3:** 2083-2090.

28. JONEC, V. & C. E. FINCH. 1975. Senescence and dopamine uptake by subcellular fractions of C57BL/6J male mouse brain. Brain Res. **91:** 197-215.

29. ZHOU, F. C., S. AUERBACH & E. C. AZMITIA. 1987. Stimulation of serotonergic neuronal maturation after fetal mesencephalic raphe transplantation into the 5,7-DHT-lesioned hippocampus of the adult rat. Ann. N.Y. Acad. Sci. This volume.

30. COTMAN, C. W. & J. V. NADLER. 1978. Reactive synaptogenesis in the hippocampus. In Neuronal Plasticity. C. W. Cotman, Ed.: 227-271. Raven Press. New York, NY.

31. HOLETS, V. T. & C. W. COTMAN. 1984. Postnatal development of the serotonin innervation of the hippocampus and dentate gyrus: Normal development and reinnervation following raphe implants. J. Comp. Neurol. **226:** 457-476.

32. AZMITIA, E. C. & P. M. WHITAKER. 1983. Formation of a glial scar following microinjection of fetal raphe neurons into the dorsal hippocampus or midbrain of the adult rat: An immunocytochemical study. Neurosci. Lett. **38:** 145-150.

33. STEINBUSCH, H. W. M., A. BEEK, A. L. FRANKHUYZEN, J. A. D. M. TONNAER, F. H. GAGE & A. BJÖRKLUND. 1987. Functional activity of raphe neurons transplanted to the hippocampus and caudate-putamen: An immunohistochemical analysis in adult and aged rats. Ann. N. Y. Acad. Sci. This volume.

34. FOSTER, G. A., M. SCHULTZBERG, A. BJÖRKLUND, F. H. GAGE & T. HÖKFELT. 1985. Fate of embryonic mesencephalic and medullary raphe neurons transplanted to the striatum, hippocampus or spinal cord of the adult rat: Analysis of 5-hydroxytryptamine, substance P and thyrotropin-releasing hormone immunoreactive cells. In Neural Grafting in the Mammalian CNS. A. Björklund & U. Stenevi, Eds.: 179-189. Elsevier. Amsterdam.

35. MCRAE-DEGUEURCE, A., M. DIDIER & J. F. PUJOL. 1981. The viability of transplants of mesencephalic raphe nuclei in the IV ventricle of the adult rat. Neurosci. Lett. **24:** 251-254.

36. LUINE, V. N., M. FRANKFURT, T. C. RAINBOW, A. BIEGON & E. C. AZMITIA. 1983. Intrahypothalamic 5,7-dihydroxytryptamine facilitates feminine sexual behavior and decreases [^{3}H]imipramine binding and 5-HT uptake. Brain Res. **264:** 344-348.

37. SEGAL, M. & E. C. AZMITIA. 1986. Fetal raphe neurons grafted into the hippocampus develop normal adult physiological properties. Brain. Res. **364:** 162-166.

38. SEGAL, M. 1987. Interactions between grafted serotonin neurons and adult host rat hippocampus. Ann. N.Y. Acad. Sci. This volume.

39. WILLIAMS, J. H. & E. C. AZMITIA. 1981. Hippocampal serotonin reuptake and nocturnal locomotor activity after microinjections of 5,7-DHT in the fornix-fimbria. Brain Res. **207:** 95-107.

40. AZMITIA, E. C. & F. C. ZHOU. 1986. Chemically induced homotypic collateral sprouting of hippocampal serotonergic afferents. In Processes of Recovery from Neural Trauma. G. M. Gilad, A. Gorio & G. W. Kreutzberg, Eds.: 129-141. Springer-Verlag. Berlin.

41. AZMITIA, E. C. 1987. In preparation.

42. AUERBACH, S., F. C. ZHOU, B. L. JACOBS & E. C. AZMITIA. 1985. Serotonin turnover in raphe neurons transplanted into rat hippocampus. Neurosci. Lett. **61:** 147-152.

43. AUERBACH, S., F. C. ZHOU, B. L. JACOBS & E. C. AZMITIA. 1987. Serotonin metabolism in raphe neurons transplanted into rat hippocampus. Ann. N.Y. Acad. Sci. This volume.

44. FRANKFURT, M. & E. C. AZMITIA. 1984. Regeneration of hypothalamic serotonergic fibers after unilateral intracerebral microinjections of 5,7-dihydroxytryptamine. Brain Res. **298:** 273-282.

45. FRANKFURT, M., K. J. RENNER, E. C. AZMITIA & V. LUINE. 1985. Intrahypothalamic 5,7-dihydroxytryptamine: Temporal analysis of effects of 5-HT content in brain nuclei and on facilitated lordosis behavior. Brain Res. **340:** 127-133.

46. LUINE, V., K. J. RENNER, M. FRANKFURT & E. C. AZMITIA. 1984. Raphe transplants into the hypothalamus of 5,7-DHT-treated female rats alters hormonal dependent sexual behavior. Science **226:** 1436-1439.

47. PRIVAT, A. 1975. Postnatal gliogenesis in the mammalian brain. Int. Rev. Cytol. **40:** 281-324.

48. WHITAKER-AZMITIA, P. M., A. RAMIREZ, L. NOREIKA, P. J. GANNON & E. C. AZMITIA. 1987. Onset and duration of astrocytic response to cells transplanted into the adult mammalian brain. Ann. N.Y. Acad. Sci. This volume.
49. WHITAKER-AZMITIA, P. M. & E. C. AZMITIA. 1987. In preparation.
50. SCHEFF, S. W., L. S. BERNARDO & C. W. COTMAN. 1980. Decline in reactive fiber growth in the dentate gyrus of aged rats compared to young adult rats following entorhinal cortex removal. Brain Res. 199: 21-38.
51. BRIZZEE, K. R. 1973. Quantitative histological studies of aging changes in cerebral cortex of rhesus monkey and albino rat with notes on effects of prolonged low-dose ionizing irradiation in the rat. Prog. Brain Res. 40: 141-160.
52. GRESIK, E. W. & E. C. AZMITIA. 1980. Age-related changes in NGF, EGF and protease in the granular convoluted tubules of the mouse submandibular gland: A morphological and immunocytochemical study. J. Gerontol. 35: 520-524.
53. GRESIK, E. W., M. J. BRENNAN & E. C. AZMITIA. 1982. Age-related changes in EGF content and protease activity in submandibular glands of male C57BL/6J. Exp. Aging Res. 8: 87-90.
54. NEEDELS, D. L., M. NIETO-SAMPEDRO, S. R. WHITTEMORE & C. W. COTMAN. 1985. Neuronotrophic activity for ciliary ganglion neurons: Induction following injury to the brain of neonatal, adult, and aged rats. Dev. Brain Res. 18: 275-284.

DISCUSSION OF THE PAPER

M. NIETO-SAMPEDRO (*University of California, Irvine, CA*): I would like to confirm that aged tissue contains neurotrophic activities as high as those in adult and young adult tissues and contains basal levels comparable to that of adult tissue of neurite promoting activity. However, after injury or after specific deafferentation of the hippocampus by entorhinal lesion, this basal activity does not change; that is, it does not increase, contrary to what happens in adult. So we believe that these two, the basal sprouting activity and the deafferentation-induced sprouting activity, are different. We have evidence for that. The deafferentation-induced activity does not change. It is not induced in the aged animal, but it is in the adult.

D. M. GASH (*University of Rochester, Rochester, NY*): That was a very nice demonstration of the survival of the mature neurons. As you know, this has been a major problem to get the mature neurons to survive in transplantation, and I was surprised to see that. Would you tell us a little bit more about your techniques. Was it simply dissecting out adult neurons and grafting them into a fetal host?

AZMITIA: We normally have two types of transplantation procedure. One is either mechanically dissociating the cells or injecting the cells as a slurry. The slurry technique was the one that we used here. What we do is dissect out the region from either the adult or the fetal tissue, do a small number of minces in a microliter of MEM, and then suck this up into a glass micropipette. It is injected as a slurry, so it is not exposed to the rigor of mechanical disassociation, but we do take pains to make sure that the tissues are at least in contact with each other. It was injected as a mixture.

C. SOTELO (*INSERM U106, CMC Foch, Suresnes*): My question was on the same problem. It is difficult for me to believe that all neurons can behave as the serotonergic neurons, but you have neurons that have very specific and very large dendritic fields like a Purkinje cell. When you try to dissociate from a postnatal day 12 cerebellum, you kill the cell immediately. So that is why I was interested in knowing what has happened with these adult neurons. Do they have the dendritic trees oriented in a single plane so that you can keep it when you try to dissociate the cell? Or can you just cut down the dendrites, and have the dendritic branches survive because they are with this fetal hippocampus?

AZMITIA: We are injecting adult dorsal raphe, so we have maybe between 500 and 1000 cells that we introduced and we see maybe 1 or 2 cells that survive this procedure. It is not the particular orientation of the cell because I think the important thing is the theoretical statement that adult neurons can, under certain very favorable conditions, survive transplantation. Furthermore, the way you feel about my serotonin cells is the same way I feel about your Purkinje cells!

I think it is probably going to be much more profitable if we start trying to see what things they do in common—to try and synthesize some of this material, especially with the large number of different cell types that can be transplanted.

SOTELO: So you are looking for general theories in biology, I understand.

AZMITIA: I knew you would.

Denervation-induced Enhancement of Graft Survival and Growth

A Trophic Hypothesis

FRED H. GAGE

University of California, San Diego
La Jolla, California

ANDERS BJÖRKLUND

University of Lund
Lund, Sweden

INTRODUCTION

Peripheral ganglionic aminergic neurons and spinal cord motoneurons depend on the presence of peripheral target tissue for differentiation and maturation.[1-5] The mechanisms regulating this response are not known. One proposal, however, is that the target tissue releases diffusible trophic factors that influence developing neurons. For both ganglionic autonomic neurons and spinal motoneurons, it has been proposed that the survival, differentiation, and axonal outgrowth of axons during development are dependent upon the retrograde transport of trophic factors produced by the target tissue.[4-9] In the adult rat, if some of the axons supplying a peripheral target tissue are experimentally interrupted, nerve processes from the remaining nerves "sprout" and reinnervate the denervated target.[10] In this situation as well, it has been postulated that the denervated target tissue releases a diffusible sprouting stimulus.[10-15]

Trophic factors that regulate neuronal survival and differentiation are also probably controlling brain development and regeneration. The existence of neurotrophic factors in the central nervous system (CNS) has been postulated, but, until recently, such factors had only been identified in peripheral tissues.[16-18] More recently, however, factors with neurotrophic properties have been identified in CNS extracts and wound fluids.[19-25] In fact, nerve growth factor (NGF) has been identified in the CNS.[26] It has been postulated that, after damage to the brain, some or all of the neurotrophic factors are available to induce a sprouting response. Several recent experiments support the possibility that diffusible trophic factors are released from the damaged brain and that they assist the survival of embryonic neurons grafted to the brain.[20,23-25]

In this paper we will review several experiments using the same model system; these experiments strongly suggest that the denervated hippocampal formation (HF) releases several trophic factors, one of which is sufficiently similar to NGF to mimic its effects on peripheral superior cervical sympathetic neurons and central cholinergic neurons implanted in the brain.

Deafferentation Procedures

Two principal surgical procedures have been employed to deafferent the HF in the grafting experiments: 1) fimbria-fornix lesion and 2) perforant path lesion.

The fimbria-fornix lesion is made by aspirating the fimbria, the dorsal fornix, the ventral hippocampal commissure, the corpus callosum, and the overlying cingulate cortex. This lesion eliminates most of the afferent brain stem projections from the locus ceruleus and dorsal and medial raphe, as well as the cholinergic forebrain projections from the medial septal area and the diagonal band of Broca. In addition, the major afferent commissural connections, from the contralateral HF, running in the ventral hippocampal commissure, are removed. This aspiration cavity extends through the septal pole of the HF exposing the vessel-rich surface overlying the anterior thalamus, which acts as a receptacle for solid grafts that are placed in the cavity abutting the damaged rostral surface of the HF.

The perforant path lesion is also an aspirative lesion, made at the level of the caudal portion of the dorsal hippocampus. The lesion extends through the occipital cortex and splenium of the corpus callosum, taking the subiculum and presubiculum, thus transecting the perforant path fibers that innervate the dorsal segments of the HF. This lesion thus eliminates a major excitatory input to the dentate gyrus through the angular bundle from the entorhinal cortex. By this procedure, 2-3 mm of vascular bed from the choroidal fissure overlying the superior and inferior colliculi is exposed. The pial vascular bed, adjacent to the HF, can also be used as a receptacle for solid grafts.

Transplantation Techniques

Two principal techniques have been used to graft fetal CNS tissue to the denervated adult HF. The first one involves the transplantation of large solid pieces of tissue to a surgically prepared transplantation cavity.[27] In this procedure good graft survival is ensured by preparing the cavity in such a way that the graft can be placed on a richly vascularized surface (for example, the pia in the choroidal fissure) that can serve as a "culturing bed" for the graft. Both the fimbria-fornix lesion and the perforant path lesion described above provide such culturing beds. These cavities are in direct communication with the lateral ventricle, which may allow for the cerebrospinal fluid (CSF) to circulate through the graft cavity and thus possibly help the graft to survive, particularly during the early postoperative period.

The second technique used in grafting CNS fetal tissue to the denervated HF involves the implantation of dissociated cell suspensions. In this technique, pieces of fetal CNS tissue are trypsinized and mechanically dissociated into a milky cell suspension. Small volumes of the suspension can then be stereotaxically injected into the desired site of the HF, using a microsyringe. The main advantage of this technique is that it allows precise and multiple placements of the cells. The technique also makes possible accurate monitoring of the number of cells injected by determining the density of cells in the suspension.

GRAFTS OF ADULT SUPERIOR CERVICAL SYMPATHETIC GANGLIA

In this experiment adult superior cervical ganglia were grafted into either the fimbria-fornix cavity[28] or into the retrosplenial cavity.[29] Although the ganglia survive well in both sites, the fiber outgrowth from the grafted sympathetic neurons was markedly different. The grafts in the fimbrial cavity extended many fibers that grew preferentially into the deafferented hippocampus, and the extension of the new adrenergic terminal network was correlated to the extent of septal deafferentation caused by the fimbrial lesion.[28] By contrast, the grafts placed in the retrosplenial cavity grew fibers only along the vessels in the cavity and the adjoining choroidal fissure, and on the surface of the adjacent part of the hippocampus and dentate gyrus. If grafting to the retrosplenial cavity was combined with a lesion of the fimbria-fornix, or with an electrolytic lesion of the medial septal area, however, the growth pattern changed dramatically. Now the entire hippocampal formation was invaded by adrenergic fibers from the graft within 1 month.[29] This effect was also seen when the fimbrial lesion was made 2 months after the ganglion had been grafted to the retrosplenial cavity, and when the fimbrial lesion preceded graft placement by 2 months.

The increased fiber outgrowth induced by fimbrial or septal lesions was also monitored biochemically, using measurements of high-affinity [^{3}H]noradrenaline uptake. Fimbrial or septal lesion caused an approximate 100-fold increase in [^{3}H]noradrenaline uptake in the hippocampal formation by 1 month, as compared to grafted rats with intact septohippocampal connections.

The growth-stimulating effect of fimbrial or septal lesions was accompanied by a trophic-like response of the grafted ganglionic neuronal cell bodies. This included a marked increase in the size of the neuronal perikarya and a marked overall increase in cell body noradrenaline content of the grafted neurons.

These various effects were specific for lesions severing the septohippocampal connections (that is, septal or fimbrial lesions), and did not occur either after lesions of the commissural input or of the perforant path input.

These effects of hippocampal deafferentation on the grafted mature sympathetic neurons, that is, increased axonal sprouting, hypertrophy, and increased noradrenaline content of the ganglionic perikarya, are similar to the NGF-induced trophic response seen in adult sympathetic neurons *in situ*.[30,31] This response is thus compatible with the idea that the adult rat hippocampus is capable of producing adrenergic neurotrophic factor(s), whose action on sympathetic neurons is similar to NGF, and that this factor is under specific control of the septal afferents to the hippocampal formation running in the fimbria-fornix.

GRAFTS OF NEONATAL SUPERIOR CERVICAL SYMPATHETIC GANGLIA TO THE HIPPOCAMPUS

In this experiment, an aspirative lesion was made unilaterally in the retrosplenial cortex in 19 adult female Sprague-Dawley rats, as described previously (FIG. 1).[32] This lesion exposes the hippocampus posterodorsally, and transects at the same time the dorsal subiculum and the perforant path axons innervating the dorsal hippocampus and dentate gyrus. In the same operation, the superior cervical ganglia (SCG) were

excised from 1-day-old rat pups and implanted (two in each cavity) in direct contact
with the exposed hippocampal surface. The cavity was filled with Gelfoam, and the
wound was closed. In 10 of the 19 implanted animals, a second aspirative lesion was
made, in the same surgical session, through the ipsilateral fimbria-fornix bundle (FIG.
1). Seven weeks after surgery, the rats were perfused and processed for catecholamine
fluorescence histochemistry. Sections were cut coronally through the implant, and the
adjacent HF and surviving ganglionic cell bodies were counted in every third section
under a fluorescence microscope.

The implanted neurons survived very poorly in the rats with intact fimbria-fornix.
By contrast, all implants in the fimbria-fornix lesion group possessed large numbers
of surviving SCG neurons. These neurons occurred singly or in clusters on the surface
of the host hippocampus or dentate gyrus. They were seen to extend processes into
the host HF where they ramified extensively, above all in the hilar zone of the dentate
gyrus (FIG. 2B).

In a second experiment, we sought to quantify biochemically the total noradrenaline
content in the transplant, including its axonal processes in the target tissue. Twelve

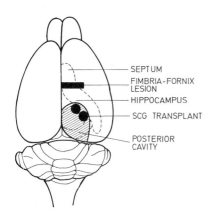

FIGURE 1. Schematic representation of the retrosplenial cortex cavity, the placement of the neonatal SCG within the cavity, and the location of
the aspirative lesion through the ipsilateral fimbria-fornix.

SEPTUM
FIMBRIA-FORNIX
LESION
HIPPOCAMPUS
SCG TRANSPLANT
POSTERIOR
CAVITY

animals were initially treated with 6-hydroxydopamine (6-OHDA) and subjected to
bilateral sympathectomy to eliminate endogenous noradrenaline, and subsequently
received neonatal ganglia transplants to the retrosplenial cavity with or without simultaneous fimbria-fornix lesion as above. The results are presented in FIGURE 3.

In the graft plus hippocampus target combined group, no transplant-derived noradrenaline was detected in rats without fimbria-fornix lesions. By contrast, transplant-
derived noradrenaline was about 30 times greater when the neonatal SCG transplants
were grafted in the presence of the fimbria-fornix lesion. In fact, the content of
transplant-derived noradrenaline in the transplant and target tissue in the presence
of target denervation was equal to the normal endogenous noradrenaline content of
the target tissue, although in the absence of target denervation there appeared to be
no significant transplant-derived noradrenaline in the transplant or the target tissue.

Fimbria-fornix transection, or lesion of the septal-diagonal band area, has previously been shown to stimulate the growth of adrenergic ganglionic fibers into the
denervated hippocampus[33–35] as well as the regeneration of the intrinsic adrenergic
locus ceruleus axons after chemically induced axotomy.[33] Both these effects have been

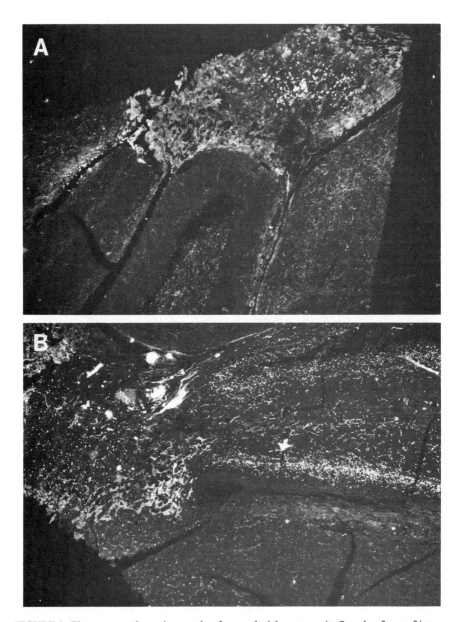

FIGURE 2. Fluorescence photomicrographs of retrosplenial cortex cavity 7 weeks after grafting of a neonatal SCG transplant. (**A**) The cavity in the absence of an ipsilateral fimbria-fornix lesion. (**B**) The cavity in the presence of an ipsilateral fimbria-fornix lesion. Original magnification for **A** and **B**: ×20; reduced to 77% of original size.

proposed to be due to the release of a neurotrophic factor (or factors) whose production normally is under the control of the cholinergic septal afferents.[33-35] In the present study, the survival of the implanted neonatal SCG neurons depended on the integrity of the fimbria-fornix bundle, which suggests that the hippocampal target factor (or factors) released by deafferentation can provide an NGF-like support for ganglionic neuronal survival. This effect seems to be specific for afferents running through the fimbria-fornix (presumably the septal cholinergic projection) since the aspirative lesion of the retrosplenial cortex, which denervates the dorsal HF of its massive perforant path input, did not have the same effect.

The survival factor or factors monitored in the present experiments may be particularly relevant with respect to the maintenance of the septal and basal forebrain cholinergic projection system and the locus ceruleus adrenergic projection system, both of which have been shown to be involved in the neurodegenerative processes associated with normal or pathological aging.[36,37]

With this in mind we conducted the following experiments.

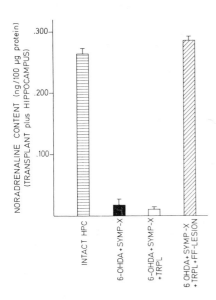

FIGURE 3. Twelve rats were depleted of all CNS noradrenaline by 6-OHDA (250 μg in 20 μl) injected into the right lateral ventricle 1 month before transplantation, and bilateral sympathectomy 5 weeks before transplantation. All 12 rats received implants of two neonatal ganglia in the retrosplenial cavity as in the previous experiment. Six of these rats received simultaneous unilateral fimbria-fornix lesions ipsilateral to the transplant. An additional group of normal, unoperated rats was taken for controls. HPC: hippocampus; SYMP-X: sympathectomy; TRPL: neonatal sympathetic ganglia transplant; FF: fimbria-fornix.

GRAFTS OF FETAL RAT BASAL FOREBRAIN TISSUE RICH IN CHOLINERGIC NEURONS

In these experiments, cell suspensions were prepared from the developing basal forebrain of donor fetuses, containing the precursor cells of the entire septal-diagonal band complex. The grafted animals received 2 μl of the cell suspensions in three separate hippocampal locations. In the same surgery session, half of the animals were subjected to a complete aspirative lesion of the fimbria-fornix and supracallosal striae.[38]

Four to 6 months after surgery, subgroups of the fimbria-fornix-lesioned and nonlesioned rats were taken for acetylcholinesterase (AChE) histochemistry. The animals were treated with diisopropylfluorophosphate (DFP) to aid in the visualization of the AChE-positive cells in the absence of neuropil staining. Cell size, cell number, and total graft volume were evaluated.

We found grafts in the hippocampus of all 14 animals that received fimbria-fornix lesions, but no grafts were found in two of the hippocampi from animals that did not receive fimbria-fornix lesions. The groups are exemplified in two grafts presented in FIGURE 4. The average graft volume measured in the animals with fimbria-fornix lesions was 1.98 mm^3. Since the average volume injected into each hippocampus was approximately 1.1 mm^3, it can be calculated that grafts in the lesioned animals were almost twice as large as the injected volume, whereas the graft size in the nonlesioned animals was reduced compared to the injected volume (FIG. 5).

The average number of AChE-positive cells counted in each of the grafts of rats that received fimbria-fornix lesions was 1457, whereas the average number in the nongrafted animals was 698. Since it was estimated that an average of about 2500 potential AChE-positive cells was injected in each hippocampus, it can be calculated that about 60% of the potential AChE-positive cells were expressed in the fimbria-fornix lesioned group, whereas only about 30% were expressed in the nonlesioned group (FIG. 5).

The average diameter along the major axis of the AChE-positive cells in the grafts in the fimbria-fornix-lesioned group was 21.7 μm, which was significantly greater than the average cell size of the nonlesioned group, that is, 17.7 μm. The diameter of 21.7 μm was close to the average diameter of AChE-positive cells in the normal adult septal-diagonal band-substantia inominata complex, which was 22.7 μm.

When the distribution of the sizes of the AChE-positive cells for the lesioned and nonlesioned groups is plotted, it can be seen that although both groups have cells throughout the range of cell sizes, the nonlesioned group has a greater number of cells in the lower end of the distribution (< 18 μm) and the lesioned group has a greater number of large cells (> 21 μm).

In order to measure the choline acetyltransferase (ChAT) activity expressed by the graft in the animals that did not receive a simultaneous fimbria-fornix lesion, an acute fimbria-fornix lesion was made 7 days before decapitation (that is, 4-6 months after grafting) to remove the endogenous ChAT activity derived from the intact septal-diagonal band projection.[38] For appropriate comparisons of the extent of ChAT expression in the graft groups, fimbria-fornix lesions were also made in nongrafted animals either at 4-6 months after grafting or at 7 days before decapitation and subsequent ChAT analysis, to match the two graft groups. ChAT activity was measured in the whole HF including the graft tissue itself. The ChAT activity for the "graft-plus-simultaneous-lesion" group was 78% of the control side, whereas the grafted group that received fimbria-fornix lesions only 7 days before decapitation had ChAT levels of only 28% of their control side. This difference was statistically different. The respective control fimbria-fornix-lesioned and nongrafted groups showed even lower ChAT activity relative to their control sides. Using these figures, the ChAT activity in the animals with long-term fimbria-fornix lesions was estimated to be threefold higher than in the animals with acute lesions.

In the control lesion experiment, there was a significant increase in ChAT activity (expressed as a percentage of that in control hippocampus) in both the rats with lesions of the retrosplenial cortex (54%) and those without lesion at the time of grafting (52%) relative to the nongrafted animals (11%). The two grafted groups, however, did not differ in their ChAT increase following grafting (that is, the graft-derived ChAT activity), in contrast to the effect seen after fimbria-fornix lesion, as described above.[38]

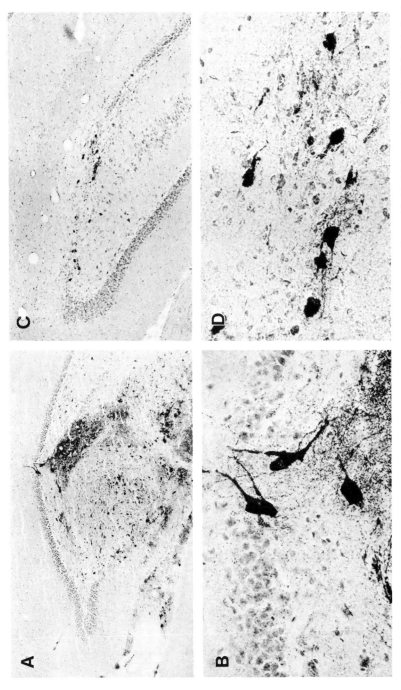

FIGURE 4. Photomicrographs prepared from AChE-stained sections of grafts in hippocampus of rats with (**A** & **B**) or without (**C** & **D**) fimbria-fornix transection. The animals were pretreated with the irreversible AChE-inhibitor DFP 4 hr before being sacrificed; this pretreatment enhances the cell body staining and eliminates virtually all staining in fibers and terminals.

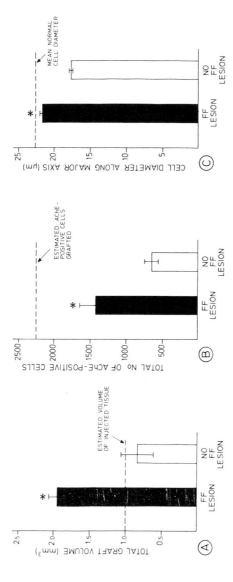

FIGURE 5. (**A**) Total graft volume from animals with or without fimbria-fornix (FF) lesion, expressed in mm³, relative to the estimated volume of tissue injected. (**B**) Total number of AChE-positive cells in transplants of DFP-treated rats with or without FF lesion, expressed relative to the estimated total number of potential AChE-positive cells grafted. (**C**) Cell diameter of AChE-positive cells along major axis in suspension grafts from DFP-treated animals with or without FF lesions, expressed in μm relative to the mean size of AChE-positive neurons in the normal septal-diagonal band complex *in situ* (*cf.* FIG. 2B). The mean ± SEM is shown for each group; each group included six to eight rats. Two independent observers measured the cell sizes of a total of 60 cells for each group; the cells were seen on randomly selected sections, which were taken from four rats in each group. Asterisks indicate significant differences between FF-lesioned and non-FF-lesioned animals (see text).

NEUROTROPHIC FACTORS IN NORMAL AND INJURED CNS TISSUE

These results support the hypothesis that denervation of the HF of its fimbria-fornix inputs results in the *in vivo* release of a neurotrophic factor (or factors) responsible for the survival-enhancing effects.

We set out to determine specifically whether the adult septal cholinergic neurons were responsive to NGF and, more directly, whether their survival could be influenced by the exogenous administration of NGF. First, we demonstrated that AChE-positive as well as noncholinergic neurons died and disappeared in the septal-diagonal band region following fimbria-fornix transection.[39] This loss amounted to 70% of the AChE-positive neurons in the medial septum and 50% of the AChE-positive neurons in the vertical limb of the diagonal band.

Next, we developed a chronic perfusion cannula system with which to deliver NGF (24 μg/ml; 10 000 trophic units/ml) to the lateral ventricle adjacent to the septal area.[40] NGF was dissolved in artificial CSF containing autologous rat serum and administered at a flow rate of 0.5 μl/hour. After a "priming" perfusion of 3 days, the fimbria-fornix was aspirated and the animal was allowed to survive with continuous perfusion of NGF through the intraventricular cannula device for an additional 2 weeks. The animals were then prepared for the visualization of cholinergic cell bodies; the number of surviving neurons in the NGF-treated animals, as determined by morphometry of both cresyl violet and AChE-positive neurons, was compared to the untreated controls. The NGF treatment prevented death of about 70% of the cholinergic neurons in the medial septum (MS) and 100% of those in the vertical limb of the diagonal band of Broca (VDB) that would have otherwise died (FIG. 6).

These results clearly demonstrate that NGF can have a protective effect on damaged cholinergic neurons that would otherwise die. At present, it is difficult to make a definitive statement concerning the specificity of the survival-promoting effect of NGF, that is, whether NGF promotes the survival of noncholinergic neurons. Cell counts indicate that the cholinergic neurons on the septal-diagonal band constitute only about 8% of the total neuronal population. Estimates based on these measurements suggest that NGF may be acting as a general neuronal survival-promoting factor on the hippocampus-projecting septal neurons.

Several neurotrophic factors have been detected in the intact CNS, including NGF[26] and the so-called brain-derived growth factor.[19] In the hippocampus, specifically, two types of factors have been postulated, one that is active on sympathetic ganglia and is blocked by anti-NGF serum, and one that is active on parasympathetic ganglia and unresponsive to anti-NGF serum.[21] Several investigators have detected trophic activity either in the denervated target or in the wound fluid[23-25] following brain damage.

Specifically, ciliary neurotrophic (CNTF) activity accumulates in Gelfoam sponges placed in entorhinal-occipital cortex lesions of the neonatal and adult rats having fimbria-fornix lesions.[25,41,42] This CNTF accumulation in the sponge is preceded by a similar CNTF accumulation in the tissue surrounding the lesion cavity, and extractable CNTF activity declines steeply and progressively farther away from the lesion. CNTF also accumulated in sponges placed in lesion cavities generated in many other brain areas. Trophic activities supporting neurons from embryonic chick spinal cord and fetal rat septal, striatal, and hippocampal tissues are also present in such gelatin sponges,[42,43] but their relationship to blood-borne peroxidases has not yet been examined. Similarly, CNS neurotrophic activity released into the CSF of human head-trauma patients, but not into the fluid of uninjured patients,[44] may also be derived from blood.

FIGURE 6. Promotion of cholinergic neuronal survival by intraventricular perfusion of NGF. The number of AChE-positive neurons present in the basal forebrain 2 weeks after the fimbria-fornix lesion is shown as a percentage of those on the contralateral unlesioned side for untreated control and for NGF-treated animals. NGF promoted survival of nearly 100% of the cholinergic neurons in both the MS and VDB.

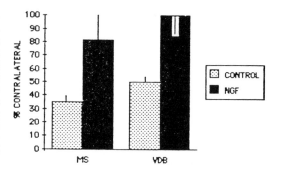

To determine whether CNTF and NGF biological activities are increased in the HF after injury, we (with M. Manthorpe, L. R. Williams, and S. Varon) selectively denervated the fimbria-fornix and measured the biological activity of the extracted denervated hippocampus for the presence of NGF and CNTF (FIG. 7).

These results suggest that both NGF and CNTF activities are elevated in the hippocampus after denervation. Our data have been confirmed for NGF activity by other investigators using different bioassay systems.[45] A cautionary note about the interpretation of the results is that, at present, it is not known whether the increase in trophic activity in the denervated tissue is a result of a target-derived factor that is increasing its product or whether the factors are increasing their availability by increasing release. In addition, depending on the dissection procedure, it is possible that some of the "wound fluid" could be included on the edges of the dissected tissue thus leading to the mistaken conclusion that the increase in factor is derived from the denervated target. In any event, this is an important approach, and it deserves additional careful attention to determine the mechanisms underlying the increased plasticity of the hippocampus after denervation.

CNTF activity may increase in injured brain tissue as a consequence of the reactive gliosis induced by chemical as well as mechanical insults.[23] Heacock et al.[46] reported that adult rat hippocampus CNTF activity increases two- to threefold within 14 days after deafferentation. Speculating that the CNTF increase may reflect the increased number of cells associated with the astroglial response, the investigators injected methotrexate (a drug that reduces proliferative gliosis) intraventricularly at the time of entorhinal lesioning. Five weeks after lesioning, the hippocampal extracts from methotrexate-treated animals had about one-half the CNTF activity of those from untreated animals. These observations are in line with in vitro studies[47,48] showing that CNTF, as well as NGF and CNS neurotrophic agents, is produced and released by cultures of purified rat brain astroglial cells.

In support of these findings, we have recently observed that there is a selective increased astroglial response in the HF following fimbria-fornix lesion (FIG. 8). This was assessed by staining with an antibody to glial fibrillary acidic protein (GFAP) at various times following the lesion.

These observations further support the possible involvement of astroglia, not only in response to a wound, but also in the subsequent trophic consequences in the denervated hippocampus.

CONCLUSION

We propose that the selective denervation of the HF leads to an increase in production and/or release of neurotrophic factors, one of which is similar in its effects to NGF. It seems clear, however, that other factors are released, and that these other factors can affect a variety of central as well as peripheral neurons. Whether selective denervation of any of the afferent systems of the hippocampus will result in a selective increase of one neurotrophic factor remains to be determined.

As a prototype of neurotrophic factors that may be responsible for some of the plasticity observed in the CNS, NGF is the best studied and characterized molecule. Thus in this summary of what is known of endogenous factors and CNS plasticity in the HF, we have focused on NGF.

The intact HF has the highest levels of NGF in the brain.[49] Radioactively labeled NGF is retrogradely transported selectively to cells in the medial septal area, some of which are cholinergic.[50] This retrograde transport is considered important for the maintenance of the cholinergic cells in the CNS. Transection of the septohippocampal fibers leads to a dramatic and rapid death of both cholinergic and noncholinergic cells in the septal area and diagonal band region.[39] These cholinergic and noncholinergic neurons are prevented from dying if they are chronically perfused with exogenous NGF.[40,51] In the hippocampus, there is a build-up of measurable biological activity for both NGF and CNTF. This build-up of neurotrophic activity coincides with the support of superior sympathetic cervical ganglia (which are dependent on NGF for their survival and growth) transplanted to the denervated hippocampus.[32] In the absence of denervation, the ganglia will not grow or survive. In addition, fetal basal forebrain neurons grafted to the hippocampus will exhibit markedly better survival and fiber outgrowth into the HF following a fimbria-fornix lesion, but not following an entorhinal lesion, thus emphasizing the selectivity of the response.[38] Finally, paralleling this increase in neurotrophic factor build-up in the hippocampus, there is an increase in glial response in regions of the hippocampus[52] in the fimbria-fornix-lesioned rats.

From this outline of data, we propose the following scenario to explain at least some of the neuroplastic responses that occur in the hippocampus.

Glial cells are the source cells of the neurotrophic factors. The cholinergic inner-

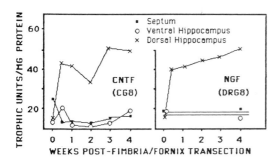

FIGURE 7. CNTF and NGF activity in deafferented septohippocampal extracts. Tissue was collected at various times after fimbria-fornix aspiration and a 10% extract prepared. The extracts were then assayed for their content of trophic activity. A two- to threefold increase in both CNTF and NGF specific activities was observed within 1 week after axotomy. (Data provided by M. Manthorpe, L. R. Williams, and S. Varon.)

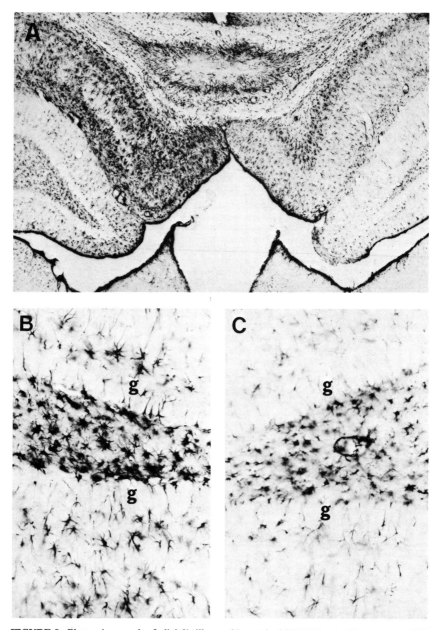

FIGURE 8. Photomicrograph of glial fibrillary acid protein (GFAP) in the hippocampus. (**A**) Left side: region ipsilateral to a fimbria-fornix lesion made 8 days earlier. Right side: region contralateral to the fimbria-fornix lesion (intact side). (**B**) Dentate hilus of hippocampal formation 8 days after an ipsilateral fimbria-fornix lesion was made. (**C**) Dentate hilus of hippocampus formation 8 days after a contralateral fimbria-fornix lesion was made. g: granule cells.

vation of the hippocampus regulates the production and release of neurotrophic factors into the HF by retrogradely transporting NGF to the cholinergic cells in the septum. These projecting cholinergic neurons use this factor for self-maintenance. If the retrograde transport system is blocked or disrupted, the lack of an NGF supply to the septal cells will result in the death of the affected neurons. Meanwhile, the glial cells respond to the deafferentation by increasing their production and release of NGF within the hippocampus, but since there is no route for transport of NGF from the hippocampus, there is an accumulation of NGF in the denervated target zone. This accumulation of NGF in the hippocampus can be detected as an increased support of the survival and fiber outgrowth of NGF-sensitive peripheral and central neurons, grafted to the denervated HF. This accumulation of trophic factor or factors in the hippocampus could also account for the so-called compensatory collateral sprouting responses seen in several monoaminergic afferent systems in the partially denervated hippocampus that occur following fimbria-fornix transection.

Fimbrial or septal lesions have been shown to induce or enhance sprouting in three different situations: 1) from perivascular sympathetic axons growing into the dentate gyrus and the CA3 area in the septal deafferented hippocampus[53,54]; 2) from the noradrenergic locus ceruleus axons after selective axotomy induced by the neurotoxic agent 5,7-dihydroxytryptamine[28]; and 3) from spared noradrenergic and cholinergic axons undergoing so-called compensatory collateral sprouting in response to the partial deafferentation induced by the fimbria-fornix lesion.[55] These growth-stimulating effects on central and peripheral adrenergic and cholinergic neurons, induced by lesioning of the septal input, resemble the effects on grafted neonatal or adult sympathetic ganglionic neurons or fetal septal neurons, summarized above, and would be most readily explained through the action of diffusible neurotrophic factors, the elaboration of which is increased as a result of the denervating lesion. The stimulatory effect on peripheral sympathetic neurons is likely to be due to the action of hippocampal NGF, or a closely related compound.

In FIGURE 9, we have depicted three alternative possible mechanisms for the afferent control of the production or availability of neurotrophic factors (NTFs) from astrocytic glial cells. In alternative A, the afferent axons (in this case the septal input) exert a direct inhibitory control over the production of an NFT (for example, NGF). Removal of this inhibition will lead to increased NTF production. In alternative B, the production of NTF is controlled by the innervated target neurons, rather than by the afferent axons directly. This implies that deafferented target neurons can induce or stimulate the production or release of a specific NTF from the adjacent glial elements. In alternative C, the NTF is normally removed by retrograde transport in the afferent neurons. Such a transport system would normally keep the extracellular concentration of the factor low, and removal of the afferent input would, consequently, lead to an increased availability of the factor at the target site. Such a retrograde transport mechanism has in fact been demonstrated for NGF[50] in the septohippocampal pathway.

There are probably several NTFs produced in the hippocampus, and they all may or may not respond in the same way to denervation. The response of these various factors to selective denervating lesions and the specificity of their actions on different neuronal types are still poorly investigated. Though at present we are beginning to gain knowledge about the cellular and molecular mechanisms underlying growth and plasticity in the HF, each new discovery uncovers a new set of questions. It is clear, however, that intracerebral grafting will provide an important *in vivo* tool that will well complement the *in vitro* tools that have been so useful in investigating cell development and plasticity.

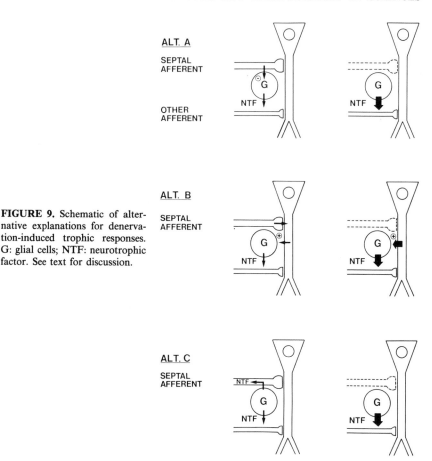

FIGURE 9. Schematic of alternative explanations for denervation-induced trophic responses. G: glial cells; NTF: neurotrophic factor. See text for discussion.

REFERENCES

1. BERG, D. K. 1984. New neuronal growth factors. Annu. Rev. Neurosci. **7:** 149-170.
2. BLACK, I. B. 1978. Regulation of autonomic development. Annu. Rev. Neurosci. **1:** 183-214.
3. COWAN, W. M., J. W. FAWCETT, D. D. M. O'LEARY & B. B. STANFIELD. 1984. Regressive events in neurogenesis. Science. **225**(4668): 1258-1265.
4. HAMBURGER, V. 1977. The development history of the motor neuron. Neurosci. Res. Prog. Bull. **15:** 1-37.
5. HENDRY, I. A. 1976. Control in the development of the vertebrate sympathetic nervous system. Rev. Neurosci. **2:** 149-178.
6. HENDRY, I. A. & J. CAMPBELL. 1976. Morphometric analysis of rat superior cervical ganglion after axotomy and nerve growth factor treatment. J. Neurocytol. **5:** 351-360.
7. HILL, M. A. & M. R. BENNETT. 1983. Cholinergic growth factor from skeletal muscle elevated following denervation. Neurosci. Lett. **35:** 31-35.
8. MCLENNAN, I. S. & I. A. HENDRY. 1978. Parasympathetic neuronal survival induced by factors from muscle. Neurosci. Lett. **10:** 269-273.

9. NISHI, R. & D. K. BERG. 1979. Survival and development of ciliary ganglion neurons grown alone in cell culture. Nature **277:** 232-234.

10. BROWN, M. C. & R. L. HOLLAND. 1979. A central role for denervated tissues in causing nerve sprouting. Nature **282:** 724-726.

11. EBENDAL, T., L. OLSON & A. SEIGER. 1983. The level of nerve growth factor (NGF) as a function of innervation. Exp. Cell Res. **148:** 311-317.

12. EBENDAL, T., L. OLSON, A. SEIGER & K. O. HEDLUND. 1980. Nerve growth factors in the rat iris. Nature **286:** 25-28.

13. HENDERSON, C. E., M. HUCHET & J. P. CHANGEUX. 1983. Denervation increases a neurite-promoting activity in extracts of skeletal muscle. Nature **302:** 609-611.

14. HOPKINS, W. G. & J. R. SLADEK. 1981. The sequential development of nodal sprouts in mouse muscles in response to nerve degeneration. J. Neurocytol. **10:** 537-556.

15. KEYNES, R. J., W. G. HOPKINS & M. C. BROWN. 1983. Sprouting of mammalian motor neurones at nodes of Ranvier: The role of the denervated motor endplate. Brain Res. **264:** 209-213.

16. HARPER, G. P. & H. THOENEN. 1980. Nerve growth factor: Biological significance, measurement, and distribution. J. Neurochem. **34**(1): 5-6.

17. LEVI-MONTALCINI, R. 1976. The nerve growth factor: Its role in growth, differentiation and function of the sympathetic adrenergic neuron. Prog. Brain Res. **45:** 235-258.

18. VARON, S. & R. ADLER. 1981. Trophic and specifying factors directed to neuronal cells. Adv. Cell. Neurobiol. **2:** 115-163.

19. BARDE, Y. A., D. EDGAR & H. THOENEN. 1982. Purification of a new neurotrophic factor from mammalian brain. EMBO J. **1:** 549-553.

20. COTMAN, C. W. & M. NIETO-SAMPEDRO. 1984. Cell biology of synaptic plasticity. Science **225:** 1287-1294.

21. CRUTCHER, K. A. & F. COLLINS. 1982. *In vitro* evidence for two distinct hippocampal growth factors: Basis for neuronal plasticity? Science **217:** 67-68.

22. MANTHORPE, M., W. LUYTEN, F. M. LONGO & S. VARON. 1983. Endogenous and exogenous factors support neuronal survival and choline acetyltransferase activity in embryonic spinal cord cultures. Brain Res. **267:** 57-66.

23. MANTHORPE, M., M. NIETO-SAMPEDRO, S. D. SKAPER, E. R. LEWIS, G. BARBIN, F. M. LONGO, C. W. COTMAN & S. VARON. 1983. Neuronotrophic activity in brain wounds of the developing rat: Correlation with implant survival in the wound cavity. Brain Res. **267:** 47-56.

24. NIETO-SAMPEDRO, M., E. R. LEWIS, C. W. COTMAN, M. MANTHORPE, S. D. SKAPER, G. BARBIN, F. M. LONGO & S. VARON. 1982. Brain injury causes a time-dependent increase in neuronotrophic activity at the lesion site. Science **2217:** 860-861.

25. NIETO-SAMPEDRO, M., M. MANTHORPE, G. BARBIN, S. VARON & C. W. COTMAN. 1983. Injury-induced neuronotrophic activity in adult rat brain: Correlation with survival of delayed implants in the wound cavity. J. Neurosci. **3:** 2219-2229.

26. KORSCHING, S. & H. THOENEN. 1984. Regulation of nerve growth factor synthesis in target tissues of the peripheral and central nervous system. Soc. Neurosci. Abstr. **10**(2): 1056.

27. STENEVI, U., A. BJÖRKLUND & N. A. SVENDGAARD. 1976. Transplantation of central and peripheral monoamine neurons to the adult rat brain: Techniques and conditions for survival. Brain Res. **114:** 1-20.

28. BJÖRKLUND, A. & U. STENEVI. 1977. Experimental reinnervation of the rat hippocampus by grafted sympathetic ganglia. I. Axonal regeneration along the hippocampal fimbria. Brain Res. **138:** 259-270.

29. BJÖRKLUND, A. & U. STENEVI. 1981. *In vivo* evidence for a hippocampal adrenergic neurotrophic factor specifically released on septal deafferentation. Brain Res. **229:** 403-428.

30. BJERRE, B., A. BJÖRKLUND & U. STENEVI. 1974. Inhibition of the regenerative growth of central noradrenergic neurons by intracerebrally administered anti-NGF serum. Brain Res. **74:** 1-18.

31. BJERRE, B., A. BJÖRKLUND & U. STENEVI. 1973. Stimulation of growth of new axonal sprouts from lesioned monoamine neurones in adult rat brain by nerve growth factor. Brain Res. **60:** 161-176.

394 ANNALS NEW YORK ACADEMY OF SCIENCES

32. GAGE, F. H., A. BJÖRKLUND & U. STENEVI. 1984. Denervation releases a neuronal survival factor in adult rat hippocampus. Nature 308: 637-639.
33. BJÖRKLUND, A. & U. STENEVI. 1977. In vivo evidence for hippocampal neuronotrophic factor specifically released on septal deafferentation. Brain Res. 229: 403-428.
34. LOY, R. & R. Y. MOORE. 1977. Anomalous innervation of the hippocampal formation by peripheral sympathetic axons following mechanical injury. Exp. Neurol. 57: 645-650.
35. STENEVI, U. & A. BJÖRKLUND. 1978. A pitfall in brain lesion studies: Growth of vascular sympathetic axons into the hippocampus of the fimbrial lesions. Neurosci. Lett. 7: 219-244.
36. COYLE, J. T., D. L. PRICE & M. R. DELONG. 1983. Alzheimer's disease: A disease of cortical cholinergic innervation. Science 219: 1184-1190.
37. BONDARIFF, W., C. Q. MOUNTJOY & M. ROTH. 1982. Loss of neurons or origin of adrenergic projection to cerebral cortex (nucleus locus coeruleus) in senile dementia. Neurology 32: 164-168.
38. GAGE, F. H. & A. BJÖRKLUND. 1986. Enhanced graft survival in the hippocampus following selective denervation. Neuroscience 17(1): 89-98.
39. GAGE, F. H., K. WICTORIN, W. FISCHER, L. R. WILLIAMS, S. VARON & A. BJÖRKLUND. 1986. Retrograde cell changes in medial septum and diagonal band following fimbria-fornix transection: Quantitative temporal analysis. Neuroscience. 1: 241-255.
40. WILLIAMS, L. R., S. VARON, G. M. PETERSON, K. WICTORIN, W. FISCHER, A. BJÖRKLUND & F. H. GAGE. Continuous infusion of nerve growth factor prevents basal forebrain neuronal death after fimbria-fornix transection. Proc. Natl. Acad. Sci. USA. 83: 9231-9235.
41. MANTHORPE, M., M. NIETO-SAMPEDRO, S. D. SKAPER, G. BARBIN, F. M. LONGO, E. R. LEWIS, C. W. COTMAN & S. VARON. 1983. Neuronotrophic activity in brain wounds of the developing rat: Correlation with implant survival in the wound cavity. Brain Res. 267: 47-56.
42. MANTHORPE, M., F. M. LONGO & S. VARON. 1982. Comparative features of spinal neuronotrophic factors in fluids collected in vitro and in vivo. J. Neurosci. Res. 8: 241-250.
43. MANTHORPE, M., S. D. SKAPER, L. R. WILLIAMS & S. VARON. 1985. Purification of adult rat sciatic nerve ciliary neuronotrophic factor. Brain Res. 367: 282-286.
44. LONGO, F. M., I. SELAK, J. ZOVICKIAN, M. MANTHORPE & S. VARON. 1984. Neuronotrophic activities in cerebrospinal fluid of head trauma patients. Exp. Neurol. 84: 207-218.
45. COLLINS, F. & K. A. CRUTCHER. 1985. Neurotrophic activity in the adult rat hippocampal formation: Regional distribution and increase after septal lesion. J. Neurosci. 5(10): 2809-2814.
46. HEACOCK, A. M., A. P. SCHONFELD & R. KATZMAN. 1984. Relationship of hippocampal trophic activity to cholinergic nerve sprouting. Soc. Neurosci. Abstr. 10: 1052.
47. RUDGE, J. S., M. MANTHORPE & S. VARON. 1985. The output of neuronotrophic and neurite-promoting agents from rat brain astroglial cells: A microculture method for screening potential regulatory molecules. Brain Res. 19: 161-172.
48. MANTHORPE, M., J. S. RUDGE & S. VARON. 1986. Astroglial cell contributions to neuronal survival and growth. In Astrocytes. S. Fedoroff, Ed. In press. Academic Press. New York, NY.
49. KORSCHING, S., G. AUBURGER, R. HEUMANN, J. SCOTT & H. THOENEN. 1985. Levels of nerve growth factor and its mRNA in the central nervous system of the rat correlate with cholinergic innervation. EMBO J. 4(6): 1389-1398.
50. SCHWAB, M. E., U. OTTEN, Y. AGID & H. THOENEN. 1979. Nerve growth factor (NGF) in the rat CNS: Absence of specific retrograde axonal transport and tyrosine hydroxylase induction in locus coeruleus and substantia nigra. Brain Res. 168: 473-483.
51. HEFTI, F. 1985. Nerve growth factor promotes survival of septal cholinergic neurons after injury. Soc. Neurosci. Abstr. 197(7): 104.
52. OLEJNICZAK, P. O., D. M. ARMSTRONG, R. D. TERRY & F. H. GAGE. 1986. Regionally specific GFAP response in hippocampus and septum following selective denervation. Soc. Neurosci. Abstr. 16: 339.
53. LOY, R. & R. Y. MOORE. 1977. Anomalous innervation of the hippocampal formation by peripheral sympathetic axons following mechanical injury. Exp. Neurol. 57: 645-650.

54. STENEVI, U. & A. BJÖRKLUND. 1978. Growth of vascular sympathetic axons into the hippocampus after lesion of the septo-hippocampal pathway: A pitfall in brain lesion studies. Neurosci. Lett. 7: 219-224.
55. GAGE, F. H., A. BJÖRKLUND & U. STENEVI. 1982. Reinnervation of the partially deafferented hippocampus by compensatory collateral sprouting from spared cholinergic and noradrenergic afferents. Brain Res. 268: 27-37.

DISCUSSION OF THE PAPER

L. KROMER (*Georgetown University, Washington, DC*): I was interested in the grafted animals that did not show behavioral recovery in the tasks. You indicated some of these had morphologically viable transplants. Was there any difference in the number of cholinergic neurons in these transplants or the innervation pattern that you could use to explain why these particular animals did not show any improvement?

BJÖRKLUND: What we did look at was the AChE fiber outgrowth. With the standard AChE staining method you cannot observe the cholinergic neurons themselves—or assess their number—but only the associated fiber outgrowth. Unrecovered animals did not differ in this respect in any obvious way from the recovered animals. So we are more inclined to believe that the cholinergic property of the grafts may be necessary for this effect to appear, but it may not be sufficient. Other conditions related to the graft integration may be important, such as the establishment of afferents to the grafts or the performance of other neuron types in the grafts that we did not observe with this anatomical technique.

M. SEGAL (*Weizmann Institute, Rehovot*): I think your data is very convincing. I just have a small conceptual problem with this. I think Dr. Bartus has one paper showing that there is a major deficit in a cholinergic receptor in the hippocampus that is in response to acetylcholine in aged hippocampus. Is that correct? Do you remember?

R. BARTUS (*American Cyanamid, Pearl River, NY*): There is a reduction in the ability of pyramidal cells in aged hippocampus to respond to iontophoretically applied acetylcholine. Not necessarily a deficit, though.

SEGAL: That is correct. Not a receptor deficit, but a decreased ability to respond to acetylcholine. Now, what would it do if you inject cholinergic neurons? Would that not change the sensitivity of the neurons to acetylcholine?

BJÖRKLUND: I can only speculate on this point. Perhaps some of the postsynaptic neuronal changes in the aged brain are reversible, so that restoration of a new functional synaptic input may be capable of improving the performance of the target neurons. If, for example, the loss of dendritic spines or the age-dependent retraction of dendritic branches, seen in hippocampal neurons in the aged brain, were reversible in this way, then the graft may, in fact, be able to improve the function and responsiveness of the host hippocampal neurons.

Norepinephrine Deficiency and Behavioral Senescence in Aged Rats

Transplanted Locus Ceruleus Neurons as an Experimental Replacement Therapy[a]

TIMOTHY J. COLLIER, DON M. GASH, AND
JOHN R. SLADEK, JR.

Department of Neurobiology and Anatomy
University of Rochester School of Medicine
Rochester, New York 14642

INTRODUCTION

Declines in norepinephrine (NE) content of specific brain regions have been detected at the biochemical level in aged primates[1–3] and rodents.[4–6] These decreases have been attributed, at least in part, to loss of brainstem NE-containing neurons in aged primates[7] and decreased transmitter content of NE neurons in aged rats.[8] Age-related noradrenergic deficits are exaggerated in Alzheimer's disease,[9–11] with the most demented patients exhibiting a decline of up to 80% in cell numbers of the locus ceruleus (LC), the pontine cell group that provides a prominent NE innervation of cortex, hippocampus, and cerebellum, among other areas.[12]

The behavioral impact of this age-related decline in NE system function is unclear. Based on previous work, however, some suggestions can be made. Because of their divergent nature, LC projections provide an anatomical substrate for modulation of information flow within multiple target systems. Electrophysiological evidence indicates that activation of the noradrenergic LC system increases the responsiveness of target neurons to other inputs, enhancing the saliency of relevant incoming signals as compared to the noise in the system.[13] Furthermore, the LC appears to be most active during behavioral states in which the organism is attending to environmental cues and initiating adaptive behavioral responses.[14] LC function also appears to influence responsiveness to stress[15] and anxiety.[16] Thus, the NE-deficient individual may exhibit deficits in selective attention to relevant environmental stimuli and adapt to environmental change less efficiently. The work described here has begun to determine whether age-related changes in NE system function can be related to specific behavioral changes, using the male Fischer-344 (F344) rat as a model system of aging. In addition, we

[a]This work was supported by Grants MH 08829 (T.J.C.), T32-AG 00107 (T.J.C.), NS 15109 (D.M.G.), and AG 00847 (J.R.S.) from the National Institutes of Health and by an Alzheimer's Disease and Related Disorders Association Faculty Scholar Award (T.J.C.).

tested whether replacement of brain NE via intraventricular LC neuron transplants may have a behaviorally therapeutic effect.

BEHAVIORAL SENESCENCE, BRAIN NE, AND THE AGED F344 RAT

One reproducible behavioral correlate of NE depletion caused by damage to the LC-dorsal NE bundle system is exaggerated reactivity to novel environmental stimuli.[17-19] NE-depleted rats exhibit overly cautious behavior, sometimes referred to as "neophobia." As a first step, we were interested in whether the natural age-related decline in brain NE content reported to occur in rats would yield behavioral neophobia reminiscent of that observed in young animals with lesions of the NE system. Thus, we screened 49 aged subjects (23 months old) and 21 young subjects (5 months old) for performance of a gustatory neophobia task.[19] Animals were adapted for 5 days to drinking from two water bottles, and consuming their entire daily fluid intake during a 30-min access session. On day 6, the water in one bottle was replaced with a palatable, but novel stimulus: a 0.1% saccharin solution. Reactivity to this novel taste was quantified by recording the percentage of total fluid intake as saccharin solution. Previous work indicates that intact young adult rats generally prefer the saccharin solution, despite its novelty, and will consume 50% or more of their intake as novel solution. Behavioral evidence from young adult subjects in our study support this finding, with 5-month-old animals consuming a mean of 57.8 ± 3.0% of their intake as saccharin solution. In contrast, 23-month-old rats tended to sample the novel stimulus, but avoid it, consuming a mean of 45.9 ± 2.1% of their intake as novel solution ($p < .01$). Indeed, aged subjects were separable into two subpopulations based on their behavior: one that exhibited responsiveness to the novel stimulus similar to that observed in young animals (18 of 49 animals, approximately 40% of the population), and a group that exhibited overly cautious behavior, scoring at least one standard deviation below the mean intake score of young adults on the gustatory test (21 of 49 animals, approximately 40% of the population). Thus, approximately 40% of the aged male F344 rats tested in this study exhibited behavior consistent with a reduction of central NE system function.

We pursued this behavioral classification of aged subjects by comparing young, aged normal, and aged neophobic rats on performance of another behavior sensitive to brain NE state: the inhibitory avoidance memory task.[20,21] In this task, subjects were placed into a brightly lighted chamber and given access to a dark chamber through an open doorway. Albino rats prefer darkness, and after a short delay, each subject entered the dark chamber. Upon entry, a mild footshock was initiated (200 μA intensity) and maintained for the duration of the learning session. Subjects learned to escape the footshock by returning to the lighted chamber, and to avoid further contact with shock by not reentering the dark chamber. All subjects were trained to a learning criterion of not entering the dark for a 2-min interval. Retention of the habit was tested 24 hr later by returning the subject to the lighted compartment, allowing access to the dark chamber, and recording the latency to enter the dark: a long latency was interpreted as a reflection of good memory for the association between darkness and footshock, a short latency was considered an indicator of poor memory.

The three experimental groups did not differ significantly on any measure of task acquisition. In contrast, retention of the task was significantly impaired in aged neophobic subjects as compared to young and behaviorally normal aged subjects (TABLE 1). Indeed, the gustatory neophobia score correlated significantly with retention performance on the avoidance task ($r(49) = .55$; $p < .01$), and grouping aged subjects that were one and two standard deviations below the mean for young animals on the gustatory test served to identify progressively more behaviorally impaired and less variable groups of aged animals. Thus, gustatory reactivity on the neophobia test appears to be a useful predictor of the quality of avoidance retention. Based on performance of these two tasks, then, a subpopulation of aged rats can be identified that are overreactive to novelty in the environment and are impaired in retention of an avoidance habit: behaviors consistent with decreased brain NE system function. It is also of interest that an equal proportion of the aged rat population exhibited no significant alteration of behavior on these tasks, suggesting that decreased NE system function is not an inevitable consequence of aging in these animals.

Following completion of behavioral testing, selected subjects from the young, aged normal, and aged neophobic groups were sacrificed and their brains processed for catecholamine histofluorescence.[22] The intensity of NE-related fluorescence in the cell bodies of the LC was quantified using microspectrofluorometry,[23] yielding an indicator of NE content in these neurons.[24] Consistent with our behavioral results, aged neophobic, memory-impaired rats exhibited a mean decline in NE histofluorescence of 18% (six subjects) as compared to young adult animals. Behaviorally normal aged rats exhibited a mean decline of 2% in fluorescence intensity (seven subjects). Thus, exaggerated reactivity to environmental novelty; impaired retention of an avoidance habit; and a modest, but reproducible, decline in LC NE content co-localize to a subpopulation of aged F344 rats.

NE REPLACEMENT VIA NEURAL TRANSPLANTS

If, as our data suggest, an age-related decline in NE content of the LC is related to impaired performance of specific behavioral tasks, then replacement of brain NE may have a therapeutic influence. Recent advances in techniques for transplantation of neurons provided an intriguing experimental approach to such neurotransmitter replacement. Accordingly, we identified a behaviorally senescent subpopulation of aged rats, based on performance of the gustatory neophobia task, and transplanted 15-16-day-gestation LC neurons into their third cerebral ventricle.[25] As a tissue control, we grafted pieces of the cerebellum (CBLM), a brain region that does not

TABLE 1. Gustatory Neophobia and Performance of the Inhibitory Avoidance Task

Experimental Group[a]	Step-through Latency[b] (sec)
Normals, 5 months old (10)	209.4 ± 36.9 (5)
Normals, 24 months old (7)	173.3 ± 38.4 (2)
Neophobics, 24 months old (12)	69.7 ± 23.9[c] (1)

[a] Number of animals in each group is shown in parentheses.
[b] Each value is a mean ± SEM. The number of animals exhibiting maximum memory performance is shown in parentheses (retention test duration: 300 sec).
[c] $F(2,26) = 5.76$, $p < .01$; Newman-Keuls test: $p < .05$ compared to both other groups.

TABLE 2. Transplanted NE Neurons and Performance of the Avoidance Task

Experimental Group[a]	Step-through Latency[b] (sec)
Unoperated, 5 months old (10)	209.4 ± 36.9
Unoperated, 24 months old (12)	69.7 ± 23.9
Received NE graft, 24 months old (6)	205.5 ± 59.9[c]
Received CBLM graft, 24 months old (5)	87.2 ± 53.7
Received NE graft, pretreated with saline, 24 months old (6)	173.5 ± 56.9
Received NE graft, pretreated with propranolol, 24 months old (7)	55.3 ± 11.3[d]
Received NE pump, 24 months old (5)	199.2 ± 62.2

[a] The number of animals in each group is shown in parentheses.
[b] Each value is a mean ± SEM.
[c] $F_{(3,29)} = 3.86$, $p < .05$; Duncan range test: $p < .05$ as compared to 24-month-old, unoperated rats.
[d] $t_{(11)} = 2.04$, $p < .05$ compared to saline controls.

contain NE neurons, into the same location in other aged subjects. Eight weeks after implantation, aged hosts were trained and tested on the inhibitory avoidance memory task.

In contrast to the poor performance normally exhibited by neophobic aged rats, subjects hosting fetal LC grafts had retention scores statistically indistinguishable from those of young animals, and significantly improved over values exhibited by unoperated aged subjects (TABLE 2, top). Aged subjects hosting cerebellar grafts showed no behavioral improvement. As before, no differences in acquisition of the task were observed. Thus, intraventricular placement of brain tissue that included the NE-containing cells of the LC enhanced retention of inhibitory avoidance in rats exhibiting behavioral signs of age-related NE depletion.

Histological examination of behaviorally effective grafts utilizing catecholamine histofluoresence revealed a few common features (FIG. 1): 1) the presence of NE-containing neurons, 2) extensive NE fiber networks within the grafts, and 3) one or more points of fusion between the graft and the host hypothalamus, with fluorescent fibers intercommunicating between graft and host at these sites.

Although NE neurons were clearly present in the grafts, other cell types also were present. This raised the possibility that some factor other than NE mediated the therapeutic influence of grafted tissue upon the aged subject's behavioral performance. Although the lack of influence of transplanted cerebellar tissue suggests that replacement of brain tissue per se is not sufficient to produce the behavioral effect, we directly addressed the influence of grafted NE neurons in two ways. First, we trained an additional 13 aged rats hosting NE-containing pontine grafts on the inhibitory avoidance task and tested the effect of NE receptor blockade on performance. Seven subjects were pretreated with the β-adrenergic receptor blocker propranolol (0.5 mg/kg, i.p., 30 min before training), and six subjects were pretreated with saline vehicle. Pretreatment with propranolol completely prevented the improvement of avoidance performance exhibited by transplant recipients receiving vehicle injections (TABLE 2, bottom). The equivalent dose of propranolol had no effect on memory performance of 5-month-old unoperated control animals. This suggests that this dose of propranolol was not sufficient to affect performance in the intact young subject. In the NE-deficient/NE-replaced aged animal, however, blockade of β-adrenergic receptors with a rela-

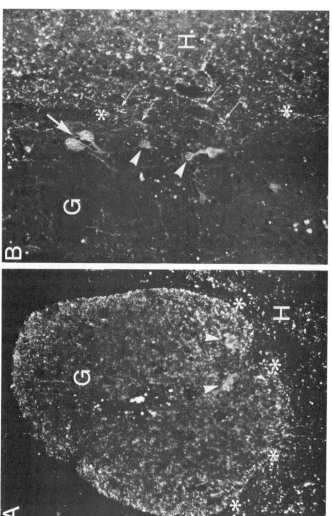

FIGURE 1. Two representative pontine tissue grafts are depicted 8 weeks after transplantation into the third ventricle of 24-month-old F344 rats. Tissue was prepared for histofluorescence of catecholamines. (**A**) Round graft (G) adhering to the floor of the third ventricle of the aged host (H) (graft-host interface is demarcated by asterisks). Note the presence of two catecholamine-containing neurons near the base of the graft (arrowheads), and the extensive network of catecholamine fibers within the graft. (**B**) Elongated graft (G) that filled the third ventricle of the host (H). In this case, the graft fused with the lateral wall of the ventricle (area between asterisks). Catecholamine fibers appear to cross the graft-host interface (small arrows). Two catecholamine cell types characteristic of the dorsal pons were visible in this graft: small, round cells typical of the LC (arrowheads) and large, stellate-like cells resembling neurons of the subceruleus (large arrow). Original magnification for **A** and **B**: ×150; reduced to 78% of original size.

tively low dose of propranolol prevented the therapeutic influence of the graft, suggesting involvement of a noradrenergic mechanism. Second, five additional aged neophobic rats were implanted with osmotic minipumps (Alzet) that continuously delivered NE into the third ventricle (10 $\mu g/\mu l$, 0.5 μl hr over 14 days). After 7 days of NE infusion, these animals were trained and tested on the avoidance task. Chronic intraventricular infusion of NE improved avoidance performance in these aged animals (TABLE 2, bottom). The combined evidence of a lack of behavioral effect of NE-free cerebellar grafts, prevention of improved avoidance performance in subjects hosting NE-containing grafts by pretreatment with a NE receptor blocker, and mimicking of the behavioral improvement by infusion of NE into the ventricle suggests that NE release from grafted neurons contributes to the observed improvement of inhibitory avoidance performance in aged rats hosting grafts.

Many questions remain unanswered concerning the mechanism by which these grafts influence behavior. It is unclear whether grafted NE neurons interact with the aged host brain via axonal connections or a humoral route through intraventricular, intraparenchymal, or intravascular diffusion of catecholamine. The finding that avoidance performance was improved in aged subjects receiving chronic intraventricular infusion of NE suggests that intraventricular release and diffusion of NE from grafted neurons may play an important role in normalizing behavior.

Further study is also required to determine the specific influence NE replacement has on avoidance behavior. Brain NE systems are believed to be involved in arousal,[26] attention,[27] and responsiveness to stress,[15] and via these mechanisms, or more directly, may influence learning and memory.[20,28] Dissociation of these factors may be difficult as they are likely to participate in most instances of learning and memory and will invariably play some role in the animal's performance. Indeed, dysfunction of physiological mechanisms regulating arousal in old age recently has been suggested as an important factor contributing to deficient memory performance in healthy aged humans.[29]

In conclusion, evidence from both rodent studies[30] and postmortem analyses of human Alzheimer's tissue[9-11] indicates that deterioration of brain NE systems may contribute to age- and dementia-related declines in cognitive performance. The present results in the F344 rat model of aging support this view, and further indicate that replacement of brain NE exerts a normalizing influence on behavioral performance. Based on prior hypotheses of LC function, reviewed briefly at the outset, it is tempting to speculate that age-related NE deficiency blurs signal-to-noise relationships in target neurons, and that NE replacement may help restore selective responsiveness to relevant environmental stimuli, thereby influencing cognitive performance. Our studies suggest that the aged brain retains the capacity to respond to NE replacement, and encourages the view that useful therapies for cognitive deficits related to aging of brain NE systems may be attainable.

REFERENCES

1. GOLDMAN-RAKIC & R. M. BROWN. 1981. Neuroscience **6:** 177-187.
2. ROBINSON, D. S. 1975. Fed. Proc. **34:** 103-107.
3. SAMORAJSKI, T. & C. ROLSTEN. 1973. *In* Progress in Brain Research. Vol. 40: Neurobiological Aspects of Maturation and Aging. D. H. Ford, Ed.: 253-265. Elsevier. Amsterdam.
4. ESTES, K. S. & J. W. SIMPKINS. 1980. Brain Res. **194:** 556-560.
5. MILLER, A. E., C. J. SHAAR & J. D. RIEGLE. 1976. Exp. Aging Res. **2:** 475-480.

6. SIMPKINS, J. W., G. P. MUELLER, H. H. HUANG & J. MEITES. 1977. Endocrinology **100:** 1672-1678.
7. VIJAYASHANKAR, N. & H. BRODY. 1979. J. Neuropathol. Exp. Neurol. **38:** 490-497.
8. SLADEK, J. R., JR. & B. C. BLANCHARD. 1981. *In* Aging. Vol. 17: Brain Neurotransmitters and Receptors in Aging and Age-Related Disorders. S. J. Enna, T. Samorajski & B. Beer, Eds.: 13-21. Raven Press. New York, NY.
9. ARAI, H., K. KOSAKA & R. IIZUKA. 1985. J. Neurochem. **43:** 388-393.
10. BONDAREFF, W., C. Q. MOUNTJOY, M. R. C. PSYCH & M. ROTH. 1982. Neurology **32:** 164-168.
11. IVERSEN, L. L., M. N. ROSSOR, G. P. REYNOLDS, R. HILLS, M. ROTH, C. Q. MOUNTJOY, S. L. FOOTE, J. H. MORRISON & F. E. BLOOM. 1983. Neurosci. Lett. **39:** 95-100.
12. LINDVALL, O. & A. BJÖRKLUND. 1978. *In* Handbook of Psychopharmacology. L. L. Iversen, S. D. Iversen & S. H. Snyder, Eds. Vol. **9:** 139-231. Plenum. New York, NY.
13. FOOTE, S. L., F. E. BLOOM & G. ASTON-JONES. 1983. Physiol. Rev. **63:** 844-914.
14. ASTON-JONES, G. 1985. Physiol. Psychol. **13:** 118-126.
15. CASSENS, G., M. ROFFMAN, A. KURUC, P. J. ORSULAK & J. J. SCHILDKRAUT. 1980. Science **209:** 1138-1140.
16. REDMOND, D. E., JR. & Y. H. HUANG. 1979. Life Sci. **25:** 2149-2162.
17. BRITTON, D. R., C. KSIR, K. THATCHER-BRITTON, D. YOUNG & G. F. KOOB. 1984. Physiol. Behav. **33:** 473-478.
18. MARTIN-IVERSON, M. T., M. PISA, E. CHAN & H. C. FIBIGER. 1982. Pharmacol. Biochem. Behav. **17:** 639-643.
19. TOMBAUGH, T. N., B. A. PAPPAS, D. C. S. ROBERTS, G. J. VICKERS & C. SZOSTAK. 1983. Brain Res. **261:** 231-242.
20. GOLD, P. E. & R. VAN BUSKIRK. 1978. Behav. Biol. **23:** 509-520.
21. STEIN, L., J. D. BELUZZI & C. D. WISE. 1975. Brain Res. **84:** 329-335.
22. HOFFMAN, D. L. & J. R. SLADEK, JR. 1973. J. Comp. Neurol. **151:** 101-112.
23. SLADEK, J. R., JR. & C. D. SLADEK. 1979. *In* Parkinson's Disease II. C. E. Finch, D. E. Potter & A. D. Kenny, Eds.: 241-250. Plenum. New York, NY.
24. LICHTENSTEIGER, W. 1971. J. Physiol. **218:** 63-84.
25. SLADEK, J. R., JR. & D. M. GASH. 1984. *In* Neural Transplants, Development and Function. J. R. Sladek, Jr. & D. M. Gash, Eds.: 243-282. Plenum. New York, NY.
26. FOOTE, S. L., G. ASTON-JONES & F. E. BLOOM. 1980. Proc. Natl. Acad. Sci. USA **77:** 3033-3037.
27. ASTON-JONES, G. & F. E. BLOOM. 1981. J. Neurosci. **1:** 887-900.
28. KETY, S. S. 1970. *In* The Neurosciences Second Study Program. F. O. Schmitt, Ed.: 324-336. Rockefeller University Press. New York, NY.
29. KUBANIS, P. & S. F. ZORNETZER. 1981. Behav. Neural Biol. **31:** 115-172.
30. ZORNETZER, S. F. 1985. Ann. N.Y. Acad. Sci. **444:** 242-254.

DISCUSSION OF THE PAPER

P. BRUNDIN (*University of Lund, Sweden*): Have you looked at the amounts of noradrenalin in any of the terminal areas that the LC projects to? Does this correlate with reductions in your aged impaired animals?

COLLIER: We have not done it yet, but we are looking at it.

BRUNDIN: Would you like to comment on the fact that you only see about a 20% reduction in fluorescence intensity whereas if you look at other systems, or specifically dopamine, you need very marked depletions to see any sort of behavioral effects?

COLLIER: I must admit that we were very surprised initially, especially since some of the lesion experiments that produce similar behavior effects are often very large, producing more than 80% depletions of forebrain NE. We were a little surprised that the 20% depletion produced a significant behavioral effect in the old animals. Although we do not know whether we are also looking at changes at the receptor level, there is some evidence from Greenberg and Weiss and others, that noradrenergic receptors in aging lose their capability to respond to a reduced input by "up-regulating." It could just be that there is some combination of a small change in cellular NE content and change at the receptor level that produces significant behavioral effects.

P. R. SANBURG (*Ohio University, Athens, OH*): You had a few young animals that showed gustatory neophobia. Did you try this in those animals?

COLLIER: There were three or four animals, and we included them in our biochemical assays. The issue is complicated a bit by a lot of noradrenergic functions expressing their effects as U-shaped functions. It turns out that when you assay NE, those few young animals that showed neophobia actually have slightly higher than normal NE levels in the LC. This was never the case with any of the old animals that showed that behavior.

M. NIETO-SAMPEDRO (*University of California, Irvine, CA*): Have you tried the effect of septal transplants?

COLLIER: We have not, but it is certainly a fine idea. The only other tissue we have transplanted is the cerebellar tissue. This tissue was used as a control.

Ultrastructural and Immunohistochemical Analysis of Fetal Mediobasal Hypothalamic Tissue Transplanted into the Aged Rat Brain[a]

A. MATSUMOTO,[b] S. MURAKAMI, AND Y. ARAI

Department of Anatomy
Juntendo University School of Medicine
Tokyo, Japan

I. NAGATSU

Department of Anatomy
Fujita Gakuen Health University
School of Medicine
Toyoake, Japan

INTRODUCTION

In recent years, intracerebral neural transplantation has been utilized to study the development and function of the central nervous system.[1-3] These studies have shown that the fetal or neonatal brain tissues can survive and develop well in the adult host brain. Evidence is accumulating that impairments of the brain functions caused by brain lesions[4-10] or genetic neuropeptide deficiency[11-14] can be recovered by the brain transplantation. In addition, grafts of fetal dopaminergic nigral[15] or cholinergic septal neurons[16] have been reported to ameliorate motor coordination or learning deficits in the aged rats. Fetal noradrenergic transplants can improve memory performance in aged rats.[17] We have demonstrated that age-dependent decline in reproductive neuroendocrine function can be reversed by transplantation of newborn mediobasal hypothalamic (MBH) tissue into the third ventricle of aged female rats.[18]

In the present study, as one step to clarify the possible correlation between the neuronal development in the brain tissue grafted into the aged brain and the functional

[a]This study was supported by Grants-in-Aid from the Ministry of Education, Culture, and Science of Japan and by the Yoshida Foundation for Science and Technology.

[b]Address for correspondence: Department of Psychology, 1283 Franz Hall, University of California at Los Angeles, Los Angeles, California 90024.

404

recovery of the pituitary-ovarian axis, ultrastructural and immunohistochemical studies on the neuronal substrates were carried out in the fetal MBH tissue transplanted into the brain of aged female rats.

MATERIALS AND METHODS

Brain Transplantation

Fourteen aged female Wistar rats (21-30 months of age) that were housed in conditions of controlled temperature (24 ± 1° C) and lighting (14:10 light:dark illumination) were used for the host animals. MBH tissue, which included the arcuate nucleus or the parietal cortex of fetal (18-20 days of gestation) or neonatal rats, was bilaterally punched out from the coronal slices (thickness: ~1.5 mm) with a stainless steel tube (inner diameter: 0.7 mm). The stainless steel tube containing neural tissues was stereotaxically placed into the floor of the third ventricle of aged female rats that had been anesthetized with Ketaral, and then the stylet was depressed to push out the grafts. At the time of the brain surgery, the state of the left ovary was inspected macroscopically by laparatomy to confirm the absence of corpora lutea. Three or 4 weeks after transplantation, the recipient aged females were sacrificed. The body, ovaries, and uterus in each animal were weighed. The brain and ovaries were examined histologically. Four brains transplanted with MBH tissue were subjected to ultrastructural and immunohistochemical analyses.

Ultrastructural Procedures

Two aged animals were anesthetized with Nembutal and were perfused through the ascending aorta with a mixture of 1% glutaraldehyde and 1% paraformaldehyde in 0.12 M phosphate buffer (PB) (pH 7.4). After perfusion, coronal hypothalamic slices of the recipient brains were postfixed in 2% OsO_4 for 2 hr at 4° C, then processed for ultrastructural examination. Thick sections of the hypothalamus were stained with toluidine blue to identify the existence of the MBH tissue grafts in the third ventricle (FIG. 1A). Ultrathin sections stained with uranyl acetate and lead citrate were examined under a JEM 1200EX electron microscope (JEOL).

Immunohistochemical Procedures

Two aged animals were anesthetized with Nembutal and perfused through the ascending aorta with 20 ml of 0.9% NaCl and subsequently with a mixture of 4% paraformaldehyde and 0.2% picric acid in 0.1 M PB (pH 7.4). The brains were removed from the skull and placed in the same fixative for 4 hr. Frozen sections were cut frontally at 50 μm and then rinsed in 0.1 M PB for 24 hr at 4° C; they were then immunostained using the avidin-biotin-peroxidase complex method (Vectastain ABC

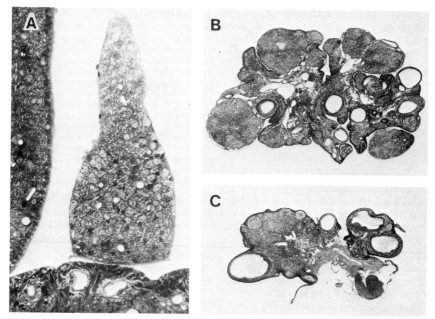

FIGURE 1. (A) MBH graft in the third ventricle of an aged female rat. (B) Ovary of an aged female rat that received an MBH graft. (C) Ovary of an intact control rat. Magnifications for **A** and for **B** and **C**: ×150 and ×12, respectively.

Kit, Vector Laboratories). The sections were incubated with tyrosine hydroxylase (TH) (dilution: 1:5000) or luteinizing hormone-releasing hormone (LHRH) (dilution: 1:2000) antiserum, which was diluted with 0.1 M PB containing 0.1% Triton X-100, for 48 hr at 4° C. After rinsing in PB, the sections were incubated with biotinylated goat antirabbit immunoglobulin G (dilution: 1:200) for 1 hr, followed by an incubation with avidin-biotinylated peroxidase complex (dilution: 1:100) for 2 hr at room temperature. The sections were finally treated with 0.0002% 3,3'-diaminobenzidine (Sigma) and 0.005% H_2O_2 in 0.05 M Tris-HCl buffer (Sigma)(pH 7.6).

RESULTS

As reported previously,[18] the ovarian weight of female rats that received MBH grafts was significantly greater than that of intact females and that of females that received cortical grafts. Ovaries of females that received MBH grafts contained follicles of various sizes and healthy appearing corpora lutea. In contrast, some follicles and masses of atrophic interstitial cells were the main components of ovaries of intact females and females that received cortical grafts. There was no significant difference in ovarian weight between the intact females and the females that received cortical grafts. The present results in ovarian weight (TABLE 1) and histology (FIGS. 1B & 1C) are similar to previous findings.[18]

Four weeks after transplantation, the MBH grafts were highly vascularized and growing in the third ventricle. All of the grafts were found to contact the ependymal layer of the third ventricle. The appearance of these grafts was similar to that of normal neural tissue (FIG. 2A). Each neural perikaryon contained a round nucleus with a prominent nucleolus and various kinds of cytoplasmic organelles, such as rough endoplasmic reticulum, mitochondria, and Golgi apparatus. The neuropil in the graft was fully occupied by axons, dendrites, and glial processes (FIG. 2B). Numerous axodendritic shaft and spine synapses were observed in the neuropil. The clear cytoplasm of dendrites was seen to contain free ribosomes, mitochondria, and neurotubules. Axon terminals were characterized by a large number of synaptic vesicles. Large granular vesicles were found to coexist with synaptic vesicles in the axon terminals. Pre- and postsynaptic specializations were thick.

In the MBH graft, a number of TH-immunoreactive neurons were demonstrated, providing evidence that these grafts contained dopaminergic neurons in the arcuate nucleus.[19,20] TH-immunoreactive somata with diameters in the range 8-12 μm were stained intensely for TH antiserum and frequently occurred in groups or clusters at the interface between the transplant and periventricular parenchyma of the host brain or just inside the surface of the graft facing on the ventricle (FIG. 3). They were multipolar and possessed well-developed processes (FIG. 4A). These processes originating from these somata were ramified well within the graft. TH-immunoreactive processes could be identified passing through the graft-host interface and penetrated the periventricular parenchyma of the host hypothalamus (FIG. 4B). A dense accumulation of TH-positive terminals was often found in the peripheral zone of the grafts (FIG. 3). The staining intensity of TH-immunoreactive terminals in the median eminence was higher in aged females bearing MBH grafts than in aged females without MBH grafts.

On the other hand, LHRH-immunoreactive neuronal perikarya could not be identified in the MBH grafts. In the recipient aged female brain, however, several LHRH-positive neuronal cell bodies could be found in the septal-preoptic region; a considerable accumulation of LHRH-positive axon terminals was also found in the median eminence.

DISCUSSION

These results of the present ultrastructural and immunohistochemical studies clearly show that the neuronal substrates of fetal MBH tissue grafted into the aged

TABLE 1. Body Weights and Organ Weights in Intact and Experimental Animals

Group	Number of Rats	Body (g)	Ovaries (mg)	Uterus (mg)
Intact control	6	299 ± 20	48.6 ± 6.4	553 ± 36
Animals with cortical grafts	5	374 ± 54	57.5 ± 3.7	644 ± 64
Animals with MBH grafts	9	384 ± 34	95.2 ± 9.6^a	796 ± 77

NOTE: Each value for weight is a mean ± SEM. Student's t test was used to determine significance.
^{a} Comparison with control: $p < .05$.

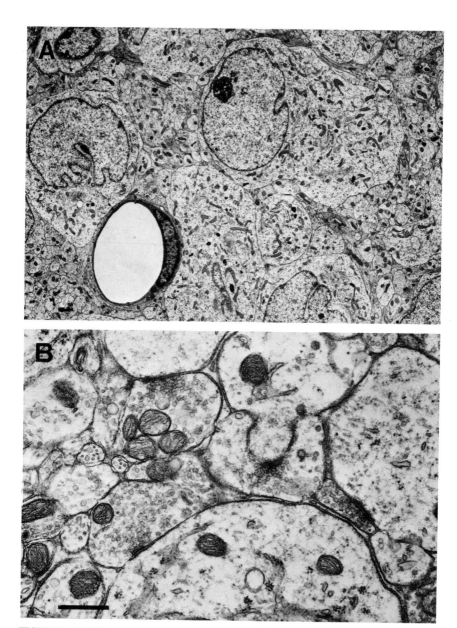

FIGURE 2. (A) Electron microgram of an MBH graft containing neuronal perikarya, neuropil, and a blood capillary. Scale bar: 1 μm. (B) Neuropil in an MBH graft. Axodendritic shaft and spine synapses are present. Scale bar: 0.5 μm. Magnifications for **A** and **B**: ×3300 and ×27 000, respectively.

brain develop and form neural connections. The MBH grafts in the aged brain contained numerous TH-immunoreactive neurons whose processes ramified within the grafts. A number of shaft and spine synapses were identified in the MBH grafts. This evidence indicates that axonal growth, dendritic branching, and spine formation occurred in the MBH tissue grafted into the aged brain during the posttransplantation period. The development of neuronal substrates grafted into the aged brain has been clarified by immunohistochemical[21] or Golgi[22] study on the neuronal morphology of the fetal hypothalamus including the supraoptic nucleus and by ultrastructural analysis on the synaptogenesis in the newborn preoptic area.[23] The fact that there were no significant changes in the neuronal morphology and synaptic population between the neural tissues grafted to the young brains and those grafted to the aged brains indicates

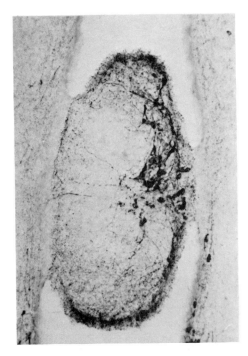

FIGURE 3. TH-immunoreactive neuronal perikarya and processes in an MBH graft. Magnification: ×88.

that the transplantation environment of the aged brain may not be substantially different from that of the young brain in the development of the grafted neural tissue.

There is evidence indicating that a significant decrease in dopaminergic activity in the tuberoinfundibular system of aged female rats could be associated with hypogonadal function and hyperprolactinemia.[24] Marked reduction in catecholaminergic synapse population was recognized in the arcuate nucleus of aged female rats.[25] The decrease in catecholaminergic activity of old females seems to be related to the age-related reduction in the efficiency of catecholaminergic neuroendocrine regulation. Systemic administration of L-dopa[26] or dopamine agonists in aged females[27] has been shown to reduce the serum prolactin level and to induce the recovery of the normal estrous cycle. Furthermore, McCann *et al.*[28] have pointed out that dopamine,

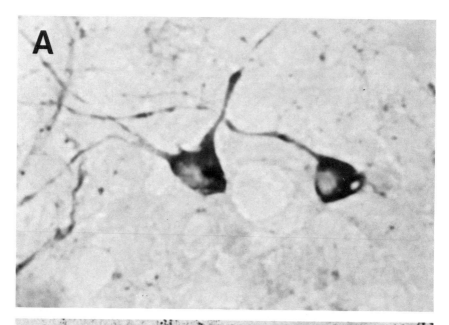

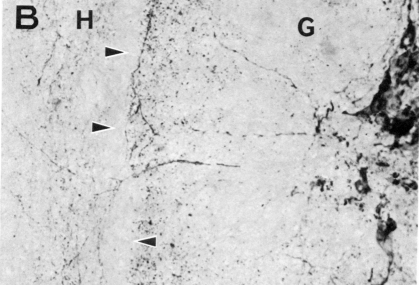

FIGURE 4. (A) TH-immunoreactive neuronal perikarya with developed processes. (B) TH-immunoreactive processes passing through the graft-host interface (arrowheads). G: graft; H: host. Original magnifications for **A** and **B**: ×880 and ×350, respectively; enlarged to 125% of original size.

in certain instances, stimulates LHRH release from the median eminence. Therefore, it is possible that TH-immunoreactive, dopaminergic neurons in the grafts may contribute to the restoration of catecholaminergic activity in females that receive MBH grafts, and thus play a stimulatory role in LHRH release. Since the LHRH-immunoreactive neurons in the MBH grafts could not be identified in the present study, it seems unlikely that the neural substrates of the grafts were the main source of LHRH in the ovulating females that receive MBH grafts. In contrast, a number of LHRH-immunoreactive neuronal perikarya and terminals could be observed in the septal-preoptic region and median eminence, respectively, in the aged host animals. The ovulatory failure in these aged females in spite of the availability of LHRH terminals in the median eminence may be due to the possible impairment of the regulatory mechanism of LHRH release. Therefore, it seems likely that the increased dopaminergic activity by MBH transplantation may be involved in activating the LHRH-producing neuronal system in the aged hypothalamus. This may be implicated in the recovery of gonadotropic function in the aged female rats that receive MBH grafts.

The presence of TH-immunoreactive neurons has been demonstrated in the fetal substantia nigra grafted into adult rats in which the nigrostrial pathway has been lesioned.[29,30] It has also been demonstrated that TH-immunoreactive neurons in the grafts can send their axons to the host striatum and make synaptic contact with the neural elements in the striatum. This suggests that synaptic connections of the grafted TH-positive neurons reinnervating the host striatum contribute to the functional recovery of motor coordination impaired by nigrostriatal pathway lesion. In the present study, TH-immunoreactive processes originating from the TH-immunoreactive neurons in the graft could be seen extending across the graft-host interface and invading the periventricular parenchyma in the aged host. It is not clear whether these processes make synaptic contact with the neural elements of the host hypothalamus or associate with the blood capillaries in the median eminence. An observed rise in the staining intensity of TH-immunoreactive terminals in the median eminence of aged female rats bearing MBH grafts (compared to the staining intensity in intact aged females) suggests that dopaminergic neurons in the grafts send their axons to the host hypothalamus and terminate around the blood capillaries in the median eminence. Further studies are needed to clarify these points.

SUMMARY

MBH tissue, which included the hypothalamic arcuate nucleus of fetal or neonatal rats, was transplanted into the third ventricle of aged (21-30-month-old) female rats. The brain and ovaries of each recipient were examined histologically 3 or 4 weeks after transplantation. Four grafted MBH tissues were examined ultrastructurally and immunohistochemically 4 weeks after transplantation. The appearance of the MBH grafts was similar to that of normal neural tissue. The neuropil in the grafts was fully occupied with numerous axons, dendrites, and glial processes. A number of axodendritic shaft and spine synapses were observed in the neuropil. Immunohistochemical analysis with antiserum to TH revealed stained (immunoreactive) neuronal perikarya and processes in the grafts. TH-immunoreactive processes originating from the TH-positive neurons in the grafts could be seen to extend across the graft-host interface. The ovaries of six out of nine females that received MBH grafts exhibited follicles of various sizes and healthy appearing corpora lutea. On the other hand, some follicles and masses of interstitial cells were prominent in the ovaries of the intact animals or controls that had received cortical grafts. In the females that received MBH grafts, the ovarian weight was significantly greater than that in the controls. These results suggest that the neural substrates in fetal MBH tissue can survive and develop well in the aged rat brain and that MBH grafts may play some role in the recovery of declined ovarian function in aged female rats.

REFERENCES

1. SLADEK, J. R., JR. & D. M. GASH, EDS. 1984. Neural Transplants: Development and Function. Plenum. New York, NY.
2. BJÖRKLUND, A. & U. STENEVI, EDS. 1985. Neural Grafting in the Mammalian CNS. Elsevier. Amsterdam.
3. WALLACE, R. B. & G. D. DAS, EDS. 1985. Neural Transplantation and Regeneration. Springer-Verlag. Berlin.
4. BJÖRKLUND, A. & U. STENEVI. 1979. Reconstruction of the nigrostriatal dopamine pathway by intracerebral nigral transplants. Brain Res. 177: 555-560.
5. PERLOW, M. J., W. J. FREED, B. J. HOFFER, A. SEIGER, L. OLSON & R. J. WYATT. 1979. Brain grafts reduce motor abnormalities produced by destruction of nigrostriatal dopamine system. Science 204: 643-647.
6. DUNNETT, S. B., W. C. LOW, S. D. IVERSEN, U. STENEVI & A. BJÖRKLUND. 1982. Septal transplants restore maze learning in rats with fornix-fimbria lesions. Brain Res. 251: 335-348.
7. LOW, W. C., P. R. LEWIS, S. T. BUNCH, S. B. DUNNETT, S. R. THOMAS, S. D. IVERSEN, A. BJÖRKLUND & U. STENEVI. 1982. Function recovery following neural transplantation of embryonic septal nuclei in adult rats with septohippocampal lesions. Nature 300: 260-262.
8. LABBE, R., A. FIRL, JR., E. J. MUFSON & D. G. STEIN. 1983. Fetal brain transplants: Reduction of cognitive deficits in rats with frontal cortex lesions. Science 221: 470-472.
9. FINE, A., S. B. DUNNETT, A. BJÖRKLUND & S. D. IVERSEN. 1985. Cholinergic ventral forebrain grafts into the neocortex improve passive avoidance memory in a rat model of Alzheimer's disease. Proc. Natl. Acad. Sci. USA 82: 5227-5230.
10. ISACSON, O., P. BRUNDIN, F. H. GAGE & A. BJÖRKLUND. 1985. Neural grafting in a rat model of Huntington's disease: Progressive neurochemical changes after neostriatal ibotenate lesions and striatal tissue grafting. Neuroscience 16: 799-817.
11. GASH, D., J. R. SLADEK, JR. & C. D. SLADEK. 1980. Functional development of grafted vasopressin neurons. Science 210: 1367-1369.
12. KRIEGER, D. T., M. J. PERLOW, M. J. GIBSON, T. F. DAVIES, E. A. ZIMMERMAN, M. FERIN & H. M. CHARLTON. 1982. Brain grafts reverse hypogonadism of gonadotropin-releasing hormone deficiency. Nature 298: 468-471.
13. GIBSON, M. J., D. T. KRIEGER, H. M. CHARLTON, E. A. ZIMMERMAN, A. J. SILVERMAN & M. J. PERLOW. 1984. Mating and pregnancy can occur in genetically hypogonadal mice with preoptic area brain grafts. Science 225: 949-951.
14. GIBSON, M. J., H. M. CHARLTON, M. J. PERLOW, E. A. ZIMMERMAN, T. F. DAVIES & D. T. KRIEGER. 1984. Preoptic area grafts in hypogonadal (hpg) female mice abolish effects of congenital hypothalamic gonadotropin-releasing hormone (GnRH) deficiency. Endocrinology 114: 1938-1940.
15. GAGE, F. H., S. B. DUNNETT, U. STENEVI & A. BJÖRKLUND. 1983. Aged rats: Recovery of motor impairments by intrastriatal nigral grafts. Science 221: 966-969.
16. GAGE, F. H., A. BJÖRKLUND, U. STENEVI, S. B. DUNNETT & P. A. T. KELLY. 1984. Intrahippocampal septal grafts ameliorate leaning impairments in aged rats. Science 225: 533-536.

17. GASH, D. M., T. J. COLLIER & J. R. SLADEK, JR. 1985. Neural transplantation: A review of recent developments and potential applications to the aged brain. Neurobiol. Aging **6:** 131-150.
18. MATSUMOTO, A., S. KOBAYASHI, S. MURAKAMI & Y. ARAI. 1984. Recovery of declined ovarian function in aged female rats by transplantation of newborn hypothalamic tissue. Proc. Jpn. Acad. **60:** 73-76.
19. VAN DEN POL, A. V., R. S. HERBST & J. F. POWELL. 1984. Tyrosine hydroxylase-immunoreactive neurons of the hypothalamus: A light and electron microscopic study. Neuroscience **13:** 1117-1156.
20. PIOTTE, M., A. BEAUDET, T. H. JOH & J. R. BRAWER. 1985. The fine structural tyrosine hydroxylase-immunoreactive neurons in rat arcuate nucleus. J. Comp. Neurol. **239:** 44-53.
21. SLADEK, J. R., JR. & D. M. GASH. 1984. Morphological and functional properties of transplanted vasopressin neurons. *In* Neural Transplants: Development and Function. J. R. Sladek, Jr. & D. M. Gash, Eds.: 243-282. Plenum. New York, NY.
22. KAPLAN, A. S., D. M. GASH, G. FLOOD & P. D. COLEMAN. 1985. A Golgi study of hypothalamic transplants in young and old host rats. Neurobiol. Aging **6:** 205-211.
23. MATSUMOTO, A., S. MURAKAMI, Y. ARAI & M. OSANAI. 1985. Synaptogenesis in the neonatal preoptic area grafted into the aged brain. Brain Res. **347:** 363-367.
24. FINCH, C. E. 1978. Reproductive senescence in rodents: Factors in the decline of fertility and loss of regular estrous cycles. *In* The Aging Reproductive System. E. L. Schneider, Ed.: 193-212. Raven Press. New York, NY.
25. MATSUMOTO, A. & Y. ARAI. 1983. Synaptic changes in the hypothalamus of old rats. *In* Integrative Neurohumoral Mechanisms. E. Endröczi, D. de Wied, L. Angelucci & U. Scapagnini, Eds.: 401-407. Elsevier. Amsterdam.
26. CLEMENS, J. A., Y. AMENOMORI, T. JENKINS & J. MEITES. 1969. Effects of hypothalamic stimulation, hormones, and drugs on ovarian function in old female rats. Proc. Soc. Exp. Biol. Med. **132:** 561-563.
27. CLEMENS, J. A. & D. R. BENNETT. 1977. Do aging changes in the preoptic area contribute to loss of cyclic endocrine function? J. Gerontol. **32:** 19-24.
28. MCCANN, S. M., M. D. LUMPKIN, O. KHORRAM, H. MIZUNUMA, X. Y. HUANG, H. K. MANGAT, W. K. SAMSON, S. R. OJEDA & A. NEGRO-VILAR. 1983. Putative synaptic transmitters controlling release of gonadotropin-releasing hormones. *In* Integrative Neurohumoral Mechanisms. E. Endröczi, D. de Wied, L. Angelucci & U. Scapagnini, Eds.: 211-225. Elsevier. Amsterdam.
29. FREUND, T. F., J. P. BOLAM, A. BJÖRKLUND, U. STENEVI, S. B. DUNNETT, J. F. POWELL & A. D. SMITH. 1985. Efferent synaptic connections of grafted dopaminergic neurons reinnervating the host neostriatum: A tyrosine hydroxylase immunocytochemical study. J. Neurosci. **3:** 603-616.
30. MAHALIK, T. J., T. E. FINGER, I. STROMBERG & L. OLSON. 1985. Substantia nigra transplants into denervated striatum of the rat: Ultrastructure of graft and host interconnections. J. Comp. Neurol. **240:** 60-70.

DISCUSSION OF THE PAPER

M. N. LEHMAN (*University of Cincinnati, Cincinnati, OH*): Have you identified any fenestrated capillaries in your medial and basal hypothalamic grafts? MATSUMOTO: I have not yet.

LEHMAN: It may provide a means for tyrosine hydroxylase elements to directly release dopamine into the hypothalamus.

MATSUMOTO: Yes. But I have not done it yet.

G. ARENDASH (*University of South Florida, Tampa, FL*): Was the age of your aged animals for transplantation about, say, 22 or 24 months? If so, there is a good chance that they had hyperprolactinemia. Did you measure any prolactin levels in those animals before or after transplantation to see if you got a reconstitution of dopaminergic inhibition of prolactin secretion?

MATSUMOTO: We have not yet measured the prolactin level.

D. STEIN (*Clark University, Worcester, MA*): There have been reports in the literature that aged female Fisher rats very often develop pituitary adenomas. Did you notice that problem in your animals? Did your transplants do anything to ameliorate that condition?

MATSUMOTO: We excluded females bearing pituitary tumors. We used only intact females.

QUESTIONER: We have induced that condition with chronic estrogen treatment in young females and find the transplants of tuberoinfundibular adrenergic neurons do in fact result in decreased pituitary weights. Our results will appear in *Neuroendocrinology*.

Anatomical and Behavioral Consequences of Cholinergic-rich Grafts to the Neocortex of Rats with Lesions of the Nucleus Basalis Magnocellularis[a]

STEPHEN B. DUNNETT

Department of Experimental Psychology
University of Cambridge
Cambridge CB2 3EB, England

CHOLINERGIC HYPOTHESIS OF DEMENTIA

It has recently been proposed that cognitive, and in particular memory, impairments associated with aging might be attributable to a decline in forebrain cholinergic function.[1-3] Several lines of evidence have been adduced in support of this hypothesis:

1) In addition to a more general age-related decline in cortical and hippocampal markers of cholinergic function, such as choline acetyltransferase (ChAT) activity, a decline in ChAT activity is particularly marked in patients dying of Alzheimer's disease.[4,5] Moreover, the postmortem decline in ChAT activity has been found to correlate with the patients' mental test scores before death.[6]

2) There is a corresponding loss[7] or atrophy[8] of the cholinergic cells of the nucleus basalis of Meynert (NBM) in Alzheimer's brains, from which originate the extrinsic cortical cholinergic innervation.

3) Anticholinergic drugs in young subjects induce functional impairments akin to the pattern of deficits manifested by demented elderly patients.[3]

4) There is some limited evidence that cholinergic drugs, such as physostigmine or choline, can enhance memory in aged subjects.[1,3]

Nevertheless, much of the evidence on the role of cholinergic systems in dementia remains indirect, and there continues to be disagreement about whether this is a primary factor in the disease etiology, or whether it is secondary to other cortical and subcortical pathology, in particular, to the development of neuritic plaques and neurofibrillary tangles.[9]

One approach to this issue is to consider whether more selective lesions of cortical or hippocampal cholinergic systems in animals yield deficits that reproduce some of the symptomatology of Alzheimer's disease. In particular, whether destruction of the

[a] These studies were supported by the Medical Research Council and the Mental Health Foundation.

415

NBM-cortical system disrupts the learning and memory capacity of experimental animals.

NBM LESIONS IN EXPERIMENTAL ANIMALS

The simplest tests of memory function in animals are provided by the passive avoidance paradigm: a normal rat will learn in a single trial to avoid a place where it has previously received an aversive experience, such as footshock. Lo Conte *et al.*[10] first showed that electrolytic lesions of the NBM induce passive avoidance memory impairments in rats, and this observation has subsequently been replicated with neurotoxic lesions of the NBM.[11,12] However, whereas passive avoidance tests are rapid and simple to run, it is difficult to attribute deficits specifically to a memory impairment rather than to other effects, such as changes in the animal's level of activation, motivational state, or discrimination and sensitivity to relevant stimuli. Therefore, subsequent studies have examined the effects of NBM lesions on more complex maze learning tasks, which are also generally disrupted.[13–16]

Several authors have distinguished between different memory systems. Of particular interest in the present context is the distinction made by Olton[17] between "working" memory, that is, specific information required for the immediate task at hand, and "reference" memory involving more general rules about the nature of stable associations in the world. Olton and colleagues had previously found that a bilateral lesion in the hippocampal system, such as a transection of the fimbria-fornix (FF), selectively disrupts working memory, leaving reference memory intact.[17] Recently, Murray and Fibiger[18] have reported the converse consequence of NBM lesions, namely that disruption of cortical cholinergic afferents impaired rats' reference memory capacity while leaving working memory intact.

Although relatively sensitive tasks are available for the assessment of an animal's learning and memory capacity, there still remains a severe problem of specificity of the lesions. In the absence of a generally available cholinergic neurotoxin, NBM lesions are most often made by infusion of excitotoxic amino acids, such as kainic acid or ibotenic acid. These toxins have the advantage, in comparison with classical lesion techniques, of being relatively selective for neuronal perikarya while sparing fibers of passage. The NBM in rats, however, is a relatively diffuse population of cells, and many other noncholinergic cell groups in the vicinity are also destroyed. In particular, ibotenic acid lesions of the NBM also produce severe regulatory, sensorimotor, and motor impairments,[16,19] which are, *a priori,* most likely to be related to damage of extrapyramidal and hypothalamic systems rather than of the NBM-cortical system itself. How then can we be sure that any of the learning and memory impairments following NBM lesions are specifically related to damage in cortical cholinergic systems?

It has been to address this issue of lesion specificity that we have begun to study the effects of cortical cholinergic grafts in rats with NBM lesions. If any of the mnemonic, learning, sensorimotor, motor, or regulatory impairments induced by the lesions can be ameliorated by grafts of cholinergic cells to the neocortex, then strong support is provided for the hypothesis that those particular impairments are attributable specifically to cortical deafferentation. Further support is provided when similar effects are not obtained from control grafts of noncholinergic tissue implanted into the same cortical sites, or of similar cholinergic tissue implanted into other sites.

VIABILITY OF CORTICAL CHOLINERGIC GRAFTS

In our first studies, unilateral lesions of the NBM have been made by stereotaxic infusion of 0.5 μl 0.06 M ibotenic acid into two sites in the vicinity of the cholinergic cells at the borders of the globus pallidus and substantia innominata. Histologically, this is accompanied by a virtually complete loss of acetylcholinesterase (AChE) staining of cells in the NBM and of fiber terminals in the ipsilateral dorsolateral neocortex (FIGS. 1A & 1B).[19,20]

Biochemical assays indicate a parallel acute decline in ChAT activity by approximately 70-80% in the ipsilateral dorsolateral cortex,[19,20] indicating a virtually complete removal of subcortical cholinergic afferents to the neocortex, since 20-25% of cortical ChAT activity is attributable to intrinsic cortical cholinergic interneurons. Three to 6 months following the lesions, cortical ChAT activity partially recovers to about 50% of normal levels.[20] This is in contrast to a study by Wenk and Olton[21] in which ChAT activity was reported to return to normal levels over 3 months; the initial lesions used in that study, however, were smaller than the ones used by us.

Graft tissue has been obtained by dissection of ventral forebrain areas from developing (E15-16) embryos (see the "standard" dissection in FIG. 5), from which are prepared dissociated cell suspensions for stereotaxic injection into the host neocortex, as has been described in detail elsewhere.[22] When the host is sacrificed several months later, the grafts are seen to survive and expand in size.[20] In Nissl-stained sections (FIGS. 1E & 1F), the morphology of the grafted cells is relatively normal, and only rarely is any gliosis seen, either within the grafts or at the graft-host border. In AChE-stained sections (FIGS. 1C & 1D), occasional densely AChE-positive cells are seen, but these are more usually masked by dense swirls of fiber staining throughout the grafts. AChE-positive fibers are invariably seen to cross the graft-host border freely, and to provide a halo of innervation into the host neocortex. Indeed, the normal laminar distribution of AChE-positive fibers in the neocortex is occasionally also reinstated,[20] but this aspect of the reinnervation has been more variable.

Dissection of areas of host neocortex proximal to the location of grafts for biochemical analysis has indicated an increase of ChAT activity to 60-70% of the normal level.[20] Thus, these grafts appear, on average, to replace between a third and a half of the extrinsic cortical cholinergic innervation, although the precise values depend on the time course of study, and on the volume, concentration, and specificity of the graft tissue (see below).

In one recent study, the fiber outgrowth from similar grafts has been examined ultrastructurally, identifying fibers of graft origin by ChAT immunocytochemistry.[23] It was found that graft-derived fibers made extensive synaptic contacts with both somatic and dendritic neuronal elements in the host brain. The contacts were of normal symmetric morphology, but the distribution of targets was abnormal, being more frequently onto pyramidal somata and less frequently onto dendrites than is seen in the intact neocortex. This intriguing observation is akin to observations of grafts both in the nigrostriatal dopamine system[24] and in the cholinergic septohippocampal system[25] and may be related to as yet unidentified mechanisms for the maximization of the functional effects of a partial reinnervation.[23,25]

FUNCTIONS OF CORTICAL CHOLINERGIC GRAFTS

Because of the severe regulatory impairments induced by bilateral ibotenic acid lesions,[16,19] our first behavioral studies have also been conducted in unilaterally lesioned

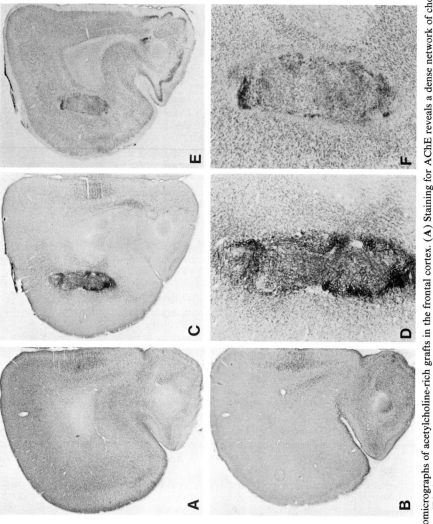

FIGURE 1. Photomicrographs of acetylcholine-rich grafts in the frontal cortex. (**A**) Staining for AChE reveals a dense network of cholinergic terminals in the intact cortex; (**B**) the cortex is extensively depleted after NBM lesions are made. Two examples of acetylcholine-rich ventral forebrain grafts in the deafferented neocortex are shown at (**C & E**) low and (**D & F**) high magnification in (**C & D**) AChE- and (**E & F**) Nissl-stained sections.

rats. Nevertheless, even unilateral NBM lesions induce impairments in passive avoidance.[10] Cholinergic grafts implanted into the deafferented dorsolateral neocortex at three sites partially ameliorated this deficit, whereas control noncholinergic grafts had no significant effect on the impairment.[26] In a second study,[27] we found a separation between the learning and retention component on this task: whereas cholinergic grafts had no effect on the impairment induced by NBM lesions in acquisition of the initial avoidance (FIG. 2A), the retention impairment 2 days later was completely reversed (FIG. 2B). The selectivity of the cholinergic grafts was confirmed by the observation that control grafts of hippocampal primordium, devoid of developing cholinergic cells, were without effect on the passive avoidance retention deficit. In the same study, it was found that the grafts again had no influence on the acquisition of a spatial navigation task in the Morris swim maze,[28] whereas the rats with cholinergic grafts were significantly improved in the precision with which they searched for the escape platform when it was removed from the pool in an extra probe trial.[27]

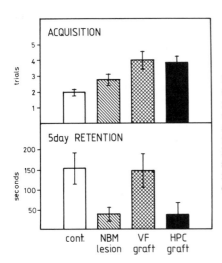

FIGURE 2. Passive avoidance acquisition (trials to criterion) and retention (latency to reenter the dark chamber) in control rats, rats with unilateral ibotenate lesions of the NBM, and rats with additional acetylcholine-rich ventral forebrain (VF) grafts or acetylcholine-poor hippocampal (HPC) grafts. The VF graft group shows a significant amelioration of the lesion-induced retention impairment. (Data from reference 27.)

Thus, these initial studies do indeed provide strong support for the relevance of cholinergic systems to some aspect of the learning or memory impairments that have been reported following NBM lesions. Nevertheless, the specificity of this conclusion is challenged in several respects:

1) The unilateral lesions were seen to also induce a range of sensorimotor impairments, some aspects of which (such as lateralized turning bias when the rat was tilted on an inclined grid) were also ameliorated by the cortical cholinergic grafts.[27] This suggests that the cortical cholinergic innervation may regulate some more general aspect of cortical function than memory per se.

2) The learning deficits induced by unilateral NBM lesions were relatively slight. For example, in the Morris water maze task, acquisition was near normal in the rats with unilateral lesions, providing little scope for assessing the effects of cortical grafts. By contrast, bilateral lesions produce a much more substantial impairment.[16] It is therefore necessary to develop a less traumatic procedure for achieving large (and hence stable) bilateral lesions of the NBM.

3) The extent of graft growth, although clear, is not very extensive. It is possible that this relates to the relatively nonspecific dissection of embryonic ventral forebrain that was used in these first studies. In parallel with the first functional studies, we have therefore attempted to improve upon the procedures for making the lesions and grafts.

IMPROVEMENTS IN LESION SPECIFICITY

In order to try to improve the NBM lesions and reduce their functional (motor and regulatory) side effects, we have compared the toxicity of ascending doses of four neurotoxic amino acids—kainic acid, ibotenic acid, n-methyl-d-aspartic acid (NMA), and quisqualic acid—according to biochemical, histological, and behavioral criteria.[19] The toxicity of these four compounds against NBM cholinergic cells, and consequently the decline in cortical ChAT activity, differed markedly (FIG. 3). At doses that produced comparable 70-75% depletions of cortical ChAT activity, unilateral injections of 0.012 M kainic acid induced far more extensive damage in a variety of local and remote subcortical nuclei than did either 0.06 M ibotenic acid or 0.12 M NMA. Nevertheless, these latter two toxins still produced more damage in areas adjacent to the NBM, such as the amygdala and zona incerta, than did 0.12 M quisqualic acid.

A similar pattern of behavioral specificity was then confirmed by making bilateral lesions with ibotenic acid, NMA, or quisqualic acid.[19] Regulatory and motor impairments induced by NMA and ibotenic acid were far more marked than the impairments induced by quisqualate. In fact, 7 of 18 rats with ibotenate lesions and 5 of 18 rats with NMA lesions died after surgery, whereas all but one of the rats with quisqualate lesions remained healthy. By contrast, in passive avoidance tests, quisqualate lesions induced as great an impairment in retention as did either ibotenate or NMA (FIG. 4).

In the light of these observations, quisqualate appears to offer the possibility of making NBM lesions that are relatively more selective for cholinergic systems than the other three toxins that were assessed.

FIGURE 3. Depletions in ChAT activity in the dorsolateral neocortex ipsilateral to neurotoxic lesions of the NBM. Four different toxins were assessed: kainic acid (KA), ibotenic acid (IBO), n-methyl-d-aspartic acid (NMA), and quisqualic acid (QUIS). Each point is based on observations in three rats. (Data from reference 19.)

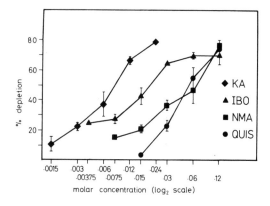

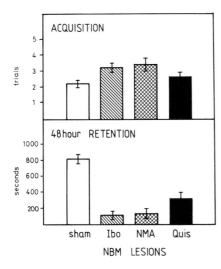

FIGURE 4. Passive avoidance acquisition and retention in sham-operated controls (sham) and rats with bilateral lesions of the NBM, induced by 0.06 M ibotenic acid (Ibo), 0.12 M *n*-methyl-*d*-aspartic acid (NMA), or 0.12 M quisqualic acid (Quis). (Data from reference 19.)

IMPROVEMENTS IN GRAFT SPECIFICITY

The second procedural improvement sought was in the specificity of the embryonic dissection of graft tissue. In a series on ontogenetic observations in the rat, Fine[29] has reported that NBM precursors are detectable as large multipolar AChE-positive neurons, situated laterally beneath the striatal eminence by E14, whereas septal precursors do not become clearly apparent as a separate population until E17.

We have therefore attempted the differential dissection of embryonic ventral forebrain in order to separate the more lateral NBM precursors from the more medial septal precursors (FIG. 5). Suspension grafts of either population of donor cells were then injected into the neocortex of rats with NBM lesions or into the hippocampus of rats with FF lesions.[30] As can be seen in FIGURE 6, grafts of both septal and NBM precursors survived, grew, and developed AChE-positive fiber connections with the host brain when transplanted to either site. The two sources of graft tissue differed in that the NBM grafts appeared to grow to a larger size, and they developed a more patchy internal organization in the AChE-stained sections than was apparent in the septal grafts. Moreover, at least in the hippocampus, the septal grafts appeared to provide a more extensive AChE-positive fiber reinnervation than the NBM grafts.

These differences between the graft tissues and targets were then quantified by tracing serial sections and computing the volumes of the grafts and of the fiber outgrowth into the host brain. FIGURE 7A shows that graft size was influenced by the two variables independently: NBM tissue grew larger than septal tissue, whichever target was selected, and the hippocampus supported more extensive growth than the neocortex, whichever graft tissue was selected. These differences can most readily be interpreted in terms of the developmental stage of the different graft tissues and the compression exerted on the grafts in cortical and periventricular sites.

More interestingly, the extent of AChE-positive fiber outgrowth was dependent on the appropriateness of the source of donor tissue (FIG. 7B). In particular, NBM tissue provided a more extensive innervation of the neocortex than did septal tissue,

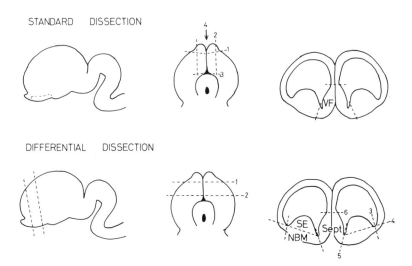

STANDARD DISSECTION

DIFFERENTIAL DISSECTION

FIGURE 5. Embryonic dissections for acetylcholine-rich graft tissue, by the standard dissection of ventral forebrain (VF), or by the differential dissection to separate septal (Sept) from NBM precursors. In the present experiments, the pieces of striatal eminence (SE) were discarded. (After reference 30.)

whereas septal tissue provided a more extensive innervation of the hippocampus than did the NBM tissue. This suggests that quite specific influences are exerted on different populations of cells to provide an appropriate reinnervation, even when they utilize the same neurotransmitter, acetylcholine.

Nevertheless, it needs to be remembered that the present dissections, although containing appropriate populations of developing cholinergic neurons, also contain many other noncholinergic cell groups. At present, we cannot separate precise populations of cells from the suspension for more selective injection. With the rapid advances in cell culture techniques that are taking place, however, this may soon be possible.

IMPROVEMENTS IN BEHAVIORAL SPECIFICITY

Although the equivalent effects of quisqualate and the other neurotoxins on passive avoidance retention, and the ameliorative effects of cortical cholinergic grafts in similar tests, support a role for cortical cholinergic systems in memory function, passive avoidance tests do not, as noted above, provide a sufficiently specific measure. We have therefore developed an operant version of delayed matching performance for rats; this test can provide a more sensitive measurement of the rate of loss of information from memory, independent of sensory, motivational, and motor changes. In the "delayed matching to position" task, rats are trained to make a "sample" response to one of two retractable levers, and, after a variable interval (during which the levers are withdrawn from the test chamber), to make a matching response for food reward to the previously sampled level (FIG. 8). The effects of bilateral NBM and FF lesions may then be compared.[31]

The FF rats performed as well as controls at the shortest delays, but performance fell off rapidly as the delay increased (FIG. 9), suggestive of a working memory deficit (recall the studies by Olton and colleagues,[17] discussed above). By contrast, the NBM lesions initially disrupted preoperative levels of performance at all delays. They were, however, then able to relearn the task to control levels over approximately 2-3 weeks (FIG. 9). This then suggests that the NBM lesions induced an impairment of retention of the task demands that they had learned preoperatively, but left intact the animals' acquisition capacity.

FURTHER STUDIES ON CORTICAL GRAFT FUNCTION

With the improvements in lesion, graft dissection, and behavioral techniques, we can now reexamine the functional consequences of cortical cholinergic grafts in rats

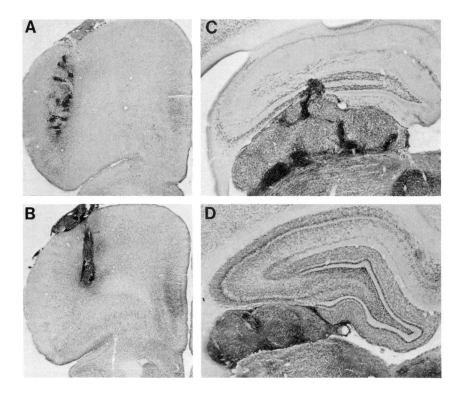

FIGURE 6. AChE-stained sections of NBM (**A & C**) or septal (**B & D**) grafts, implanted into the frontal cortex of rats with NBM lesions (**A & B**) or into the hippocampus of rats with FF lesions (**C & D**).

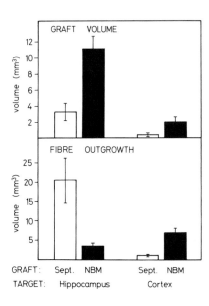

FIGURE 7. Volumes of the grafts and of the AChE-positive fiber outgrowth in rats that received either septal or NBM graft tissue, implanted either into the deafferented hippocampus or into the deafferented frontal cortex. (Data from reference 30.)

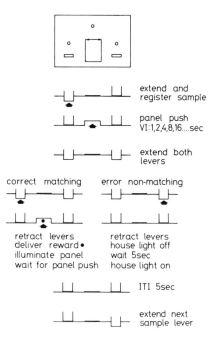

FIGURE 8. Schematic diagram of the operant delayed matching paradigm. At the top is shown the side wall of the operant chamber, with a central food well covered with a transparent perspex flap panel and with a retractable lever on either side. Three stimulus lights above each lever and the panel were not used. Each stage of a trial is illustrated, viewed from above, with responses of the animal indicated by a solid arrow. VI: variable interval delay that takes one of the values 1, 2, 4, 8, 16, or 32 sec at random. ITI: intertrial interval.

with NBM lesions. The effects of the differential embryonic dissections have not yet been examined, but in an unpublished study, the delayed matching task has recently been used to assess the capacity of cholinergic grafts into the neocortex of rats with bilateral quisqualate lesions.

Thirty-four rats were trained on the delayed matching, and then 19 received bilateral NBM lesions with 0.12 M quisqualic acid. Eight of the lesioned rats then received six grafts (using the standard dissection), injected in six deposits in the dorsolateral neocortex at three rostrocaudal levels on each side. All rats were then retested 3 months later. As shown in FIGURE 10, the deficits induced by the lesions were less severe than those seen in the former experiment, probably because of the long recovery period that was necessary to provide time for graft growth and rein-

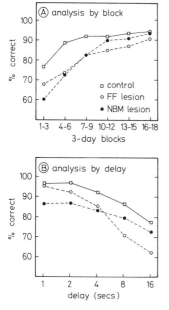

FIGURE 9. Delayed matching performance by control rats and by rats with bilateral FF or NBM lesions. The same performance data is shown first in terms of successive 3-day blocks of trials, averaging the different delay intervals (A), and second in terms of the different delay intervals, averaging the different test days (B). (Data from reference 31.)

nervation following lesion and transplantation surgery. The NBM lesion deficit, however, is still highly significant, and is directly comparable with the previous observations: the deficit is initially present at all delay intervals and recovers over approximately 3 weeks of retraining. By contrast, the lesioned rats with grafts were able to perform at control levels for all delays after the first 3 days of testing (FIG. 10).

At the completion of the operant tests, the rats were also tested for passive avoidance to compare with the previous results. As previously, bilateral NBM lesions with quisqualic acid did not produce any deficits in acquisition, but the lesioned rats showed a large retention impairment 2 days later (FIG. 11). The retention deficit was significantly reduced by the grafts, but in this experiment the grafted animals did not improve completely, that is, return to control levels of performance.

FUNCTIONS OF CORTICAL CHOLINERGIC SYSTEMS

The present studies provide strong support for the involvement of cholinergic NBM-cortical systems in certain aspects of cognitive performance. In disentangling the precise contribution, the absence of deficits following quisqualate lesions in some behavioral measures is as informative as the recovery induced by cortical grafts in others. Thus the rats with bilateral quisqualate lesions, and extensive depletions of cortical ChAT activity, were unimpaired in acquiring the passive avoidance criterion on the training days, although dramatic impairment was seen when retention was tested 2-5 days later. Similarly, in the delayed matching tests, the NBM lesions disrupted retention of the previously learned task even at the shortest delays, although they were able to relearn the contingencies within 2-3 weeks. Moreover, in contrast to the rats with FF lesions, the NBM rats showed a normal rate of forgetting at increasing delays, indicating that the short-term "working" component of memory remained intact.

Together, these observations suggest that NBM lesions disrupt the retention or retrieval of previously learned associations, rather than a learning impairment per se. The amelioration of these deficits by intracortical grafts of cholinergic-rich tissue, suggests that the lesion deficit is due to disruption of cortical cholinergic afferents. Additionally, given that recovery was seen in animals where the grafts are positioned in an ectopic location, it seems unlikely that the intrinsic NBM-cortical system is involved in relaying specific information. Rather, it suggests that the cholinergic inputs regulate neocortical function in a relatively nonspecific manner. Since all areas of neocortex receive an extensive cholinergic innervation, it is not surprising that other, noncognitive functions were also ameliorated by the grafts, such as several aspects of

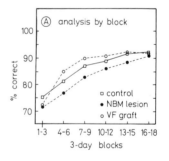

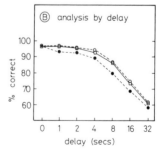

FIGURE 10. Delayed matching performance by control rats, rats with bilateral NBM lesions, and rats with lesions plus intracortical acetylcholine-rich grafts. As in FIGURE 9, the same performance data is shown first in terms of successive 3-day blocks of trials, averaging the different delay intervals (A), and second in terms of the different delay intervals, averaging the different test days (B). The impairment in the lesioned rats is small but significant, and is reversed by the grafts to control levels. (Unpublished data.)

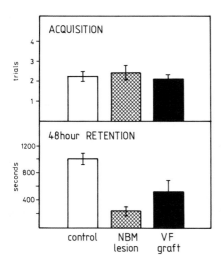

FIGURE 11. Passive avoidance acquisition and retention in the control, NBM lesion, and acetylcholine-rich graft rats, previously tested in the delayed matching task. The grafted rats show a significant amelioration of the lesion-induced retention deficit, but are still impaired in comparison with normal control performance. (Unpublished data.)

motor and sensorimotor performance.[27] An aspect of graft function that has not yet been investigated is the importance of graft placement, since it seems likely that the precise pattern of cortical deafferentation and reafferentation will have profound effects on the profile of deficits manifested by the rats.

CONCLUSIONS

Although most studies of intracerebral transplants have been primarily interested in the mechanisms of development and regeneration, and the capacity of the central nervous system for plasticity and recovery, this technique also provides a powerful complement to lesion and stimulation procedures for studying the neural basis of behavior. The present studies exemplify this principle, using grafts to manipulate central neurotransmitter systems with a specificity that cannot readily be achieved by contemporary lesion techniques alone.

ACKNOWLEDGMENTS

I wish to thank the stimulation and collaboration provided by my colleagues: Professors A. Björklund and I. Q. Whishaw; Drs. S. D. Iversen, T. W. Robbins, A. Fine, and D. Clark; and C. N. Ryan, G. Toniolo, S. T. Bunch, and G. Jones.

REFERENCES

1. BARTUS, R. T., R. L. DEAN, B. BEER & A. S. LIPPA. 1982. The cholinergic hypothesis of geriatric memory dysfunction. Science 217: 408-417.
2. COYLE, J. T., D. L. PRICE & M. R. DELONG. 1983. Alzheimer's disease: A disorder of cortical cholinergic innervation. Science 219: 1184-1190.
3. DRACHMAN, D. A. & B. J. SAHAKIAN. 1980. Memory, aging and pharmacosystems. In The Psychobiology of Aging: Problems and Perspectives. D. Stein, Ed.: 347-368. Elsevier/North-Holland. Amsterdam.
4. BOWEN, D. M., C. B. SMITH, P. WHITE & A. N. DAVISON. 1976. Neurotransmitter-related enzymes and indices of hypoxia in senile dementia and other abiotrophies. Brain 99: 459-496.
5. DAVIES, P. & A. J. F. MALONEY. 1976. Selective loss of central cholinergic neurons in Alzheimer's disease. Lancet ii: 1403.
6. PERRY, E. K., B. E. TOMLINSON, G. BLESSED, K. BERGMANN, P. H. GIBSON & R. H. PERRY. 1978. Correlation of cholinergic abnormalities with senile plaques and mental test scores in senile dementia. Br. Med. J. 2: 1457-1459.
7. WHITEHOUSE, P. J., D. L. PRICE, R. G. STRUBLE, A. W. CLARK, J. T. COYLE & M. R. DELONG. 1982. Alzheimer's disease and senile dementia: Loss of neurons in the basal forebrain. Science 215: 1237-1239.
8. PEARSON, R. C. A., M. V. SOFRONIEW, A. C. CUELLO, T. P. S. POWELL, F. ECKENSTEIN, M. M. ESIRI & G. K. WILCOCK. 1983. Persistence of cholinergic neurons in the basal nucleus in a brain with senile dementia of the Alzheimer's type demonstrated by immunohistochemical staining for choline acetyltransferase. Brain Res. 289: 375-379.
9. PERRY, R. H. 1986. Recent advances in neuropathology. In Alzheimer's Disease and Related Disorders. M. Roth & L. L. Iversen, Eds. Br. Med. Bull. 42: 34-41.
10. LO CONTE, G., L. BARTHOLINI, F. CASAMENTI, I. MARCONCINI-PEPEU & G. PEPEU. 1982. Lesions of cholinergic forebrain nuclei: Changes in avoidance behavior and scopolamine actions. Pharmacol. Biochem. Behav. 17: 933-937.
11. FLICKER, C., R. L. DEAN, S. K. FISHER & R. T. BARTUS. 1983. Behavioral and neurochemical effects following neurotoxic lesions of a major cholinergic input to the cerebral cortex in the rat. Pharmacol. Biochem. Behav. 18: 973-981.
12. FRIEDMAN, E., B. LERER & J. KUSTER. 1983. Loss of cholinergic neurons in the rat neocortex produces deficits in passive avoidance learning. Pharmacol. Biochem. Behav. 19: 309-312.
13. SALAMONE, J. D., P. M. BEART, J. E. ALPERT & S. D. IVERSEN. 1984. Impairment in T-maze reinforced alternation performance following nucleus basalis magnocellularis lesions in rats. Behav. Brain Res. 13: 63-70.
14. HEPLER, D. J., G. L. WENK, B. L. CRIBBS, D. S. OLTON & J. T. COYLE. 1985. Memory impairment following basal forebrain lesions. Brain Res. 346: 8-14.
15. LERER, B., J. WARNER, E. FRIEDMAN, G. VINCENT & E. GAMZU. 1985. Cortical cholinergic impairment and behavioral deficits produced by kainic acid lesions of rat magnocellular basal forebrain. Behav. Neurosci. 99: 661-677.
16. WHISHAW, I. Q., W. T. O'CONNOR & S. B. DUNNETT. 1985. Disruption of central cholinergic systems in the rat by basal forebrain lesions or atropine: Effects on feeding, sensorimotor behavior, locomotor activity and spatial navigation. Behav. Brain. Res. 17: 103-115.
17. OLTON, D. S. 1983. Memory function and the hippocampus. In The Neurobiology of the Hippocampus. W. Seifert, Ed.: 335-373. Academic Press. New York, NY.
18. MURRAY, C. L. & H. C. FIBIGER. 1985. Learning and memory deficits after lesions of the nucleus basalis magnocellularis: Reversal by physostigmine. Neuroscience 14: 1025-1032.
19. DUNNETT, S. B., I. Q. WHISHAW, G. JONES & S. T. BUNCH. 1987. Behavioural, biochemical and histological effects of different neurotoxic amino acids injected into the nucleus basalis magnocellularis of rats. Neuroscience 20: in press.
20. FINE, A., S. B. DUNNETT, A. BJÖRKLUND, D. CLARKE & S. D. IVERSEN. 1985. Transplantation of embryonic ventral forebrain neurons to the neocortex of rats with lesions of nucleus basalis magnocellularis. I. Biochemical and anatomical observations. Neuroscience 16: 769-786.

21. WENK, G. L. & D. S. OLTON. 1984. Recovery of neocortical choline acetyltransferase activity following ibotenic acid injection into the nucleus basalis of Meynert in rats. Brain Res. 293: 184-186.
22. BJÖRKLUND, A., U. STENEVI, R. H. SCHMIDT, S. B. DUNNETT & F. H. GAGE. 1983. Intracerebral grafting of neuronal cell suspensions. I. Introduction and general methods of preparation. Acta Physiol. Scand. Suppl. 522: 1-7.
23. CLARKE, D. J. & S. B. DUNNETT. 1986. Ultrastructural organization of choline acetyltransferase-immunoreactive fibers innervating the neocortex from embryonic ventral forebrain grafts. J. Comp. Neurol. 250: 192-205.
24. FREUND, T., J. P. BOLAM, A. BJÖRKLUND, U. STENEVI, S. B. DUNNETT, J. F. POWELL & A. D. SMITH. 1985. Efferent synaptic connections of grafted dopaminergic neurons reinnervating the host neostriatum: A tyrosine hydroxylase immunocytochemical study. J. Neurosci. 5: 603-616.
25. CLARKE, D. J., F. H. GAGE & A. BJÖRKLUND. 1986. Formation of cholinergic synapses by intrahippocampal septal grafts as revealed by choline acetyltransferase immunohistochemistry. Brain Res. 369: 151-162.
26. FINE, A., S. B. DUNNETT, A. BJÖRKLUND & S. D. IVERSEN. 1985. Cholinergic ventral forebrain grafts into the neocortex improve passive avoidance memory in a rat model of Alzheimer's disease. Proc. Natl. Acad. Sci. USA 82: 5227-5230.
27. DUNNETT, S. B., G. TONIOLO, A. FINE, C. N. RYAN, A. BJÖRKLUND & S. D. IVERSEN. 1985. Transplantation of embryonic ventral forebrain neurons to the neocortex of rats with lesions of nucleus basalis magnocellularis. II. Sensorimotor and learning impairments. Neuroscience 16: 787-797.
28. MORRIS, R. G. M. 1981. Spatial localization does not require the presence of local cues. Learn. Motiv. 12: 239-260.
29. FINE, A. 1985. Cholinergic basal forebrain development in rat. Neurosci. Lett. (Suppl. 21): S72.
30. DUNNETT, S. B., I. Q. WHISHAW, S. T. BUNCH & A. FINE. 1986. Acetylcholine-rich neuronal grafts in the forebrain of rats: Effects of environmental enrichment, neonatal noradrenaline depletion, host transplantation site, and regional source of embryonic donor cells on graft size and acetylcholinesterase-positive fibre outgrowth. Brain Res. 378: 357-373.
31. DUNNETT, S. B. 1985. Comparative effects of cholinergic drugs and nucleus basalis or fimbria-fornix lesions on delayed matching in rats. Psychopharmacology 87: 357-363.

DISCUSSION OF THE PAPER

W. LOW (*Indiana University, Indianapolis, IN*): Do you see any sparing of the nucleus basalis nerve cells? Do you see any renervation by spared nerve cells?

DUNNETT: Not so far as we know. When we looked at the electron microscopical level, which was done by Dr. Clarke in Oxford, there appeared to be a virtually complete loss even 3 to 6 months after lesion of synaptic contacts in the deep layers of the neocortex. There are some spared terminals in the superficial layers even immediately after the lesion. Whether this is attributable to intrinsic neurons, we do not know. But, consequently, the detailed analysis of the extent of the lesion and the pattern of the graft has been assessed in terms of innervation in the deep cortical layers.

B. HOROWITZ (*National Institutes of Health, Bethesda, MD*): Have you looked at any age-related changes having done this in both young and old rats?

DUNNETT: No. The studies have been conducted in parallel to the ones by Dr.

Björklund and Dr. Gage. We have not yet looked at this particular task in old rats per se, and so far I have consistently used young adult females.

J. H. KORDOWER (*University of Rochester, Rochester, NY*): In postcommisural regions of the brain inclusive of nucleus basalis, there are numerous AChE-positive but not ChAT-positive cells. Are these contained within your graft? And, if so, how do you dissociate them from the cholinergic neurons?

DUNNETT: I use AChE staining for routine assessment of the grafts and in particular to assess the extent of the pattern applied throughout the region. We have also done the ChAT-positive cells with Dr. Clarke, and we see exactly the same pattern of survival of cells in the graft and fiber outgrowth, although at the low magnification level the images are not as straightforward as with the AChE.

Transplantation of Nucleus Basalis Magnocellularis Cholinergic Neurons into the Cholinergic-depleted Cerebral Cortex

Morphological and Behavioral Effects[a]

GARY W. ARENDASH AND PETER R. MOUTON

Division of Physiology and Development
Department of Biology
University of South Florida
Tampa, Florida 33620

INTRODUCTION

A fundamental role for central nervous system cholinergic dysfunction in the severe memory deficits characteristic of senile dementia of the Alzheimer's type (SDAT) has been clearly established.[1,2] In this regard, marked reductions in choline acetyltransferase (ChAT) and acetylcholinesterase (AChE) activities within the cortex of SDAT brains have been consistently observed.[1,3,4] Since the principal source of cholinergic innervation to the neocortex is the nucleus basalis of Meynert (NBM) within the basal forebrain and since the brains of SDAT patients are characterized by a degeneration or atrophy of such cholinergic neurons within the NBM,[5–7] it has been suggested that the cortical cholinergic hypofunction and memory deficiencies of SDAT may be due, in large part, to a degenerative/dysfunctional "NBM-to-cortex" cholinergic pathway.[2] Indeed, some evidence indicates that degenerative changes in cortical cholinergic terminals are involved in the pathogenesis of neuritic plaques,[8] which constitute a neuropathological marker for SDAT. Further emphasizing the importance of the NBM-to-cortex cholinergic pathway are recently discovered correlations between cell death within the NBM of SDAT patients, the degree of their dementia, and the density of neuritic plaques in the neocortex at autopsy.[9] Thus, the death or dysfunction of neurons constituting this central nervous system cholinergic pathway may be of critical importance in the pathogenesis and symptomology of SDAT.

[a] This work was supported by Grant HD 17933 from the National Institutes of Health, Grant 83-001 from the Alzheimer's Disease and Related Disease Association, and a grant from the American Foundation for Aging Research.

Since the rat has an analogous forebrain cholinergic pathway,[10,11] we have been interested, first, in characterizing the biochemical, neurohistological, and behavioral deficits induced by destroying this pathway and, second, in challenging the ability of cholinergic transplants to reverse or alleviate such deficits.

THE nBM-LESIONED RAT

Providing the primary cholinergic innervation to the rat neocortex is a group of large neurons in the nucleus basalis magnocellularis (nBM)[12] located within the ventromedial aspects of the globus pallidus (FIG. 1). In adult Sprague-Dawley rats, excitotoxic lesioning of the nBM with ibotenic acid (5 μg in 1 μl phosphate-buffered saline at two nBM sites) decreases cortical ChAT activity by 40-50% at 6 weeks after lesioning (FIG. 2). In fact, we found a positive correlation ($r = .98$) between the percentage of nBM destruction (as indicated by AChE staining) and the percentage decrease in anterior cortex ChAT activity at this 6-week time point. Additionally, the neocortex of nBM-lesioned rats showed substantially reduced AChE staining (FIG. 1).

These decreases in cortical ChAT activity and AChE staining, both of which are characteristic of SDAT brains, appear to be permanent and due to destruction of the

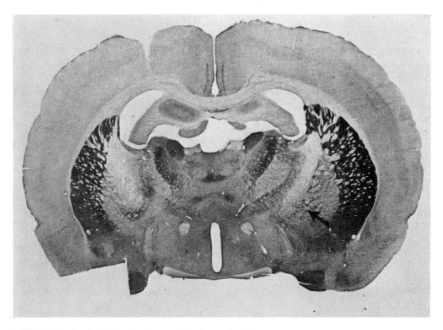

FIGURE 1. An AChE-stained coronal brain section from an animal given a unilateral ibotenic acid injection into the left nBM 1½ months before sacrifice. The arrow indicates the dark-staining normal nBM on the control side. Note the reduced AChE-positive staining in the neocortex on the nBM-lesioned side.

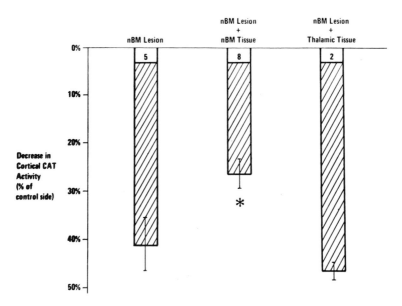

FIGURE 2. Percentage decreases in anterior cortex ChAT activity at approximately 1½ months after either unilateral nBM lesioning or after transplantation into the cortex ipsilateral to nBM lesioning. The asterisk indicates results that are significantly different ($p < .05$) from those of the nBM lesion group.

"nBM-to-cortex" cholinergic pathway. Furthermore, we have found nBM-lesioned rats to be severely deficient in a variety of tests for learning and memory abilities, including passive avoidance, two-way active avoidance, Lashley III maze learning, and 17-arm radial maze performance.[13,14] Thus, the nBM-lesioned rat may be an appropriate animal model for the neocortical cholinergic hypofunction and cognitive deficiencies of SDAT.

nBM CELL SUSPENSION TRANSPLANTS

Since nBM-lesioned animals exhibit cortical cholinergic hypofunction and are learning/memory deficient, the possible alleviation of these biochemical and behavioral deficits by cholinergic-rich nBM cell suspension transplants was investigated. Recipients were adult males who had been given unilateral or bilateral ibotenic acid lesions of the nBM 1-2 weeks earlier. The nBM or thalamic (control) cell suspensions were prepared from dissected fetal brains on day 18 of gestation according to methodology we have previously used.[13]

Bilaterally lesioned rats received eight cell suspension deposits of 2 μl each within the frontoparietal cortex (four on each side); animals with unilateral nBM lesions received four cell suspension deposits within the cortex ipsilateral to the lesion.

Recipients bearing unilateral nBM lesions plus transplants were sacrificed 1½ months later, whereas those with bilateral lesions and transplants were behaviorally tested for learning/memory abilities before sacrifice at least $5\frac{1}{2}$ months after transplantation. Some brains were processed for Nissl and AChE staining,[15] whereas others had the neocortex removed (for ChAT activity determination[16]) before histological processing.

HISTOLOGICAL ANALYSIS OF nBM TRANSPLANTS

Cortically placed nBM cell suspension transplants were relatively easy to discern in AChE-stained brain sections. At $1\frac{1}{2}$ months after transplantation, such cholinergic-rich cell suspensions showed intense AChE staining, which was due to the presence of AChE-positive cell bodies and fibers in the immediate vicinity of transplantation (FIG. 3). Very limited, if any, AChE-positive fiber outgrowth was observed from nBM tissue transplants into adjacent neocortical areas of the recipients at this $1\frac{1}{2}$-month time point. In sharp contrast, nBM cell suspension transplants in recipients that were allowed to survive $5\frac{1}{2}$ months after grafting showed considerable AChE-positive fiber outgrowth into extensive cortical regions (FIGS. 4 & 5), thus alleviating the nBM lesion-induced decrease in cortical AChE staining. Usually, this fiber outgrowth proceeded down the lateral concavity of the neocortex and was sometimes most intense within deeper cortical layers (FIG. 5) that had, before lesioning, received substantial cholinergic innervation from the recipient's nBM (FIG. 1).

In light of the apparently extensive reinnervation of the neocortex by AChE-positive fibers from long-term nBM transplants, it was of interest to specifically identify cholinergic perikarya within such transplants. Therefore, nBM-lesioned rats that had been given nBM suspension transplants 6 months earlier were injected (i.m.) with diisopropylfluorophosphate (DFP) several hours before sacrifice. Since DFP is an irreversible inhibiter of AChE, only cholinergic neurons will stain intensely for AChE if animals are sacrificed several hours after such treatment.

Through this methodology, transplanted cholinergic neurons were found within cortically placed nBM suspension grafts at 6 months after transplantation (FIG. 6). Labeled cells were generally found in the periphery of these grafts, at the interface between the graft and host parenchyma. In several instances, dendrites from such cells were seen to spread into the host neocortex. The transplanted AChE-positive neurons were large and morphologically similar to basal forebrain cholinergic neurons.[12] Thus, transplanted nBM cholinergic neurons would appear capable of long-term survival after cortical transplantation. Although not characterized in the present study, a migration of cortically placed nBM (cholinergic) neurons to distant subcortical loci is possible and is currently being investigated.

BIOCHEMICAL EFFECTS OF nBM TRANSPLANTS

At $1\frac{1}{2}$ months after unilateral nBM lesioning, anterior cortex ChAT activity was seen to have decreased on the lesioned side by about 41% (FIG. 2); this decrease was attributable to the destruction of the neurons constituting the nBM-to-cortex cholinergic pathway. For those animals given unilateral nBM suspension transplants into the cortex shortly after ipsilateral nBM lesioning, however, anterior cortex ChAT

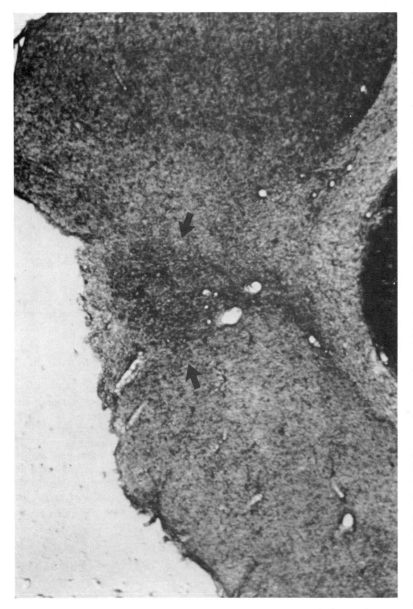

FIGURE 3. An intense AChE-stained nBM suspension transplant within the neocortex of an nBM-lesioned recipient at 1½ months after transplantation. The arrows indicate transplant-host interfaces. Original magnification: ×63; reduced to 86% of original size.

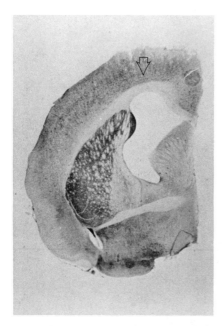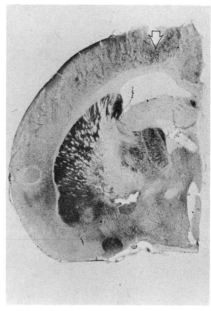

FIGURE 4. AChE-stained half-brain sections from two nBM-lesioned animals. Each animal was given nBM suspension transplants into the cortex 5½ months before sacrifice. Note the extensive AChE-positive staining within dorsal and lateral neocortical regions. The arrows indicate approximate locations of nBM suspension infusion.

activity was seen to have decreased by only about 26% compared to levels on the unlesioned contralateral side. This attenuated decrease in anterior cortex ChAT activity by nBM suspension transplants was probably attributable to the cholinergic neurons within such grafts. As indicated in the previous section, large basal forebrain-like cholinergic neurons reside within cortically placed nBM transplants.

The enhanced cortical ChAT activity in nBM-transplanted animals appears to be specific for the cholinergic-rich nBM suspension grafts since cortically placed grafts of thalamic (noncholinergic) cell suspensions were ineffective in enhancing cortical ChAT activity in several nBM-lesioned recipients (FIG. 2). To minimize any variations in ChAT activity that might accompany variations in lesion location, all animals included in the above cortical ChAT activity comparisons had at least a 70% destruction of the nBM according to analysis of AChE-stained brain sections.

LEARNING AND MEMORY IN TRANSPLANT RECIPIENTS

From histological and biochemical standpoints, nBM suspensions in nBM-lesioned rats are capable of alleviating cortical AChE staining deficits and increasing cortical ChAT activity, respectively. Such cholinergic-rich transplants may also have the ability to enhance learning and memory processes in lesioned recipients. As previously indicated, rats bearing bilateral ibotenic acid lesions of the nBM were found to be behaviorally deficient in a variety of learning/memory tasks including passive avoidance, active avoidance, and Lashley III maze learning. Such cognitive deficits might be induced, in large part, by eliminating the nBM-to-cortex cholinergic pathway; if so, cholinergic-rich nBM suspensions might enhance the cognitive performance of nBM-lesioned rats. In this context, results from the above three tests of learning/ memory function in transplant recipients will be briefly presented.

The passive avoidance task proceeds as follows: an animal is placed in a lighted compartment; a guillotine door is raised to expose a dark compartment (rats, which prefer dark environments, invariably enter the dark compartment with a latency of only a few seconds); the door is lowered and a mild 2-sec footshock is applied before the animal is removed from the dark chamber; finally, the animal is returned to the lighted compartment three times—1 min, 24 hr, and 48 hr after the shock trial—to test for learning/memory of the shock. Rats are never shocked again after the shock trial, even if they enter the dark chamber.

Most sham-lesioned rats remembered the shock throughout the three postshock trials: they either did not enter the dark chamber when the door was raised or had a high latency before doing so. Rats with bilateral nBM lesions, however, were learning/memory deficient (that is, had short latencies before entering the dark chamber) during each of the postshock trials. In fact, most nBM-lesioned rats entered the dark chamber during the 1-min postshock trial, thus indicating a rather substantial

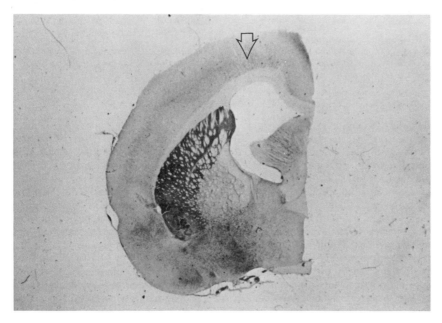

FIGURE 5. An AChE-stained brain section from an nBM-lesioned rat given nBM suspension transplants into the cortex $5\frac{1}{2}$ months before sacrifice. Note that, despite the lack of AChE-positive staining in the recipient's nBM (induced by ibotenic acid lesioning), inner layers of the neocortex stain fairly intensely because of the presence of multiple nBM suspension grafts within the cortex. The arrow indicates the approximate location of an nBM suspension infusion.

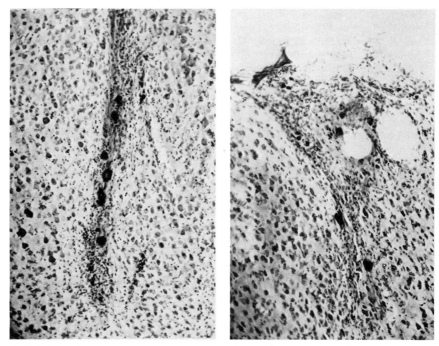

FIGURE 6. Photomicrographs of brain sections, processed for DFP-AChE pharmacohisto-chemistry (counterstained with Nissl), showing the frontoparietal cortex of a recipient at two coronal levels. Visualized are dark-staining cholinergic neurons within two different nBM suspension transplants at these coronal levels.

learning dysfunction or short-term memory dysfunction or both. Those nBM-lesioned animals that had received multiple nBM suspension transplants, however, appeared to have enhanced learning/memory during this 1-min postshock trial in that their latencies were no different from those of sham-lesioned control rats and significantly greater ($p < .01$) than those of rats with nBM lesions alone. This behavioral effect at 1 min may be specific for nBM (cholinergic-rich) transplants because lesioned recipients with thalamic (noncholinergic) transplants had latencies significantly less than those of sham-lesioned rats ($p < .05$) and not significantly different from those of rats given nBM lesions alone. Irrespective of whether lesioned animals had been given nBM or thalamic suspension transplants, however, no enhanced memory (that is, greater latencies) of the shock trial was observed at the 24 hr and 48 hr postshock trials compared to animals with nBM lesions alone. These data suggest that nBM suspension transplants may enhance the learning or short-term memory aspects or both of passive avoidance behavior but not the long-term memory components associated with this task.

After passive avoidance testing, rats were tested for two-way active avoidance behavior in a shuttle box; that is, rats were tested for their ability to learn to avoid a footshock by moving from one side of the box to the other side within 4 sec after hearing a 1-sec tone. Rats were given 10 trials per day and tested for 30 days to "acquire" or learn this conditioned avoidance response (CAR).

A group of sham-lesioned rats was tested: the frequency with which the CAR was exhibited increased gradually over the test period until, by the end of testing, rats were exhibiting the CAR 60% of the time. The nBM-lesioned rats that received thalamic suspension transplants exhibited essentially no acquisition: the CAR frequency was 20% at the beginning of the test and never increased. Thus, thalamic transplants clearly could not enhance the poor learning abilities of nBM-lesioned rats in this task.[13] Those nBM-lesioned animals that received nBM (cholinergic-rich) suspension implants, however, showed learning ability that was not statistically different from that exhibited by the sham-lesioned control animals. The rats that received nBM transplants exhibited the CAR 40% of the time by the end of testing.

Acquisition training was followed by 10 days of "extinction" testing (10 trials per day), during which the tone was not followed by a shock, even if the animal remained stationary. Those animals that showed a slow rate of extinction (that is, continued showing high numbers of CARs) were thought to have superior memory retention of the avoidance behavior. This was clearly the case for sham-lesioned animals: the frequency with which they exhibited the CAR gradually decreased throughout extinction testing (FIG. 7). The sham-lesioned animals had significantly higher extinction scores than the thalamic transplant recipients, which never acquired the CAR to begin with. In sharp contrast, animals with nBM suspension transplants showed improving performance during much of the extinction testing period (FIG. 7); their performance was, in fact, not statistically different from that of sham-lesioned control animals over the 10-day testing period. Thus, these results on active avoidance

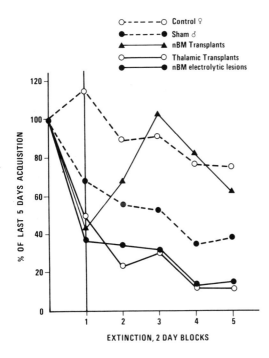

FIGURE 7. Extinction performance during two-way active avoidance testing, expressed as a percentage of the last 5 days of acquisition. The nBM and thalamic transplant groups had previously received bilateral ibotenic acid lesions of the nBM.

testing from an initial group of transplant recipients appeared to indicate that nBM (cholinergic) transplants have the ability to enhance learning and memory performance during shuttle box testing. More recent two-way active avoidance results, however, which were taken from another, larger group of transplant recipients (Arendash *et al.*, unpublished observations), failed to demonstrate an nBM transplant-induced enhancement of learning (acquisition) or memory retention (extinction) compared to thalamic transplant recipients. Neither nBM nor thalamic transplant groups showed improvement in acquisition compared to nBM-lesioned animals. Therefore, our initial results from this test must, at best, be interpreted with caution.

In a third behavioral test, transplant recipients were placed in the start box of a Lashley III maze, which included six alleys. To get a food reward at the end of the maze, weight-reduced recipients had to turn alternately upon going through each of six doors separating the six alleys. Thus, animals could have made alternation errors (turning the wrong way) or door errors (going past a door they should have entered) or both. There were no statistical differences for either type of error between the nBM and thalamic transplant groups during the 25 days of this test. Therefore, no specific enhancement of maze performance was observed for nBM (cholinergic)-transplanted animals compared to thalamic (noncholinergic)-transplanted animals.

Summarizing the behavioral results, it appears that nBM transplants may have the ability to enhance learning or short-term memory processing or both in passive avoidance behavior, although initial nBM transplant-induced enhancements in learning/memory during active avoidance testing could not be replicated. Furthermore, no specific improvement in Lashley III maze performance seemed to be induced by nBM transplants.

DISCUSSION AND CONCLUSIONS

Considerable biochemical and pharmacological evidence supports a fundamental role for central nervous system cholinergic neurons in memory processing.[1,2] Apparently, both major cholinergic systems, the septohippocampal pathway and the nBM-to-cortex pathway, are important for normal memory abilities in that elimination or disruption of either pathway induces substantial cognitive deficits in experimental animals.[13,14,17–19]

Already well documented is the ability of cholinergic-rich septal grafts to enhance hippocampal cholinergic markers and improve spatial learning/memory abilities in fornix-transected rats.[19,20] Similarly, the cholinergic-depleted neocortex of nBM-lesioned rats would appear to be a suitable implantation site for challenging the ability of cholinergic-rich nBM suspensions to alleviate the cortical cholinergic marker deficiencies and learning/memory dysfunction characteristic of the nBM-lesioned rat.

Because extensive areas of neocortex were depleted of their extrinsic cholinergic innervation by nBM lesioning in this study, multiple cortical implants of cholinergic-rich nBM suspension were clearly required if the highest probability for cholinergic reinnervation and improved behavioral performance was to be provided. From a neurohistological standpoint, AChE-positive fiber outgrowth from such nBM suspension transplants was not evident at $1\frac{1}{2}$ months after transplantation, but was extensive throughout much of the frontoparietal cortex within $5\frac{1}{2}$ months after grafting. Within nBM transplants, the identification of cholinergic neurons similar in morphology to those normally present in the basal forebrain suggests that at least some, and perhaps much, of the AChE-positive fiber outgrowth from these transplants was cholinergic in nature. Whether or not such fibers establish classical synaptic connections with the recipient's cortical neurons is not known at present. It is interesting, however, to note that a recent electron microscopy study indicates that ChAT-immunoreactive synapses, presumably from cholinergic neurons within septal implants, establish synaptic connections with cell bodies and dendrites of host hippocampal neurons.[21]

Biochemically, nBM suspension transplants appeared to have the ability to at least partially compensate for the decreased cortical ChAT activity found after nBM lesioning. It should be noted that the entire anterior cortex was assayed for ChAT activity, not just the cortical regions surrounding infusion areas. In this context, a transplant-induced prevention of one-third the decrease in cortical ChAT activity normally associated with nBM lesioning (at $1\frac{1}{2}$ months) indicates that cholinergic neurons within nBM transplants were surviving in reasonable numbers and functioning metabolically. In an earlier study, Björklund et al.[20] found septal suspension transplants, placed within the cholinergic-depleted hippocampus, capable of restoring hippocampal ChAT activity to near normal within 6 months after grafting. Although cortical ChAT activity determinations were made in the present study at $5\frac{1}{2}$ months after cortical transplantation of either nBM or thalamic suspensions, no conclusions could be reached concerning any transplant effects on cortical ChAT activity because subcortical tissues were unavailable for histological verification of nBM lesion effectiveness. Nonetheless, the nBM transplant-induced enhancement of cortical ChAT activity at $1\frac{1}{2}$ months suggests that cholinergic-rich nBM transplants can have a biochemical impact on the cholinergic-denervated cortex.

The behavioral performance of nBM transplant recipients in several tasks of learning and memory abilities was encouraging in several respects, though difficult to interpret in others. Certainly, elimination of the nBM-to-cortex cholinergic pathway through nBM excitotoxic lesioning induces profound deficiencies in a variety of cognitive tasks,[13,14,17] providing an opportunity for cholinergic transplants to have a significant behavioral impact. Cholinergic-rich nBM transplants did, in fact, appear to enhance learning or short-term memory or both in nBM-lesioned recipients during passive avoidance testing at 3 months after transplantation.

Several reasons could explain why our earlier study showed nBM transplant-induced enhancements in the acquisition and retention of active avoidance behavior[13] whereas a later study, in which a second group of animals was tested, did not. First, the second group of graft recipients received two 5-μg infusions of ibotenic acid into each nBM compared to only one infusion bilaterally for each graft recipient in the first group; thus, more substantial neuronal losses within and around the region of the nBM were probably realized in the second group. Second, active avoidance testing for the second group was begun later after lesioning/transplantation and was done during a time when nBM lesion-induced degenerative changes begin to occur in both the neocortex and hippocampus (Arendash et al., unpublished observations).

If the behavioral enhancements seen during passive and active avoidance are due to functioning cholinergic neurons within nBM transplants, acetylcholine release by such transplanted neurons may occur in either of two ways to activate postsynaptic cholinergic receptors: 1) through a nonspecific, diffusionary release of acetylcholine or 2) through establishment of synaptic connectivity with recipient neurons, perhaps filling cortical synaptic spaces that had previously been occupied by cholinergic neurons of nBM origin. As for the mechanism of acetylcholine's action to possibly enhance cognitive function, acetylcholine may be a general "activator" of brain mechanisms facilitatory to the establishment of new learning/memory circuitry. Acetylcholine is, in fact, excitatory to cortical and hippocampal neurons,[22,23] probably by inducing the closure of a specific subset of voltage-sensitive potassium channels via muscarinic transmission.[22,24] Such modulation of excitability by acetylcholine could be exerted over prolonged periods of time through generation of slow excitatory postsynaptic potentials.[22,24]

Future cholinergic transplant studies in nBM-lesioned rats must continue to utilize a variety of avoidance and spatial tasks to more clearly define potential cognitive effects of cholinergic-rich nBM grafts, as well as the specificity of any behavioral effects observed for nBM grafts. Perhaps more robust behavioral effects induced by such nBM transplants would be observed if the lesioned nBM, and not the neocortex, were used as a transplantation site.

Studies designed to investigate the biochemical, neurohistological, and behavioral impact of cholinergic-rich suspensions in nBM-lesioned recipients would appear to have particular relevance for SDAT, in which central nervous system cholinergic dysfunction is probably involved in the disease's pathogenesis and symptomology.[1,2] Since the biochemical and behavioral deficits induced by nBM lesioning mimic those of SDAT to a considerable degree, the continued use of nBM-lesioned recipients in cholinergic transplant studies is warranted. It is hoped that such studies will not only elucidate more fully the involvement of cholinergic neurotransmission in learning and memory processes, but will provide substantial and consistent improvements in such cognitive functions as well.

REFERENCES

1. BARTUS, R., R. DEAN & B. BEER. 1982. The cholinergic hypothesis of geriatric memory dysfunction. Science 217: 408-417.
2. COYLE, J., D. PRICE & M. DELONG. 1983. Alzheimer's disease: A disorder of cortical cholinergic innervation. Science 219: 1184-1190.
3. BOWEN, D., N. SIMS, J. BENTON, G. CURZON, A. DAVISON, D. NEARY & D. THOMAS. 1981. Treatment of Alzheimer's disease: A cautionary note. N. Engl. J. Med. 305: 1016.
4. ROSSOR, M., N. GARRETT, A. JOHNSON, C. MOUNTJOY, M. ROTH & L. IVERSEN. 1982. A postmortem study of the cholinergic and GABA systems in senile dementia. Brain 105: 313-330.
5. WHITEHOUSE, P., D. PRICE, R. STRUBLE, A. CLARK, J. COYLE & M. DELONG. 1982. Alzheimer's disease and senile dementia: Loss of neurons in the basal forebrain. Science 215: 1237-1239.
6. PEARSON, R., M. SOFRONIEW, A. CUELLO, T. POWELL, F. ECKENSTEIN, R. ESIRI & G. WILCOCK. 1983. Persistence of cholinergic neurons in the basal nucleus in a brain with senile dementia of the Alzheimer's type demonstrated by immunohistochemical staining for choline acetyltransferase. Brain Res. 289: 375-379.
7. NAGAI, T., P. MCGEER, J. PENG, E. MCGEER & C. DOLMAN. 1983. Choline acetyltransferase immunohistochemistry in brains of Alzheimer's disease patients and controls. Neurosci. Lett. 36: 195-199.
8. STRUBLE, R., L. CORK, P. WHITEHOUSE & D. PRICE. 1982. Cholinergic innervation in neuritic plaques. Science 216: 413-415.
9. JACOBS, R., N. FARIVAR & L. BUTCHER. 1984. Loss of somata nucleus basalis is correlated positively with magnitude of dementia, severity of pathology, and age of onset of Alzheimer's Disease. Paper presented at the Fourteenth Annual Meeting of the Society for Neuroscience. Anaheim, CA.
10. LEHMANN, J., J. NAGY, S. ATMADJA & H. C. FIBIGER. 1980. The nucleus basalis magnocellularis: The origin of a cholinergic projection to the neocortex of the rat. Neuroscience 5: 1161-1174.
11. JOHNSTON, M., M. MCKINNEY & J. T. COYLE. 1981. Neocortical cholinergic innervation: A description of extrinsic and intrinsic components in the rat. Exp. Brain Res. 43: 159-172.

12. SATOH, K., D. ARMSTRONG & H. C. FIBIGER. 1983. A comparison of the distribution of central cholinergic neurons as demonstrated by acetylcholinesterase pharmacohistochemistry and choline acetyltransferase immunohistochemistry. Brain Res. Bull. **11:** 693-720.
13. ARENDASH, G., P. STRONG & P. MOUTON. 1985. Intracerebral transplantation of cholinergic neurons in a new animal model for Alzheimer's disease. *In* Senile Dementia of the Alzheimer's Type. J. T. Hutton & A. D. Kenny, Eds.: 351-376. Alan R. Liss. New York, NY.
14. MURRAY, C. L. & H. C. FIBIGER. 1985. Learning and memory dificits after lesions of the nucleus basalis magnocellularis: Reversal by physostigmine. Neuroscience **14:** 1025-1032.
15. KARNOVSKY, M. & L. ROOTS. 1964. A "direct-coloring" thiocholine method for cholinesterases. J. Histochem. Cytochem. **12:** 219-221.
16. FONNUM, F. 1969. Radiochemical microassays for the determination of choline acetyltransferase and acetylcholinesterase activities. Biochem. J. **115:** 465-472.
17. FLICKER, C., R. DEAN, D. WATKINS, S. FISCHER & R. BARTUS. 1983. Behavioral and neurochemical effects following neurotoxic lesions of a major cholinergic input to the cerebral cortex in the rat. Pharm. Biochem. Behav. **18:** 973-981.
18. WALKER, J. & D. OLTON. 1984. Fimbria-fornix lesions impair spatial working memory but not cognitive mapping. Behav. Neurosci. **98:** 226-242.
19. DUNNETT, S., W. LOW, S. IVERSEN, U. STENEVI & A. BJÖRKLUND. 1982. Septal transplants restore maze learning in rats with fornix-fimbria lesions. Brain Res. **251:** 335-348.
20. BJÖRKLUND, A., F. GAGE, R. SCHMIDT, U. STENEVI & S. DUNNETT. 1983. Recovery of choline acetyltransferase activity and acetylcholine synthesis in the denervated hippocampus reinnervated by septal suspension implants. Acta Physiol. Scand. Suppl. **522:** 59-66.
21. CLARK, D. & A. BJÖRKLUND. 1986. Formation of cholinergic synapses by intrahippocampal septal grafts as revealed by choline acetyltransferase immunocytochemistry. Brain Res. **369:** 151-162.
22. COLE, A. & R. NICOLL. 1984. Characterization of a slow cholinergic postsynaptic potential recorded *in vitro* from rat hippocampal pyramidal cells. J. Physiol. **352:** 173-188.
23. KRNJEVIC, K., R. PUMAIN & L. RENAUD. 1971. The mechanism of excitation of acetylcholine in the cerebral cortex. J. Physiol. **215:** 247-268.
24. BROWN, D. 1983. Slow cholinergic excitation: A mechanism for increasing neuronal excitability. Trend Neurosci. August: 302-307.

DISCUSSION OF THE PAPER

L. KROMER (*Georgetown University, Washington, DC*): One question about the ChAT determinations in the cortex in both animals that received lesions and animals with transplants: What kind of dissection and what regions of the cortex did you use to measure your enzyme levels?

ARENDASH: We took basically about 70% of the anterior cortex from midline on down to about the rhinal fissure.

KROMER: And did this tissue actually contain the transplanted region itself?

ARENDASH: Yes.

KROMER: So all of your increased ChAT activity could be due solely to ChAT within the transplant and not to outgrowth and the surrounding cortex?

ARENDASH: We really do not know. But we have not just punched out the tissue immediately around the transplant. In fact we were biasing ourselves in the opposite direction by taking so much additional tissue.

Morphological and Behavioral Characteristics of Embryonic Brain Tissue Transplants in Adult, Brain-damaged Subjects[a]

DONALD G. STEIN AND ELLIOTT J. MUFSON[b]

Department of Psychology
Clark University
Worcester, Massachusetts
and
Department of Neurology
Beth Israel Hospital
Boston, Massachusetts

MORPHOLOGIC FEATURES OF FETAL FRONTAL TRANSPLANTS

During the last several years, there has been a resurgence of interest in the ability of implanted fetal central nervous system (CNS) tissue to promote anatomical restoration and return of function to brain-damaged mammals.[1] The parameters underlying functional recovery, however, are not well defined. One important question is whether brain grafts develop morphological characteristics seen in normal intact issue. A second is whether anatomical reorganization with specificity of connections is required for behavioral recovery. Recent studies have provided strong evidence that grafts can correct some of the behavioral impairments resulting from destruction to the adult host brain.[2-6] Experiments conducted in our laboratory show that the learning deficits in spatial alternation resulting from bilateral destruction of the medial frontal cortex are reduced in rats with embryonic frontal cortex grafts.[7] Furthermore, E19 frontal cortex transplanted into animals with bilateral occipital cortex damage partially restores the ability of these animals to perform a brightness discrimination task.[8]

In order to gain greater insight into the factors that may influence functional recovery, it is important to describe the morphologic features of CNS grafts and to determine whether their structural characteristics are required for recovery of function, especially after cortical injuries involving areas that are thought to mediate complex

[a]Portions of the research described in this paper were supported by Contract DGS1-84 with the American Paralysis Association, Contract BPNB 1 RO1 MH39514-01 with the National Institute of Mental Health, the ADRDA Faculty Scholar Award (E. J. M.), Grant NIA AG05134 from the Alzheimer's Research Center, and Clark University.

[b]Present address: Institute for Biogerontology, 13220 North 105th Avenue, Sun City, Arizona 85351.

behaviors. The purpose of this study was to analyze the histologic features of fetal neocortex grafts that we have previously shown to enhance behavioral recovery.

The present anatomical evaluations are based on male Sprague-Dawley (Charles River) rats that were approximately 105 days of age and sustaining bilateral medial frontal cortex aspiration lesions before receiving fetal cortex implants. Seven days after the initial aspiration surgery, the rats were anesthetized and, on this day, according to procedures described previously,[7] received transplants of frontal cortex taken from Sprague-Dawley donors on day 19 of gestation. With a metal rod (tip diameter: 1.0 mm) attached to a 1.0-ml syringe, two pieces of the donor tissue representing frontal cortex from each hemisphere (~ 6 mm^3), bathed in Ringer's solution, were extruded from the syringe approximately 0.5 mm into the wound cavity.

Two months after implantation, rats were perfused with 0.1% glutaraldehyde (TABB)-4% paraformaldehyde (Fisher), 0.1 glutaraldehyde (Kodak)-2% paraformaldehyde (Aldrich), 1% paraformaldehyde-1.25% glutaraldehyde in 0.1 M phosphate buffer (pH 7.4), or 10% formalin. The histological procedures included acetylcholinesterase (AChE) histochemistry, choline acetyltransferase (ChAT) immunohistochemistry, Nissl stains, concurrent Nissl-AChE preparations, Loyez stains, and cytochrome oxidase histochemistry. The methodological details are described in several reports.[9-14]

Microscopic evaluation of Nissl-stained tissue showed that the implantation cavity included mainly the medial frontal cortex (FIG. 1). Formation of the wound cavity produced some damage to the caudate nucleus and the olfactory bulb, however; there was no apparent involvement of the septal region. The transplants from embryonic frontal cortex seen in the implantation cavity were either embedded in the parenchyma of the host brain, forming a continuous bridge connecting the injured hemispheres, or came to lie in the subarachnoid space connected by a tissue stalk to the host cortex (FIGS. 2 & 3).

Light microscopic examination of the graft-host interface showed continuity as well as regions marked by apparent glial proliferation (FIGS. 2 & 3). Border regions separating the graft and host were often observed adjacent to a zone of low neuronal cell density resembling a molecular layer (FIGS. 2B & 3A). We also found marked variation in the internal organization of the grafts. In some cases, the transplant was composed of several cellular islands with no preferential positioning or lamination of neurons (FIG. 2A). In contrast, grafts that were more homogeneous in composition had the appearance of a pseudolaminar organization (FIG. 3A). In these grafts, separate cell aggregates organized in a partial laminar fashion were surrounded by a cellular zone resembling the molecular layer of intact cortex. Nissl-stained tissue demonstrated that the grafts contained large pyramidal and nonpyramidal neurons (FIG. 3B). We also observed binuclear perikarya, neurons with multiple nucleoli, as well as glia scattered throughout the implants (FIG. 3B). In grafted tissue processed with the Loyez stain, we observed bundles of myelinated fibers. The most consistent location of myelinated fiber tracts was along either the interface separating graft subsectors or the host and the graft (FIG. 4). Some areas of the grafts contained narrow fiber tracts that coursed parallel to the long axis of the implant, whereas in other regions fascicles formed swirl-like fiber arrays (FIG. 4A). Furthermore, all implants stained for the enzyme AChE exhibited positive fibers and cell bodies (FIGS. 5 & 6). Control sections treated with butyrylthiocholine were negative for cellular or axonal staining. Unlike normal adult rat cortex, there was no clear laminar organization of AChE. Furthermore, the staining was not uniform within or between grafts. In addition, enzyme-containing fibers were observed crossing the graft-host interface (FIGS. 5A & 5B) as well as within tissue stalks connecting the graft and the host (FIG. 6B). Thionin-counterstained, AChE-reacted grafted tissue revealed that only a few neurons were

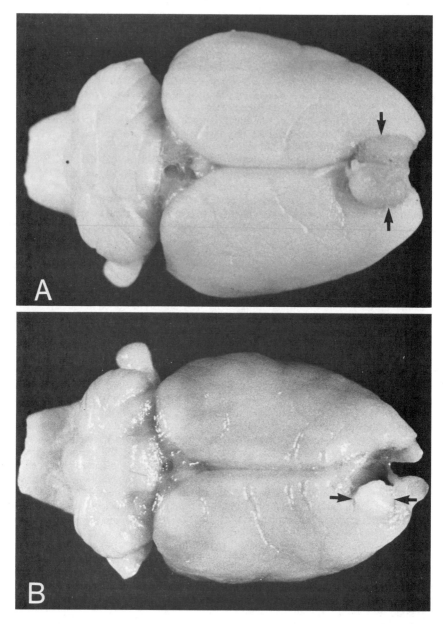

FIGURE 1. Dorsal surface view of two rat brains showing (**A**) bilateral and (**B**) unilateral cortex implants (arrows) positioned within the damaged frontal cortex of the host brain. Original magnifications for **A** and **B**: ×5 and ×4, respectively; figure reduced to 96% of original size.

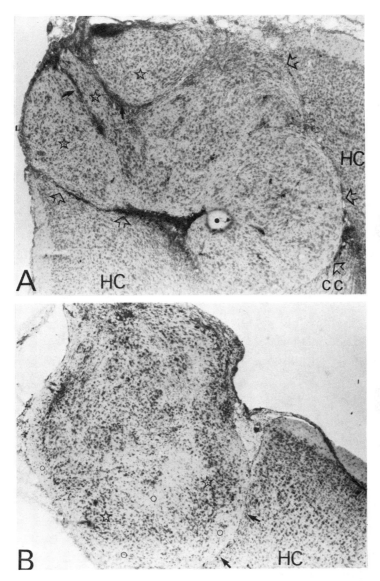

FIGURE 2. Photomicrographs of cresyl violet-stained coronal sections of fetal cortex implants. (**A**) High-power micrograph of the left graft shown in FIGURE 1A. The graft was partially embedded within the parenchyma of the host brain and consists of several lobules (stars) separated by glial scarring (black arrows). Note the nonlaminar arrangement of the graft as compared to the adjacent host cortex (HC). The graft-host border is indicated by open arrows. The black dot indicates a vacuolar space in the graft. Dorsal is toward the left and medial is toward the top. (**B**) Coronal section showing a fetal cortex graft attached to the host cortex. The grafted fetal cortex has a pseudolaminar organization. Note the molecular-like region (open circles) surrounding a zone of neurons arranged in a laminar fashion (open stars). The graft-host border is indicated by black arrows. Dorsal is toward the top and medial is toward the left. Original magnification: ×50; reduced to 61% of original size.

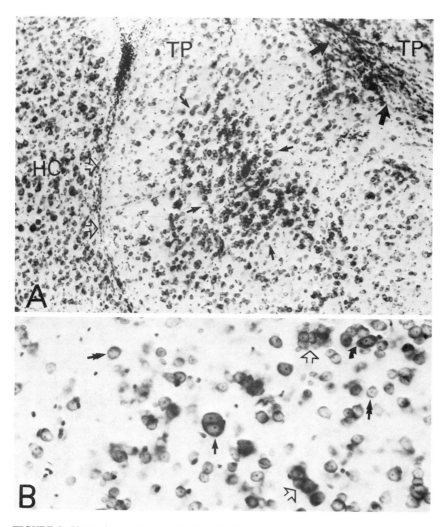

FIGURE 3. Photomicrographs of celloidin-embedded, cresyl violet-stained grafted tissue. (**A**) Transplant (TP) containing a cluster of neurons (small black arrows) surrounded by a relatively cell-free, molecular-like zone. Virtually no glial scarring is seen along the graft-host interface (open arrows). Heavy glial formation separates subdivisions of this transplant (wide black arrows). (**B**) Cresyl violet-stained fetal cortex tissue showing pyramidal-type neurons (curved arrow), small clusters of neurons (open arrow), neurons containing multiple nucleoli (double arrows), and a double-appearing neuron within a single membrane (small black arrow). Original magnifications for **A** and **B**: ×100 and ×200, respectively; figure reduced to 67% of original size.

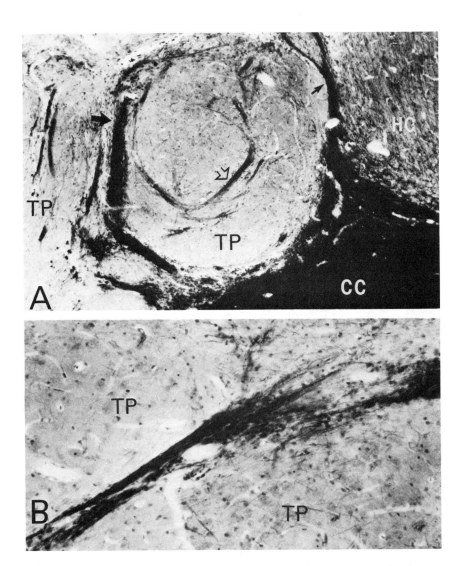

FIGURE 4. Photomicrographs of transplanted tissue stained using the Loyez method for mye-linated fibers. (**A**) Dense accumulation of myelinated fibers (black arrows) along the exterior surface of an implant. Note the bifurcation of a bundle of myelinated fibers (small black arrow) prior to encircling a piece of the implant. Swirls (open arrows) and pencil-thin bundles (curved arrow) of myelinated fibers may be seen coursing within a transplant. (**B**) Myelinated fiber tract coursing between the border region separating subdivisions of a graft. The ends of these tracts branch to form small fascicles before entering the individual transplant lobes. Original magnification: ×50; reduced to 67% of original size.

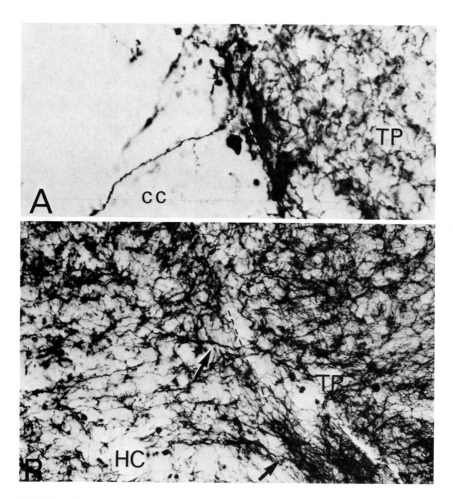

FIGURE 5. Photomicrographs showing the histochemical demonstration of AChE in grafted cortex. (**A**) AChE staining in a transplant that developed adjacent to the corpus callosum (CC). Note the AChE-positive fibers within the corpus callosum coursing toward the implant. White dots indicate the graft-host interface. (**B**) Intense AChE-positive fiber staining in both the host cortex (HC) and adjacent transplant (TP). Positive axons may be seen crossing the border between the host and the transplant (arrows). Original magnification for **A**: ×100; reduced to 70% of original size.

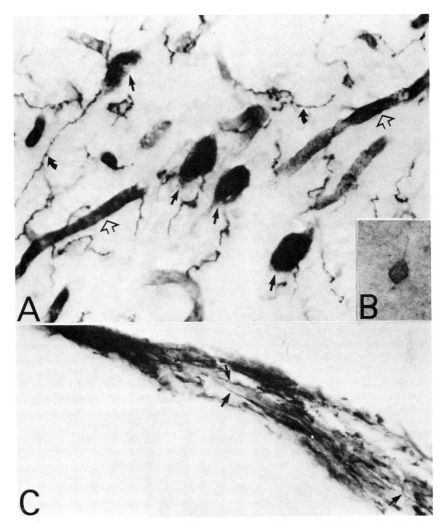

FIGURE 6. (**A**) Photomicrograph of fetal cortex-grafted tissue stained for AChE showing AChE-reactive fibers (curved arrows), neurons (black arrows), and butyrylcholinesterase-positive blood vessels (open arrows). (**B**) Grafted cortical neuron immunohistochemistry stained for ChAT. (**C**) AChE-positive fibers (arrows) coursing within a transplant stalk. Original magnifications for **A** and for **B** and **C**: ×100 and ×200, respectively; figure reduced to 71% of original size.

AChE positive within the implant. AChE-stained fibers were also observed to surround AChE-positive blood vessels (FIG. 6A). This vascular staining was seen in tissue reacted with butyrylthiocholine and acetylthiocholine, indicating that these vessels were butyrylcholinesterase positive. In addition, tissue stained with the monoclonal antibody AB8 for the cholinergic enzyme ChAT revealed only a few positive neurons and axons. Control sections employing nonspecific rat immunoglobulin G in place of the AB8 were negative. These grafted ChAT-immunoreactive neurons were small bipolar cell bodies located primarily in the periphery of each implant (FIG. 6B). This is in marked contrast to the widespread distribution of AChE-positive neurons seen within the grafts.

Staining for the mitochondrial enzyme cytochrome oxidase, which has been suggested to correlate with cell metabolism,[12] revealed that graft metabolic activity was not homogeneous. For example, in the graft shown in FIGURE 7, areas of intense activity were located in its lateral portion as compared to the less intense and more homogeneous reactivity seen in its medial sector. Cytochrome oxidase-reacted tissue counterstained with thionin revealed that the activity patches often corresponded to areas containing circumscribed aggregates of neurons. Since grafted fetal cortex does not appear uniformly active, the zones of highest metabolism may have a greater concentration of neurons or receive greater synaptic input, as suggested by Sharp and Gonzalez.[15] It is also possible that these areas of intense physiological activity produce a neurotrophic substance or substances critical for behavioral recovery.

The present study has demonstrated that E19 frontal cortex implanted into a bilateral frontal cortex wound cavity can survive and differentiate for at least 2 months. Although the grafts of frontal cortex developed adjacent to damaged cortex, they did not exhibit a normal morphological appearance. Instead, the grafts showed a disorganized architectonic arrangement. Despite this lack of normal cortical organization, the implants contained many of the morphologic characteristics of mature cortex. For example, the grafts contained neurons of various sizes, long myelinated axons, AChE- and ChAT-positive fibers and perikarya, and distinct regions of metabolic activity. In fact, some transplants exhibited a crude internal organization with features similar to normal cortical structure, as previously described.[15–18] Furthermore, large pyramidal neurons were scattered among nonpyramidal perikarya in the implants similar to those reported by others.[7,15–18] The nonpyramidal neurons observed in our grafts may correspond to the stellate, spiny, or aspiny perikarya described in Golgi-impregnated tissue from cortical implants.[17,18] As described by Alexandrova and Polezhaev,[19] distributed among these normal-looking perikarya were cell bodies with multiple nucleoli as well as binuclear-appearing neurons. Since most mature neurons have a single nucleolus as compared to the numerous nucleoli that are often seen in developing neurons,[20] it is possible that some of the neuronal perikarya in the grafts may not have responded to or lacked the signals that guide differentiation of young neurons.

Another morphological feature of our cortical grafts is the expression of extensive myelinated axonal bundles. Our findings demonstrated that the heaviest bands of myelinated axons were located along the external regions of the graft similar to that reported in brainstem implants,[21] suggesting that the mechanism or mechanisms guiding the development of myelinated axons in fetal cortical and brainstem grafts may be potentially similar. For instance, in this volume several investigations demonstrate the importance of glial cell proliferation as a matrix for the migration of axons. Interestingly, many of the large myelinated fiber bundles seen in our material were located in areas of extensive glial activity. Therefore, these observations may provide clues as to the processes underlying the normal maturation of long axonal pathways in the CNS of mammals.

ChAT and AChE staining revealed positive fibers and cell bodies distributed within the grafts. ChAT-reacted tissue revealed only a very few perikarya located at the periphery as compared to the more numerous and widely distributed AChE-positive neurons seen in grafts. Interestingly, the distribution of AChE-reactive perikarya has been shown to be widespread throughout all cortical lamina, whereas ChAT-positive neurons are found mainly in the more superficial cortical layers.[11] Perhaps the differential normal cortical distribution of these cell types is reflected in our cortical grafts.

The AChE activity observed in the cortical grafts may have developed intrinsically after implantation or originated from extrinsic sources. Developmental histochemical investigations of rodent cortical AChE indicate that there are very few positive fibers in the newborn, although intense enzyme activity appears by the end of the first postnatal week.[22] AChE-containing perikarya, however, have been described in the

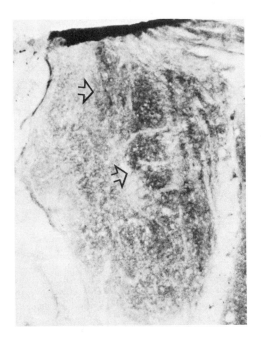

FIGURE 7. Coronal section of grafted fetal cortex showing variations in endogenous cytochrome oxidase activity. Note the dark patches of enzymatic activity (open arrows) located in the medial as compared to the lower levels of activity in the more lateral portions of the graft. Dorsal is toward the top and medial is toward the right. The dark strip across the top is a fold in the tissue. Original magnification: ×10; reduced to 85% of original size.

cortex of newborn rats.[22] Thus, the possibility exists that at least part of the AChE staining observed in the present grafts originated from AChE-positive intrinsic cortical neurons, but it is more likely that there was fiber ingrowth arising from extratransplant areas.

The major extrinsic source of cortical cholinergic input arises from the cholinergic neurons located within the nucleus basalis (Ch4),[9] whereas a minor cortical cholinergic innervation originates from the brainstem cholinergic neurons of the pedunculopontine (Ch5) or the lateral dorsal tegmental (Ch6) nuclei.[23] It is possible, therefore, that the cholinergic axons originating from these cholinergic neuron groups grew to innervate the maturing cortical implant. Interestingly, reinnervation of denervated hippocampus has been demonstrated by AChE and ChAT histochemistry following implantation of embryonic cholinergic septal neurons into animals with damage to the septohippocampal cholinergic pathways.[24] The reinnervation of hippocampus presents in a laminar fashion as opposed to the nonlaminar pattern seen in our neocortical grafts,[25] although AChE is distributed in a layered fashion in adult rodent cortex.[26] Perhaps there are intrinsic developmental neurobiological differences between neo- and allocortex (or in the transplantation procedures used) that may account for these observations. Such results have led to the suggestion that regeneration of axotomized brain perikarya can be initiated by a piece of deafferented embryonic CNS tissue.[27] It has also been shown, however, that trophic factors can influence the growth and survival of various types of neurons and nonneuronal tissue including cholinergic perikarya and implanted adult chromaffin cells.[28] Therefore, it is possible that grafted fetal cortex releases a trophic substance that may promote axonal sprouting or sparing of neurons that would ordinarily die as a result of the injury.

With respect to behavior after frontal cortex grafts, the present as well as previous results[7,8] indicate that normal morphological organization of implanted cortex may not be a necessary prerequisite for restoration of behavioral performance. In fact, we have found that fetal frontal cortex implants are also capable of reducing visual learning impairments in animals with occipital cortex damage, whereas transplanted occipital cortex tissue was less effective in producing recovery of brightness discrimination compared to frontal cortex grafts.[8] These investigations suggest that behavioral improvement may be the result of nonstructural factors related to the grafted tissue. Perhaps fetal cortex grafts induce functional enhancement by the production of some as yet unknown trophic substance.

BEHAVIORAL FEATURES OF FETAL BRAIN TISSUE TRANSPLANTS IN ADULT RATS WITH CORTICAL LESIONS

In the preceding section of this paper, we showed that there are some characteristics of transplanted fetal brain tissue that resemble normal CNS structure. For the most part, however, the implanted tissue does not grow into the typical morphology and structure of the adult organism. Yet, despite the disordered and abnormal cellular relationships seen in the transplants, they are capable of at least partially restoring behavioral capacities to adult recipients that have suffered bilateral brain injuries. We have already shown that implants of fetal frontal cortex taken from embryos on day 21 of gestation can enhance the acquisition of spatial alternation learning in adult rats with frontal cortex injuries.[7]

Our findings should not be that surprising: many investigators, including the contributors to this volume, have shown that injections of dissociated fetal cells can enhance recovery when placed into or near damaged areas of the brain.[29] Although few would argue that integrity of structure is required for mediating functional recovery after the injection of cells, some investigators have suggested that behavioral recovery requires at least the physical integration of the cells with the host brain.[30] Migration of neurons from transplant into host tissue, extension of processes, and synaptic contacts on host dendrites are some of the kinds of integration thought necessary.[31]

Converging lines of evidence argue against the notion that the structural anatomy of neuronal tissue must be maintained in order to promote any type of behavioral recovery. First, as noted above, suspensions of cells can enhance recovery when they have been chemically and mechanically dissociated and then injected into the cerebral ventricles. Second, systemic or intracerebral administration of trophic substances such as GM1 gangliosides[32] or nerve growth factors[33] result in significant behavioral recovery after different types of brain injuries, despite a lack of neuronal replacement. Third, recent work reported in this volume by Nieto-Sampedro and Cotman[34] has shown that injury-induced neurotrophic factors or implants of purified and isolated glial cells can enhance behavioral recovery.

If nonspecific factors such as the trophic substances mentioned above can facilitate recovery, what role then, do the transplants of fetal tissue play? Are specific, neuronal relationships or specific connections necessary to promote functional recovery in all cases? In our laboratory, we decided to explore this problem in several ways. To test the specificity hypothesis, we asked whether implants of embryonic frontal cortex into the damaged occipital cortex of adults could enhance recovery of visual performance. We chose to study restoration of sensory capacity because it is generally thought that damage to the visual system results in profound deficits with virtually no capacity for recovery. Certainly, if specificity of neural connections is important for visual performance, it would be unlikely that the deranged histological features we observed in our embryonic frontal tissue transplants would enhance functional recovery. If, however, implants of embryonic frontal tissue into the damaged occipital cortex of an adult animal could promote recovery, the argument that it is dependent upon specific, anatomical characteristics or connections or both would be seriously weakened.

In our first study,[8] we used 35 male Sprague-Dawley rats that were approximately 100 days of age at the beginning of the experiment. Twenty-seven animals received bilateral aspiration lesions of the occipital cortex, and eight rats served as unoperated controls. After a 1-week postoperative recovery period, the rats with visual cortex lesions were given implants of E19 fetal brain tissue taken from either occipital cortex ($N = 9$) or frontal cortex ($N = 9$). The fetal tissue was obtained using the same procedures we had employed in previous investigations[7] and described in the first part of this paper, except for the fact that we took both anterior and posterior neocortex for transplantation. One group of brain-damaged rats did not receive any transplants, and they served as lesion controls. The fourth control group of animals was anesthetized and had their scalps reopened and resutured at the time the lesion groups received the implants of fetal tissue.

Two weeks after transplantation, all of the animals began testing on a black-versus-white brightness discrimination task followed by a pattern discrimination problem requiring the rats to choose between alternating, horizontal or vertical, black-and-white stripes.[8] In this experiment, implants of frontal, but not occipital fetal cortex facilitated the learning of a brightness discrimination task in adult rats with occipital cortex damage (FIG. 8). Despite significant improvement in the ability of the animals with implants of frontal tissue to learn the brightness discrimination, they did not perform nearly as well as intact controls, and they were as impaired as the lesion-only controls on the pattern discrimination task. We were surprised to find that the frontal but not the occipital implants facilitated recovery of the brightness discrimination even though both types of tissue grew substantially in the host brain lesion cavity.

In interpreting these data, one can argue that the E19 occipital tissue was more differentiated than the frontal cortex at the time of implantation, and that implants of younger occipital tissue might have been more effective in promoting recovery. Although that may indeed be the case, the finding does not detract from the fact that frontal tissue was able to mediate partial restoration of brightness discrimination capacity in animals that would ordinarily be profoundly impaired as a result of the visual cortex removals.

It was also interesting to note that, following injections of wheat-germ agglutinated

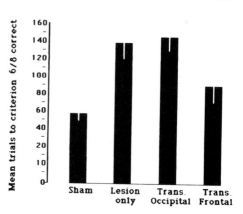

FIGURE 8. Mean trials to criterion (6/8 correct) on brightness discrimination learning task. Animals with implants of frontal cortex are significantly better than both the lesion only and occipital transplant groups.

horseradish peroxidase (HRP) into the transplants, we did not see any retrograde label in the host brain tissue. In one case of leakage of HRP into host tissue, however, we found labeled neurons in the lateral geniculate nucleus; this finding indicated the failure of the HRP reaction in the transplant tissue was not due to artifacts in the reaction.

In considering these findings, it is difficult to argue that neuromorphological specificity and anatomical integration with the host tissue constitute a requisite for promoting functional recovery in cortically brain-damaged adult subjects. It is possible, however, to argue that, as a task, brightness discrimination is not very sophisticated; animals could use subcortical structures to learn the response eventually. Accordingly, we decided to replicate our work by examining the capacity of animals with occipital cortex lesions and implants of embryonic frontal or occipital cortex to learn a brightness discrimination and to discriminate between two kinds of patterns of black-and-white stripes. Following a suggestion by Dr. Fred H. Gage, we pretreated some of our transplant recipients with five injections of 25 mg/kg of the immunosuppressant drug cyclosporin A to reduce the possibility of transplant rejection due to the brain's limited immune response to foreign tissue.

Because albino rats are not visually proficient, we decided to use adult, male, Long-Evans, hooded rats in the second experiment reported here. The surgical procedures were identical to those employed in our previous studies.[7,8] Seven days after the initial injury, three groups of eight animals each received transplants of E19 frontal or occipital cortex directly into the area of injury. As a control for the cyclosporin A, one group with occipital transplants received injections of olive oil. Animals with frontal transplants received only injections of olive oil because they had shown recovery in the first experiment.

All of the animals first began testing on the two-choice brightness discrimination, shock avoidance task 22 days after the initial cortical injury. The animals were given eight trials each day for 20 consecutive days. Following this training, the rats had a 2-week rest period and then began training on a more difficult discrimination task that required them to distinguish between oblique black-and-white alternating stripes (///\\\ ). At the end of this period, the rats were given an additional 20 days of testing on horizontal or vertical black-and-white stripes with avoidance of mild footshock as reinforcement for learning.

As in our previous experiment, we were able to demonstrate that the implants of fetal frontal cortex into the damaged occipital cortex of adult animals enhanced recovery of brightness discrimination ability (FIG. 9). In addition, our results showed, for the first time, that the implants could also improve the brain-damaged rats performance on the horizontal-vertical and the oblique stripe pattern discrimination task. In the group with lesions alone, only one rat was able to learn the task within the time frame of the testing whereas 80% of the rats with frontal transplants and 75% of the rats with occipital transplants were able to perform this task.

In contrast to our first experiment, we now report that the animals with occipital cortex lesions showed recovery of both brightness and pattern discrimination ability when pretreated with cyclosporin A.

Although the occipital transplants were effective, it is worth emphasizing that, once again, the implants of embryonic frontal cortex tissue into the damaged occipital cortex of an adult recipient could facilitate brightness and pattern discrimination. Under such circumstances, it is difficult to conclude that specificity of connections or the presence of homologous tissue (that is, occipital to occipital) is required to obtain some degree of functional recovery after brain injury.

In the present study, examination of the brain tissue showed, in comparison to our first study, that the lesions were large. The damage extended from the medial wall to the posterior cortex anterior to the posterior region of somatosensory cortex. In the dorsal-ventral plane, the lesions removed all of area 18, 17 and 18a, and there was damage to the splenium of the corpus callosum and dorsal hippocampus. We were surprised to find that several months after surgery only a few of the transplants survived and grew in the host cortex. In those cases, the transplants had fewer neurons and more glia than those observed in our previous study.

If, as it now seems, the long-term anatomical integrity of solid fetal brain tissue transplants or their homology to mature cortex are not required to promote recovery, what then, are some of the factors that affect the capacity of transplants to influence recovery from brain damage? From a clinical perspective, one question that needs to be considered is whether the interval between injury and introduction of the transplants is a factor. To study this question, we employed 72 100-day-old male Sprague-Dawley rats. Fifty-eight of the animals received bilateral aspiration lesions of frontal cortex, and the remainder served as sham-operated controls. At 7, 14, 30, and 60 days after the cortical removals, four of the groups ($N = 8$ for each group) were given implants

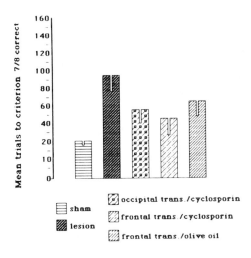

FIGURE 9. Mean trials to criterion (7/8 correct) on a horizontal/vertical, black-and-white, striped pattern discrimination problem. In this experiment all of the fetal brain tissue grafts succeeded in enhancing performance in comparison to rats with occipital cortex lesions alone.

of fetal frontal cortex taken from embryos at day 19 of gestation. All of the lesion or sham controls received a second "sham" operation to control for surgical stress, anesthesia, etc.

Ten days after the transplant operations, squads of rats began testing on the spatial alternation task we used previously.[7] We observed that implants of fetal brain tissue at 7 and 14 days after initial injury could significantly improve acquisition of the spatial task although the animals with transplants did not perform as well as intact controls. The groups of rats receiving the transplants of fetal tissue 30 and 60 days after injury were as impaired as their counterparts with lesions alone (FIG. 10).

Our data from this experiment can be taken to suggest that there is a specific "window of opportunity" during which transplants of embryonic brain tissue can be used to facilitate behavioral recovery from brain injury. It appears that, at least for damage to the frontal cortex, this opportunity lasts for about 2 weeks. During this time, transplants can be used to promote functional recovery. In fact, this period is quite advantageous in comparison to other treatments that are given to promote

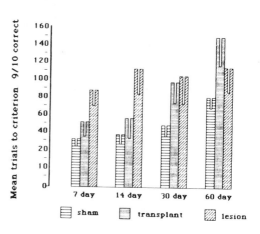

FIGURE 10. Mean trials to criterion (9/10 correct) on spatial alternation learning in rats with frontal cortex lesions given fetal brain tissue implants (E19) at 7, 14, 30, and 60 days after their initial injury. Rats given transplants at 7 and 14 days after injury showed improved performance with respect to animals with lesions only. Transplants made at 30 and 60 days after operation were without effect.

recovery. For example, there is evidence to suggest that intracerebral injections of nerve growth factor are effective only when administered within 1 hr after brain damage.[35] Ganglioside injections, although having the advantage of being injected systemically (intraperitoneally or subcutaneously), seem to be most effective when given within 1-4 hr after trauma.[36] In this context then, implantation of embryonic tissue as a therapy for brain injury may have some advantage because there is more time following injury during which the treatments could be effective.

When we examined the brains from the various groups of animals, we were not surprised to see that the implants of fetal tissue in the 30 and 60 groups were negligible: these groups showed no recovery in comparison to animals with lesions alone. We were surprised, however, when rats in the group that had received implants 14 days after operation, and showed substantial behavioral recovery of spatial alternation, had few surviving transplants. In contrast, the transplants made at 7 days all survived, were relatively large, and developed as described in the first section of this paper.

Given these data, our observations are consistent with reports that fetal brain tissue transplants may work by releasing neurotrophic factors that sustain neurons (or glia) in the host brain.[37] Moreover, since the 14-day group did show substantial recovery in the absence of viable transplants, it may be that the effects of embryonic tissue on recovery are mediated relatively early in the posttraumatic phase of the injury and that the tissue itself (or specific connections between transplant and host) may not always be necessary for maintaining long-term functional recovery. One way to examine this question is to test the animals long after the transplants have been made. Recently, Dunnett and his colleagues[38] replicated our initial results with frontal transplants, but they then went on to show that the spatial alternation deficits returned within 3-4 months in animals with transplants. This is a critical finding because the extent and duration of recovery following brain implants must be substantial if brain tissue implants are to be given serious consideration in a clinical or therapeutic context.[39]

With respect to the question of brain damage and recovery, we now know that there are many factors that can contribute to restitution of function.[40] Although there has been much progress, the specific mechanisms by which fetal brain tissue transplants mediate recovery are not completely understood. Indeed, in some circumstances, factors that are not immediately apparent can contribute to the success or failure of transplants to promote functional recovery.

One such factor is the hormonal state of the organism at the time of injury and transplant. Recent experiments at Clark University indicate that the hormonal state of female rats influences behavioral recovery following frontal cortex injury.

Michael Attella examined the problem of whether circulating levels of progesterone could influence recovery of function of spatial alternation in female rats who had received bilateral injury to the frontal cortex. To influence circulating estradiol and progesterone, Attella rendered two groups of females pseudopregnant by application of both daily vaginal stimulation and dilute silver nitrate solution to the nasal mucosa. One pseudopregnant group was subjected to bilateral medial frontal cortex injury and one group served as an intact control. Two groups of females were allowed normal estrus cycling. One group was then given frontal lesions, and the other served as a normal cycling, intact control.

Two weeks after all surgery had been completed, the animals began testing for retention of preoperatively learned spatial alternation. As FIG. 11 shows, intact animals are completely unaffected in their retention performance regardless of whether they are allowed to cycle normally or are rendered pseudopregnant. In marked contrast, however, the animals that were permitted to cycle normally at the time of surgery and thereafter were profoundly more impaired than animals with higher levels of progesterone caused by the pseudopregnancy condition. We observed this severe deficit on all of our measures of postoperative retention performance.

What are the implications of such findings for transplantation research? One immediate question that comes to mind is as follows: What are the influences of hormonal levels and sex on the replication of our findings as well as those of others? Attella's results suggest that normal cycling actually may render female brain-injured animals far more impaired in their spatial learning performance than pseudopregnant females. Such factors should be given serious consideration when attempting to replicate the behavioral consequences of transplanted neural tissue.

The conclusion to be drawn from our experiments and those of our colleagues working to facilitate recovery from brain injury is that the phenomenon is quite complex and probably involves both neuronal and nonneuronal mechanisms. For instance, when working with the anatomy of fetal tissue transplants, it is tempting to assume that specific neuronal connections between the host brain must be necessary to observe behavioral consequences, but we have already provided and cited evidence to show that this may not always be the case. Instead of forming specific, neural connections, transplants could work by releasing neurotransmitters or neurotrophic factors that exert their effects by activating already present, but relatively ineffective pathways that are related to the damaged system.[41] Under the right physiological conditions, such as deafferentation of a sensory system or transection of afferents from a finger or limb, these "latent" pathways appear within minutes after the injury (that is, long before sprouting or growth of neurons and their processes could take place). Latent pathways and synapses can be demonstrated by recording the shift in the receptive fields of individual neurons in the CNS[42] from one part of the body to another. If such pathways are implicated in behavioral recovery, fetal tissue transplants and administration of neurotrophic substances (or transmitter replacement) could work by providing the chemical input necessary to stimulate their operation, and this might be accomplished without the need for specific connections between the transplant and the host brain.

Although this hypothesis is quite speculative, the activation of "silent" pathways by neurotrophic factors could be one of the mechanisms by which nonspecific transplants, or transplants that do not last for a long time in the host brain, exert their effects.

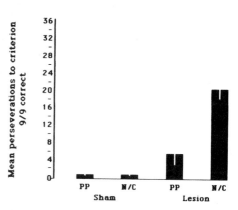

FIGURE 11. Postoperative retention performance in normal cycling, pseudopregnant, female rats with frontal cortex lesions. Pseudopregnant females are significantly better in retention than normal cycling counterparts. The estrus cycle has no effect on performance of intact rats.

Despite the growing interest in recovery from brain injury, we are really just beginning to understand and appreciate some of the parameters that are involved in the process of repair and restoration of function after brain injury. Although we all have predilections that guide our thinking and research, the complexity of CNS functioning practically guarantees that no single approach is likely to provide a "magic bullet" that will cure all aspects of brain damage. Although our task may be more difficult, we might rejoice in the fact that so many possibilities to promote CNS plasticity do exist.

ACKNOWLEDGMENTS

We would also like to express our appreciation to Arthur Firl, Randy Labbe, Amy Nattinville, and Mike Attella for their assistance in the conduct of this experiment.

REFERENCES

1. BJÖRKLUND, A. & U. STENEVI. 1984. Intracerebral nigral implants: Neuronal replacement and reconstruction of damaged circuitries. Annu. Rev. Neurosci. **7:** 279-308.
2. FREED, W. J., M. J. PERLOW, F. KAROUM, A. SEIGER, L. OLSON, B. J. HOFFER & R. J. WYATT. 1980. Restoration of dopaminergic function by grafting of fetal rat substantia nigra to caudate nucleus: Long-term behavioral, biochemical, and histochemical studies. Ann. Neurosci. **8:** 510-520.
3. BJÖRKLUND, A. & U. STENEVI. 1979. Reconstruction of the nigrostriatal dopamine pathway by intracerebral nigral transplants. Brain Res. **177:** 555-560.
4. DUNNETT, S. B., W. C. LOW, S. D. IVERSEN, U. STENEVI & A. BJÖRKLUND. 1982. Septal transplants restore maze learning in rats with fornix-fimbria lesions. Brain Res. **251:** 335-348.
5. GAGE, F. H., A. BJÖRKLUND, U. STENEVI, S. B. DUNNETT & P. A. T. KELLY. 1984. Intrahippocampal septal grafts ameliorate learning impairments in aged rats. Science **225:** 533-536.
6. FINE, A., S. B. DUNNETT, A. BJÖRKLUND & S. D. IVERSON. 1985. Cholinergic ventral forebrain grafts into the neocortex improve passive avoidance memory in a rat model of Alzheimer's disease. Proc. Natl. Acad. Sci. U.S.A. **82:** 5227-5230.
7. LABBE, R., A. FIRL, JR., E. J. MUFSON & D. G. STEIN. 1983. Fetal brain transplants: Reduction of cognitive deficits in rats with frontal cortex lesions. Science **221:** 470-472.
8. STEIN, D. G., R. LABBE, A. FIRL, JR. & E. J. MUFSON. 1985. Behavioral recovery following implantation of fetal tissue into mature rats with bilateral cortical lesions. *In* Neural Grafting in the Mammalian CNS. A. Björklund & U. Stenevi, Eds.: 605-614. Elsevier. Amsterdam.
9. MESULAM, M. M., E. J. MUFSON, A. I. LEVEY & B. H. WAINER. 1983. Cholinergic innervation of cortex by the basal forebrain: Cytochemistry and cortical connection of the septal area, diagonal band nuclei, nucleus basalis (substantia innominata), and hypothalamus in the rhesus monkey. J. Comp. Neurol. **214:** 170-197.
10. MUFSON, E. J., T. L. MARTIN, D. C. MASH, B. H. WAINER & M. M. MESULAM. 1986. Cholinergic projections from the parabigeminal nucleus (Ch8) to the superior colliculus in the mouse: A combined analysis of horseradish peroxidase transport and choline acetyltransferase immunohistochemistry. Brain Res. **370:** 144-148.
11. LEVEY, A. I., B. H. WAINER, D. B. RYE, E. J. MUFSON & M. M. MESULAM. 1984. Choline acetyltransferase-immunoreactive neurons intrinsic to rodent cortex and distinction from acetylcholinesterase-positive neurons. Neuroscience **13:** 341-353.
12. WONG-RILEY, M. T. T. 1979. Changes in the visual system of monocularly sutured or enucleated cats demonstrated with cytochrome oxidase histochemistry. Brain Res. **171:** 11-28.
13. STERNBERGER, L. A. 1979. Immunocytochemistry. 2nd ed.: 104-169. John Wiley & Sons. New York, NY.
14. HEDREEN, J. C., S. J. BACON & D. L. PRICE. 1985. A modified histochemical technique to visualize acetylcholinesterase-containing axons. J. Histochem. Cytochem. **30:** 134-140.
15. SHARP, F. R. & M. F. GONZALEZ. 1984. Fetal frontal cortex transplant [^{14}C]2-deoxyglucose uptake and histology: Survival in cavities of host rat brain motor cortex. Neurology **34:** 1305-1311.
16. JAEGER, C. B. & R. D. LUND. 1980. Transplantation of embryonic occipital cortex to the tectal region of newborn rats: A light microscopic study of organization and connectivity of the transplants. J. Comp. Neurol. **194:** 571-597.
17. DAS, G. D., B. H. HALLAS & K. G. DAS. 1980. Transplantation of brain tissue in the brain of rat. I. Growth characteristics of transplants from embryos of different ages. Am. J. Anat. **158:** 135-145.
18. FLOETER, M. U. & E. J. JONES. 1984. Connections made by transplants to cerebral cortex of rat brains damaged *in utero*. J. Neurosci. **4:** 141-150.
19. ALEXANDROVA, M. A. & L. V. POLEZHAEV. 1984. Transplantation of various regions of embryonic brain tissue into the brain of adults. J. Hirnforsch. **25:** 89-97.

20. JACOBSON, M. 1978. Differentiation, Growth and Maturation of Neurons: Developmental Neurobiology: 115-180. Plenum. New York, NY.
21. KROMER, L. F., A. BJÖRKLUND & U. STENEVI. 1983. Intracephalic embryonic neural implants in the adult rat brain. I. Growth and mature organization of brainstem, cerebellar, and hippocampal implants. J. Comp. Neurol. 218: 433-459.
22. KRISTT, D. A. 1979. Development of neocortical circuitry: Histochemical localization of acetylcholinesterase in relation to cell layers of rat somatosensory cortex. J. Comp. Neurol. 186: 1-16.
23. MUFSON, E. J., A. I. LEVEY, B. H. WAINER & M. M. MESULAM. 1982. Cholinergic projections from the mesencephalic tegmentum to neocortex in rhesus monkey. Abstr. Soc. Neurosci. 8: 965.
24. KROMER, L. F., A. BJÖRKLUND & U. STENEVI. 1981. Innervation of embryonic hippocampal implants by regenerating axons of cholinergic septal neurons in the adult rat. Brain Res. 210: 153-171.
25. COTMAN, C. W. 1984. Specificity of termination fields formed in developing hippocampus by fibers from transplants. In Neural Transplants. J. R. Sladek, Jr. & D. M. Gash, Eds.: 305-324. Plenum. New York, NY.
26. JOHNSTON, M. V., M. MCKENNEY & J. T. COYLE. 1981. Neocortical cholinergic innervation: A description of extrinsic and intrinsic components in the rat. Exp. Brain Res. 43: 159-172.
27. STENEVI, U., A. BJÖRKLUND & L. F. KROMER. 1984. Use of CNS implants to promote regeneration of central axons across denervating lesions in the adult rat brain. In Neural Transplants. J. R. Sladek, Jr. & D. M. Gash, Eds.: 325-360. Plenum. New York, NY.
28. HEFTI, F., J. HARTIKKA & W. FIRCH. 1985. Gangliosides alter morphology and growth of astrocytes and increase the activity of choline acetyltransferase in cultures of dissociated septal cells. J. Neurosci. 5: 2086-2094.
29. BRUNDIN, P., O. ISACSON, F. H. GAGE, U. STENEVI & A. BJÖRKLUND. 1985. Intracerebral grafts of neuronal cell suspensions. In Neural Grafting in the Mammalian CNS. A. Björklund & U. Stenevi, Eds.: 51-60. Elsevier. Amsterdam.
30. SOTELO, C. & R. M. ALVARADO-MALLART. 1985. Cerebellar transplants: Immunocytochemical study of the specificity of Purkinje cells' inputs and outputs. In Neural Grafting in Mammalian CNS. A. Björklund & U. Stenevi, Eds.: 205-216. Elsevier. Amsterdam.
31. CLARKE, D. 1986. Cholinergic synapses after basal forebrain transplantation into young and aged hippocampus. Ann. N.Y. Acad. Sci. This volume.
32. SABEL, B., G. DUNBAR & D. G. STEIN. 1984. Gangliosides minimize behavioral deficits and enhance structural repair after brain injury. J. Neurosci. Res. 12: 429-443.
33. HART, T., N. CHAIMAS, R. MOORE & D. G. STEIN. 1978. Effects of nerve growth factor on behavioral recovery following caudate nucleus lesions in rats. Brain Res. Bull. 3: 245-250.
34. NIETO-SAMPEDRO, M. & C. COTMAN. 1986. Production of neurotrophic factors by conditioning lesion before transplantation. Ann. N.Y. Acad. Sci. This volume.
35. STENEVI, U., B. BJERRE, A. BJÖRKLUND & W. MOBLEY. 1974. Effects of localized intracerebral injections of nerve growth factor on the regenerative growth of lesioned central nonadrenergic neurons. Brain Res. 69: 217-234.
36. LI, Y. S., S. P. MAHADEK, M. M. RAPPORT & S. E. KARPIAK. Acute effects of GM1 ganglioside: Reduction in both behavioral asymmetry and loss of Na$^+$, K-ATPase after nigrostriatal transection. Brain Res. In press.
37. CUNNINGHAM, T. 1986. Specific trophic effects of transplanted target cells on host cells of different ages. Ann. N.Y. Acad. Sci. This volume.
38. DUNNETT, S. B., C. N. RYAN, P. D. LEVIN, M. REYNOLDS & S. T. BUNCH. 1987. Functional consequences of embryonic neocortex transplanted to rats with prefrontal cortex lesions. In preparation.
39. BACKLUND, E.-O., L. OLSON, Å. SEIGER & O. LINDVALL. 1987. Toward a transplantation therapy in Parkinson's disease: A progress report from continuing clinical experiments. Ann. N.Y. Acad. Sci. This volume.
40. FINGER, S. & D. G. STEIN. 1982. Brain Damage and Recovery: Research and Clinical Perspectives. Academic Press. New York, NY.

41. WALL, P. D. 1977. The presence of ineffective synapses and the circumstances which unmask them. Philos. Trans. R. Soc. London, Ser. B. **278:** 361-372.
42. MERZENICH, M. M., J. H. KAAS, J. T. WALL, M. SUR, R. J. NELSON & D. J. FELLEMAN. 1983. Progression of change following median nerve section in the cortical representation of the hand in areas 3b and I in adult owl and squirrel monkeys. Neuroscience **10:** 639-665.

DISCUSSION OF THE PAPER

D. M. GASH (*University of Rochester, Rochester, NY*): Looking at your data, I was not sure whether cyclosporin A had a positive effect or not. I did not see all your controls, for instance. Did you find that cyclosporin A on the occipital transplants did indeed give you the most amelioration?

STEIN: Exactly. It seems that the cyclosporin A compared to olive oil injections had no impact whatsoever on the frontal transplants, but did seem to ameliorate recovery in animals that had been given the occipital transplants.

GASH: Your slides did not show the olive oil control.

STEIN: No, and that is because we did not do it. We remembered—and it is always easy to have an explanation in hindsight—that in our first study we did not see any effects whatsoever from the occipital transplants. We were trying to see specifically if we could have an effect in the occipital region. We thought the frontal cortex would work. In retrospect, we should have had the appropriate control and had it in the group for the frontal cortex experiments.

J. P. MCALLISTER (*Temple University, Philadelphia, PA*): Do you have any other observations on your striatal lesions with the ganglioside and transplants specifically in terms of locomotor behavior or sensory motor behavior?

STEIN: Yes, we do. First, we did not do striatal transplants, and we did not do a combined ganglioside-transplant study. This is strictly with intrasystemic injections of gangliosides. Gangliosides worked after an entorhinal cortex lesion. In Karpiak's hands, they work after nigrostriatal transections. Gangliosides appear to do two things. First, they appear to reduce cerebral edema immediately after injury. Second, they seem to promote sparing of neurons in the substantia nigra and in the ventral tegmental area. You can get that effect with roughly 15 days of intraperitoneal injections of this substance. We also noted that in an earlier study that direct injection of 125 biological units of NGF per side of 2.5s NGF directly into the caudate nucleus immediately after injury produces substantial recovery on a spatial reversal test.

One of the things we found with these ganglioside injections or with NGF is that the time interval that you have, let us call it a window of opportunity after injury, is much more restricted than with the transplants. At least we know we can get functional recovery 14 days after injury. We see that if you wait 4 or 6 hours after our ganglioside treatments, they lose their ability to have any effect. Evidently these are important differences, or so it seems so far.

QUESTIONER: I had the impression from one of the slides shown early in your presentation that at 60 days the animals receiving transplants were significantly worse than those that did not get the transplants.

STEIN: They were not significantly worse.

QUESTIONER: They just looked like that.

STEIN: No, just variance.

S. B. DUNNETT (*Cambridge University, England*): I was intrigued that in the study you reported that the survival was very poor with a 30- to 60-day delay. At what age was the fetal donor tissue taken?

STEIN: This is a critical variable. The animals were E20, so we have not gone back to see whether younger tissue or adding more tissue, for example, would have had better consequences. These are basically E20 animals, and I think it is a legitimate question to know what would happen if we used younger tissue. I think it is an empirical question that has to be addressed.

DUNNETT: The younger tissue does survive just as well at 30 days.

STEIN: I think you have to deal with strain differences as well as some procedural differences. We really had terrible survival with longer delays, and quite good survival in the 7-day group, so I do not think it is something we are doing wrong per se in our laboratory. I do not have a better answer for you at this time. We did, however, go back in our long-surviving animals and make a small priming lesion to see if in fact the animals with the second priming lesion would do better. We did not get statistically significant results. I hate to say this, but it looked as if the priming lesion aided transplant survival somewhat and tended to make the animals perform better. But with only 10 animals per group, we did not have enough to achieve statistical significance with an analysis of variance.

M. K. HAMMOCK (*George Washington University, Washington, DC*): When did you first notice apparent improvement in function after your transplantation?

STEIN: We begin testing about 7 days after the implants are placed into the brain. It is probably unlikely that you are going to get much in the way of host transplant outgrowth and ingrowth, although we see that in our transplants. We begin to see the animals separating if you plot them out over time and look at the day-by-day analysis of the number of errors, for example, in the maze. You begin to see differences emerge at about the 8th and 10th day or even earlier, so it is quite early on. And with gangliosides you see similar effects.

HAMMOCK: Your photographs seem to show isolated islands of transplanted tissue. What physiologic modus operandi could give this apparent improvement?

STEIN: We have also seen isolated islands in adjacent sections. I think it is very much like what other people have said at this meeting yesterday: what is probably going on is that the transplants are releasing neurotrophic factors, as yet unspecified, which probably work to promote neuronal survival in the remaining host brain. I always feel uncomfortable as a psychologist talking about a specific target area. We have tried to count cells in different projection areas, but one of the things that you have to realize is that even on a task as "simple" as, say, a spatial alternation problem, you are dealing with a number of different sensory and motor capacities. It really is a very difficult kind of problem to determine exactly what the specific locus of that behavior is and where the fundamental changes and brain organization might be taking place that lead to the restitution of these relatively complex behaviors.

Summary and Discussion

R. T. Bartus (*American Cyanamid Company, Pearl River, NY*): I would like to thank all the speakers for their scintillating and provocative talks, for tolerating our iron fist, and for keeping our schedule.

Given the way we have pushed everybody along this afternoon, I am now a little embarrassed to spend time myself. However, the conference organizers have asked me, as someone not directly involved in the research discussed in this session, to provide some "fresh insights," a general overview of the significance of the research, and an unbiased opinion of how future work should progress. Dr. Butler and I will each make some comments; we hope they will be provocative enough to stimulate some discussion.

My first impression is that the expectations that have been raised by progress in this area over the past decade are analogous to the expectations raised by the progress of the New York Mets during the same period. Both brain transplantation research and the rebuilding of the Mets did not attract much attention at first; however, both in this research and for the Mets, small successes began to accumulate over the years and interest began to grow. When people began to be excited over the possibilities, their expectations seemed to be justified by even more successes. It seemed that everyone, except for the most critical skeptics, began to have great expectations. Even the press became caught up in the excitement.

But, alas, as success has continued expectations have become so great that in certain ways we have come full circle. Every complication and every new, unexplained wrinkle is now perceived to be some sort of failure. Perhaps it is just that too many of us have expected too much too soon.

Leaving this demonstration of how unrealistic expectations can lead to disappointment as a backdrop, I would like to give an overview of the work and how it may progress in the future. But first let me say how impressed I am by the progress and the elegance of the work that has been presented here. This work represents one of the most exciting areas of neurobiology, and I have to admit to being just a little jealous of those more intimately involved. It is rather fun, however, to see what is going on. I am intrigued and excited about the possibilities, not only with regard to the understanding and formulation of more basic and fundamental principles of what neural function is all about, but with regard to possible therapeutic benefits.

At the risk of oversimplifying and of being presumptuous about the purposes of the people actually doing the work, I would say that there are four general areas of interest. The first area is the accumulation of basic experimental information regarding neural function. Of course, there is tremendous evidence that this approach has already been useful. The survival of neural tissue that could remain viable and functional over periods of time would have been unthinkable until recently—as recent as my years in graduate school. But these properties have been well established, as the studies presented at this conference have demonstrated. We have also seen work that has defined and quantified the factors influencing survival. This is very important work, and it has increased and will continue to increase our insight into how the nervous system really works.

The second area is the identification of new subjects of inquiry—spin-offs from attempts to implant brain tissue into the nervous system. Two new subjects have already emerged: neural trophic factors and the migration and function of astrocytes. Neural trophic factors and their specificities alone represent a whole new realm of inquiry, one that is independent of actually using brain tissue as a means of correcting function of studying changes in the brain. The migration and the function of astrocytes have been largely ignored, except by small islands of investigators. It is an interesting area, however, and I will be curious to see the results obtained by people studying whether functional recovery may be induced by simply transplanting astrocytes themselves.

The third area is something I would call replacement therapy. One kind of replacement therapy—brain tissue transplantation—could provide a means of correcting age-related deficits and other sorts of neural degenerative problems.

Tissue transplantation may seem the best way to restore lost neural transmitter function for several reasons: you may have a more specific site of action; you may have a degree of biological self-control over neural transmitter release because of autoreceptors; you may be able to minimize the adverse effects of transplantation by taking advantage of this specificity and self-control; and you may have, in a particular graft, a piece of tissue containing actual multiple neural transmitters. Tissue transplantation could offer the most biologically relevant way of replacing whatever may be lost.

Unfortunately, we do not really know what the risks and benefits of tissue transplantation are in comparison to other treatments. Until we do, we will not be able to adequately weigh the moral, ethical, and legal issues raised by this technique. Direct comparisons of the kind performed by Dr. Collier and his colleagues would be very useful. They found, much to their disappointment, that an Alza pump was just as effective as tissue grafts. I do not think tissue transplantation should be applied to humans until we can demonstrate that this technique has some clear advantages as a means of replacement therapy.

The fourth issue—the "Big Daddy" of the whole thing—is functional reinnervation. We have heard a number of concepts being thrown around about functional transplantation and have been told of there being some sort of functional reinnervation of the lesion site. Assertions such as these have yet to be adequately scrutinized, and I must say, at the risk of sounding like an adversary, that some results seem to have been cavalierly interpreted.

What has really captured the imagination of the neural science community is the idea that you may actually be able to repair a damaged brain. This is the area that is the most difficult to study; this is the area, if my impressions of what I have heard today and read in the literature are correct, that investigators have yet to address directly. Certainly, careful analyses of whether tissue survives and remains functionally viable are necessary, and interesting in themselves, but these analyses are not sufficient. What would be more impressive is if the analyses also demonstrated whether recovery of biological functions is due to functional innervation. There are many difficulties with this type of analysis. For example, Dr. Azmitia has shown that certain factors exist which may be missing in aged brain, thus providing recovery of some functions but not others. You may be able to have the tissue survive but not provide behavioral recovery. The demonstration by Björklund and Gage of a possible difference in response to drug treatment at least allows for the tantalizing possibility that the tissue graft may be doing more than simply providing a biologic Alza pump. But it would be interesting to know whether or not the complete dose-response is shifted versus only a single dose being affected. Additionally, is the response to drugs merely quantitatively different or is it qualitatively different, as might be expected from functional reinnervation?

The problems of functional reinnervation, difficult as they are, need to be addressed more directly and more aggressively by this research community. Evidence of morphological reinnervation does not satisfy the question of functional reinnervation. People have shown that synapses in reinnervated tissue are qualitatively different from those that would normally be seen. Evidence of morphological reinnervation merely satisfies the first important step in trying to demonstrate the existence of functional reinnervation.

Recovery of behavior is an important objective, but, once accomplished, would still not provide proof of functional reinnervation. Functional reinnervation seems to be influenced by many different factors, some of which have been mentioned today. For example, behavior can spontaneously recover without any transplant at all. Additionally, transplanted astrocytes or neurotrophic factors systemically floating through the body can produce improvement in some behaviors. Although it should be our ultimate goal, functional recovery should not be taken as evidence of functional reinnervation.

Dr. Segal's work with electrophysiology provides a very elegant opportunity to look at these things more clearly. We need not be content with taking a retina and implanting it on the superior colliculus, although obviously this was done for many clear and important reasons. But in terms of functional reinnervation, I would like to see someone create a lesion in the superior colliculus, show a clear visual deficit, put neonatal superior colliculus tissue into the brain, stimulate the eyeball, and show the evoked response in the cortex. That would be functional reinnervation! Of course, we are a long way from doing this, but something of the kind will have to be accomplished if we are going to satisfy this last issue.

There are a lot of controls that could be done: a lesion of the graft site after recovery could be interesting. What sort of effects might we see? If Don Stein is correct in some of his surmises, and if I am correct in what he is surmising, we might see there is no loss in function after creating a lesion in the graft. If we find that function persists, we will have to change the way we think about these things. I have already mentioned that the use of astrocytes and drugs as tools or as relative controls will be necessary.

The whole role of neurochemistry has been ignored in this area, not only postsynaptically to the graft. People have elegantly shown that there is a nice innervation between the axons of the graft and the cell bodies of the host. What about the other side of that functional reinnervation? What about the cell bodies of the graft being reinnervated by the axons of the host? I am not sure how many people are really looking at this. It is a critical necessity for demonstrating functional reinnervation. In summary, the progress accomplished in this area has been genuinely impressive, and the contribution to neuroscience quite significant. At the same time, a tremendous amount of work remains to be done.

R. BUTLER (*Mount Sinai School of Medicine, New York, NY*): I join Dr. Bartus in congratulating the organizers of what has been an excellent set of presentations this afternoon. Like Dr. Bartus, I am not part of this research community: it is the reason I was asked to speak here. I am a gerontologist, a psychiatrist, and a former director of a large research enterprise.

Although rodent models were stressed in this session, it is worth noting that research on possibly uniquely human diseases such as Alzheimer's disease may require nonhuman primate models. We should take advantage of every opportunity to again invoke the Institute of Laboratory Animal Resources of the National Academy of Sciences to look at a variety of animal models for relevant processes and disabilities that bear upon aging. This work needs to be brought to the attention of people in this particular research community.

Moreover, the absence of definitive biomarkers of aging may help to confound some of the work that would endeavor to deal with models of aging, dementia, and neurodegenerative diseases.

No pun intended, but the differentiation of aging and disease really is a gray area!

With regard to differentiation, to what degree is it a quantitative matter? To what degree is there a qualitative difference? How much does one become the other? In a given quantitative step, does aging or accelerated aging become disease or disability?

It certainly seems clear, both from the discussions today and from the data and writings that are available, that we can no longer think of Alzheimer's disease as a single neurodeficiency disease, or as a single-site disease, but as a multiple-site, multiple neurotransmittor deficiency disease.

It struck me this afternoon that many people seemed to describe aging as the result of some kind of deficiency. Many decrements that occur with age were mentioned, but it seemed no one was adventurous enough to look at aging as a multiple pack of processes, and not as a single process. It might be worth bringing to your attention an important symposium we are helping to cosponsor with the American Museum of Natural History, the National Institute on Aging, and the Mount Sinai School of Medicine. It will be held from the 3rd to the 6th of June, and will bring together various biologists in the field of aging. We hope to begin to look more seriously at utilizing the new recombinant DNA and hybridoma technologies, to reexamine a variety of theories of aging, and to see what the future directions might be.

All of these comments meant to be responsive to the differentiation that was discussed this afternoon. Perhaps some of the knowledge we will gain from studying the biochemistry of aging and the biochemistry of repairability will help us to better understand differentiation, growth, aging, and ultimate death. We may come to write about gerontogenes as much as we write about oncogenes.

I would like, in addition to making remarks from the clinical perspective, to make a few remarks from the perspective of health and science policy. Personally, I find it somewhat unattractive to talk about "wars" on things—the war on cancer or the war on Alzheimer's disease. I do not like to oversell science. However, it is worth looking back on the impact of the war on cancer and noting the degree to which our understanding of cell biology and molecular biology has been dramatically enhanced since 1972. And it may simply be a matter of need, particularly in this era of Gramm-Rudman-Hollings, that we have to focus upon a few neurodegenerative diseases and make them national health science priorities in order to garner the type of research funds that we need in order to study and advance basic neurobiology. We really are at a stage where we can begin to build a great body of knowledge, but we must attract adequate support for the basic science of neurobiology.

Perhaps Dr. Stein's presence helped to stimulate these thoughts. He did, after all, help create the National Coalition for Science and Technology, and all of us, whatever we do, would benefit from a greater commitment to the support of science. We rely on a continuous infusion of trained people and on the availability of resources—primate colonies, rodent colonies, cell lines in Camden at the Institute of Medical Research—wherever we need to do what we aspire to do.

I would conclude by saying that although we now have a solid body of knowledge with which to work, we do seem to be a way yet from intervening in ways that would bring hope to people.

R. J. WYATT (*National Institute of Health, Washington, DC*): I think the major issue for grafting—and this is really in response to Dr. Butler's comments—is the issue of definition of function. Function is not an ERG and it is not an electromyogram and it is not a reinnervation of the graft by reciprocal axons. Function is vitality and the ability to move. To function is to be able to think and to be able to sense. This is an important definition, and one that should be kept fairly clean.

M. SEGAL (*Weizmann Institute, Rehovot, Israel*): I have come out of this session a little bit puzzled; I do not quite understand how these things actually work. For example, Dr. Collier finds a 20% decrease in norepinephrine content in the locus ceruleus. Anybody who has created lesions in the locus ceruleus knows that unless you cut 95% of locus ceruleus you do not get a behavioral deficit. You do not. Now you look at aging animals, and they show a 20% difference in norepinephrine content. And in the presentation on the cholinergic system there was about a 20% decrease in cholinergic innervation of the hippocampus. In these two animal models, you take a piece of tissue and you reinnervate or you innervate—you do something—and you get a tremendous behavioral recovery.

Dr. Arendash talked about injections into the cortex. He found a very small recovery of cholinesterase and 5 to 6 square millimeters of reinnervated tissue in the cortex. About 10% of the entire cortex was reinnervated, and he found good behavioral recovery. But implantation itself causes damage. All the pictures we have seen today show damage in the cortex. What is happening here? I am really puzzled. All of the talks in this session presented results that are just contrary to my idea of how this thing should go.

G. ARENDASH (*University of South Florida, Tampa, FL*): I could speak, perhaps, about the cholinergic system. Although it is true, as I presented, that by 1½ months one does not have extensive outgrowth of the cholinergic fibers, one does have outgrowth by 6 months. We do multiple transplants by making eight injections into the frontal parietal cortex. The innervation that results is rather extensive, and can completely eliminate the cholinergic deficit, which is on the order of 50% in the cortex. I disagree that there is substantial damage induced by the Hamilton microliter syringe, even if as many as eight injections are made. In any event, damaged cortex would represent a small amount of the total cortical area. If we were transplanting into the substantia nigra or some other small structure, we would have to be more concerned about damaged tissue. When trying to innervate a structure as large as the cortex, however, the amount of damage is acceptable.

S. B. DUNNETT (*University of Cambridge, England*): You have to distinguish between the volume of the injection and the volume of the graft after it has grown. The injection volume is quite small. If you made lesions this size you would see very little damage. However, a graft several months older would be larger. If you made lesions this size you would probably have a very disruptive influence.

I should also say the extent of outgrowth is greater than you are suggesting. For any one graft, one usually makes a conservative estimate of size: a 1 millimeter radius, for example. The area of the graft may actually be 4 millimeters. Multiply this area by the number of grafts—six in my case, eight for Dr. Arendash—and you would find that your grafts may have extended to quite a big area. Having said this, I still find it amazing that these things work. I have to wonder with you.

T. COLLIER (*University of Rochester Medical School, Rochester, NY*): I agree that it seems strange that a 20% deficit could create the effect. I must tell you again, however, that this deficit is a measure of relative intensity, and that I do not really know biochemically if it is actually a larger measure or, for that matter, a smaller one. There is pretty strong evidence that the noradrenergic receptors in the aged brain are changing their ability to react to deficits, and it could be that a small deficit in transmitters coupled with the receptor change is going to produce the equivalent of a lesion-induced deficit.

A. BJÖRKLUND (*University of Lund, Sweden*): I would like to talk about the danger of having simplistic views about these things. I must confess that when we started this research I thought the only way we would be able to influence function would be to concentrate on functions that had simple mechanisms; that is, I thought we might be able to influence simple mechanisms by crude means. Rotational behavior in the rat after a unilateral dopamine lesion would qualify. This behavior could be seen as an example of a mass effect, and could be understood within the context of our knowledge of the dopamine system.

We have seen that you can remove tissue from the cortex and then implant cortical tissue into the cortex. Dr. Nieto-Sampedro has shown that you can put Gelfoam into cortical wounds, fluid, or glia. Dr. Kimble has published results that show you can remove tissue from the hippocampus and then implant fetal hippocampal tissue. In each of these examples, tissue implantation can be seen to have an effect. Of course, one is lost if one assumed the mechanism was the same for all the effects. It will be a challenge for us to introduce these confusing issues and still promote understanding of our work. We may be dealing with a whole range of mechanisms influencing brain function and the plasticity of brain circuitry. Perhaps part of the secret here is that we are misunderstanding some basic properties of brain circuitry; that is, it may be an oversimplification to say that brain circuitry is very much dependent upon stable wiring and that the functional properties as revealed in behavior, for example, reflect the state or function of modifiable circuits where the possibilities to influence the performance of these circuits are manyfold. There are various ways we can attain a similar goal. This may explain why, for example, glial mechanisms may work in the same general direction as transmitter mechanisms or possible rewiring or reconnectivity mechanisms.

BARTUS: That is an excellent point. Sufficient data has been presented at this meeting alone to suggest that this sort of thing is going on. Dr. Stein has presented results that indicate many of these deficits recover over time and that recovery may be facilitated by neurotrophic factors. Certainly, drugs can affect recovery. The mechanism for the replacement therapy neurotransmitters is probably different from that for the neurotrophic factors. And then there is the question of whether brain tissue itself provides something unique other than the neurotransmitters or the neurotrophic factors. These things need to be addressed aggressively. This is the one area covered in this very exciting and positive meeting that I could feel negative about. No one seems to be trying to figure out why it is we get these behavioral effects. We can implant tissue, and sure, it is alive. Look at the beautiful pictures. We got this behavioral effect. But why? No one seems to be serious about answering this question.

D. STEIN (*Clark University, Worcester, MA*): I would like to respond to your point about the specificity of connections. Some investigators are beginning to analyze an entirely different paradigm to explain this specificity. We do not think about this much from our anatomical perspective or from our psychological perspective, but we all think that we must have new, ingrowing connections or fibers replacing those that have been lost. Some very elegant and beautiful work has been done by Dr. Merzenic and his colleagues at the University of California at San Francisco. They have demonstrated that there is an almost instantaneous change when you make a lesion of the digits. They have looked at the change in receptor fields from specific removals of digits or stimulation of digits. It is very similar to the work of Patrick Wall, who has demonstrated that there are latent synapses or relatively ineffective or inefficient pathways that can become activated almost instantaneously upon the denervation of a given system. Some of the substances we are introducing may be activating these relatively ineffective or latent pathways.

Now this is not something for those of us who tend to look at stained tissue or use myoclonal antibody immunohistochemistry. We are not going to see this kind of an effect by looking for sprouting or degeneration, but it may very well be a hypothesis to consider. Substances introduced by transplants or by other means may in fact be activating these additional pathways. These redundant pathways, because of development and genetics, may be suppressed while the primary pathways function. In the absence of these primary pathways, however, the redundant pathways may come into play. There is a lot of evidence along these lines.

F. H. GAGE (*University of California at San Diego, La Jolla, CA*): Another issue is that a lot of the deficits we have looked at recover spontaneously. In order to study graft-induced recovery of function, people have had to first create functional deficits by making fairly large lesions. Human pathology is such that in many cases you need to make very large lesions to create significant functional deficits. Therefore, in order to get a recovery, you may not need a complete restoration of the system. You may just have to bring the system above the threshold for the particular function you are looking at. A related issue is the level of analysis. In our functional analyses, we are usually satisfied with looking at transplants. We see spectacular recovery. But if we examine any of these models a little bit further, we find that they are not completely recovered. They show dramatic deficits. If we look at our models close enough to see these deficits, we may see how a graft can induce functional recovery and yet leave a deficit—this would tell us about the specificity in the function of the graft. Perhaps some other component of the graft would become evident if we tried another level of analysis. The level of analysis we choose could determine what functional recovery may reveal.

D. GOLDOWITZ (*Thomas Jefferson University, Philadelphia, PA*): I emphatically second Dr. Butler's challenge to the neuroscientists in this room to provide more basic neuroscience research in addition to studying clinical implications. If we go back to Dr. Bartus's analogy with the Mets, I can bring up an analogy with another New York team: the Yankees. Unfortunately, scientists can "buy" phenomena the way the Yankees buy players. The Yankees can buy a Winfield, and they can buy a Henderson, but they will still have a team that does nothing. As opposed to the Mets, who have become champion contenders because they built from their farm teams and cultivated substantial fielders and hitters. The basic sciences can benefit from this kind of approach.

D. M. GASH (*University of Rochester School of Medicine, Rochester, NY*): I wanted to point out that for anyone interested in reading some literature like that presented by Dr. Marie Gibson, we have paradigms for recovery of function in the neuroendocrine system that are easier than the paradigms for memory and learning. For example, our work on vasopressor-deficient rats shows that the only way you can see functional recovery is to transplant vasopressor neurons. These establish very specific connections with other targets: organs, blood vessels, and the median eminence. With our model and with Dr. Gibson's work on gonadotrophin-deficient mice, we can look very closely at specificity.

A lot of progress is being made, and this progress is possible because of the work that has been done in basic science. Many fundamentals have already been derived from work in basic science—our work, Dr. Björkland's work, and the work done by the other contributors here. Let us not write this off. We do have a substantial body of work to look back on.

BARTUS: I agree Dr. Gash, and I certainly hope that neither of us implied that we were writing anything off.

Intracerebral Grafting of Dopamine Neurons

Experimental Basis for Clinical Trials in Patients with Parkinson's Disease[a]

P. BRUNDIN,[b,c] R. E. STRECKER,[c] O. LINDVALL,[c,d]
O. ISACSON,[c] O. G. NILSSON,[c] G. BARBIN,[e]
A. PROCHIANTZ,[e] C. FORNI,[f] A. NIEOULLON,[f]
H. WIDNER,[d,g] F. H. GAGE,[h] AND A. BJÖRKLUND[c]

[c]*Department of Histology*
University of Lund
and
[d]*Department of Neurology*
University Hospital of Lund
Lund, Sweden
[e]*College de France*
Group NB, INSERM U114
Paris, France
[f]*Unité de Neurochimie*
CNRS
Marseille, France
[g]*Department of Clinical Immunology*
Karolinska Institute
Huddinge, Sweden
[h]*Department of Neurosciences*
University of California at San Diego
La Jolla, California

[a]This work was supported by Grant 04X-3874 from the Swedish Medical Research Council, by Grants AG-3766 and NS-6705 from the National Institute of Health and Aging, and by the European Science Foundation.

[b]Address for correspondence: Department of Histology, University of Lund, Biskopsgaten 5, S-223 62 Lund, Sweden.

INTRODUCTION

The possibility that dopamine (DA) neurons could be grafted to patients with Parkinson's disease (PD) in an attempt to alleviate the parkinsonian symptoms was discussed already in the late seventies when the first reports of successful functional DA neuron grafts in rats appeared.[1,2] Recent advances with grafting of DA neurons in primates[3,4] and between different species,[5,6] in combination with an accumulation of data demonstrating that neural grafts can be functional in several different brain systems,[7] has greatly increased the clinical interest and served as an impetus to explore the clinical possibilities of DA neuron grafting. There have already been clinical trials showing that adrenal medullary tissue can be grafted to the basal ganglia of PD patients, giving rise to minor and transient beneficial effects, without causing any adverse effects.[8-10] Although the results with adrenal medullary tissue have so far not been too encouraging, reverting to neurons as donor tissue will not necessarily provide a simple solution, as obviously there remain many unsolved problems facing the clinical application of neural grafting. Some of the problems are general to neural grafting in humans, and others can be held to be more specific to the features of the disease. This review points to some recent experimental results in animals that touch upon unsolved issues relevant to the possible future neural grafting in PD, either in a directly practical way or from a more theoretical viewpoint.

PD: CLINICAL FEATURES AND IMPORTANCE OF NEW THERAPEUTIC APPROACHES

PD in its classical form constitutes about 90% of all cases of symptomatic parkinsonism. In the general population, it has a prevalence of approximately 1 in 1000, and, as the disease shows increasing prevalence with increasing age, as many as 1 in 100 over 50 years of age have been estimated to be suffering from PD.[11]

Initial symptoms may be mild, but the disease invariably progresses and eventually disables the patient. The classical triad of motor symptoms includes hypokinesia, rigidity, and tremor. In an advanced stage of the disease, the patient displays extreme poverty of movement, postural abnormalities, a mask-like facial expression, a monotonous voice, and, because of muscular rigidity, an inability to relax even when resting. Signs of dementia, which cannot be attributed merely to normal aging, occur in a higher proportion of PD patients than in the general population.[12,13]

The pathological finding that has been most emphasized is the severe degeneration of DA neurons in the substantia nigra pars compacta,[13,14] leading to severe depletions of DA in the caudate nucleus and, in particular, the putamen.[15] There is also evidence indicating that the mesocortical DA system is affected by the disease, although to a lesser degree.[16] Furthermore, it is important to point out that the locus ceruleus and basal nucleus of Meynert usually exhibit cell loss, and levels of transmitters other than DA are altered in several different regions of the brain.[13,17-20] There is no real knowledge of the etiology of idiopathic PD and, therefore, little hope at present of finding a way of preventing the disease before it actually occurs, or of slowing down the progressive degeneration of DA neurons.

Today the main treatment strategy is replacement therapy for the lost DA transmission, either by the DA precursor L-dopa or by a directly acting DA receptor agonist, such as bromocriptine. Both these approaches, in general used in combination, can initially give a major symptomatic relief. Generally, the beneficial effects of the drug treatment subside after a few years, and major side effects, such as dyskinesias and "on-off" phenomena, appear. Hence the treatment currently available, although a blessing compared to when there was no treatment available, still leaves a majority of PD patients severely disabled. Therefore, it is of great importance to seek new therapeutic strategies for a disease that is very distressing for the patient and that is likely to become a greater health problem in society with increased life expectancy. At least in theory, the most attractive treatment would also involve replacement therapy, but then the more radical approach of replacing the actual missing cells by neural grafting.

EXPERIMENTAL STUDIES WITH DA NEURON GRAFTS

The DA system in the rat is well suited for the study of functional effects of neural grafts for several reasons. The normal anatomy of the system is well known, and the survival and growth of grafts can easily be studied because of the existence of specific histochemical, and more recently immunohistochemical, techniques that allow the visualization of catecholamine-containing neurons. Furthermore, because of the existence of the relatively specific neurotoxin 6-hydroxydopamine (6-OHDA), the DA-lesioned rat has provided a useful experimental model, which benefits from the availability of good, quantifiable behavioral correlates and the availability of well-characterized drugs that act on the DA system.[21] It is then not surprising that the first series of studies demonstrating functional effects of neural grafts were conducted in rats with unilateral 6-OHDA lesions of the nigrostriatal pathway.[1,2] The initial studies showed that fetal DA neurons could survive intracerebral grafting and reverse deficits in drug-induced motor behaviors, and that the functional capacity of the grafts was apparently dependent on their exact location in the caudate-putamen and their ability to generate axonal fibers that grew into the host brain.[22,23] At about the same time, it was also found that solid DA transplants could restore deficits in sensorimotor orientation and ameliorate akinesia under spontaneous conditions.[24,25] Since then, several studies have demonstrated the functionality of DA neuron grafts in different models (for a review, see reference 26), and defined more precisely the optimal conditions for transplant survival and function. This review will discuss only a few of these recent studies in an attempt to highlight how the experimental work can contribute in different ways to the development of a transplantation therapy in PD.

POTENTIAL PROBLEMS IN CLINICAL NEURAL GRAFTING TO PD PATIENTS

There are several types of problems that face clinical neural grafting in PD: some of them are mainly technical or methodological and basically require the translation of experience from the animal experimental field to the human situation. Other issues are more strictly biological and concern, for example, the innate constraints of the cells to be grafted and the functional limitations of the parkinsonian brain. Many of the latter issues are so complex, or are so difficult to approach experimentally, that an answer may be impossible to find without actually performing the clinical trials. Basically, one can divide all the unsolved issues into two principal categories: those concerning the donor tissue specifically, and those involving the recipient, that is, the parkinsonian patient.

SOURCES OF DA NEURON-RICH DONOR TISSUE

Animal studies have shown that good survival of transplanted DA neurons is obtained only with fetal donor tissue. There are also certain constraints on how old the fetal ventral mesencephalic DA neurons may be when grafted if good survival is to be obtained, and these constraints vary depending on the technique used and the age of the transplant recipient. When grafting cell suspensions to adult rat recipients, we have found that graft survival is very good when the donor fetuses are of 13-15 days gestational age, whereas fetuses that are a mere 24 hr older have, using our standard trypsin incubation dissociation protocol, given rise to poor graft survival.[27,28] If solid grafts are used, however, and are placed in pre-made surgical cavities in the cortex overlying the neostriatum, fetal mesencephalic DA neurons will survive even if 17 days has passed since conception.[29] When grafting to human brain, the donor tissue must most likely be prepared in the form of either dissociated single cells or small tissue aggregates, as they would have to be implanted with fine surgical instruments in order to minimize damage to the surrounding brain tissue. If human fetal tissue is to be considered, and a dissociated cell suspension or a tissue fragment technique utilized, findings in rodents suggest that the ideal donor material may be obtained 9-11 weeks after conception. This is based on results with the dissociation technique, which indicate that the neurons survive best if they are prepared not later than around the time when they become postmitotic, which, according to morphological studies in the nigrostriatal DA system of human fetuses, is probably around the aforementioned time.[30] The use of human fetuses in clinical grafting would, however, raise several kinds of problems.

First, one can question whether it is ethically justifiable to use aborted human fetal tissue at all for transplantation purposes, and one may argue that central nervous system (CNS) tissue, in particular, should not be used as donor tissue in transplantation therapy. However, the ethical questions concerning the use of human fetal tissue for grafting purposes are beyond the scope of this review.

Second, the use of human fetal tissue could lead to immunological rejection because the donor and recipient will not be genetically similar, as they are in most experimental rodent studies. The immunological problems, and possible ways to avoid them, are discussed at some length in a later section.

Third, the availability of human fetal tissue is limited both with regard to the amount of suitable tissue one can obtain at a given time and also with regard to the predictability of when a suitable donor will appear. This latter problem may be possible to approach using *in vitro* techniques to store or enrich neuronal tissue. We have previously found that fetal rat basal forebrain tissue can be stored in a simple cryoprotectant at $+4°$ C for 5 days and then, after dissociation, still survive implantation into the hippocampus.[31] Using a more refined approach with dissociated cultures containing mesencephalic DA neurons, we found, in an initial study, that the DA neurons would survive grafting when redissociated after 6 days in culture and after having spent an additional 2 days in suspension, when transported between France and Sweden.[32] Recently, we have extended these findings and studied the survival and function of DA neurons that were grafted after either 2 or 7 days in culture. We compared the fate of these grafts with transplants prepared freshly from fetal donors of ages that were equivalent to the age of the cells that had been maintained *in vitro* for 2 and 7 days, respectively. Functional grafts were only observed in rats receiving freshly prepared tissue from 14-day-old fetuses and 16-day-old fetuses, and in rats receiving grafts of cells maintained for 2 days in culture (FIG. 1). Upon histological analysis, surviving DA neurons were found in relatively large numbers (FIG. 2) in all the rats from the groups that exhibited behavioral compensation. Small numbers (4-20) of DA neurons were also found to have survived in grafts prepared from tissue maintained *in vitro* for 7 days, and in the "age-matched" grafts, freshly prepared from 20-day-old fetuses, there were at most only 6 DA neurons found in a graft. The good graft survival from 16-day-old donors was unexpected, as it is not seen when we graft using our routine dissociation procedure.[28] In this experiment, the tissue was dissociated using a protocol similar to that used for preparation of the *in vitro* cultures, which involved a longer incubation in trypsin and a less vigorous multiple-step mechanical dissociation method. Moreover, a wider gauge cannula than used previously was utilized (inner diameter: 0.25 mm, compared to 0.11 mm in previous studies) for the graft injection, allowing larger clumps of undissociated tissue to be injected. This particular observation indicates that the restrictions on donor age may not be as absolute as they first appeared, and that with more refined techniques dissociated tissue grafts from even older donors may survive. In summary, the results indicate that DA neurons can readily be maintained in culture for a limited time and still survive intracerebral grafting, but also that the maturation of the neurons that occurs *in vitro* probably makes them more sensitive to the grafting procedure.

SURVIVAL, GROWTH, AND FUNCTIONAL CORRELATES OF GRAFTED DA NEURONS

Using the cell suspension technique, in the order of 1 in 1000 to 1 in 100 of all the cells injected will survive in the graft as DA-containing neurons.[28] Of course, only a minority of the cells injected are actually destined to become producers of DA. Based on data routinely obtained in our laboratory, and studies indicating that the rat mesencephalon contains approximately 30 000-40 000 DA neurons,[33] we estimate that up to 10% of the future DA neurons dissected from the fetus actually survive grafting with the cell suspension technique. In mature ventral mesencephalic grafts, we have observed that approximately 1 in 500 of the cell bodies with a nuclear diameter greater than 12-15 μm (presumed neurons) contain DA (unpublished observation). In this context, it is interesting to compare the number of DA neurons required in a graft to attain behavioral effects in rodents with the actual number of DA neurons that normally innervate the neostriatum. Studies in rats and mice now point to the threshold number of DA neurons necessary to obtain a reduction in amphetamine-induced rotation in the unilaterally 6-OHDA-lesioned rodent as being on the order of 1-2% of the number of DA neurons in the rodent's nigrostriatal pathway.[28,34] Possible reasons for the seemingly low number of grafted neurons needed for functional effects include the following: the host striatal neurons are supersensitive to DA after the 6-OHDA lesion; each grafted DA neuron has an increased DA turnover[35,36];

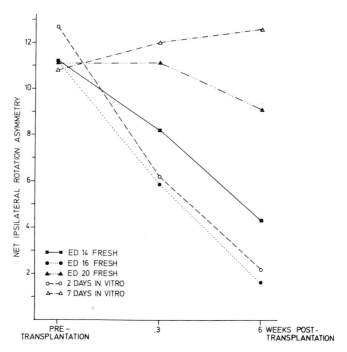

FIGURE 1. Effects of different types of neural grafts on motor asymmetry as assessed in an amphetamine-induced (5 mg/kg, i.p.) rotation test at different times after transplantation. "Net ipsilateral rotation asymmetry" scores were obtained by subtracting turns contralateral to 6-OHDA lesion from those made ipsilateral to lesion. "Fresh" (filled symbols) signifies groups receiving freshly prepared ventral mesencephalic cell suspensions of the donor age stated. Open symbols represent groups that received tissue cultured for either 2 or 7 days. ($N = 7$ for all groups except "2 days *in vitro*," for which $N = 6$; ED: embryonic day.)

amphetamine causes an abnormal situation that increases the efficacy of the system; only reinnervation of a small critical zone of the neostriatum may be necessary for reversal of the studied deficit in rotational behavior.[26] The normal human nigrostriatal pathway comprises 200 000–400 000 DA neurons,[37] and, if these figures are also relevant in the clinical setting, as few as 2000–8000 surviving DA neurons could be sufficient to give rise to functional effects in humans. One should be cautious, however, when drawing parallels between experimental data and the clinical situation for the PD patient when discussing cell numbers. First, it is not well documented that L-dopa-treated PD patients are supersensitive to DA in the neostriatum,[38] although such a supersensitivity has been reported in untreated patients.[39] Second, the rotation tests in rodents are performed under amphetamine stimulation, a situation that might not be feasible to maintain in the daily life of a PD patient.

DA neurons are able to *survive* in several different sites in the rat CNS. These sites include the neostriatum, nucleus accumbens, septum, prefrontal and parietal cortices, hippocampus, tectum, cerebellum, lateral ventricle, lateral hypothalamus, and substantia nigra.[1,2,27,40-44] Although all these sites support survival of the DA neurons, the fiber outgrowth of the grafted neurons tends to be confined to the graft itself unless the implant is placed in a region that normally is innervated by DA. The prime example of such a "target area" is of course the neostriatum. In the rat neostriatum, grafted DA neurons have been seen to extend a dense network of axonal processes up to 1.5-2.0 mm away from the actual implant, into the host brain.[40]

We have recently investigated the survival and growth of DA neurons when grafted to the neostriatum, as a cell suspension, mixed together with fetal target cells from the striatal primordium.[45] There is a large body of evidence from *in vitro* studies indicating that striatal target cells alter several parameters of DA neuron growth and function when they are co-cultured in the same dish.[46,47] We found that the addition of fetal striatal cells increased the area of dense outgrowth of DA fibers without significantly affecting survival of the grafted DA neurons or the DA content in the grafts and, finally, without causing any major effect on their functionality, as assessed behaviorally.[45] Interestingly, when the same kind of "co-grafts" were injected into the hippocampus (a nontarget region for DA neurons), the addition of striatal cells gave rise to a significant increase in graft DA content (FIG. 3). The principal difference in the biochemical results when implanting co-grafts in the neostriatum versus the hippocampus can be explained by the fact that in the study utilizing the neostriatum as transplantation site the grafts containing mesencephalic tissue already had access to target neurons in the adult host striatum, and the addition of fetal target cells probably only affected the pattern of the fiber outgrowth. These studies, in addition to those demonstrating a paucity of fiber outgrowth from DA grafts placed in nontarget regions,[40] all emphasize the importance of the transplantation site in the regulation of graft DA fiber outgrowth. The factor or factors in the neostriatum that stimulate DA fiber outgrowth from the grafted neurons do not seem to be species specific because mouse DA neurons implanted in the rat neostriatum also exhibit extensive axonal outgrowth (discussed further below).[6]

Another illustration of a region-specific graft innervation of DA fibers can be found when mesencephalic grafts are injected into the septum. DA fibers extending from such grafts form a unique basket-like innervation around host septal neurons (unpublished observation) in a fashion similar to that found in the normal rat.[48] Similar

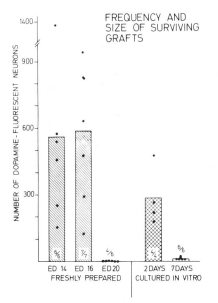

FIGURE 2. Number of DA-fluorescent neurons found in the grafts at subsequent histological analysis. Each dot represents one rat, and the bars show group means. The number at the bottom of each bar indicates the proportion of analyzed rats that had surviving DA neurons in that group.

observations of basket-like innervation patterns have been reported, using DA immunohistochemistry, when mesencephalic grafts aimed at the nucleus accumbens have leaked into the adjacent septum.[42,49]

The size of the axonal network is of particular interest when discussing the extent of reinnervation that one would desire when grafting to the neostriatum of PD patients. The human neostriatum is obviously several times larger than the rat caudate-putamen, and the question arises whether a grafted human fetal DA neuron retains the capacity to extend axons several centimeters long, as it does normally, or whether the grafting procedure itself damages the neuron and limits its growth capacity to a few millimeters, regardless of its species origin and "normal" length of axonal tree. This issue can, to a certain extent, be approached experimentally by grafting DA neurons from larger animals to the neostriatum of rats and studying whether the extent of DA fiber outgrowth, or more specifically the length of fibers, is greater than that obtained with rat DA neurons. Although the aforementioned data speak in favor of the host CNS regional environment governing the genesis of axonal outgrowth from grafted DA neurons, it is clearly possible that the "target stimulus" is only required to turn on the development of fibers and that properties intrinsic to the neuron itself ultimately govern the final size of the axonal network.

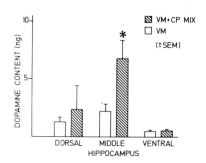

FIGURE 3. Total DA content in three different regions of the hippocampus ($N = 6$) that received grafts of either pure ventral mesencephalic cell suspensions (VM) or a mixture of mesencephalic cells and striatal target calls (VM + CP MIX). The hosts first received intraventricular injections of 6-OHDA to deplete endogenous catecholamines. *: $p < .05$ (Student's t test).

In the PD patient, the most extensive depletion of DA occurs in the putamen (around 95% depletion), whereas the caudate nucleus retains some 50% of its DA, even in advanced cases of PD.[15] These data, in addition to anatomical studies in animals showing that the putamen is more closely related to motor structures in the brain,[50] suggest that the putamen is the most suitable target for neural grafting in PD patients. Indeed, in the most recent study with adrenal autografts in PD patients, which resulted in some transient functional effects, the implants were made in the putamen.[9,10] Consistent with the experimental data, the putamen also ought to provide a suitable site to stimulate fiber outgrowth from the grafts. Studies involving intrastriatal mesencephalic transplants in aged rats have shown that the aged striatum also supports fiber outgrowth from grafted DA neurons,[51,52] although aged rats are documented to have reduced receptor densities in the striatum,[53] and that DA neuron grafts can ameliorate age-related impairments.[52] This is a particularly important finding in view of the majority of PD patients being over the age of 50.[11] Although there are clear indications that the putamen is a suitable site for grafting in the PD patient, the distinct heterogeneity of function in the striatal complex calls for a word of caution and suggests that the exact location of the graft within the striatal complex may be of critical importance. Early graft studies clearly showed that DA transplants to the dorsal and ventrolateral striatum would support recovery of different aspects of the unilateral 6-OHDA-induced behavioral syndrome.[22,23,25,54] Recently, we have seen that

DA grafts placed in a 6-OHDA-lesioned nucleus accumbens of a rat with a mesostriatal 6-OHDA lesion on the same side will, paradoxically, induce an increase in the speed of amphetamine-induced ipsilateral rotation,[55] whereas previous work has shown that suspension grafts placed further dorsolateral in the striatal complex in the same hemisphere attenuate or totally eliminate the rotational behavior.[54] This also suggests that in the clinical situation, small variations in the placement of a surviving graft, or an exceedingly restricted zone of reinnervation, may give rise to disparate functional effects or could result in there being no functional effects at all. Possibly the clinical transplantation surgery can be conducted under local anesthesia, making it possible to first stimulate the intended graft site, either electrically or with DA receptor agonists, to elucidate which functions may eventually be affected by a transplant at that particular site. Furthermore, as PD patients can exhibit different symptomatic profiles, small variations in transplantation site could therefore be made in accordance with the clinical picture of the individual patient.

SPONTANEOUS ACTIVITY OF DA GRAFTS: NEURONAL FIRING, DA METABOLISM, AND RELEASE

Even if the problem of finding DA-producing donor neurons suitable for clinical grafting could be solved, and a functionally adequate number of DA neurons were implanted at a suitable site, there still remains the issue of to what extent the neurons will be spontaneously active in the PD patient after grafting.

There is accumulating evidence from experimental studies showing that DA neuron grafts are spontaneously active. Solid grafts of fetal mesencephalic tissue have been shown to contain neurons with spontaneous firing patterns reminiscent of those seen in normal adult rat nigral DA neurons.[56,57] In addition, there is evidence that solid transplants of fetal mesencephalic tissue depress the firing rate of host striatal neurons, and that this effect is more pronounced close to the graft where the reinnervation is most dense.[58] This is consistent with measurement of DA metabolism in the graft-reinnervated neostriatum,[35,36] indicating that the grafted DA neurons have an active turnover of the transmitter, even at rates above normal.

More direct evidence for spontaneous DA release from fetal mesencephalic grafts comes from studies utilizing techniques that monitor transmitter release *in vivo*. Using the intracerebral dialysis technique, it was possible to monitor, from multiple intrastriatal implants of mesencephalic cell suspension, a spontaneous release of DA that reached a mean of 40% of normal striatal levels, as compared to the > 90% reduction seen in rats with 6-OHDA lesions alone.[59] After the local administration of amphetamine, the release increased approximately 14-fold; this increased release is similar to the response found in the normal striatum. In a more recent study, we have found that the spontaneous DA release can be restored to normal levels in regions of the striatum by DA neuron grafts.[60] Subsequently, these grafts were found to contain severalfold higher numbers of DA neurons, ranging between 2000 and 5000 per host, than the prior study. In this second dialysis study, the grafts were challenged by the directly acting DA receptor agonist apomorphine, which in a normal striatum causes a decrease in DA release,[61] to see whether they possessed some normal physiological characteristics. Although the grafts appeared less sensitive to the effect of apomorphine, they did respond with a decrease in DA release, providing evidence that the activity of the grafted DA neurons can, potentially, be regulated via autoreceptors or via a host-graft feedback loop.

To study when the appearance of DA release occurs after transplantation, carbon paste voltammetry electrodes were implanted in the striatum 1 week after the transplantation of mesencephalic cell suspensions.[62] Although the signal in 6-OHDA-lesioned rats remained depressed and never exceeded 5% of normal, a substantial recovery of signal was seen in the grafted rats. This increase in voltammetric signal appeared in a sudden manner 5-8 weeks after grafting, which is around 3-4 weeks after the time when amphetamine-induced rotation usually begins to be affected by mesencephalic cell suspension grafts. In the best cases, the signal amplitude reached the levels of normal striatum, and, at subsequent histological analysis, the grafts were found to be of the same size as those in the latter dialysis study (see above and FIG. 4) in which approximately normal striatal DA release was monitored in the grafts. The late increase in signal amplitude, several weeks after the time when final status of functionality under amphetamine-stimulated conditions normally is reached, suggests that the evolution of spontaneous release is a prolonged process and that the functionality of the amphetamine-induced DA release is dependent on a threshold effect beyond which an additional increase in DA release capacity will not be reflected in additional functional effects. In a clinical situation, therefore, where the spontaneous release may be the most important in the functional context, one might expect an improvement of spontaneous behavior long after the appearance of the first effects that can be detected by pharmacological stimulation.

Another important issue is whether the spontaneous activity of the grafted DA neurons can somehow be regulated in a synaptic fashion by the host brain. Electron microscopic immunocytochemistry[63,64] has shown that the graft-derived DA fibers form abundant and partly accurate synaptic contacts with the striatal projection neurons of the host. There is, however, to date only sparse evidence for afferents from host neurons to intracerebral nigral grafts. In an electrophysiological study, using solid nigral grafts placed in a cavity overlying the neostriatum, neurons within the grafts have been found to respond to stimulation of the frontal cortex and lower brainstem of the host.[57] In addition, there is electron microscopic evidence for dendrites from grafted neurons extending into the host striatum and receiving synaptic inputs from the host neurons that conceivably could play a role in regulating the activity of the grafted neurons.[63]

SPONTANEOUS ACTIVITY OF DA GRAFTS: BEHAVIORAL STUDIES

Extensive experimental evidence has shown that drug-induced behaviors are affected by DA neuron grafts,[26] but there are fewer examples of functional effects in spontaneous behavioral situations. In rats with age-related motor impairments, DA neuron implants have been found to improve performance in a spontaneous motor coordination test without affecting locomotor activity.[53] In rats with 6-OHDA lesions, early graft studies showed that DA neurons could reverse spontaneous side bias and reinstate the ability to orient to sensory stimuli contralateral to a 6-OHDA lesion.[24,25,54] This involves simple reflex-like responses, but it has recently been shown that more complex spontaneous motor tasks can also be affected by DA grafts. Specifically, rats have been trained in a conditioned rotation paradigm, which involves the water-deprived rat learning to perform body turns in a particular direction to receive a reward of sucrose water. Rats with extensive lesions of the mesostriatal pathway are unable to perform this learned motor response in a direction away from the lesion,[65]

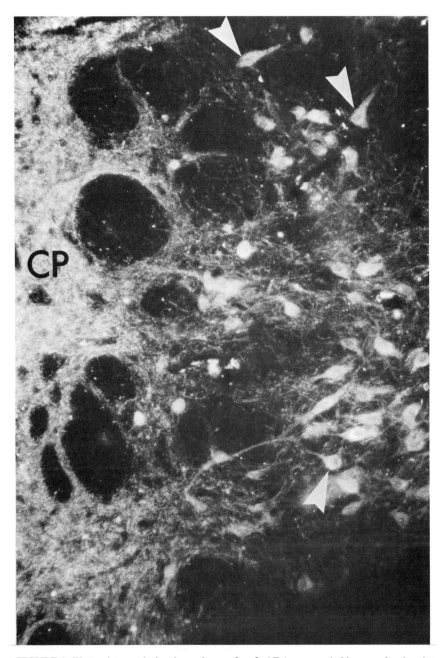

FIGURE 4. Photomicrograph showing a cluster of grafted DA neurons (white arrowheads point to examples of perikarya) densely innervating the host caudate-putamen (CP) in a rat included in the voltammetry experiment discussed in the text.

whereas lesioned rats with DA grafts can learn the turning behavior, albeit at a slower rate than controls and without ever reaching control performance within the time period they were trained.[66] We have also seen that rats with large grafts that show complete compensation of both apomorphine- and amphetamine-induced rotation are markedly impaired compared to normal controls in the conditioned turning task (unpublished observations). This disparity may exist because different striatal regions need to be reinnervated for the different kinds of behavior, as has been demonstrated for turning behavior and sensorimotor orientation,[26] or because the grafts, possibly by lacking the appropriate afferent and efferent connections, are unable to function accurately in more complex behaviors. Nevertheless, these findings call for caution when interpreting data from behavioral studies using DA grafts because rats that are completely normalized in their drug-induced turning bias may still retain major asymmetric neurological deficits in a task that requires similar motoric movements. This highlights the possibility that in the clinical situation symptoms with similar characteristics may be affected to different degrees and, moreover, that it may be necessary to drive the grafts by pharmacological stimulation to affect some aspects of the parkinsonian syndrome.

FUNCTIONAL LIMITATIONS OF DA NEURON GRAFTS

Among the many reports that demonstrate how DA neuron grafts can affect or reverse the behavioral deficits induced by 6-OHDA lesions in the rat DA system, there are a few reports of how DA neuron grafts have failed to or have only partially affected the lesion-induced deficits (for example, the conditioned rotation data mentioned above). Probably there also exist several unpublished studies in which surviving mesencephalic transplants have not been found to affect the studied behavioral parameters; these studies would have never reached the literature. Experiments that have revealed functional limitations of DA neuron grafts are interesting to discuss with regard to whether the limitations are biological or technical and to how they may relate to a future clinical application of DA neural grafts in PD.

Rats with large bilateral lesions of the mesotelencephalic DA system will, in addition to motoric symptoms, exhibit severe impairments in eating and drinking behaviors (aphagia and adipsia).[67] Single or multiple implants of mesencephalic tissue in various forebrain regions have been found to significantly affect the motoric symptoms in such rats, but, at the same time, have been found to give rise to only minor changes in the aphagia and adipsia (unpublished observations).[68,69]

When rats are subject to bilateral lesions that particularly affect the mesolimbocortical DA system and partially spare the mesostriatal DA system, they are able to eat and drink but exhibit several regulatory motoric and cognitive symptoms, such as deficits in hoarding behavior. DA neuron grafts have been shown to completely reverse these deficits, but only when the rats are challenged with a low dose of amphetamine and not in a spontaneous situation.[42] This indicates that although the grafts may contain the neurochemical or anatomical substrates or both to reverse the functional deficit, they will not do this without being "artificially" activated. In a similar model, with rats that have lesions of the mesolimbocortical DA system, we have recently studied the effects of DA neuron transplants on the rats' performance in the Morris water maze. The lesion gives rise to severe impairments in the rat's ability to find an escape platform located under the water surface in a circular pool filled with opaque water. The lesioned rats basically show none of the search behavior that a normal rat exhibits and also display marked decreases in swim speed. In continuing experiments, we have observed that mesencephalic cell suspensions implanted in the nucleus accumbens and striatum are able to restore the swim speed in some of the grafted animals, whereas their ability to locate the escape platform may remain unaffected (unpublished observation). This indicates that the behavioral deficit seen in the watermaze after extensive 6-OHDA lesions in the mesolimbocortical system consists of several components that can be independently affected. The limitation of the behavioral recovery after grafting may in this particular instance be due to the fact that none of the grafts were aimed at the neocortical regions that were also deprived of their DA innervation. Alternately, the information processing required for the animal to acquire the spatial navigation task may be more complex than the neural processes governing swimming ability or speed, and thus may not be possible to affect with DA neural grafts.

The underlying reasons for the functional limitations of the grafts can only be speculated upon. As mentioned previously, there may be biological constraints, such as those related to the connectivity of the grafts. Paucity or lack of host afferents and some abnormal efferent graft connections have been advocated in electron microscopic studies of solid nigral grafts.[63,64] In some cases, the absence of effects may simply be related to either too few DA neurons having been implanted or to inadequate graft placement. As will be discussed later, these two points are very important to clarify the human clinical situation. In addition, it should be pointed out that a subgroup of PD patients shows symptoms of dementia that may be related to a cholinergic deficit in the basal nucleus of Meynert and, therefore, may not be amenable to treatment by DA neuron grafts.

IMMUNOLOGICAL ASPECTS OF GRAFTING DA NEURONS

Several studies, dating back to the first half of this century, have demonstrated that grafts of immunologically incompatible tissue to the brain are not rejected with the same frequency or as soon after grafting as they are when placed in another location in the body.[70] These findings led Medawar to introduce the concept of the brain as an immunologically privileged transplantation site.[71]

The large majority of neural grafting studies have been conducted using donors and recipients that have been of a similar strain of rodent, and have thus avoided any major immunological barriers. For reasons of brevity, the discussions in this paper concerning neural grafting across immunological barriers will be limited to experiments involving transplants of fetal mesencephalon. Although the exact limitations of and the mechanisms underlying the immunological privilege of the brain are not known, the empirical finding that fetal DA-containing neurons could survive grafting between species[5] has raised hopes that maybe in a future clinical application one could graft nervous tissue from genetically dissimilar individuals without immunosuppression. More recent data, however, has stressed that although there is partial protection of immunologically incompatible DA neurons when grafted to the brain, the use of immunosuppressive treatment can greatly increase the functional effects, the survival frequency, and the size of xenografts.[6] Specifically, we studied the effects of the immunosuppressive drug cyclosporin A on the survival of mouse DA neurons grafted, using the cell suspension method, to the 6-OHDA-denervated rat striatum. All of the immunosuppressed rats exhibited behaviorally functional grafts and large numbers of surviving DA neurons 6 weeks after transplantation, whereas only 3 out of 7 of the nonimmunosuppressed rats possessed small surviving grafts.[6] Two rats in the cyclosporin A-treated group were studied a further 4 and 14 weeks, respectively, after termination of the 6-week immunosuppression period. Both these rats retained large grafts that were rich in DA neurons and that remained functional.

This finding, in addition to the known extraordinary immunologically privileged nature of the brain, prompted us to investigate whether short-term cyclosporin A treatment could support long-term survival of intracerebral DA grafts. Using the same model, we grafted fetal mouse mesencephalic tissue to rats that received no immunosuppression, or were allocated to either a 10-day or a 21-day cyclosporin treatment scheme. Three weeks after transplantation, several rats in the 10- and 21-day cyclosporin groups showed, as expected, evidence of surviving functional transplants (FIG. 5). After 6 weeks, however, only three rats out of nine in the 10-day treatment group still showed a major functional graft effect (FIG. 5B), whereas four rats seemed to have at least partially rejected their grafts between the 3- and 6-week tests (FIG. 5C). In the 21-day treatment group, 7 out of 10 rats showed clear signs of functioning transplants 6 weeks after transplantation, but this figure was only 4 out of 9 at the 6-month time point (FIG. 5D). In summary, it still remains to be established whether a short-term immunosuppressive treatment can support long-term survival of intracerebral fetal neural grafts. Notably, it has been hypothesized that the time taken for the closure of the ruptured blood-brain barrier after transplantation surgery might represent a critical time period after which immunosuppression is not necessary. Recently, we have looked at the leakage of macromolecules across the blood-brain barrier after intrastriatal neural cell suspension injection and found that the leakage in the striatum already ceases to be detectable 5-6 days after surgery (unpublished observation). This suggests that even when the blood-brain barrier is intact to macromolecules, foreign antigens can be detected by the immune system and eradicated from the brain.

Recent neural grafting experiments in primates[3,4] are of special immunologic relevance to the human clinical situation. In the primate experiments, fetal CNS tissue has been grafted without immunosuppression between individuals that were genetically dissimilar and that still showed prolonged survival. Several studies have demonstrated that CNS tissue under normal conditions bears low levels of both major and minor transplantation antigens,[72,73] and thus is of low immunogenicity; furthermore, one may speculate that when grafting CNS tissue within species that have a more prolonged fetal development than rodents, the cells are not mature enough to express their antigens until the acute inflammatory response associated with the transplantation surgery, which can induce such an expression, has subsided.

GRAFTS OF HUMAN FETAL DA NEURONS TO THE RAT BRAIN

We have recently initiated a series of studies to explore the characteristics of fetal human CNS tissue when transplanted to the brains of immunosuppressed rats. With this approach, we hope to establish optimal parameters for donor age, dissection, and tissue preparation for survival of mesencephalic DA neurons; to estimate the DA neuron survival frequency; and to study the functional capacity of DA neurons.

We have grafted ventral mesencephalic tissue, from fetuses obtained at routine hospital abortions, to the 6-OHDA-denervated rat striatum. In a first study, we obtained CNS tissue from a 16-week-old fetus and prepared it according to the cell suspension technique. The cells were intrastriatally injected into rats given daily cyclosporin A injections. At histological analysis after 5 weeks, there were traces of the cannula tract in all the animals, but none of the rats showed any evidence of a surviving implant.

In a second study, we grafted in a similar fashion tissue from an 11-week-old fetus. Each rat received 4 μl of cell suspension intrastriatally (equivalent to approximately 100 000 viable cells). These rats were perfused for catecholamine histochemistry 6-12 weeks after grafting. All six of the graft recipients contained surviving transplants, and the number of DA neurons was counted in five of them and found to range between 14 and 74 (mean: 44). In one rat, which was perfused 6 weeks after grafting, fluorescent fibers were found to radiate into the dorsal host striatum from DA neurons (72 in total) that had a somewhat immature bipolar appearance.

In a continuing study, we have grafted mesencephalic tissue from a 9-week-old fetus. The behavior of the five graft recipients (FIGS. 6 & 7) showed no evidence of graft function 8 weeks after transplantation. When rat or mouse fetal DA neurons are grafted, the functional effects in the amphetamine-induced rotation test are usually fully established by that time. Interestingly, when tested 12.5 weeks after transplantation, although the rats maintained a relatively high turning score in the direction ipsilateral to their lesions (FIG. 6), four out of five rats were suddenly able to perform some turning in a direction away from their lesions (FIG. 7), especially during the early part of the test session. In a recent study performed with DA grafts in 6-OHDA-lesioned mice, we found that turning in a direction contralateral to the lesion may be a very sensitive indicator of graft function and that this turning behavior could be correlated with survival of grafted DA neurons.[34] Thus, a study performed in mice gave some information that is very relevant to the analysis of the functional capacity of grafted human neurons. When tested 3 weeks later, four out of the five rats with human mesencephalic tissue grafts did indeed also show a marked decrease in their ipsilateral turning score and a further increase in contralateral turning (FIG. 7). Several studies have shown that unilaterally 6-OHDA-lesioned rats, when selected according to our behavior criterion of a complete lesion, do not spontaneously recover.[35] The reduced turning response seen in these grafted rats can therefore be taken as a strong indication that fetal human DA neurons have the capacity to function after intracerebral grafting. One should note that the appearance of functional effects occurred when the human cells were about 21-24 weeks old (counted from the estimated day of conception), when their development may still be proceeding.

Although these preliminary observations raise some hopes that human fetal tissue could be used for grafting to PD patients, they have also emphasized some important technical factors. First, it would seem that when using the cell suspension technique the upper limit for suitable donor age is definitely less than 16 weeks (counting from the estimated day of conception). Second, in a clinical situation, any major functional effects would be expected to appear much later than in studies using rodent donor tissue.

POTENTIAL UNDESIRABLE EFFECTS OR COMPLICATIONS OF INTRACEREBRAL NEURAL GRAFTS IN PD PATIENTS

When implanting neural tissue in the basal ganglia of a human, it is possible that the surgical trauma involved causes brain damage (for example, through hemorrhage) that could give rise to functional deficits. The clinical trials with grafts of adrenal medulla however, have not demonstrated any adverse effects of the stereotaxic im-

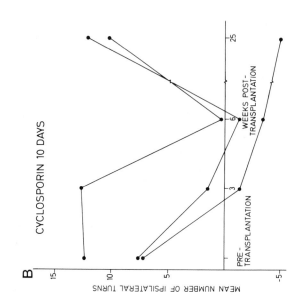

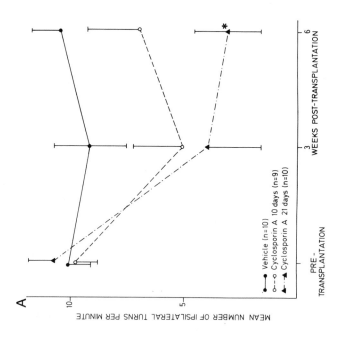

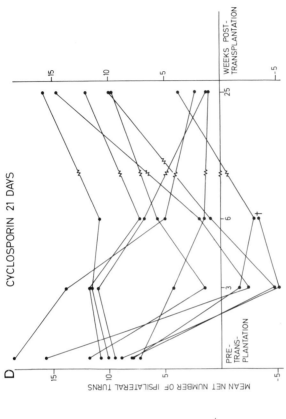

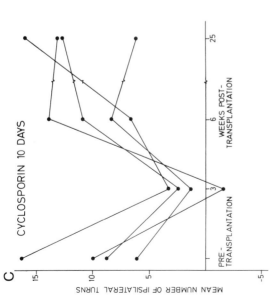

FIGURE 5. Effects of mouse neural grafts on motor asymmetry in rats as assessed in an amphetamine-induced (5 mg/kg, i.p.) rotation test at different times after transplantation. Rats were either treated with the immunosuppressive drug cyclosporin A (10 mg/kg each day), for 10 (**A, B & C**) or 21 (**A & D**) days, or were given vehicle injections (**A**). (**A**) Group means illustrated. *: $p < .05$ (ANOVA with post hoc Newman-Keuls' test). (**B**) Examples of the motor asymmetry of individual rats in the 10-day cyclosporin A group that still showed functional grafts after 6 weeks. (**C**) Examples of motor asymmetry of individual rats in the 10-day cyclosporin A group that showed functional grafts after 3 weeks and that apparently were rejected after 6 weeks. (**D**) The motor asymmetry of all the individual rats in the 21-day cyclosporin A group. Note that only four rats still show evidence of surviving grafts after 25 weeks.

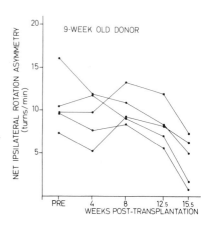

FIGURE 6. Effects of human neural grafts, obtained from a 9-week-old donor, on motor asymmetry in rats as assessed in an amphetamine-induced (5 mg/kg, i.p.) rotation test at different times after transplantation. All the rats were treated with daily injections of cyclosporin A (10 mg/kg each day).

plantation,[8-10] and the implantation of neural tissue is not likely to be more deleterious for the patient.

If a graft survives the initial transplantation surgery, several unwanted sequale are conceivable. First, a graft that is slightly misplaced, or grows uncontrollably into brain regions adjacent to the striatum, could form abnormal connections that could affect the PD patient in a negative fashion. Nevertheless, in view of the target specificity of grafted DA neurons in rodents,[40] it seems unlikely that the human grafted DA neurons would give rise to a major innervation of areas outside the normal DA termination fields.

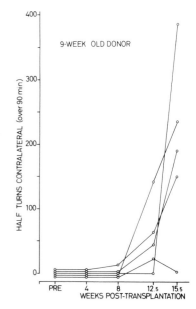

FIGURE 7. Effects of human neural grafts, obtained from an 9-week-old donor, on the number of full body turns performed in a direction contralateral to the lesion over 90 min at different time points after transplantation.

Second, a graft innervating the striatum could give rise to unwanted movements (dyskinesias), analogous to those found as a side effect of pharmacological DA replacement therapy. There is evidence from experimental studies that under amphetamine stimulation DA grafts can be "overactive" and cause rats with unilateral 6-OHDA lesions to actively rotate only in a direction away from the transplanted side.[74] It is unclear, however, whether such exaggerated graft effects can occur in the spontaneously behaving animal.

Third, DA neurons in a surviving graft may be affected by the unknown underlying disease process in PD and gradually degenerate as a result. Indeed, serum from PD patients has, in preliminary studies, been suggested to contain a factor that inhibits the survival or development of DA neurons *in vitro*.[75]

Still, with these potential undesirable effects in mind, the compelling evidence that fetal DA neurons can survive transplantation in experimental animals and reverse behavior deficits encourages efforts toward the development of a clinical application of neural grafting in PD patients.

ACKNOWLEDGMENTS

We would like to express our sincere gratitude to several members of technical staff of the Department of Histology who have assisted in the recent studies. The staff includes J. Berglund, B. Falck, A. Flasch, K. Fogelström, K. Friberg, B. Haraldsson, U. Jarl, C. Jönsson, Y. Jönsson, R. Mårtensson, A. Persson, and G. Stridsberg. We are also very grateful to Professor B. Åstedt and members of staff of the Department of Gynecology at the University Hospital of Lund for providing human fetal material. Cyclosporin A was supplied by Sandoz Ltd., Täby, Sweden.

REFERENCES

1. BJÖRKLUND, A. & U. STENEVI. 1979. Reconstruction of the nigrostriatal pathway by intracerebral nigral transplants. Brain Res. 177: 555-560.
2. PERLOW, M. J., W. J. FREED, B. J. HOFFER, Å. SEIGER, L. OLSON & R. J. WYATT. 1979. Brain grafts reduce motor abnormalities produced by destruction of nigrostriatal dopamine system. Science 204: 643-647.
3. SLADEK, J. R., JR., T. J. COLLIER, S. N. HABER, A. Y. DEUTCH, J. D. ELSWORTH, R. H. ROTH & D. E. REDMOND, JR. 1987. Reversal of parkinsonism by fetal nerve transplants in primate brain. Ann. N.Y. Acad. Sci. This volume.
4. BAKAY, R. A. E., D. L. BARRON, M. S. FIANDACA, P. M. IUVONE, A. SCHIFF & D. C. COLLINS. 1987. Biochemical and behavioral correction of MPTP Parkinson-like syndrome by fetal cell transplantation. Ann. N.Y. Acad. Sci. This volume.
5. BJÖRKLUND, A., U. STENEVI, S. B. DUNNETT & F. H. GAGE. 1982. Cross-species grafting in a rat model of Parkinson's disease. Nature 298: 652-654.
6. BRUNDIN, P., O. G. NILSSON, F. H. GAGE & A. BJÖRKLUND. 1985. Cyclosporin A increases survival of cross-species intrastriatal grafts of embryonic dopamine-containing neurons. Exp. Brain Res. 60: 204-208.
7. BJÖRKLUND, A. & U. STENEVI. 1984. Intracerebral neural implants: Neuronal replacement and reconstruction of damaged circuitries. Annu. Rev. Neurosci. 7: 279-308.

8. BACKLUND, E.-O., P.-O. GRANBERG, B. HAMBERGER, G. SEDVALL, Å. SEIGER & L. OLSON. 1985. Transplantation of adrenal medullary tissue to striatum in parkinsonism. *In* Neural Grafting in the Mammalian CNS. A. Björklund & U. Stenevi, Eds.: 551-556. Elsevier. Amsterdam.

9. LINDVALL, O., E.-O. BACKLUND, L. FARDE, G. SEDVALL, R. FREEDMAN, B. HOFFER, A. NOBIN, Å. SEIGER & L. OLSON. 1986. Transplantation in Parkinson's disease: Two cases of adrenal medullary grafts to putamen. Submitted for publication.

10. BACKLUND, E.-O., L. OLSON, Å. SEIGER & O. LINDVALL. 1987. Toward a transplantation therapy in Parkinson's diseas: A progress report from continuing clinical experiments. Ann. N.Y. Acad. Sci. This volume.

11. KESSLER, I. I. 1978. Parkinson's disease an epidemiologic perspective. Adv. Neurol. **19:** 355-383.

12. LIEBERMAN, A., M. DZIATOLOWSKI, M. KUPERSMITH, M. SERBY, A. GOODGOLD, J. KOREIN & M. GOLDSTEIN. 1979. Dementia in Parkinson's disease. Ann. Neurol. **6:** 355-359.

13. GASPAR, P. & F. GRAY. 1984. Dementia in idiopathic Parkinson's disease: A neuropathological study of 32 cases. Acta Neuropathol. **64:** 43-52.

14. FORNO, L. S. 1982. Pathology of Parkinson's disease. *In* Movement Disorders. C. D. Marsden & S. Fahn, Eds.: 25-40. Butterworths. London.

15. NYBERG, P., A. NORDBERG, P. WESTER & B. WINBLAD. 1983. Dopaminergic deficiency is more pronounced in putamen than in nucleus caudatus in Parkinson's disease. Neurochem. Pathol. **1:** 193-202.

16. JAVOY-AGID, F. & Y. AGID. 1980. Is the mesocortical dopamine system involved in Parkinson's disease? Neurology **30:** 1326-1330.

17. MANN, D. M. A. & P. O. YATES. 1983. Pathological basis for neurotransmitter changes in Parkinson's disease. Neuropathol. Appl. Neurobiol. **9:** 3-19.

18. ARENDT, T., V. BIGL, A. ARENDT & A. TENNSTEDT. 1983. Loss of neurons in the nucleus basalis of Meynert in Alzheimer's disease, paralysis agitans and Korsakoff's disease. Acta Neuropathol. **61:** 101-108.

19. CANDY, J. M., R. H. PERRY, E. K. PERRY, D. IRVING, G. BLESSED, A. F. FAIRBURN & B. E. TOMLINSON. 1983. Pathological changes in the nucleus of Meynert in Alzheimer's and Parkinson's diseases. J. Neurol. Sci. **54:** 277-289.

20. JAVOY-AGID, F., M. RUBERG, H. TAQUET, B. BOKOBZA, Y. AGID, P. GASPAR, B. BERGER, J. N'GUYEN-LEGROS, C. ALVAREZ, F. GRAY, J. J. HAUW, B. SCATTON & L. ROUQUIER. 1983. Biochemical neuropathology of Parkinson's disease. Adv. Neurol. **40:** 189-198.

21. UNGERSTEDT, U. & G. W. ARBUTHNOTT. 1970. Quantitative recording of rotational behavior in rats after 6-hydroxydopamine lesions of the nigrostriatal dopamine system. Brain Res. **24:** 485-493.

22. BJÖRKLUND, A., S. B. DUNNETT, U. STENEVI, M. E. LEWIS & S. D. IVERSEN. 1980. Reinnervation of the denervated striatum by substantia nigra transplants: Functional consequences as revealed by pharmacological and sensorimotor testing. Brain Res. **199:** 307-333.

23. DUNNETT, S. B., A. BJÖRKLUND, U. STENEVI & S. D. IVERSEN. 1981. Behavioral recovery following transplantation of substantia nigra in rats subjected to 6-OHDA lesions of the nigrostriatal pathway. I. Unilateral lesions. Brain Res. **215:** 147-161.

24. BJÖRKLUND, A., U. STENEVI, S. B. DUNNETT & S. D. IVERSEN. 1981. Functional reactivation of the deafferented neostriatum by nigral transplants. Nature **289:** 497-499.

25. DUNNETT, S. B., A. BJÖRKLUND, U. STENEVI & S. D. IVERSEN. 1981. Grafts of embryonic substantia nigra reinnervating the ventrolateral striatum ameliorate sensorimotor impairments and akinesia in rats with 6-OHDA lesions of the nigrostriatal pathway. Brain Res. **229:** 209-217.

26. DUNNETT, S. B., A. BJÖRKLUND, F. H. GAGE & U. STENEVI. 1985. Transplantation of mesencephalic dopamine neurons to the striatum of adult rats. *In* Neural Grafting in the Mammalian CNS. A. Björklund & U. Stenevi, Eds.: 451-469. Elsevier. Amsterdam.

27. BJÖRKLUND, A., R. H. SCHMIDT & U. STENEVI. 1980. Functional reinnervation of the neostriatum in the adult rat by use of intraparenchymal grafting of dissociated cell suspensions from the substantia nigra. Cell Tissue Res. **212:** 39-45.

28. BRUNDIN, P., O. ISACSON & A. BJÖRKLUND. 1985. Monitoring of cell viability in suspensions of embryonic CNS tissue and its use as a criterion for intracerebral graft survival. Brain Res. **331:** 251-259.
29. STENEVI, U., A. BJÖRKLUND & S. B. DUNNETT. 1980. Functional innervation of the denervated neostriatum by nigral transplants. Peptides **1**(Suppl. 1): 111-116.
30. OLSON, L., L. O. BOREUS & Å. SEIGER. 1973. Histochemical demonstration and mapping of 5-hydroxytryptamine- and catecholamine-containing neuron systems in the fetal brain. Z. Anat. Entwicklungsgesch. **139:** 259-282.
31. GAGE, F. H., P. BRUNDIN, O. ISACSON & A. BJÖRKLUND. 1985. Rat fetal brain tissue grafts survive and innervate host brain following five-day pregraft tissue storage. Neurosci. Lett. **60:** 133-137.
32. BRUNDIN, P., G. BARBIN, O. ISACSON, M. MALLAT, B. CHAMAK, A. PROCHIANTZ, F. H. GAGE & A. BJÖRKLUND. 1985. Survival of intracerebrally grafted rat dopamine neurons previously cultured *in vitro*. Neurosci. Lett. **61:** 79-84.
33. BJÖRKLUND, A. & O. LINDVALL. 1984. Dopamine-containing systems in the CNS. *In* Handbook of Chemical Neuroanatomy. Vol. 2. Classical Transmitters in the CNS. A. Björklund, T. Hökfelt & M. J. Kuhar, Eds.: 55-122. Elsevier. Amsterdam.
34. BRUNDIN, P., O. ISACSON, F. H. GAGE, A. PROCHIANTZ & A. BJÖRKLUND. 1986. The 6-hydroxydopamine-lesioned mouse as a model for assessing functional effects of neuronal grafting. Brain Res. **366:** 346-349.
35. SCHMIDT, R. H., M. INGVAR, O. LINDVALL, U. STENEVI & A. BJÖRKLUND. 1982. Functional activity of substantia nigra grafts reinnervating the striatum: Neurotransmitter metabolism and [^{14}C]2-deoxy-D-glucose autoradiography. J. Neurochem. **38:** 737-748.
36. SCHMIDT, R. H., A. BJÖRKLUND, U. STENEVI, S. B. DUNNETT & F. H. GAGE. 1983. Intracerebral grafting of neuronal cell suspensions. III. Activity of intrastriatal nigral suspension implants as assessed by measurements of dopamine synthesis and metabolism. Acta Physiol. Scand. Suppl. **522:** 19-28.
37. MCGEER, P. L., E. L. MCGEER & J. S. SUZUKI. 1977. Aging and extrapyramidal function. Arch. Neurol. **34:** 33-35.
38. REISINE, T. D., J. Z. FIELDS, H. I. YAMAMURA, E. D. BIRD, E. SPOKES, P. S. SCHREINER & S. I. ENNA. 1977. Neurotransmitter alterations in Parkinson's disease. Life Sci. **21:** 335-344.
39. HORNYKIEWICZ, O. 1982. Imbalance of brain monoamines and clinical disorders. Prog. Brain Res. **55:** 419-429.
40. BJÖRKLUND, A., U. STENEVI, R. H. SCHMIDT, S. B. DUNNETT & F. H. GAGE. 1983. Intracerebral grafting of neuronal cell suspensions. I. Survival and growth of nigral cell suspensions implanted in different brain sites. Acta Physiol. Scand. Suppl. **522:** 9-18.
41. FREED, W. J., M. J. PERLOW, F. KAROUM, Å. SEIGER, L. OLSON, B. J. HOFFER & R. J. WYATT. 1980. Restoration of dopaminergic function by grafting of fetal substantia nigra to the caudate nucleus: Long-term behavioral, biochemical and histochemical studies. Ann. Neurol. **8:** 510-519.
42. HERMAN, J.-P., K. CHOULLI, M. GEFFARD, D. NADAUD, K. TAGHZUOTI & M. LE MOAL. 1986. Reinnervation of the nucleus accumbens and frontal cortex of the rat by dopaminergic grafts and effects on hoarding behavior. Brain Res. **372:** 210-216.
43. DUNNETT, S. B., S. T. BUNCH, F. H. GAGE & A. BJÖRKLUND. 1984. Dopamine-rich transplants in rats with 6-OHDA lesions of the ventral tegmental area: Effects on spontaneous and drug-induced locomotor activity. Behav. Brain Res. **13:** 71-82.
44. JAEGER, C. B. 1985. Cytoarchitectonics of substantia nigra grafts: A light and electron micropic study of immunocytochemically identified dopaminergic neurons and fibrous astrocytes. J. Comp. Neurol. **231:** 121-135.
45. BRUNDIN, P., O. ISACSON, F. H. GAGE & A. BJÖRKLUND. 1986. Intrastriatal grafting of dopamine-containing neuronal cell suspensions: Effects of mixing with target or non-target cells. Dev. Brain Res. **24:** 77-84.
46. PROCHIANTZ, A., U. DI PORZIO, A. KATO, B. BERGER & J. GLOWINSKI. 1979. *In vitro* maturation of mesencephalic dopaminergic neurons from mouse embryos is enhanced in presence of their striatal target cells. Proc. Natl. Acad. Sci. USA **76:** 5387-5391.
47. CHAMAK, B., A. FELLOUS, A. TOUATI, G. BARBIN & A. PROCHIANTZ. 1987. Are neu-

roastroglial neuronotrophic interactions regionally specified? Ann. N.Y. Acad. Sci. This volume.

48. LINDVALL, O. 1975. Mesencephalic dopaminergic afferents to the lateral septal nucleus in the rat. Brain Res. **87:** 89-95.

49. CHOULLI, K., J.-P. HERMAN, D. NADAUD, K. TAGHZUOTI, H. SIMON & M. LE MOAL. 1986. Behavioral recovery following 6-OHDA lesion of the nucleus accumbens and intra-accumbens implantation of dopaminergic grafts. In New Concepts in Alzheimer's Disease. M. Briley, A. Kato & M. Weber, Eds. Macmillan. London.

50. BJÖRKLUND, A. & O. LINDVALL. 1986. Catecholaminergic brainstem regulatory systems. In Handbook of Physiology: The Nervous System. Vol. 4. Intrinsic Regulatory Systems in the Brain. F. E. Bloom, Ed.: 155-235. American Physiological Society. Bethesda, MD.

51. GAGE, F. H., A. BJÖRKLUND, U. STENEVI & S. B. DUNNETT. 1983. Intracerebral grafting of neuronal cell suspensions. VIII. Cell survival and axonal outgrowth of dopaminergic and cholinergic cells in the aged brain. Acta Physiol. Scand. Suppl. **522:** 67-75.

52. GAGE, F. H., S. B. DUNNETT, U. STENEVI & A. BJÖRKLUND. 1983. Aged rats: Recovery of motor impairments by intrastriatal nigral grafts. Science **221:** 966-969.

53. AGNATI, L. F., K. FUXE, F. BENEFATI, G. TOFFANO, M. CIMINO, N. BATTISTINI, L. CALZA & E. MERLO PICH. 1984. Studies on aging processes. Acta Physiol. Scand. Suppl. **532:** 45-61.

54. DUNNETT, S. B., A. BJÖRKLUND, R. H. SCHMIDT, U. STENEVI & S. D. IVERSEN. 1983. Intracerebral grafting of neuronal cell suspensions. IV. Behavioral recovery in rats with unilateral 6-OHDA lesions following implantation of nigral cell suspension in different brain sites. Acta Physiol. Scand. Suppl. **522:** 29-37.

55. POULSEN, E., P. BRUNDIN, R. E. STRECKER & A. BJÖRKLUND. 1987. Fetal dopamine neurons implanted unilaterally into the nucleus accumbens drive amphetamine-induced locomotion and circling. Ann. N.Y. Acad. Sci. This volume.

56. WUERTHELE, S. M., W. J. FREED, L. OLSON, J. MORIHISA, L. SPOOR, R. J. WYATT & B. J. HOFFER. 1981. Effect of dopamine agonists and antagonists on the electrical activity of substantia nigra neurons transplanted into the lateral ventricle of the rat. Exp. Brain Res. **44:** 1-10.

57. ARBUTHNOTT, G., S. B. DUNNETT & N. MACLEOD. 1985. Electrophysiological recording from nigral transplants in the rat. Neurosci. Lett. **57:** 205-210.

58. STRÖMBERG, I., S. JOHNSON, B. J. HOFFER & L. OLSON. 1985. Reinnervation of the dopamine-denervated striatum by substantia nigra transplants: Immunohistochemical and electrophysiological correlates. Neuroscience **14:** 981-990.

59. ZETTERSTRÖM, T., P. BRUNDIN, F. H. GAGE, T. SHARP, O. ISACSON, S. B. DUNNETT, U. UNGERSTEDT & A. BJÖRKLUND. 1986. Spontaneous release of dopamine from intrastriatal nigral grafts as monitored by the intracerebral dialysis technique. Brain Res. **362:** 344-349.

60. STRECKER, R. E., T. SHARP, P. BRUNDIN, T. ZETTERSTRÖM, U. UNGERSTEDT & A. BJÖRKLUND. 1986. Autoregulation of dopamine release and metabolism by intrastriatal nigral grafts as revealed by intrastriatal dialysis. Neuroscience. In press.

61. ZETTERSTRÖM, T. & UNGERSTEDT. 1984. Effects of apomorphine on the in vivo release of dopamine and its metabolites, studied by brain dialysis. Eur. J. Pharmacol. **97:** 29-36.

62. FORNI, C., P. BRUNDIN, R. E. STRECKER, S. EL GANOUNI, A. BJÖRKLUND & A. NIEOULLON. 1987. Long-term monitoring of dopamine release by in vivo voltammetry during reinnervation of the denervated striatum by mesencephalic grafts. Submitted for publication.

63. MAHALIK, T. J., T. E. FINGER, I. STRÖMBERG & L. OLSON. 1985. Substantia nigra transplants into denervated striatum of the rat: Ultrastructure of graft and host interconnections. J. Comp. Neurol. **240:** 60-70.

64. FREUND, T. F., J. P. BOLAM, A. BJÖRKLUND, U. STENEVI, S. B. DUNNETT, J. F. POWELL & A. D. SMITH. 1985. Efferent synaptic connections of grafted dopaminergic neurons reinnervating the host neostriatum: A tyrosine hydroxylase immunocytochemical study. J. Neurosci. **5:** 603-616.

65. DUNNETT, S. B. & A. BJÖRKLUND. 1983. Conditioned turning in rats: Dopaminergic involvement in the initiation of movement rather than the movement itself. Neurosci. Lett. **41:** 173-178.

66. DUNNETT, S. B., I. Q. WHISAW, G. H. JONES & O. ISACSON. 1986. Effects of dopamine-rich grafts on conditioned rotation in rats with unilateral 6-OHDA lesions. Neurosci. Lett. **68:** 127-133.
67. UNGERSTEDT, U. 1971. Aphagia and adipsia after 6-hydroxydopamine-induced degeneration of the nigrostriatal dopamine system. Acta Physiol. Scand. Suppl. **367:** 95-124.
68. DUNNETT, S. B., A. BJÖRKLUND, U. STENEVI & S. D. IVERSEN. 1981. Behavioral recovery following transplantation of substantia nigra in rats subject to 6-OHDA lesions of the nigrostriatal pathway. II. Bilateral lesions. Brain Res. **229:** 457-470.
69. DUNNETT, S. B., A. BJÖRKLUND, R. H. SCHMIDT, U. STENEVI & S. D. IVERSEN. 1983. Intracerebral grafting of neuronal cell suspensions. V. Behavioral recovery in rats with bilateral 6-OHDA lesions following implantation of nigral cell suspensions. Acta Physiol. Scand. Suppl. **522:** 39-47.
70. BARKER, C. F. & R. E. BILLINGHAM. 1977. Immunologically privileged sites. Adv. Immunol. **25:** 1-54.
71. MEDAWAR, P. B. 1948. Immunity to homologous grafted skin. III. The fate of skin homografts transplanted to the brain, to subcutaneous tissue, and to the anterior chamber of the eye. Br. J. Exp. Pathol. **29:** 58-69.
72. WONG, G. H. W., P. F. BARTLETT, I. CLARK-LEWIS, F. BATTYE & J. W. SCHRADER. 1984. Inducible expression of H-2 and Ia antigens on brain cells. Nature **310:** 688-691.
73. TRAUGOTT, U., L. SCHEINBERG & C. RAINE. 1985. On the presence of Ia-positive endothelial cells and astrocytes in multiple sclerosis lesions and its relevance to antigen presentation. J. Neuroimmunol. **8:** 1-14.
74. HERMAN, J.-P., K. CHOULLI & M. LE MOAL. 1985. Hyper-reactivity to amphetamine in rats with dopaminergic grafts. Exp. Brain Res. **60:** 521-526.
75. LEON, A., R. DAL TOSO, D. PRESTI, S. MAZZONI, D. VINCENZI & G. TOFFANO. 1985. Sera from parkinsonian patients contain inhibitory activity for the development of fetal mesencephalic dopaminergic neurons in culture. J. Neurochem. **44**(Suppl.): S13.

DISCUSSION OF THE PAPER

L. KROMER (*Georgetown University, Washington, DC*): It is really interesting that there is such a delay in the effect with these human embryonic tissue grafts. I know you have not looked at the histology, but some of the studies indicate that the recipient may be stimulating maturation of the presynaptic element. Would you care to speculate a little bit about what the time course may be and if this could be happening in your situation?

BRUNDIN: We looked at those animals that received the 11-week-old donor tissue. I mentioned we perfused one after 5½ weeks. These neurons do not look mature in the sense that they do not have a multipolar appearance. They are bipolar and very small. Maybe grafting to a target region will induce fiber outgrowth, but the cell will retain its internal clock with respect to fiber outgrowth.

J. M. GORELL (*Henry Ford Hospital, Detroit, MI*): How long do you believe it would take to have continued immunosuppression of the recipient to maintain the survivability and functionality of the grafts from the fetal donor?

BRUNDIN: Today we do not have any solid evidence of anything else but permanent immunosuppression being adequate. We have some pilots suggesting that 6 weeks of immunosuppression in a rodent might produce long-term survival, and we know that 10 days is not enough.

GORELL: And what is the potential price to pay in terms of immune-related diseases?

BRUNDIN: In the case of cyclosporin A, the potential price is fairly small if you use a modern dose regime with a low dose. There are problems with kidney toxicity in some cases. There are problems with hypertrophy of the gums, for instance, but the risk of getting what you call opportunistic infections is supposed to be relatively small with cyclosporin A treatment. The experience comes from renal grafts and heart transplants where people are on immune suppression for the rest of their lives.

M. RITTER (*Associated Press, New York, NY*): I understand from your paper that the fetal tissue came from therapeutic abortions. You said that ethical considerations might prevent this from being a source for therapeutic transplants. What do you mean by that? What considerations are you talking about?

BRUNDIN: We know that many people in the general public would question the use of any human fetal tissue for transplantation purposes. The brain is considered different from the rest of the body in the sense of the cells having some special property. This might make transplantation of brain cells a more controversial ethical question. In Sweden, human fetal tissue has been used in attempts to cure diabetes mellitus. For example, Langerhans' islets have been grafted. It is not a totally new field.

I think transplantation of fetal tissue is something that has to be discussed in public because we researchers may have a very special view. We may have a very clear view that we think this is ethically justifiable, but the general public might not share this view. The responsibility for making these judgments should be shared by everyone, not just by the researchers.

There is one other thing I think one should weigh in any ethical question: the cost versus the benefits. We are not trying to cure some minor cosmetic feature in a human being, we are trying to cure a devastating disease. If it was a question of grafting little bits of skin to make people look more beautiful, I do not think it would be ethically justifiable—from any point of view.

Behavioral Effects of Intraaccumbens Transplants in Rats with Lesions of the Mesocorticolimbic Dopamine System

K. CHOULLI, J. P. HERMAN,[a] N. ABROUS,
AND M. LE MOAL

Laboratoire de Psychobiologie des Comportements Adaptatifs
Institut National de la Santé
et de la Recherche Médicale Unité 259
Université Bordeaux II
33077 Bordeaux Cedex, France

INTRODUCTION

One problem concerning neural grafts is determining whether neurons implanted into the host nervous system, among established neuronal circuitries, can sustain some meaningful physiological function. The answer to this question, however, depends on the system studied. The general opinion, given the methods we have at present, is that some functional role may be achieved with neuronal systems having no precise information processing role and without a very precise and specific wiring (for a recent discussion, see reference 1). One of the systems belonging to this category is the one consisting of the mesotelencephalic dopaminergic neurons. The first reports have shown that after the lesion of the dopaminergic innervation of the striatum, intrastriatal dopaminergic grafts can indeed compensate for some of the deficits resulting from the lesion.[2-4] During the last 2 years, we have studied the ability of intraaccumbens dopaminergic grafts to restore functions after lesions of the mesocorticolimbic dopaminergic system. Our first results indicated that such grafts may have some, although limited, functional capacity after the local lesion of the dopaminergic terminals of the nucleus accumbens.[5,6] In the present study, we extended our original study to include further functional models. Furthermore, we tested whether the recoveries observed with the intraaccumbens grafts after the local lesion of the nucleus accumbens could also be found after a more extensive initial lesion, that is, after the destruction of the whole mesocorticolimbic dopaminergic system by lesioning at the cell body level.

[a]To whom correspondence should be addressed.

METHODOLOGICAL ASPECTS

The dopaminergic innervation of the nucleus accumbens of male rats was lesioned by injecting 6-hydroxydopamine (6-OHDA) either directly into the nucleus accumbens (Acc group) or into the cell body region (A10 area) of the ventral mesencephalic tegmentum (A10 group). The injection of the neurotoxin into the nucleus accumbens destroys the dopaminergic terminals in this structure as well as in the anteromedial striatum, frontal cortex, and septum,[6] whereas the lesion of the cell bodies destroys the whole mesocorticolimbic system. After having submitted the animals to some behavioral tests, grafting into the nucleus accumbens was performed 4 weeks after the initial lesion. Grafts consisted of a cellular suspension prepared from mesencephali of E14 rat embryos [6] injected stereotaxically into the nucleus accumbens. Behavioral tests were performed at various time points after grafting.

BEHAVIORAL STUDY OF THE FUNCTIONAL CAPACITIES OF INTRAACCUMBENS DOPAMINERGIC GRAFTS

Drug-induced Behaviors

The lesion of the dopaminergic innervation of the nucleus accumbens provokes a loss of the locomotor stimulation brought about by d-amphetamine, an indirectly acting dopaminergic agonist.[7,8] This deficit is present in both groups of lesioned animals when tested a short time after the lesion (FIG. 1). When tested 3 months after the initial lesion (that is, 2 months after grafting), a disappearance of the deficit could be noted in the animals that had a local lesion in the nucleus accumbens, whereas a deficit persisted in the group that had a mesencephalic lesion. Grafted animals of both lesion groups were markedly stimulated by the drug, and in fact this stimulation was significantly higher than that observed either for lesioned or even for control animals. Such a hyperreactivity of the grafted animals has been documented before[9] and has been attributed to a defective regulation of the activity of grafted neurons. It is noticeable that the grafted animals of the A10 group seem to be even more sensible to the action of d-amphetamine than those of the Acc group. This could be tentatively attributed to the denervation of the amygdala in the A10 group, as it has been shown previously that the lesion of the dopaminergic innervation of this structure enhances the behavioral action of d-amphetamine.[10] On the other hand, this group displays a higher postsynaptic receptor hypersensitivity (see below). This heightened hypersensitivity could also be involved in the enhanced response of these animals to d-amphetamine.

The destruction of the dopaminergic terminals of the nucleus accumbens provokes the appearance of the postsynaptic dopamine receptor hypersensitivity, which can be demonstrated by measuring the locomotor response of the lesioned animals to small doses of apomorphine, a direct dopamine receptor agonist. As shown in FIGURE 2, this response was still enhanced 3 months after the initial lesion in both lesioned groups. The intraaccumbens graft was unable to reverse this hypersensitivity in either group, although an insignificant decrease could be noticed in the grafted animals of the Acc group.

Spontaneous Behaviors

The action of the graft has been tested on two types of spontaneous behavior, exploratory activity and hoarding behavior, that are known to be disrupted after lesions of the kind we used.[11,12]

Exploratory activity during a 15-min period was measured by counting the number of times animals poked their noses through holes made around the wall of a circular open field. As shown in FIGURE 3, this activity was depressed in experimental animals immediately after the lesion, regardless of the type of lesion. Furthermore, the graft had no influence on this behavior as measured 2 months after transplantation.

In previous experiments, we have shown that a transient recovery of exploratory

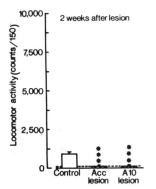 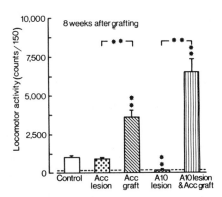

FIGURE 1. Effect of *d*-amphetamine sulfate (1.5 mg/kg, i.p.) on locomotor activity before and after implantation of dopaminergic grafts into the nucleus accumbens. The dashed line represents locomotor activity after saline injection. The labeling on this figure is the same as that seen on subsequent figures: Control: control, nonlesioned animals; Acc lesion: animals with a local 6-OHDA lesion of the nucleus accumbens; Acc graft: animals with a dopaminergic graft implanted into the nucleus accumbens after a local, intraaccumbens lesion; A10 lesion: animals with a 6-OHDA lesion of the ventral mesencephalic tegmentum; A10 lesion & Acc graft: animals with a dopaminergic graft implanted into the nucleus accumbens after a mesencephalic lesion. Each bar represents a mean ± SEM ($N = 8$-12). *: $p < .05$; **: $p < .01$; ***: $p < .005$ (compared to the control level).

activity could be induced for grafted animals with lesions of the nucleus accumbens if the grafted neurons were stimulated by a small dose of *d*-amphetamine at the time of testing.[5] We repeated this procedure in the present experiment 4 months after the initial lesion, by testing the behavior of the animals following pretreatment with saline or *d*-amphetamine (0.2 mg/kg, i.p., 10 min) (FIGS. 4B & 5B). At that time the lesioned controls of the Acc group, but not those of the A10 group, had recovered from the initial deficit. The grafted animals of both groups still presented deficient exploratory activity when tested without drug treatment. With the *d*-amphetamine pretreatment, grafted animals of the Acc group performed at the same level as intact controls (FIG. 4B), whereas the same treatment had no influence on the exploratory activity of the grafted animals of the A10 group (FIG. 5B). It is noticeable that the level of locomotor activation induced by this dose of *d*-amphetamine was higher for

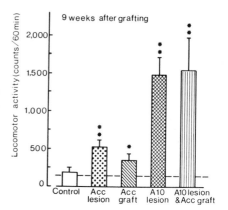

FIGURE 2. Effect of apomorphine (0.1 mg/kg, s.c.) on locomotor activity 2 months after grafting.

the grafted animals of the A10 group than that seen for the grafted animals of the Acc group (FIGS. 4A & 5A). This last observation indicates that the restoration of the exploratory behavior after stimulation by d-amphetamine was not a mere consequence of the locomotor activation brought about by the treatment.

The same procedure was followed for testing hoarding behavior. This behavior was seen to be depressed 1 to 4 months after the local lesion of the nucleus accumbens.[12,13] When tested 5 months after the lesion (as in the study described here), however, the behavioral deficit disappeared in the lesioned control animals of the Acc group (FIG. 4C) and persisted in the A10 control group (FIG. 5C). One may see how the reversal of the hoarding behavior deficit was similar to the reversal of the exploratory behavior deficit: grafted animals of both experimental groups displayed the hoarding deficit in the absence of drug treatment, but a d-amphetamine-induced reversal was only seen in grafted animals of the Acc group (FIGS. 4C & 5C).

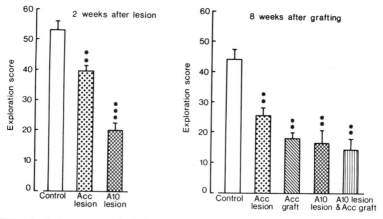

FIGURE 3. Exploratory activity before and after implantation of dopaminergic grafts into the nucleus accumbens.

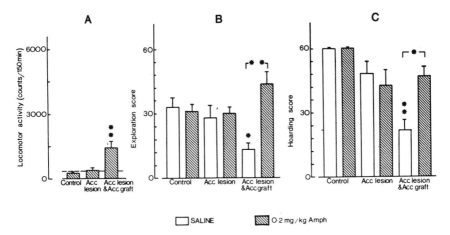

FIGURE 4. Effect of *d*-amphetamine (0.2 mg/kg, i.p.) on locomotor activity (**A**), exploratory activity (**B**), and hoarding behavior (**C**) 3 months after the implantation of dopaminergic graft into the nucleus accumbens lesioned with 6-OHDA.

Acquired Behaviors

Schedule-induced polydipsia was investigated by putting the food-deprived animals on a restricted feeding schedule (one food pellet delivered every 60 sec) and recording the amount of water drunk during the 30-min experimental session. Under these conditions, control animals rapidly acquire excessive drinking behavior (FIG. 6). The development of this behavior was attenuated in the lesioned control animals of the

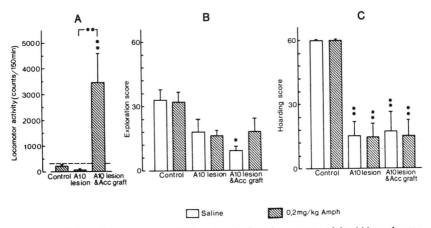

FIGURE 5. Effect of *d*-amphetamine (0.2 mg/kg, i.p.) on locomotor activity (**A**), exploratory activity (**B**), and hoarding behavior (**C**) 3 months after the implantation of dopaminergic grafts into the nucleus accumbens (the ventral mesencephalic tegmentum had been lesioned with 6-OHDA before grafting).

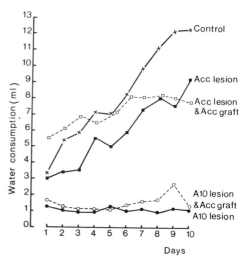

FIGURE 6. Acquisition of schedule-induced polydipsia 5 months after the implantation of dopaminergic grafts into the nucleus accumbens.

Acc group and was totally blocked by the mesencephalic lesion in the A10 group. The presence of the dopaminergic graft in the nucleus accumbens had no influence on this deficit in either lesion model. In fact, grafted animals of the Acc group did not develop any polydipsic behavior at all, despite a higher initial water consumption during the experimental session (but not in their home cage). This was in contrast to the acquisition of such a behavior in the lesioned control animals of the Acc group.

The second acquired behavior tested was that of the spatial navigation in the Morris water maze. In the test, the animals were put in a tank filled with water and had to find a platform hidden under the water by using spatial cues of the environment to orientate themselves. Control animals learned to locate the platform by the second day of the test (FIGS. 7 & 8) whereas neither lesioned nor grafted animals were able to learn to escape during the experimental period. Some differences in the behavioral pattern of the experimental animals, however, could be noted. Animals of the Acc group swam vigorously but randomly all over the surface of the tank, finding the platform occasionally by chance (FIG. 9). On the other hand, animals of the A10 group tended to swim slowly, and were frequently seen immobile on the surface of the water. Moreover, they followed the perimeter of the tank, without swimming to the open surface (FIG. 10). These behavioral patterns were left unchanged by the graft as well. In contrast to its effect in the exploration or hoarding tests, d-amphetamine pretreatment (0.2 mg/kg) did not help the grafted animals to locate the platform. Grafted animals of both lesion groups shifted instead to rapid and sustained swimming around the perimeter of the water tank (FIGS. 9 & 10).

ANATOMY OF INTRAACCUMBENS DOPAMINERGIC GRAFTS

At the end of the above behavioral study, some of the animals were sacrificed and the grafts examined by an immunohistochemical approach, using an antibody raised against tyrosine hydroxylase. The appearance of the graft was similar for the grafted animals of the Acc group and for animals of the A10 group (FIG. 11). Dopaminergic neurons were found all over the nucleus accumbens and also along the injection cannula in the anteromedial striatum. These neurons were located preferentially at the periphery of the graft and gave rise to a rich reinnervation of the adjacent areas, with fibers extending between 1 and 1.5 mm.

BIOCHEMICAL STUDIES OF THE DOPAMINERGIC GRAFTS

The behavioral studies have shown that in order to reveal a functional effect of the graft, implanted dopaminergic neurons have to be stimulated by a small dose of *d*-amphetamine. This requirement could be due to the fact that the grafted neurons, being placed in a nonphysiologic location (that is, into a terminal area of the meso-corticolimbic system), would not be subject to physiological modulations of their activity. We tested the existence of two such modulations: feedback regulation and activation by a physiological stimulus, namely footshock stress.

Dopaminergic neurons are known to be subject to a feedback regulation which may be disclosed by measuring the activity of such neurons after a treatment of the animals with a dopaminergic receptor blocker.[13] We administered haloperidol to control animals and to animals bearing an intrastriatal dopaminergic graft, and measured the dopaminergic activity in the striatum by taking the DOPAC:DA ratio as an indicator of this activity.[14] The results shown in TABLE 1 indicate that the activity of the grafted neurons was increased following the treatment, and that the increase resembles that seen for the dopaminergic neurons of control animals. This points toward the existence of some feedback regulation of the activity of the grafted dopaminergic neurons. This regulation, however, most probably involves a regulation by presynaptic receptors rather than interneuronal feedback, as a similar activation has been described for dopaminergic neurons implanted into the lateral ventricle.[15]

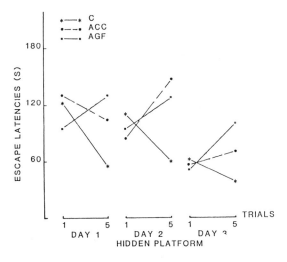

FIGURE 7. Place navigation task. Time course of the latency to escape onto the platform, 6 months after grafting into the nucleus accumbens following its lesion with 6-OHDA.

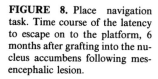

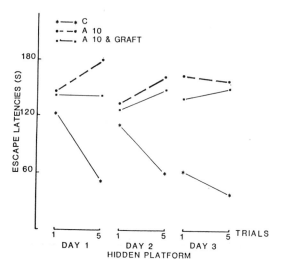

FIGURE 8. Place navigation task. Time course of the latency to escape on to the platform, 6 months after grafting into the nucleus accumbens following mesencephalic lesion.

The second model explored was that of the activation of the dopaminergic neurons by electric footshock. This activation may be measured in the terminal areas of the mesocorticolimbic system.[16] Control animals and animals bearing a 6-OHDA lesion of the A10 area and grafted subsequently with dopaminergic neurons into the nucleus accumbens were subjected to 20 min of electric footshock stress, and the dopaminergic activity in the nucleus accumbens was measured at the end of the stress session. The results show (FIG. 12) that although exposure to stress significantly elevated the DOPAC:DA ratio in the nucleus accumbens of the control animals, it had no influence on dopaminergic activity in the grafted nucleus accumbens. This result indicates that, in accordance with our hypothesis, the grafted neurons are not subject to physiological interneuronal modulation of their activity.

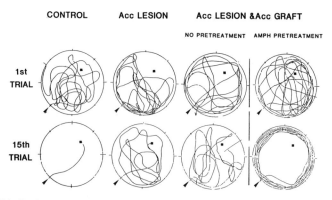

FIGURE 9. Evolution of the swimming pattern in the Morris water maze between the first and last trial after local nucleus accumbens lesion. *d*-Amphetamine pretreatment (0.2 mg/kg) was given only on the last day; in that case the 1st trial represented corresponds to the 11th experimental trial. The black dot represents the platform; the arrow shows the starting point.

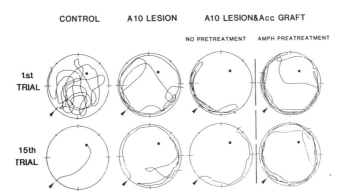

FIGURE 10. Evolution of the swimming pattern in the Morris water maze between the first and last trial, following mesencephalic lesion. For details see FIGURE 9.

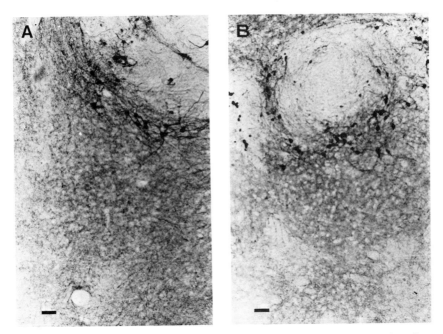

FIGURE 11. Appearance of the intraaccumbens dopaminergic graft 6 months after implantation in an animal that had previously been subjected to a local nucleus accumbens lesion (**A**) or to mesencephalic lesion (**B**). Immunohistochemical procedure using an antibody raised against tyrosine hydroxylase. Each bar represents 50 μ.

CONCLUSION

In summary, the results indicate the following: 1) After the local lesion of the nucleus accumbens, but not after the lesion of the A10 area, a spontaneous gradual recovery from some behavioral deficits could be observed. 2) No such spontaneous reversal of deficits was found for grafted animals. 3) Nevertheless, the grafted animals could display some recovery when implanted neurons were stimulated by d-amphetamine; however, this action of the graft was limited in that it could be observed only for some behavioral models and only for animals of the Acc group.

The disappearance of some of the behavioral deficits provoked by the lesion of the dopaminergic neurons has been previously noted for lesions involving the nigrostriatal system.[17,18] In the present case, this recovery may be mediated by a reinnervation of the previously lesioned nucleus accumbens by dopaminergic neurons having survived after the lesion. Two observations point in this direction: 1) No reversal of deficits was seen in animals with lesions of the dopaminergic cell bodies in the ventral mesencephalon, indicating that the presence of these cells is required for the recovery. 2) If animals with local lesions to the nucleus accumbens are subjected to a second intraaccumbens 6-OHDA injection, the initial deficits reappear.[19] It must be noted that some behavioral deficits (such as deficits of acquired behaviors or of movement initiation) persisted, and showed no signs of diminishing, throughout the experimental period.

The present observations concerning the lack of spontaneous recovery for the grafted animals of the Acc group are in contrast with the observed restoration of normal behavior for lesioned controls, and confirm our previous observations made with similar grafts. These results indicate that the intraaccumbens graft may counteract endogenous processes leading to functional recovery. The mechanisms of this inhibition are unclear at present. The graft itself could provoke a secondary lesion at the site of implantation. This secondary lesion, however, probably does not cause the observed inhibition, as the grafted animals, which were given pharmacological stimulation, were able to transiently display a recovery. On the other hand, the presence of a rich graft-

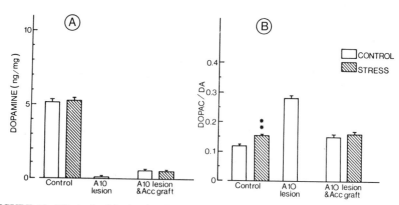

FIGURE 12. Effect of a 20-min electrical footshock on the dopamine level (**A**) and on the DOPAC:DA ratio (**B**) in the nucleus accumbens of control or lesioned animals and in animals with dopaminergic grafts implanted into the nucleus accumbens. **: $p < .01$ (compared to the nonshock condition).

TABLE 1. Effect of Haloperidol on the DOPAC:DA Ratio in the Striatum

	DOPAC:DA Ratio	
Treatment	Control Striatum	Grafted Striatum
Saline	0.080 ± 0.009	0.148 ± 0.012
Haloperidol (0.5 mg/kg, 60 min)	0.270 ± 0.010^a	0.317 ± 0.020^a

NOTE: Each value represents a mean $\pm$ SEM ($N = 5$-8).
$^a p < .005$ compared to saline treatment.

originated innervation of the nucleus accumbens could inhibit the reinnervation of this structure by dopaminergic fibers of the host, thus leading to the observed lack of spontaneous reversal of deficits. Further experiments, however, are needed to confirm the existence of such a competition.

Intraaccumbens dopaminergic grafts were nevertheless able to reinstate some function after the lesion of the dopaminergic innervation of the nucleus accumbens. This recovery, however, was limited in several respects. First, in order to be revealed, the implanted neurons had to be stimulated by a low dose of *d*-amphetamine. A tentative explanation for this requirement could be, that given their ectopic, nonphysiological location, the activity of the neurons would not be modulated in response to environmental stimuli. In fact, such a lack of modulation was indicated by the lack of activation of the grafted neurons by stress. Second, recovery could only be demonstrated for some behavioral models, such as locomotor activity, exploration, or hoarding, whereas other deficits were not influenced by the presence of the graft even when stimulated by *d*-amphetamine. This fact could be related to the complexity of the behavioral task or to an insufficient degree of reinnervation provided by the graft or both. Moreover, recovery from a deficit other than that of *d*-amphetamine-induced locomotor activation was not observed with grafts after the lesion of the whole mesocorticolimbic dopaminergic pathway. This indicates that even for the compensation of more simple behavioral deficits, such as an exploratory behavior deficit, a reinnervation of the nucleus accumbens by the graft is a necessary but insufficient condition. Further studies are under way in which multiple grafts are being implanted into the various terminal areas of the mesocorticolimbic system to reveal whether recovery follows the simultaneous reinnervation of several areas after the A10 lesion.

REFERENCES

1. FREED, W. J. 1985. Neurobiol. Aging **6:** 153-156.
2. FREED, W. J., M. J. PERLOW, F. SEIGER, L. OLSON, B. HOFFER & R. J. WYATT. 1980. Ann. Neurol. **8:** 510-519.
3. BJÖRKLUND, A., S. B. DUNNETT, U. STENEVI, M. E. LEWIS & S. D. IVERSEN. 1980. Brain Res. **199:** 307-333.
4. DUNNETT, S. B., A. BJÖRKLUND, R. H. SCHMIDT, U. STENEVI & S. D. IVERSEN. 1983. Acta Physiol. Scand. Suppl. **522:** 29-37.
5. HERMAN, J. P., D. NADAUD, K. CHOULLI, K. TAGHZOUTI, H. SIMON & M. LE MOAL. 1985. *In* Neural Grafting in the Mammalian CNS. A. Björklund & U. Stenevi, Eds.: 519-527. Elsevier. Amsterdam.

6. HERMAN, J. P., K. CHOULLI, M. GEFFARD, D. NADAUD, K. TAGHZOUTI & M. LE MOAL. 1986. Brain Res. **372**: 210-216.
7. KELLY, P. H., E. M. JOYCE, K. I. MINNEMAN & O. PHILLIPSON. 1977. Brain Res. **122**: 382-387.
8. KOOB, G. F., L. STINUS & M. LE MOAL. 1981. Behav. Brain Res. **3**: 341-359.
9. HERMAN, J. P., K. CHOULLI & M. LE MOAL. 1985. Exp. Brain Res. **60**: 521-526.
10. LOUILOT, A., K. TAGHZOUTI, J. M. DEMINIÈRE, H. SIMON & M. LE MOAL. 1987. *In* Neurotransmitter Interaction. M. Sandler, C. Feuerstein & B. Scatton, Eds.: 193-204. Raven Press. New York, NY.
11. TAGHZOUTI, K., H. SIMON, A. LOUILOT, J. P. HERMAN & M. LE MOAL. 1985. Brain Res. **344**: 9-20.
12. KELLEY, A. E. & L. STINUS. 1985. Behav. Neurosci. **99**: 531-545.
13. CARLSSON, A., W. KEHR, M. LINDQUIST, T. MAGNUSSON & C. V. ATACK. 1982. Pharmacol. Rev. **24**: 371-384.
14. ROTH, R. H., C. MURRIN & R. J. WALTER. 1976. Eur. J. Pharmacol. **36**: 163-171.
15. WUERTHELE, S. M., W. J. FREED, L. OLSON, J. MORIHISA, L. SPOOR, R. J. WYATT & B. HOFFER. 1981. Exp. Brain Res. **44**: 1-10.
16. HERMAN, J. P., D. GUILLONNEAU, R. DANTZER, B. SCATTON, L. SEMERDJIAN-ROUQUIER & M. LE MOAL. 1982. Life Sci. **30**: 2207-2214.
17. ZIGMOND, M. J. & E. M. STRICKER. 1973. Science **182**: 713-720.
18. NEVE, K. E., M. R. KOZLOWSKI & J. F. MARSHALL. 1982. Brain Res. **244**: 33-44.
19. HERMAN, J. P., K. CHOULLI, D. NADAUD, K. TAGHZOUTI, H. SIMON & M. LE MOAL. 1986. *In* New Concepts in Alzheimer's Disease. H. Briley, A. Kato & M. Weber, Eds.: 265-279. Macmillan. London.

DISCUSSION OF THE PAPER

H. BERNSTEIN-GORAL (*Downstate Medical Center, State University of New York, Stony Brook, NY*): In your first studies concerning locomotor response to amphetamine with your nucleus accumbens lesions, you did not give your dose of amphetamine. Did you see any stereotypic behavior that may indicate a shift in your dose response curve?

HERMAN: The dose was 1.5 milligrams per kilogram body weight. At this dose we have not seen any stereotypic behavior. On the other hand, we do see a shift in the dose response curve in that the grafted animals are much more sensitive to amphetamine. They respond to a dose of amphetamine as small as 0.1 milligrams per kilogram body weight, a dose that has no effect at all in the normal animal.

A. BJÖRKLUND (*University of Lund, Sweden*): The local accumbens lesion will also affect areas away from the local injection site because of the axons passing through. Have you considered that the cortical areas in frontal cortex will be denervated? Could you put that into the context of interpreting your lesion data?

HERMAN: It is true that we have a lesion of the frontal cortex innervation, too, but these grafts reinnervate the frontal cortex as well when put into the very anterior level of the nucleus accumbens. I think that we have got reinnervation of both the structures, perhaps less total for the frontal cortex than for the nucleus accumbens.

BJÖRKLUND: Could it be that the amphetamine effect is mediated more by the very sparse inputs to parts of the cortex rather than the accumbens? Or that the efficiency of the innervation may be important to consider, and that these behaviors depend on the coordinated function over wider areas of the limbic cortical region?

HERMAN: Yes. I think these are real possibilities.

BJÖRKLUND: Do you know what local 6-OHDA into the frontal cortex would do in the behavioral tasks?

HERMAN: No. We have not tried it.

A. W. DECKEL (*Johns Hopkins University School of Medicine, Baltimore, MD*): My paper is about an effect strikingly similar to the amphetamine effect in a different system. In the striatum with fetal striatal transplants, we found that one correlate to that hyperactivity had to do with quantitative aspects of the transplantation methodology. How many cells you put in there, for example. Did you look at surviving graft size, the number of cells, or whether any quantitative measures of your graft itself correlated with your behavioral outcomes?

HERMAN: We have looked at the histology of all these animals, and we have had different survival rates. We had two rats that had rather poorly surviving grafts that showed poor behavioral recovery. But for all the others the range of dopaminergic cells was between 5000 and 20 000. There was no real correlation between the degree of behavioral recovery and the number of surviving cells that we could see for the latter animals.

DECKEL: You mean you tested for correlations between dopaminergic cell counts and behavioral outcome and found none?

HERMAN: We found no real correlation. It looks as if recovery would appear above a threshold level of reinnervation and would not vary then with variations of the degree of reinnervation above that level.

Voltammetric Analysis of Nigral Graft Function[a]

BARRY J. HOFFER,[b,c] GREG A. GERHARDT,[c,d]
GREG M. ROSE,[c,e] INGRID STRÖMBERG,[f]
AND LARS OLSON[f]

[c]Department of Pharmacology
and
[d]Department of Psychiatry
University of Colorado Health Sciences Center
Denver, Colorado
[e]Department of Medical Research
Veterans Administration Medical Center
Denver, Colorado
[f]Department of Histology
Karolinska Institute
Stockholm, Sweden

INTRODUCTION

Transplantation of immature brain tissue into the developing and adult central nervous system has attracted much attention, both as a tool for studying brain development,[1,2] and as a potential approach for repairing damaged neuronal circuits.[1,3–5] As presented by several contributors to this volume, intraventricular, intracavity, or dissociated intraparenchymal grafts of the fetal substantia nigra region, placed into striatum that has been depleted of dopamine (DA) by 6-hydroxydopamine (6-OHDA) pretreatment, can restore many of the behavioral dysfunctions induced by such a denervation.[6,7] Since the substantia nigra transplants produce DA-containing nerve fibers that invade adjacent areas of host striatum, it has been postulated that restoration of behavioral function is the result of this reinnervation of the damaged host striatum by nerve fibers from the graft. There has been little direct evidence thus far, however, to suggest that ingrowing nerve fibers from the grafts actually release neurotransmitters.

In recent years, it has become possible to measure changes in the extracellular levels of the monoamine neurotransmitters and their metabolites in the brain using

[a]This work was supported by Grants 14X-03185, 14P-5867, and K84-14V-6998 from the Swedish Medical Research Council; by Grants NS-09199, AG-04418, AG-06434, and ES-02011 from the U. S. Public Health Service; and by the Veterans Administration Medical Research Service.

[b]Address for correspondence: Department of Pharmacology, Box C236, University of Colorado Health Sciences Center, 4200 East Ninth Avenue, Denver, Colorado 80262.

510

in vivo electrochemical methods.[8,9] Improvements in recording electrode technology have greatly increased the selectivity of such methods, and thus have reduced some of the previous ambiguity as to the identity of the detected electroactive species.[10–15] Most of the previously reported studies employing *in vivo* electrochemistry, however, have focused on neurochemical sequelae after parenteral administration of drugs.[16–23] Because of individual differences in metabolism, this method may not be well suited for quantitative mapping in transplant-reinnervated animals; in addition, the long-lasting effect of even a single drug injection often precludes studying response reproducibility in an anesthetized animal.

A promising resolution to the problems of parenteral drug use has involved coupling local application of KCl via pressure ejection with *in vivo* electrochemical techniques as a means of studying release from monoamine nerve terminals *in situ*. In the present studies, we have sought to delineate several critical aspects of local application of KCl combined with *in vivo* electrochemical recording, in order to establish its utility as a means of activating monoaminergic nerve terminals *in situ* and studying presynaptic release. A detailed description of the methodology, as well as the electrode evaluation required to carry out this technique, will be presented first. Subsequently, the dose-response relationship between the amount of KCl ejected and the concentration of released electroactive species will be described. The possibility that Na^+, another monovalent cation, could induce similar releases was investigated as a control for bolus effects. The K^+-induced releases were recorded from several brain regions in an effort to correlate signal amplitudes with known densities of monoaminergic innervation. The influence of DA reuptake blockade on response magnitude was also evaluated.

In the second portion of our work to be presented, we wished to determine if K^+-induced neurotransmitter release could be demonstrated in DA-depleted rat caudate nucleus that had been reinnervated by DA-containing fibers originating from substantia nigra transplants. The magnitude, time course, and spatial distribution of K^+-evoked releases were utilized as parameters to indicate the presence of fiber ingrowth from the transplant, as well as to assess the functional nature of the innervation. To provide standards for comparison, various types of control striata, detailed below, were also studied, as were striata from animals that had received 6-OHDA lesions but were not subsequently grafted.

METHODS

Denervations and Transplantations

Adult female albino rats (Sprague-Dawley) were anesthetized with halothane and received a unilateral injection of 6-OHDA (8 μg in 4 μl of Ringer's solution) into the ascending nigrostriatal pathway. This procedure causes massive and permanent degeneration of dopaminergic terminals in the caudate nucleus on the injected side. The degree of denervation was confirmed by measuring the amount of contralateral rotational behavior that was elicited by intraperitoneal apomorphine injection (0.1 mg/kg).[24] All animals used as hosts for subsequent transplantation were judged, on the basis of behavioral testing, to have had a complete unilateral DA denervation.

Thirty to 60 days after the 6-OHDA treatment, host animals were again anesthetized and placed in a stereotaxic frame. The bone overlying the anterior cortex was removed, and, using aspiration, a cavity was prepared through the cortex and corpus callosum to expose the dorsal surface of the striatum on the denervated side. According to the "delayed cavity" protocol,[25] the rats were left to recover for another 1-2 months. They were then reanesthetized with halothane and again placed in the stereotaxic frame. The cavity was exposed and its lower half filled with six pieces of the substantia nigra area, prepared from fetal rats with a crown-to-rump length of 16-20 mm, dissected as described elsewhere.[26] The cavity was then covered with Gelfoam and the skin over the skull sutured together. Animals were housed in group cages, were exposed to a 12-hr light-dark cycle, received food and water *ad libitum*, and required no special postoperative treatments.

Acute Animal Preparation for Electrochemistry

Rats were anesthetized with chloral hydrate (400 mg/kg, i.p., in distilled water), intubated, and placed in a stereotaxic frame. Anesthetic levels were maintained using subsequent 100-150 mg/kg doses as needed. The animals rested on a heating pad; body temperature was kept at 37° C as indicated by a rectal thermometer. The skull overlying the anterior cortex was removed bilaterally. Reference and auxiliary electrodes (described below) were inserted into brain regions remote from the recording site and cemented into place using dental acrylic.

Electrochemical Methods

The electrochemical working electrodes used in these experiments were of the Nafion-coated graphite epoxy capillary (GEC) type. These were fabricated, calibrated, and characterized for selectivity and response time as previously described.[15,27] All calibrations were performed at room temperature using solutions prepared with 0.1 M phosphate-buffered saline (pH 7.4). Electrodes used for experimentation showed excellent linearity over a DA concentration range from 0.25 to 15.0 μM (FIG. 1); calibrations were performed in solutions that contained 250 μM ascorbic acid to mimic brain extracellular levels.[28] All electrodes used for experimentation had a selectivity for DA versus ascorbic acid of greater than 100:1. The electrodes were also tested with solutions containing 50 μM uric acid and were found to exhibit poor sensitivity for this potentially confounding substance.[29] We have previously shown that, in rat brain, these electrodes are insensitive to locally applied anionic monoamine metabolites such as 3,4-dihydroxyphenylacetic acid (DOPAC).[15] Electrode tip diameters were typically 50-200 μ. An Ag/AgCl wire served as the reference electrode and an Ag wire was used as the auxiliary electrode.

Electrochemical measurements were performed using a modified version of a microcomputer-controlled chronoamperometry apparatus.[30] A block diagram of the recording system is seen in FIGURE 2A. An oxidation potential of +0.55 V with respect to the reference was applied to the GEC electrode for 1 sec (FIG. 2B). It has been demonstrated that this voltage is below the threshold required to alter the excitability of striatal neurons.[31] The resulting oxidation current was digitally integrated during the final 500 msec. A delay of 5 sec was employed between measurements; the GEC electrode was maintained at a resting potential of 0.0 V during this interval.

Micropipette-GEC Electrode Assemblies

The K^+-evoked local releases were carried out using rigid micropipette-GEC electrode assemblies. Single- or double-barreled micropipettes, used for ejection of KCl or other solutions, were prepared from 1-mm O.D. fiber-filled glass capillaries using a vertical electrode puller. Single-barreled micropipettes and one barrel of the double-barreled pipettes were filled with a solution containing 120 mM KCl and 2.5

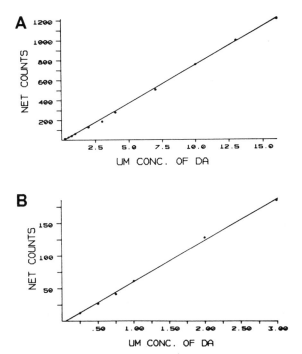

FIGURE 1. (**A**) Calibration curve for a Nafion-coated GEC electrode. Only electrodes that showed a very high degree of linearity (linear regression correlation factor $\geq .997$) were used in the experiments. (**B**) Expanded portion of the calibration curve demonstrating that the electrodes maintain their linearity at very low DA concentrations.

mM $CaCl_2$, or with normal saline (154 mM NaCl). The second barrel of the double-barreled micropipettes was filled with a 50 μM solution of nomifensine maleate (Hoechst-Roussel) dissolved in saline. After filling, the micropipette tips were bumped to a final inside diameter of 10-12 μ. The GEC and the K^+-containing micropipette were then fastened together, with a tip separation of 280-320 μ, using sticky wax. Local application of all agents *in situ* was accomplished using the technique of pressure ejection.[32]

Experimental Protocols

Experiments were initiated with the insertion of an electrode assembly into a selected region of the brain. Electrochemical measurements were performed every 5 sec to establish a baseline response. Once a steady-state signal was achieved, the effect of local application of KCl or other pressure-ejected solutions was studied. Pressure pulses applied to the K^+-containing micropipette ranged from 5-30 psi for durations of 5-10 sec. Upon observation of a K^+-evoked electrochemical response, ejection pressure was increased by 2.5-5.0 psi, and the ejection was repeated. Ejection pressure continued to be increased until a maximal signal was observed. At still higher ejection pressures, only a depression of the baseline signal was recorded. This depression was presumably due to local dilution of the electroactive species by the KCl bolus (see

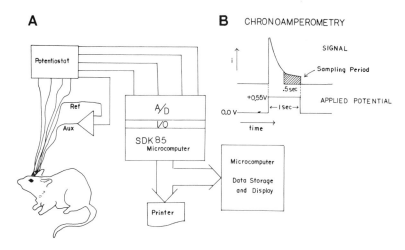

FIGURE 2. (A) Basic block diagram of the *in vivo* electrochemical recording apparatus. **(B)** Voltage and current waveforms from the chronoamperometric recordings are illustrated.

below). Electrochemical measurements were continued following the application of the pressure pulse until the recorded response returned to a baseline value. Signals were expressed as micromolar changes from baseline, calculated using the *in vitro* calibration curve determined for each GEC electrode.

Local K^+ stimulations were carried out in five different types of striatal tissue. Normal rat striatum, as well as the untreated sides of 6-OHDA-treated animals and 6-OHDA treated rats that received substantia nigra transplants, served as control tissue. The striata of 6-OHDA-treated animals was examined to provide information on residual signals recorded in the absence of the dopaminergic afferents to the caudate nucleus. Finally, 6-OHDA-denervated striatum that had received fetal substantia nigra grafts was investigated. The control sides of the 6-OHDA-treated and the transplanted rats were always studied first to establish the characteristics of each electrode assembly. To test for any time-dependent changes in the performance of a given electrode assembly, however, control side loci were again studied at time points later in the experiment. For averaged data, variability was expressed as the standard error of the mean (SEM). Statistical comparisons were made using the two-tailed Student's t test.

Histology

At the conclusion of the recording session, animals were overdosed with chloral hydrate and intracardially perfused with 100 ml of 0.9% NaCl, followed by 500 ml of 10% formalin in phosphate buffer (pH 7.4). The brain was removed and placed in the formalin solution for at least 24 hr, after which sucrose (30% w/v) was added to the fluid. Once the brain had sunk, it was quickly frozen, and 50-μ-thick sections were made. The sections were mounted on gelatin-coated slides and allowed to dry. After this, they were counterstained with cresyl violet; dehydrated; cleared; and mounted, using Permount, with coverslips. Recording sites were identified by localizing a given electrode track; for grafted striata, these were then classified according to their location as proximal to (≤ 1 mm) or distal from (> 1 mm) the transplant.

In a separate group of 6-OHDA-treated rats that received substantia nigra transplants, immunohistochemical localization of tyrosine hydroxylase-like reactivity was carried out using the indirect immunofluorescence method[33,34] in order to visualize the pattern of reinnervation. In addition, catecholamines were visualized by Falck-Hillarp fluorescence histochemistry[35,36] using freeze-dried, paraffin-embedded tissues.[37]

RESULTS

Control Experiments

Relationship between KCl Ejection and the Magnitude of Evoked Release

Only a limited range of "dose dependence" was observed for a given K^+-containing micropipette. Below the threshold pressure, no change in the electrochemical signal was elicited by application of a pressure pulse. As the threshold was reached, a small release (generally < 1.5 μM) of the electroactive species was observed. If the ejection pressure was increased only slightly from the threshold, a much larger release was evoked; typical releases are seen in FIGURE 3. At 15-25 psi above threshold, however, the initial response to the KCl bolus was a rapid and transient decline in the electrochemical signal. This phenomenon was probably the result of excessive application of the KCl solution, which caused a dilution of the basal level of electroactive species present at the tip of the recording electrode (see also Specificity Controls, below). The decline in the electrochemical signal was followed by an increase that had a peak amplitude that was often attenuated. In addition, the signal was occasionally observed to rapidly decline well below the initial baseline. A complete description of the dose dependence of the K^+-evoked releases has been previously reported.[38]

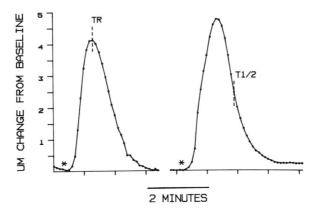

FIGURE 3. Reproducibility of K^+-evoked releases of electroactive species from the caudate nucleus of the rat. The second trace was obtained after a delay of 20 min. The TR and T1/2 designations refer to the rise time and half decay times of the signals. The timing of the KCl applications is indicated by the asterisks above the traces.

Thus, KCl ejection pressures 5-10 psi above threshold were selected for routine use in subsequent experiments presented here. Under these conditions, it was estimated that the volume of KCl delivered into the extracellular space did not exceed 100 nl.[32] In several cases, however, we were able to observe the effect of the sudden injection of an estimated several microliters of the KCl solution, caused by accidental breakage of the microelectrode tip in the brain. In these instances, the electrochemical signal very rapidly increased to peak values that were three- to fourfold greater than were seen under any other circumstances.[38] The evoked releases were also prolonged in duration compared to those normally seen. These unusually large releases could not be reproduced at the same site (see Reproducibility, below).

Characteristics of K^+-evoked Releases from Rat Striatum

A depth profile was constructed for the K^+-evoked releases recorded from control striata. The profile, shown in FIGURE 4, was based upon histologically verified electrode placements 0.0-1.5 mm anterior and 2.5-3.5 mm lateral to bregma ($N = 94$, 6-23 releases per site). There was a trend toward a gradual reduction in the releases evoked in more ventral regions of the striatum; a significant difference was found between the most dorsal (4.0 mm) and the most ventral (6.0 mm) site ($p < .05$).

Reproducibility of the K^+-evoked Releases

The evoked signals were found to be reproducible at a given site within the caudate nucleus. We generally observed that 15-20 min were necessary between KCl applications. The variation in release magnitudes after a 20-min time delay between applications was less than 10%. Reproducible signals observed in the rat striatum after a 20-min time delay are shown in FIGURE 3. About 80% of the attempts to obtain multiple releases from the same site were successful. Nearly all of the failures were attributable to plugging of the pressure micropipette tip; in cases where this difficulty was not immediately encountered, as many as six repeated stimulations could be achieved, with minimum variability in the recorded signals.

Specificity Controls

The specificity of K^+ in inducing releases of electroactive species was assessed by substituting normal saline (154 mM NaCl) for the KCl solution. The pressure parameters employed, as well as the characteristics of the electrode array, were identical to those used for the applications of the KCl solution. Local application of the NaCl solution in rat caudate nucleus ($N = 8$) consistently produced a decrease in the electrochemical baseline with a subsequent return to the preapplication levels; an increase was never observed. An example of the recorded signal following NaCl application is shown in FIGURE 5A.

The K^+-evoked releases were also recorded from sites dorsal or ventral to the caudate nucleus; these data are summarized in TABLE 1. Releases obtained from the cerebral cortex or nucleus accumbens had consistently smaller amplitudes than those obtained from the striatum. At other sites, the electrochemical signal declined following the application of KCl and then slowly returned to the preapplication baseline without any increase. An example of this phenomenon is shown in FIGURE 5B. Subsequent histological examination of such recording sites showed that, in 27 of 31 cases, the electrode array had been accidentally placed into the corpus callosum or anterior commissure.

Effects of Reuptake Blockade on the K^+-evoked Releases

The reproducible characteristics of the releases allowed pharmacological manipulations to further determine the identity of the detected electroactive species following

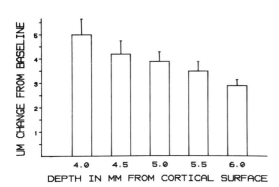

FIGURE 4. Bar graph of average K^+-evoked release magnitudes recorded from different depths (6-23 releases per site) of the rat caudate nucleus.

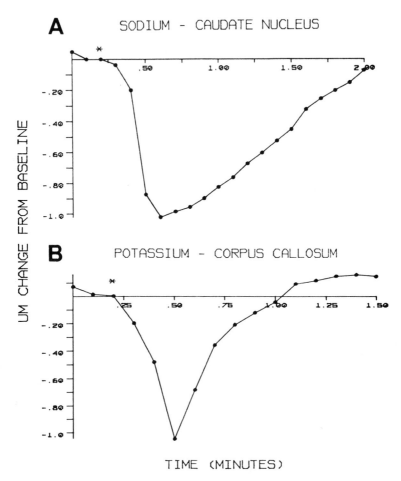

FIGURE 5. (A) Normal saline (154 mM NaCl) ejection adjacent to a Nafion-coated electrode in the caudate nucleus of the rat. (B) The K^+-evoked "release" recorded from a histologically verified placement of the electrode array into the corpus callosum of a rat. The timing of the applications are indicated by the asterisks above both traces. In both cases, only a transient depression of the signal was observed.

KCl application. Using double-barreled micropipettes coupled with the Nafion-coated GEC electrodes (see Methods), we studied the effects of the dopaminergic reuptake blocker, nomifensine, upon the signals observed in rat striatum. In these cases, an initial application of KCl was made to determine the magnitude of the evoked release from a given site. Following a 20-min time delay, nomifensine was ejected from the second barrel of the pipette (2.5-5.0 psi for 20-40 sec). Immediately afterwards, a second application of KCl was effected. When using the double-barreled micropipettes, there was no significant increase in the average release obtained from the application of KCl alone. A statistically significant increase in the K^+-evoked signal was observed, however, after nomifensine pretreatment. FIGURE 6 illustrates the effects of nomifensine on the K^+-evoked signals. The average change from baseline was 4.9 ± 0.3 μM under the control condition, versus 8.3 ± 0.7 μM following nomifensine pretreatment ($p < .001$, $N = 11$). The time course of the K^+-evoked signal was also altered by the nomifensine treatment. An average 43% increase in the baseline-to-baseline time course of the signal was observed ($p < .05$).

In Vivo *Electrochemistry of 6-OHDA-lesioned and Grafted Striata*

Magnitudes of K^+-evoked Releases

Of special significance for studies on grafts was the maintenance of linearity at concentrations of DA of less than 1.0 μM (FIG. 1), for this allowed reliable determination of K^+-evoked release in both the normal and 6-OHDA-treated caudate nucleus. The mean release magnitudes for all recorded sites are shown in FIGURE 7. The three bars on the left of the figure represent the control groups: striata of normal animals (NC), striata contralateral to the denervated caudate nucleus of rats that received only 6-OHDA treatment (6OHC), and striata contralateral to the grafted side of transplant animals (TPC). The differences among these three control groups were not statistically significant ($p > .2$). At the right of the figure are three more bars, which show the release magnitudes obtained from experimentally manipulated striata. The first of these represents the mean value recorded from sites histologically determined to be ≤ 1.0 mm from the graft in the caudate nucleus of rats that received substantia nigra transplants (TPP); the second bar represents the mean for sites recorded within the same caudates, but at distances > 1.5 mm from the graft (TPD); the last bar shows the mean value for K^+-evoked releases from the denervated striata of animals that received only 6-OHDA treatment (6OH).

The difference between the TPP group and the three control groups was only significant for the 6OHC case ($p < .05$). The TPD and 6OH groups, however, differed from both the control groups and the TPP group ($p < .001$ for all). There was no significant difference between the TPD and 6OH groups.

TABLE 1. Regional Dependence of the K^+-evoked Signals Recorded in the Rat Brain

Brain Region	Average K^+-evoked Signal[a]	N
Cerebral cortex	1.2 ± 0.2	14
Corpus callosum	0.1 ± 0.1[b]	19
Caudate nucleus	4.2 ± 0.5	86
Anterior commissure	0.1 ± 0.1[c]	12
Nucleus accumbens	2.6 ± 0.4	32

[a] Each of the values for K^+-evoked release is expressed as an average micromolar signal observed using DA *in vitro* calibration curves. Variability is expressed as SEM.
[b] Only 3 of the 19 release attempts yielded measurable release.
[c] Only 1 of the 12 release attempts yielded measurable release.

FIGURE 6. The effects of the catecholamine reuptake blocker, nomifensine, on the K$^+$-evoked signals recorded from the caudate nucleus of the rat. The +NOM curve represents the K$^+$-evoked signal observed after local pretreatment with nomifensine from the second barrel of the micropipette. The control curve was recorded from the same region of the striatum 20 min before the application of the reuptake blocker. The asterisk indicates the applications of the KCl solution.

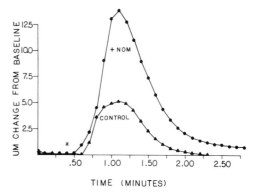

TIME (MINUTES)

Spatial Relationship of K$^+$-evoked Releases

The relationship between the magnitude of K$^+$-evoked release and the proximity of a given recording site to a transplant is shown for an individual animal in FIGURE 8. The left portion of the figure is a diagram of the anatomical placement of the transplant at the base of a cavity on the dorsal surface of the caudate nucleus. This graft was located about 1 mm anterior to bregma. An electrode track just beneath the transplant, extending in depth from 4.0 to 6.0 mm below the brain surface, is also shown. The bar graph on the right shows the magnitude of K$^+$-evoked releases obtained at the depths indicated. The release from the dorsal site, nearest the transplant, was significantly greater than releases from more ventral sites. This type of dorsoventral gradient was seen in all five transplanted animals. In a similar vein, marked antero-

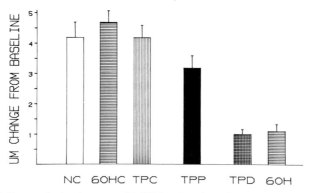

FIGURE 7. Bar graph showing mean ($\pm$ SEM) values for K$^+$-evoked releases obtained from control and experimentally manipulated striata. The bars on the left show the values from the three control groups: NC: normal caudate ($N = 86$); 6OHC: control side of rats that received only unilateral 6-OHDA lesions ($N = 29$); TPC: control side of rats that received unilateral 6-OHDA lesions and subsequent substantia nigra transplants ($N = 59$). The bars on the right show the values obtained from striatal sites proximal to (≤ 1.0 mm) (TPP; $N = 51$) and distal from (> 1.0 mm) (TPD; $N = 27$) a transplant, and from the 6-OHDA-denervated caudate (6OH; $N = 38$). See the text for details and statistical analysis.

posterior gradients were seen in three of these rats. Electrode penetrations greater than 1.0 mm anterior or posterior to a transplant manifested far less release than was obtained from tracks just beneath a graft (see also the work by Rose *et al.*[39]).

Temporal Dynamics of the K+-evoked Signals

Experimental manipulations resulted in changes in the time course of K+-evoked releases observed in the caudate nucleus as well. Typical releases from control; 6-

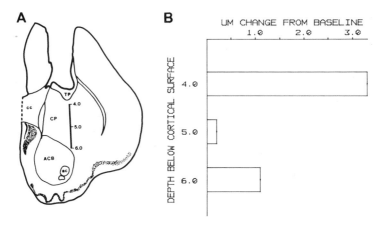

FIGURE 8. Relationship between the proximity of the striatal recording site and release magnitude. (**A**) Diagram of a substantia nigra transplant (TP) at the base of a cavity that reaches the dorsal surface of the caudate nucleus (CP). A recording track is also shown, indicating depths below cortical surface where K+-evoked releases were induced. (**B**) Horizontal bars indicate the release magnitudes at each of these points. Note that the largest release was obtained from the site proximal to the transplant. ACB: nucleus accumbens; cc: corpus callosum; ac: anterior commissure.

OHDA-treated; and 6-OHDA-treated, transplant-reinnervated striata are illustrated in FIGURE 9; KCl ejection is indicated by the asterisk in each case. The time course of the releases was quantified by measuring both the time to peak response (TR) as well as one-half the time required for the response to return to baseline following the application of the KCl bolus (T1/2). These data are presented in TABLE 2.

As can be seen from this table, the release time courses from the three control groups were quite consistent and did not differ statistically from each other. Releases obtained from the caudate nucleus of 6-OHDA-treated rats, either without or distal to a transplant, had significantly shorter rise times. Releases obtained from the striata adjacent to the graft, however, had essentially normal time courses. Thus, the duration of K+-evoked releases qualitatively paralleled release magnitude.

DISCUSSION

The present results demonstrate the utility of coupling local application of KCl with *in vivo* electrochemical detection as a means of studying release and reuptake from monoamine nerve terminals *in situ*. This conclusion is supported by the findings that the K^+-evoked signals were reversible, partially dose dependent, and reproducible. The K^+ effect is specific in that the releases were associated with rat brain regions that contained monoamine nerve terminals and that NaCl application did not produce similar effects. Finally, we have demonstrated that the technique can be coupled with local drug application methods to study the effects of an agent that alters reuptake processes.

The evoked releases from the striatum were reproducible only if an adequate delay time was interposed between stimulations. The reproducibility of the K^+-evoked releases is also an indication of the relatively noninvasive nature of this technique. Interestingly, the "refractory" period for rat caudate nucleus was the same as has been reported for obtaining reproducible electrochemical signals after electrical stimulation of monoaminergic afferents to this structure.[40]

Nafion-coated GEC electrodes were used to minimize possible signal interference from monoamine metabolites and ascorbic acid; we also determined that these electrodes were insensitive to another potential interferent, uric acid (see Methods). Unfortunately, the electrodes do not discriminate between DA, serotonin, and norepinephrine at the oxidation potential currently employed. A recent study,[41] however, has determined the relative concentrations in the rat striatum of these three neurotransmitters, in the order listed above, to be, on the average, 100:8:2; thus, serotonin and norepinephrine should provide only a minor contribution to the K^+-evoked

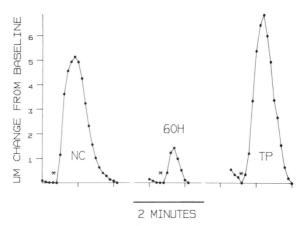

FIGURE 9. Examples of the magnitude and time course of K^+-evoked releases obtained from normal caudate nucleus (NC); 6-OHDA-denervated caudate (6OH); and 6-OHDA-denervated, transplanted caudate (TP). The latter release was obtained from a site within 1.0 mm of a substantia nigra graft. Note that following 6-OHDA treatment both the magnitude and time course of K^+-evoked releases are reduced compared to control. Adjacent to a substantia nigra transplant, however, normal release parameters are observed. Each asterisk indicates the timing of a KCl application.

TABLE 2. Time Course of K$^+$-evoked Releases

	TR (sec)	T1/2 (sec)	N
Control groups			
Normal	45 ± 3.3	81 ± 5.3	45
Transplant	43 ± 2.4	72 ± 7.2	17
6-OHDA	38 ± 5.2	67 ± 7.7	17
Experimental groups			
Transplant			
Proximal	40 ± 4.8	78 ± 7.2	14
Distal	25 ± 2.9^a	38 ± 3.5^b	10
6-OHDA	29 ± 5.9	47 ± 9.6	10

NOTE: No significant difference was found between any two control groups ($p >$ .1), between any of the control groups and the proximal to the transplant group ($p >$ .2), or between the 6-OHDA experimental group and the distal to transplant group ($p >$ .4).

^{a} $p <$ .05 versus the proximal to transplant group; $p <$ .01 versus any of the control groups.
^{b} $p <$ .001 versus the proximal to transplant group or versus any of the control groups.

electrochemical signals recorded here. Potentiation of release magnitudes and time courses following application of the reuptake blocker nomifensine also suggest that the electrochemical signal is derived from DA-containing nerve terminals, as serotonin reuptake mechanisms are hardly affected by nomifensine.[42] The recording of only very small signals from confirmed electrode placements into corpus callosum or anterior commissure is also consistent with the absence of DA nerve terminals in these regions. A high level of extracellular ascorbic acid has been reported in the corpus callosum[42]; it did not, however, contribute to K$^+$-evoked signals in the present studies. Thus, the data obtained with the Nafion-coated electrodes, as well as the pharmacological and anatomical data, support the hypothesis that the major component of the K$^+$-evoked electrochemical signals is DA.

A second important finding of the present series of experiments is that monoamines can be released in almost normal quantities from a DA-denervated striatum that has been reinnervated by transplants of fetal substantia nigra. The patterning of K$^+$-evoked release magnitudes correlated well with the previously reported distribution of outgrowing graft-derived fibers as visualized using fluorescence histochemistry or tyrosine hydroxylase immunocytochemistry.[1,34,44] In addition to reductions in magnitude, significant differences in the time course of K$^+$-evoked releases from the striata were observed after 6-OHDA treatment; these differences were not present in areas of the caudate proximal to a transplant.

Although suggesting that organotypic release of DA does occur from substantia nigra transplant-derived nerve fibers, the present results do not establish the existence of synapses between efferents from the graft and the host caudate neurons; recent ultrastructural studies, however, have supported this possibility.[45] Moreover, we have recently found that locally applied phencyclidine, an indirect DA agonist that acts presynaptically to either cause transmitter release or block its reuptake, was much more effective in altering the spontaneous firing rate of caudate neurons proximal to substantia nigra transplants in 6-OHDA-treated rats.[34] This finding, taken together with the results of the present study, would strongly suggest that DA, released from substantia nigra transplant afferents to host striatal neurons, provides a functional input to the caudate neurons.

In conclusion, the present findings, together with information provided by histochemical, electrophysiological, and behavioral studies, support the postulate that substantia nigra transplants ameliorate the dysfunction observed following 6-OHDA treatment by providing a specific DA input to the host caudate nucleus. In future studies, we plan to determine if such transplant-derived dopaminergic inputs are also endogenously activated during relevant behaviors in unanesthetized animals.

REFERENCES

1. BJÖRKLUND, A. & U. STENEVI. 1984. Intracerebral neural implants: Neuronal replacement and reconstruction of damaged circuitries. Annu. Rev. Neurosci. **7:** 279-308.
2. OLSON, L., A. BJÖRKLUND & B. HOFFER. 1984. Camera bulbi anterior: New vistas on a classical locus for neural tissue transplantation. *In* Neuronal Transplants, Development, and Function. J. R. Sladek, Jr. & D. M. Gash, Eds.: 125-166. Plenum. New York, NY.
3. BJÖRKLUND, A. & U. STENEVI. 1979. Reconstruction of the nigrostriatal dopamine pathway by intracerebral nigral transplants. Brain Res. **177:** 555-560.
4. OLSON, L., E. BACKLUND, W. FREED, M. HERRERA-MARSCHITZ, B. HOFFER, A. SEIGER & I STRÖMBERG. 1985. Transplantation of monoamine-producing cell systems *in oculo* and intracranially: Experiments in search of a treatment for Parkinson's disease. Ann. N. Y. Acad. Sci. **457:** 105-126.
5. PERLOW, M., W. FREED, B. HOFFER, A. SEIGER, L. OLSON & R. WYATT. 1979. Brain grafts reduce motor abnormalities produced by CNS damage. Science **204:** 643-647.
6. DUNNETT, S. B., A. BJÖRKLUND & U. STENEVI. 1983. Dopamine-rich transplants in experimental parkinsonism. Trends Neurosci. **6:** 266-269.
7. FREED, W. J., B. J. HOFFER, L. OLSON & R. J. WYATT. 1984. Transplantation of catecholamine-containing tissues to restore the functional capacity of the damaged nigrostriatal system. *In* Neuronal Transplants, Development, and Function. J. R. Sladek, Jr. & D. M. Gash, Eds.: 377-406. Plenum. New York, NY.
8. ADAMS, R. N. & C. A. MARSDEN. 1982. Electrochemical detection methods for monoamine measurements *in vitro* and *in vivo. In* Handbook of Pharmacology. L. L. Iverson. S. S. Iverson & S. H. Snyder, Eds. Vol. **15:** 1-74. Plenum. New York, NY.
9. MARSDEN, C. A., M. P. BRAZELL & N. T. MAIDMENT. 1984. An introduction to *in vivo* electrochemistry. *In* Measurement of Neurotransmitter Release *in Vivo*. C. A. Marsden, Ed.: 127-152. John Wiley & Sons. Chichester.
10. GONON, F. G., C. M. FOMBARLET, M. J. BUDA & J. F. PUJOL. 1981. Electrochemical treatment of pyrolytic carbon fiber electrodes. Anal. Chem. **53:** 1386-1389.
11. GONON, F., M. BUDA & J. F. PUJOL. 1984. Treated carbon fiber electrodes for measuring catechols and ascorbic acid. *In* Measurement of Neurotransmitter Release *in Vivo*. C. A. Marsden, Ed.: 153-171. John Wiley & Sons. Chichester.
12. MARCENAC, F. & F. GONON. 1985. Fast *in vivo* monitoring of dopamine release in the rat brain with differential pulse amperometry. Anal. Chem. **57:** 1778-1779.
13. EWING, A. G., R. M. WIGHTMAN, & M. A. DAYTON. 1982. *In vivo* voltammetry with electrodes that discriminate between dopamine and ascorbate. Brain Res. **249:** 361-370.
14. BLAHA, C. D. & R. F. LANE. 1983. Selective voltammetric measurement of brain catecholamines at chemically modified graphite paste electrodes. Brain Res. Bull. **10:** 861-864.
15. GERHARDT, G. A., A. F. OKE, G. NAGY, B. MOGHADDAM & R. N. ADAMS. 1984. Nafion-coated electrodes with high selectivity for CNS electrochemistry. Brain Res. **290:** 390-395.
16. LANE, R. F., A. T. HUBBARD & C. D. BLAHA. 1978. Brain dopaminergic neurons: *In vivo* electrochemical information concerning storage, metabolism and release processes. Bioelectr. Bioeng. **5:** 504-525.
17. HUFF, R., R. N. ADAMS & C. O. RUTLEDGE. 1979. Amphetamine dose-dependent changes of *in vivo* electrochemical signals in rat caudate. Brain Res. **173:** 369-372.

18. GONON, F., M. BUDA, R. CESPUGLIO, M. JOUVET & J. F. PUJOL. 1980. *In vivo* electrochemical detection of catechols in the neostriatum of anesthetized rats: Dopamine or DOPAC? Nature (London) **286:** 902-904.

19. HEFTI, F. & E. MELAMED. 1981. Dopamine release in rat striatum after administration of L-dopa as studied with *in vivo* electrochemistry. Brain Res. **225:** 333-346.

20. MOS, J., H. J. BROXTERMAN & W. P. VAN BENNEKOM. 1981. *In vivo* voltammetric investigations into the action of HA-966 on central dopaminergic neurons. Brain Res. **207:** 465-470.

21. KENNETT, G. A. & M. H. JOSEPH. 1982. Does *in vivo* voltammetry in the hippocampus measure 5-HT release? Brain Res. **236:** 305-316.

22. O'NEILL, R. D., R. A. GRÜNWALD, M. FILLEME & W. J. ALBERY. 1982. Linear sweep voltammetry with carbon paste electrodes in the rat striatum. Neuroscience **79:** 1945-1954.

23. HOWARD-BUTCHER, S., C. D. BLAHA & R. F. Lane. 1984. A comparison of the CNS stimulants with phencyclidine on dopamine release using *in vivo* voltammetry. Brain Res. Bull. **13:** 497-501.

24. UNGERSTEDT, U., T. LJUNGBERG, B. HOFFER & G. SIGGINS. 1975. Dopamine supersensitivity in the striatum. Adv. Neurol. **9:** 57-65.

25. STENEVI, U., A. BJÖRKLUND & N.-A. SVENDGAARD. 1976. Transplantation of central and peripheral monoamine neurons to the adult rat brain: Techniques and conditions for survival. Brain Res. **14:** 1-20.

26. SEIGER, A. & L. OLSON. 1977. Quantitation of fiber growth in transplanted central monoamine neurons. Cell Tissue Res. **179:** 285-316.

27. NAGY, G., G. A. GERHARDT, A. F. OKE, M. E. RICE, R. N. ADAMS, R. B. MOORE III, M. N. SZENTIRMAY & C. R. MARTIN. 1985. Ion exchange and transport of neurotransmitters in Nafion films on conventional and microelectrode surfaces. J. Electroanal. Chem. **188:** 85-94.

28. SCHENK, J. O., E. MILLER, R. GADDIS & R. N. ADAMS. 1982. Homeostatic control of ascorbate concentration in CNS extracellular fluid. Brain Res. **253:** 353-356.

29. CRESPI, F., T. SHARP, N. MAIDMENT & C. A. MARSDEN. 1983. Differential pulse voltammetry *in vivo:* Evidence that uric acid contributes to the indole oxidation peak. Neurosci. Lett. **43:** 203-207.

30. CHENG, H.-Y., W. WHITE & R. N. ADAMS. 1980. Microprocessor-controlled apparatus for *in vivo* electrochemical measurement. Anal. Chem **52:** 2445-2448.

31. HEFTI, F. & D. FELIX. 1982. Chronoamperometry *in vivo:* Does it interfere with spontaneous neuronal activity in the brain? J. Neurosci. Methods **7:** 151-156.

32. PALMER, M. R., S. M. WUERTHELE & B. J. HOFFER. 1980. Physical and physiological characteristics of micropressure ejection of drugs from multibarreled pipettes. Neuropharmacology **19:** 931-938.

33. COONS, A. H. 1958. Fluorescent antibody methods. *In* General Cytochemical Methods. J. F. Danielli, Ed.: 399-422. Academic Press. New York, NY.

34. STRÖMBERG, I., S. JOHNSON, B. HOFFER & L. OLSON. 1985. Reinnervation of dopamine-denervated striatum by substantia nigra transplants: Immunohistochemical and electrophysiological correlates. Neuroscience **14**(4): 981-990.

35. CORRODI, H. & G. JONSSON. 1967. The formaldehyde fluorescence method for the histochemical demonstration of biogenic amines: A review on the methodology. J. Histochem. Cytochem. **15:** 65-78.

36. FALCK, B., N.-A. HILLARP, G. THIEME & A. TORP. 1962. Fluorescence of catecholamines and related compounds condensed with formaldehyde. J. Histochem. Cytochem. **10:** 348-354.

37. OLSON, L. & U. UNGERSTEDT. 1970. A simple high capacity freeze-drier for histochemical use. Histochemie **22:** 8-19.

38. GERHARDT, G. A., G. M. ROSE & B. J. HOFFER. 1986. Release of monoamines from striatum of rat and mouse evoked by local application of potassium: Evaluation of a new *in vivo* electrochemical technique. J. Neurochem. **46:** 842-850.

39. ROSE, G., G. GERHARDT, I. STRÖMBERG, L. OLSON & B. HOFFER. 1985. Monoamine release from dopamine-depleted rat caudate nucleus reinnervated by substantia nigra transplants: An *in vivo* electrochemical study. Brain Res. **341:** 92-100.

40. EWING, A. G., J. C. BIGELOW & R. M. WIGHTMAN. 1983. Direct *in vivo* monitoring of dopamine released from two striatal compartments in the rat. Science **221:** 169-171.
41. SCHENK, J. O., E. MILLER, M. E. RICE & R. N. ADAMS. 1983. Chronoamperometry in brain slices: Quantitative evaluation of *in vivo* electrochemistry. Brain Res. **277:** 1-8.
42. TUOMISTO, J. 1977. Nomifensine and its derivatives as possible tools for studying amine uptake. Eur. J. Pharmacol. **42:** 101-106.
43. STAMFORD, J. A., Z. L. KRUK & J. MILLAR. 1984. Regional differences in extracellular ascorbic acid levels in the rat brain determined by high-speed cyclic voltammetry. Brain Res. **299:** 289-295.
44. SCHULTZBERG, M., S. B. DUNNETT, A. BJÖRKLUND, U. STENEVI, T. HÖKFELT, G. J. DOCKRAYS & M. GOLDSTEIN. 1984. Dopamine-and cholecystokinin-immunoreactive neurons in mesencephalic grafts reinnervating the neostriatum: Evidence for selective growth regulation. Neuroscience **12:** 17-32.
45. MAHALIK, T. J., T. E. FINGER, I. STRÖMBERG & L. OLSON. 1985. Substantia nigra transplants into denervated striatum of the rat: Ultrastructure of graft to host interconnections. J. Comp. Neurol. **240:** 60-70.

DISCUSSION OF THE PAPER

QUESTIONER: Aside from the use of reuptake blockers and specific presynaptic receptor blockers, I would like to ask you about other ways to increase the specificity for overcoming the major problem: knowing what is really being released chemically.

GERHARDT: Philosophically, I have to state that there is a fundamental limit with any *in situ* technique. You have to learn how to use your tools. The electrophysiologists have been doing this for 20 or 30 years now and have characterized their system. I can only show you so many times in a beaker where we pressure-eject ascorbate and DOPAC next to our electrodes. The bottom line is how do you know what it is you are measuring. There are some experimental approaches for providing further chemical proof of the species adjacent to the electrode. These things are left up to the electrochemistry types like myself. We are working on further enhancing the selectivity of these recordings to take advantage of the inherent chemistry of the molecules.

C. NICHOLSON (*New York University, New York, NY*): Obviously this is a very exciting technique. It is extremely elegant—the use of K^+ to release DA and other compounds. But we know that in real life the brain does not use this as a means of releasing these compounds. Could you say what the prospects are for using your electrochemical techniques to investigate functional reinnervation by real pathways and functional release?

GERHARDT: We find in an intact animal that is anesthetized that the caudate is a very quiet area. Cell firing rates are low, and you do not see a lot of DA. In a freely moving animal, everyone is wondering whether the *in vivo* electrochemistry is going to be able to pick up neurotransmissions from a behavioral event. One of the things that we really did not understand a long time ago was the fact that reuptake processes are very active. In a normal undrugged animal the results are incredible. You can pressure eject a little bit of DA into the extracellular space in the striatum and it is gone! And this is not just diffusion: uptake is very capable of taking back up DA into cells adjacent to other terminals that have released DA. You have seen my K^+ signals.

Although it is slow in the sense of electrophysiology, it is still a relatively rapid event. I think in time, in a freely moving animal, if we turn our gains up high enough and approach the problems in a logical fashion, we are going to see some indication of true physiological release.

Are Neuronotrophic Neuron-Astrocyte Interactions Regionally Specified?[a]

B. CHAMAK, A. FELLOUS, A. AUTILLO-TOUATI,
G. BARBIN, AND A. PROCHIANTZ

Chaire de Neuropharmacologie
Institut National de la Santé
et de la Recherche Médicale Unité 114
Collège de France
75231 Paris Cedex 05, France

INTRODUCTION

For the last few years, our laboratory has been involved in the study of specific neuron-neuron interactions between the mesencephalic dopaminergic neurons and their target cells from the striatum. We have demonstrated that the growth cones of the dopaminergic neurons do specifically recognize their target cells and that the establishment of reciprocal interactions between dopaminergic and striatal neurons is accompanied by an increased ability of the monoaminergic cells to take up and synthesize dopamine.[1-4]

More recently, our focus of interest has shifted toward the specificity of neuron-astrocyte interactions. Some evidence has been provided showing that the morphological traits of dopaminergic neurons differ when these cells are allowed to develop on astrocyte monolayers derived from the mesencephalon or from the striatum.[5]

Following this observation, we would like to discuss here the possibility that astrocytes from different brain regions have a specific trophic influence on the neurons from the same region.

RESULTS

Dopaminergic Neurons Grown on Mesencephalic or Striatal Astrocytes Are Morphologically Different

FIGURE 1 presents two different aspects of mesencephalic dopaminergic neurons visualized by autoradiography after [³H]dopamine uptake.[2] The linear nonbranched

[a] This work was supported by grants from the Institut National de la Santé et de la Recherche Médicale, the Ministère de la Recherche et de la Technologie (84 C 1315), and the Rhône Poulenc Santé.

528

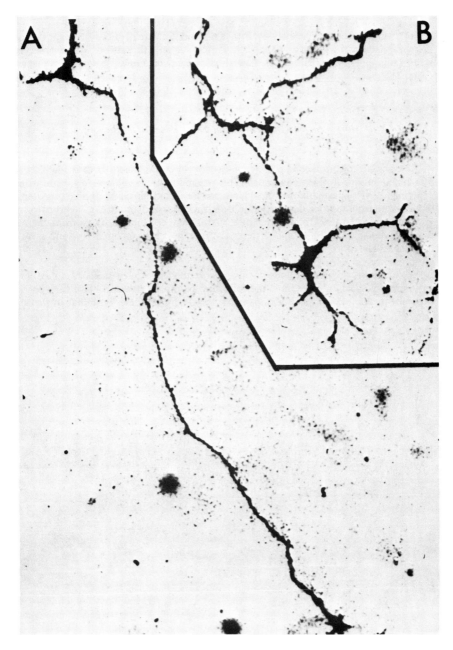

FIGURE 1. Mesencephalic dopaminergic neurons visualized by autoradiography after [³H]dopamine uptake. (A) The linear nonbranched type of neurite is observed on Gmes and Gstr. (B) The more complex and branched neurites are observed on Gmes exclusively. Neurons from 13-day-old mouse embryos are cultured for 2 days on preestablished 3-week-old glial monolayers.[5]

neuron (FIG. 1A) represents the major type present after 2 days on striatal astrocytes (Gstr). Both types, nonbranched (FIG. 1A) and branched (FIG. 1B), coexist on mesencephalic astrocytes (Gmes). Such a different growth pattern is also observed when dopaminergic explants are allowed to develop on Gmes or Gstr monolayers (FIG. 2).

This Morphological Differentiation Is an Instructive Phenomenon

The absence of branched neurons on Gstr could be explained by their inability to attach and survive in these conditions. This possibility was examined in the following experiment: Mesencephalic neurons (Nmes) were plated on Gmes and Gstr. After 2 days, the morphology of dopaminergic cells was analyzed (control). Neurons from sister cultures (Nmes/Gmes and Nmes/Gstr) were trypsinized away from the astrocytes, replated on Gmes and Gstr in the four possible combinations, and grown for 2 days. The morphology of dopaminergic neurons was then examined. The results are presented in TABLE 1.

In this table, the nondeveloped neurons were too small to be safely classified into any morphological category, but the following points seem clear: 1) In the control experiment, the total number of dopaminergic neurons on Gmes is similar to that on

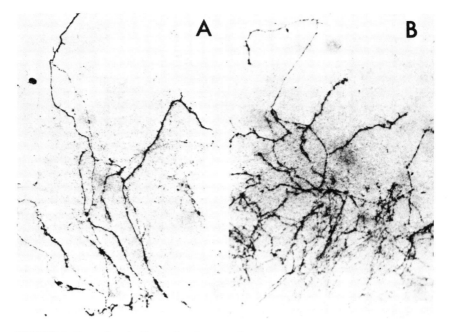

FIGURE 2. Dopaminergic fibers migrating out of a mesencephalic explant seeded for 2 days on (**A**) striatal or (**B**) mesencephalic astroglial monolayers. Note the different patterns of growth between the two neuron-astrocyte co-cultures.

TABLE 1. Modification of the Morphology of Dopaminergic Neurons upon Their Being Transferred from One Glial Monolayer to Another

| | First Glial Monolayer | | | | | |
| | Mesencephalic | | | Striatal | | |
	Branched	Linear	Nondeveloped	Branched	Linear	Nondeveloped
Second Glial Monolayer						
None (control)	705 (51)	458 (33)	196 (14)	(0)	1103 (86)	167 (14)
Mesencephalic	199 (32)	215 (34)	209 (34)	147 (38)	137 (35)	104 (27)
Striatal	5 (1)	347 (71)	137 (28)	(0)	253 (83)	52 (17)

NOTE: Percentages are shown in parentheses.

Gstr (1359 and 1270, respectively). 2) Neurons previously grown on Gstr can exhibit the branched phenotype after transfer on Gmes.

These two points do not support a selective attachment and survival of the branched phenotype on Gmes. They strongly suggest that the same neuron can adopt either morphology in response to the astrocytic influence.

Is Direct Contact with the Astrocyte Important?

The presence of the two morphologically distinct populations on Gmes indicates that morphogenetic induction is probably mediated through direct contact with the astrocytes. It also suggests that the Gmes population is heterogeneous, with one subpopulation only being able to induce the branched phenotype.

This nondiffusible nature of the signal was further investigated in the experiment schematized in FIGURE 3. The morphologies of the dopaminergic neurons on Gmes and Gstr are not modified by the common culture medium (FIG. 4).

Ultrastructural Aspect of Dopaminergic Neurons on Gmes and Gstr

The ultrastructure of the dopaminergic neurons grown for 2 days on Gmes and Gstr was examined by electron microscopy. The thin and nonbranched fibers are similar to very immature axons. They mainly contain microtubules and mitochondria; their diameter (0.12-0.50 μm) remains constant over their entire length; and they are devoid of ribosomes (FIG. 5A). On Gmes, a new type of neurite is present that contains ribosomes (FIG. 5B), shows several branching points, and tapers when the distance to the cell body increases. In addition, it seems that the level of maturation of dopaminergic cell bodies, as estimated by the size of the Golgi zone and the nucleocytoplasmic ratio, is higher on Gmes than on Gstr (Touati *et al.*, unpublished results).

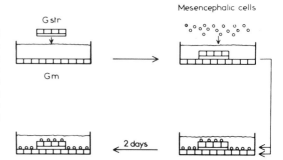

FIGURE 3. Gstr grown for 3 weeks on a 16-mm² glass coverslips and Gmes are presented to dissociated embryonic mesencephalic neurons. After 2 days, the morphologies of the dopaminergic neurons are analyzed by autoradiography after [³H]dopamine uptake.

It therefore appears that there is a specific maturation of some dopaminergic neurons on Gmes, and that this maturation is characterized by an enhanced development of the cell body and by the outgrowth of the dendritic arborization.

In the course of this ultrastructural study, we were struck by the fact that mesencephalic nondopaminergic neurons present in the cultures on Gmes and Gstr were morphologically similar to dopaminergic neurons. This led us to examine the morphological traits of striatal neurons on both monolayers. This study (to be published elsewhere) demonstrates that striatal neurons develop better and grow an extensive dendritic arborization on Gstr but not on Gmes. We can therefore propose that as far as the mesencephalon and the striatum are concerned, the maturation of central neurons is dependent upon the association of their cell bodies with astrocytes from the same region (homotopic astrocytes).

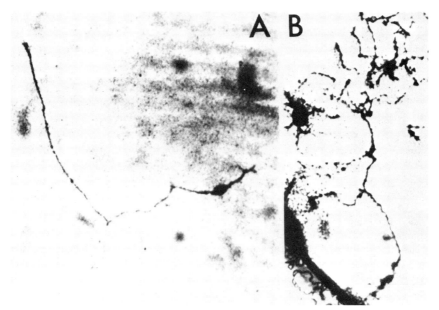

FIGURE 4. Result of the experiment schematized in FIGURE 3. (A) Linear dopaminergic neuron on the Gstr. (B) Branched dopaminergic neuron on Gmes.

DISCUSSION

It is known that astroglial cells provide a unique substratum for neuritic growth.[6-8] Several recent reports have also pointed out the heterogeneity of the astrocytic population based on specific markers or on specific behaviors of neurons, such as the ability of granule cells to migrate on Bergmann glia but not on flat stellate astrocytes.[9,10]

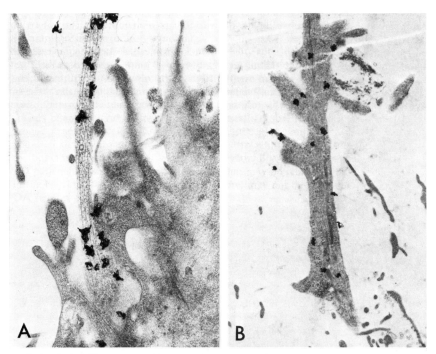

FIGURE 5. (A) Ultrastructural features of a dopaminergic axon-like fiber in contact with Gstr. (B) Ultrastructural features of a dopaminergic dendrite-like fiber in contact with Gmes. The glial cells are not in the plane of the section. Note the presence of numerous ribosomes. Original magnifications for **A** and **B**: $\times 20\,000$ and $\times 10\,000$, respectively; figure reduced to 65% of original size.

We propose here another example of astrocyte heterogeneity revealed by the enhanced development of neurons grown on homotopic versus heterotopic astrocytes. This enhancement is mainly characterized by a dramatic dendritic outgrowth. The dendritic development is shown at the ultrastructural level; it is also shown by immunocytochemical studies using a specific antibody against the microtubule-associated protein 2 (FIG. 6).[11]

The mechanism by which this dendritic outgrowth is induced is still unclear. Two hypotheses can be envisaged. First, this phenomenon is the consequence of the influence of local trophic factors on the physiology of homotopic neurons. Second, at the surface of the astrocytes, there exist specific cues that allow or inhibit dendritic growth cone adhesion and dendrite elongation according to the homotopic or the heterotopic nature of the neuronal cell body.

Indeed, the observation that specific neuron-neuron and neuron-astrocyte interactions play a role in the maturation of subpopulations of neurons is of interest for the study of the behavior of embryonic dopaminergic neurons after they have been transplanted into adult denervated striata. Brundin *et al.* have recently demonstrated that co-grafting mesencephalic dopaminergic neurons with embryonic striatal cells exerts a stimulatory effect on their morphological development and accelerates the behavioral recovery of the animals.[12] It will be of interest to investigate whether prior cultivation of the dopaminergic neurons with neurons and astrocytes from the mesencephalon or the striatum modifies the reinnervation pattern and the behavioral recovery. A first step toward this analysis has been the demonstration that dopaminergic neurons can be kept in culture for 1 week, trypsinized, and reimplanted without significant loss of their ability to restore nearly normal motor behavior to rats.[13]

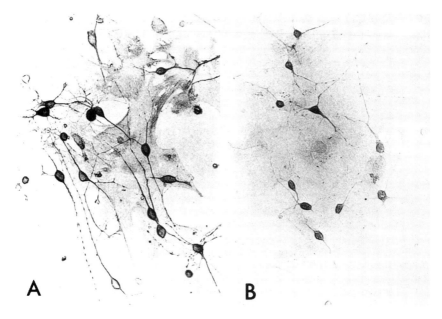

FIGURE 6. Microtubule-associated protein 2 immunoreactivity of mesencephalic embryonic (13-day-old) neurons grown for 2 days on 3-week-old (**A**) Gmes or (**B**) Gstr.

REFERENCES

1. PROCHIANTZ, A., U. DI PORZIO, A. KATO, B. BERGER & J. GLOWINSKI. 1979. *In vitro* maturation of mesencephalic dopaminergic neurons from mouse embryos is enhanced in the presence of their target cells. Proc. Natl. Acad. Sci. USA **76:** 5387-5391.
2. DI PORZIO, U., M.-C. DAGUET, J. GLOWINSKI & A. PROCHIANTZ. 1980. Effect of striatal cells on *in vitro* maturation of mesencephalic dopaminergic neurons grown in serum-free conditions. Nature **288:** 370-373.

3. PROCHIANTZ, A., M.-C. DAGUET, A. HERBERT & J. GLOWINSKI. 1981. Specific stimulation of *in vitro* maturation of mesencephalic dopaminergic neurons by striatal membranes. Nature **293:** 570-572.

4. DENIS-DONINI, S., J. GLOWINSKI & A. PROCHIANTZ. 1983. Specific influence of striatal target neurons on the *in vitro* outgrowth of mesencephalic dopaminergic neurites: A morphological quantitative study. J. Neurosci. **3:** 2292-2299.

5. DENIS-DONINI, S., J. GLOWINSKI & A. PROCHIANTZ. 1984. Glial heterogeneity might define the three-dimensional shape of mouse mesencephalic dopaminergic neurons. Nature **303:** 641-643.

6. NOBLE, M., J. FOK-SEANG & J. COHEN. 1984. Glia are a unique substrate for the *in vitro* growth of central nervous system neurons. J. Neurosci. **4:** 1892-1903.

7. FALLON, J. R. 1985. Prefrontal outgrowth of central nervous system neurites on astrocytes and Schwann cells as compared to nonglial cells *in vitro*. J. Cell Biol. **110:** 198-207.

8. MALLAT, M., V. MOURA NETO, F. GROS, J. GLOWINSKI & A. PROCHIANTZ. 1986. Two simian virus 40 (SV40)-transformed cell lines from the mouse striatum and mesencephalon presenting astrocytic characters. II. Interactions with mesencephalic neurons. Dev. Brain Res. **26:** 23-31.

9. RAFF, M. D., E. R. ABNEY, J. COHEN, R. LINDSAY & M. NOBLE. 1983. Two types of astrocytes in culture of developing rat white matter: Differences in morphology, surface gangliosides and growth characteristics. J. Neurosci. **3:** 1289-1300.

10. HATTEN, M. E., R. K. H. LIEM & C. MASON. 1984. Two forms of astroglia interact differently with cerebellar neurons *in vitro*. J. Cell Biol. **98:** 193-204.

11. CHAMAK, B., A. FELLOUS, J. GLOWINSKI & A. PROCHIANTZ. 1987. MAP2 expression and neuritic outgrowth and branching are co-regulated through region-specific neuroastroglial interactions. J. Neurosci. In press.

12. BRUNDIN, P., O. ISACSON, F. H. GAGE & A. BJÖRKLUND. 1986. Intrastriatal grafting of dopamine-containing neuronal cell suspensions: Effects of mixing target or nontarget cells. Dev. Brain Res. **24:** 77-84.

13. BRUNDIN, P., G. BARBIN, O. ISACSON, M. MALLAT, B. CHAMAK, A. PROCHIANTZ, F. H. GAGE & A. BJÖRKLUND. 1985. Survival of intracerebrally grafted rat dopamine neurons previously cultured *in vitro*. Neurosci. Lett. **61:** 79-84.

DISCUSSION OF THE PAPER

P. WHITAKER-AZMITIA (*State University of New York, Stony Brook, NY*): When one does astrocyte cultures, they are normally from newborn animals, are they not?

PROCHIANTZ: We tried animals between E15 and 1 week PN. During this time we could not see any difference: they were still able to do whatever we wanted them to do.

WHITAKER-AZMITIA: Normally from embryonic day 14 to 16 rats you do not get a lot of GFAP-staining cells. Is it possible that when one is doing transplants you would have much better survival of the grafts if you used astrocytes that were, say, 2 weeks older than the neurons you were transplanting? The growth factor production is better in those older astrocytes than in the younger ones.

PROCHIANTZ: This is what we do *in vitro*. We take a cell out of the animal to make the astrocytes and let them grow for 2 or 3 weeks in culture so as to get monolayers. We do not know whether 3-week-old astrocytes in culture are similar to 2-week-old astrocytes *in vivo*. I tend to believe not: we do not have the normal influence.

But we have reactive astrocytes in culture for 2 or 3 weeks, and then we add the embryonic neurons on top of them. So indeed it would be very nice to take these 3-week-old astrocytes and transplant them *in vivo* with the embryonic neurons.

C. B. JAEGER (*New York University Medical Center, New York, NY*): What is the percentage of immature astrocytes in the mesencephalic astrocyte culture? You mentioned 20% in the striatal culture.

PROCHIANTZ: The percentage is the same in either culture. Mesencephalic and striatal astrocytes look very much alike in culture.

JAEGER: Can you make them mature in culture?

PROCHIANTZ: Yes, it is very obvious that when you put neurons on the astrocyte they change a lot. The bundles get much thicker and there is no specificity. If you take whatever population of neurons on whatever population of astrocytes you are studying, you get the same kind of maturation.

L. KROMER (*Georgetown University, Washington, DC*): The question I was interested in is have you grown any of these neurons on astrocyte monolayers where the astrocytes themselves have been killed to see if the membranes that are left can have the same effect?

PROCHIANTZ: We have tried, but we have had no success so far. I must say that the only success we may have by partly killing the astrocytes is to submit them to osmotic shocks, which do not kill the astrocytes completely, but at least block protein synthesis. Killing the astrocytes would make them detach. We tried to heat them, we tried to fix them with formaldehyde—all the tricks. Nothing worked.

J. SILVER (*Case Western Reserve University, Cleveland, OH*): Did you examine the role of adhesion phenomena in your system? Are axons sticking more tightly to one type versus another? Have you examined this or considered this in your philosophy?

PROCHIANTZ: We would like to do that. We would like to have growth cone populations from dendrites and axons and see what sticks to the astrocytes, but we do not have the tools to do that now.

C. SOTELO (*INSERM U106, CMC Foch, Suresnes*): I like the experiments with the MAPs. But I do not understand exactly when you stain the cells on the different astrocytes with the MAPs. You see sometimes positive, sometimes negative staining. If all these cells have processes, do you look with phase contrast or something like it?

PROCHIANTZ: Some of the population of cells have no processes at all. The top line in the drawing I showed had cells with no processes. We saw nondeveloped cells, so we cannot say what kind of processes are going to develop. The number of nondeveloped cells without processes is higher on the heterotypic astrocyte than the homotypic ones. Whether this is an accident or whether this means that there is less maturation factor in the nonmatching astrocyte, I do not know. The MAPs provide only an indirect way of seeing processes.

SOTELO: Are the astrocytes inducing the formation of processes or not? When you do not have processes, you do not have MAPs.

PROCHIANTZ: Yes, this is possible. Though MAPs is a tricky marker, too. It is a marker for two things: first, for the maturation of a cell and, second, for dendritic outgrowth. We do not know whether dendritic outgrowth is the first event that might trigger maturation or whether the maturation of cells precedes and somehow causes the dendritic outgrowth. Another possibility, which I tend to believe, is that maturation and dendritic outgrowth are separate effects.

Striatal Neural Transplants in the Ibotenic Acid-lesioned Rat Neostriatum

Cellular and Functional Aspects

O. ISACSON,[a,b] M. PRITZEL,[c] D. DAWBARN,[d]
P. BRUNDIN,[b] P. A. T. KELLY,[e] L. WIKLUND,[f]
P. C. EMSON,[g] F. H. GAGE,[h] S. B. DUNNETT,[i]
AND A. BJÖRKLUND[b]

[b]*Department of Histology*
University of Lund
S-223 62 Lund, Sweden

[c]*Institute of Anatomy and Special Embryology*
CH-1700 Fribourg, Switzerland

[d]*Department of Medicine*
University of Bristol
Bristol BS2 8HW, England

[e]*Department of Physiology*
University of Cardiff
Cardiff CF1 1XL, Wales

[f]*Département de Neurophysiologie Appliquée, CNRS*
91190 Gif-sur-Yvette, France

[g]*AFRC Institute of Animal Physiology*
Cambridge CB2 4HT, England

[h]*Department of Neurosciences*
University of California at San Diego
La Jolla, California 92093

[i]*Department of Experimental Psychology*
Cambridge University
Cambridge CB2 3EB, England

INTRODUCTION

In attempts to further develop the understanding of the morphology, function, and plasticity of the striatal neural circuitry, we have induced neuronal damage by

[a]Present address: Department of Anatomy, Downing Site, Cambridge University, Cambridge CB2 3EB, England.

the excitotoxin, ibotenic acid (IA), in the rat neostriatum (NS). The IA lesion of the NS causes extensive neuronal cell loss in this structure, with many similarities to the neuropathology seen in Huntington's disease. Implantation of striatal neural precursor cells, obtained from fetal striatum, into the previously damaged NS or its major projection areas, has provided a novel approach for the investigation of how the implanted neuroblasts and developing neurons can adapt to a transplant condition and to what extent the implanted fetal striatal tissue can be incorporated in a functional way in a damaged adult host neuronal circuitry.[cf. 1]

Grafts of immature striatal tissue can survive well in NS in which lesions have been created with IA, that is, in IA-lesioned NS.[2–12] Moreover, the striatal grafts have been shown to be capable of normalizing the locomotor hyperactivity characteristically seen after striatal IA lesions[3–8,12] and to partly compensate for the increased metabolic activity induced by the IA lesion in parts of the extrapyramidal system.[3] Recently, we have also found that cognitive impairments, as seen in a defective performance of the IA-lesioned animals in so-called delayed alternation tasks,[13–15] can be markedly ameliorated by the intrastriatal striatal grafts.[5]

This paper will summarize this work and present the results of recent studies of striatal transplants using morphological, biochemical, and behavioral techniques.

LESION AND GRAFTING PROCEDURE

IA (Sigma or Biosearch Products) (20 μg/μl in phosphate buffer, with pH adjusted to 7) was injected at four sites in the head of the NS. At each site, 0.25 μl (equivalent to 5 μg IA) was injected.[3,4] Some of the animals received unilateral IA lesions, whereas others, which were used in behavioral experiments (see below), received bilateral lesions in the anteromedial striatum (10 μg IA per hemisphere).[5]

Four to 6 days after the IA lesion, the rats received striatal implants into the part of the NS with the lesion (coordinates as above) using the cell suspension technique.[2,4,16] Tissue was obtained from the striatal primordia dissected from fetuses of 14-15-day gestational age (crown-to-rump length: 12-14 mm, from the same breeder's stock of Sprague-Dawley rats as the recipient animals). The striatal primordia, protruding from the wall of the lateral ventricle, were reached via an incision through the overlying cortex. They were carefully cut out from both hemispheres and later incubated in 0.1% trypsin (Sigma, crude type II) dissolved in a 0.6% glucose-saline medium. The tissue was dissociated into a milky cell suspension, which ultimately contained approximately two to four striatal primordia per 10 μl of medium. Finally, 1.00-1.25 μl of the cell suspension was injected over 3-5 min at each of the IA lesion sites.

RESULTS

General Morphology, Immunohistochemistry, and Receptor Binding following the Striatal IA Lesion

One week after the lesion, very few surviving neurons were found in the head of the NS in the rats with IA lesions,[4] where the bulk of tissue had a gliotic appearance with a massive astrocytic reaction. There was minor atrophy of the NS, seen as a small dilation of the lateral ventricle. A thin, selectively spared zone was seen in the dorsomedial NS, in addition to the relatively spared areas in the uninjected tail of the NS. The nucleus accumbens appeared unaffected in the vast majority of cases. The globus pallidus (GP) and substantia nigra (SN) exhibited no apparent shrinkage or cell damage at 1 week. In the neocortex, there was variable and local cell damage or necrosis at the sites of needle penetration. Rats processed for catecholamine histofluorescence had apparently normal fluorescence intensity of fibers in the striatum and related areas, with small patchy losses of fluorescence at the sites of the needle tips, probably signifying nonspecific damage at the injection sites.

The extent of the striatal lesion acutely after the IA injection was also evaluated immunohistochemically using antibodies directed against Met-enkephalin (ME) and substance P (SP),[11] which are known to be contained in the striatal efferents projecting to the GP and SN pars reticulata (SNr), respectively.[17,18] ME-like immunoreactivity was markedly reduced in the GP ipsilateral to the striatal lesion as compared with the control side. Likewise, there was a marked reduction in the density of SP-immunoreactive fibers in the SN ipsilateral to the lesion compared with the nonlesioned contralateral side.

Four to 20 weeks after the lesion, cresyl violet and acetylcholinesterase (AChE) staining indicated a marked volume atrophy of the injected head of the NS, amounting to about 40-70% (FIG. 1a) of the nonatrophied contralateral side, with packed fiber bundles mainly assembled in the lateral part of the lesioned area. At this postoperative period, the GP and the SNr were clearly shrunken, but without obvious gliosis or pathological changes. The shrinkage was clearly less in the caudal NS (that is, the tail) than in the rostral NS. Rats with IA lesions processed for catecholamine histofluorescence showed intensely fluorescent fibers between densely packed myelinated fiber bundles of the atrophic rostral NS (*cf.* FIG. 4). In the atrophied parts of the gray matter (that is, the areas of extensive neuronal cell loss), the dopamine fiber density was similar to that normally seen; it was, however, markedly reduced at the injection sites (*cf.* FIG. 4). This suggests that the total dopamine terminal network was actually reduced within the neuron-depleted NS area.[4]

Receptor autoradiography of muscarinic, opiate, and dopamine receptors in the lesioned rats showed a near total absence of binding in the central area of the lesion, comprising 90-95% of the total volume of the head of the caudate-putamen (CP). A density of receptors similar to that in the intact contralateral side was observed in the spared tail and in the lateral and medial rims of the NS.[11]

Neurochemical Analysis of the IA Lesion

Within 1 week, the IA lesion caused a 70-85% reduction in glutamate decarboxylase (GAD) activity (FIG. 2a),[4] an indirect marker for GABA neurons contained in the NS, and there was a similar reduction of the cholinergic neuronal marker, choline acetyltransferase (ChAT). The progressive recovery seen in the specific activity of GAD and ChAT in the lesioned part of the NS (from about 15-30% of control at 1 week to about 40-60% of control at 20 weeks after lesion) (FIG. 2a) is largely, if not exclusively, due to the shrinking of the lesioned NS to about half its normal volume within the same period.[4] Our studies show that the total enzyme activity level of the lesioned NS remains virtually unchanged, between 15 and 25% of control, over the 20-week experimental period, which speaks against any significant regeneration or sprouting of spared neurons in the IA-lesioned striatum.

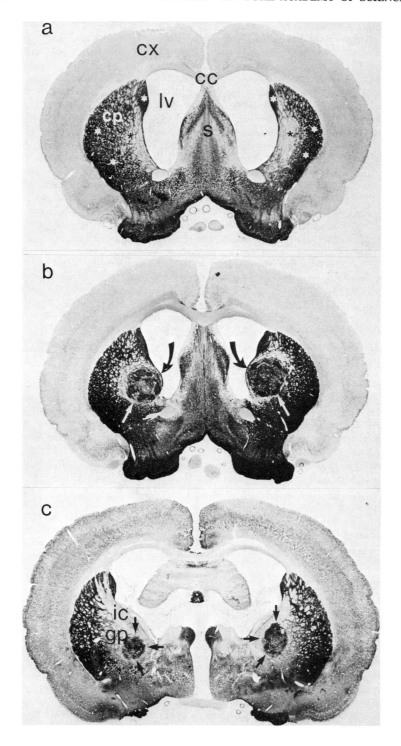

Striatal dopamine levels (FIG. 2b) underwent a progressive reduction in the IA-lesioned area, but with a slower time course than GAD or ChAT. Our results seem consistent with the idea that the dopaminergic afferents are acutely spared by the IA lesion, but that they undergo gradual regressive changes over the subsequent weeks, so that the total dopamine content in the lesioned rostral NS is reduced by about 80% at 20 weeks after the lesion. This change in dopamine was not seen in those portions of the striatum that had not received lesions or had received only partial lesions.

The nearly complete neuronal depletion in the head of the NS, achieved with the present IA lesion, was accompanied by marked (35-70%) reductions in GAD activity in the two principal striatal efferent targets, GP and SN, and there were no signs of recovery over the 20-week experimental period, except in transplanted animals (see below). This is consistent with a substantial destruction of both the striatopallidal and the striatonigral projection neurons in the animals with IA lesions, resulting in a profound GABA-ergic deafferentation of these two structures.[4]

General Morphology, Immunohistochemistry, and Receptor Binding of Striatal Transplants

Using regular cell body staining (cresyl violet), the distribution of neuronal perikarya was found to be even throughout the graft, although detailed quantification showed that the density of medium-to-large cells ($> 10 \mu$m) was increased. AChE staining showed deeply stained neuropil distributed in a patch-like pattern, in the transplants.[4,11] These patches were much more distinct than any found in the contralateral normal striatum. Immunohistochemical staining of the striatal grafts was performed with antisera raised against some of the neuropeptides that normally occur in the striatum, including SP, ME, cholecystokinin, neuropeptide Y, and somatostatin. They were all detected immunohistochemically in the striatal transplants.[11] Antisera against SP and ME revealed stained cell bodies and terminal networks that were distributed in a patchy manner. Staining with antisera against neuropeptide Y and somatostatin showed distinct cell bodies evenly distributed throughout the entire striatal graft. In addition, cholecystokinin-immunoreactive cell bodies were found in the graft.

The AChE-positive, ME-positive, and SP-positive fibers all showed an uneven, patchy distribution in the grafts (*cf.* FIGS. 1b, 1c & 5). Since neither the cresyl violet staining of the overall cell distribution nor the neuropeptide Y- and somatostatin-immunoreactive fibers and cell bodies exhibited this feature, it seems improbable that the patchiness was an artifact. Rather, the uneven distribution of the neurochemical markers may reflect the normal compartmentalization that is known to occur in the intact striatum.

FIGURE 1. Photomicrographs of sections from three rats. Each section was stained for AChE. (**a**) Section from a rat from the lesion-only group (without grafts), at the level of the caudate-putamen (cp). The central, neuron-depleted area of the lesion (packed with myelinated fiber bundles) is indicated by a black star, whereas relatively spared areas are indicated by white stars. (**b**) Section from a rat from the CP graft group. The grafts, indicated by arrows, are located within the central area of the lesion. (**c**) Section from a rat from the GP graft group, at the level of the GP. The grafts (arrows) are located within the medial part of the globus pallidus (gp) adjacent to the internal capsule (ic). cx: neocortex; cc: corpus callosum.

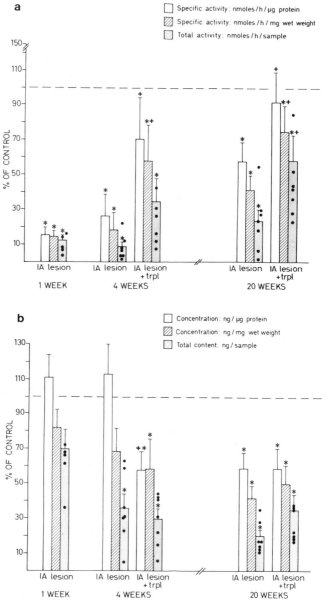

FIGURE 2. GAD activity (**a**) and dopamine content (**b**) in the rostral IA-lesioned CP region dissected at different times after the lesion and grafting. Means ± SEM expressed as percent of control. Specific enzyme activity was calculated both in terms of activity per μg protein (open columns) and mg wet weight (hatched columns). In addition, the total activity of the rostral CP region was calculated (stippled columns). Individual values for total enzyme activity or total dopamine content are shown as black dots. ANOVA with post hoc Newman-Keuls: ⋆: $p >$ .05 (different from controls); +: $p <$ .005 (different from lesion only); no symbol: $p <$ .05. (Data from reference 4.)

Interestingly, the so-called striosomal patterns have been shown to change during the course of development. Thus, during the fetal and neonatal period, patches of high AChE staining intensity coincide with patches of high ME staining intensity[19] and with patches of high muscarinic receptor binding.[20,21] Also, opiate receptor patches have been shown to coincide with dopamine histofluorescence in the neonatal rat.[22,23] Some of these early developmental characteristics are consistent with the staining patterns observed in the striatal transplants,[11] where zones of high AChE staining intensity coincided with patches of high ME immunoreactivity and (although to a lesser degree) with zones of high SP immunoreactivity. The patches of AChE also corresponded well with the dopamine D_2 receptor distribution in the graft. Opiate receptor patches, as revealed by [^{3}H]diprenorphine binding, appeared only within areas of AChE staining. The nature of the relationship between dopamine receptors and striosomes has not to our knowledge been investigated autoradiographically during development. Muscarinic receptors in the graft, by contrast, were more homogeneously distributed than in the fetal striatum and thus more closely resembled the receptor distribution of the mature striatum.

Neurochemical Analysis of the Striatal Grafts in the IA-lesioned Striatum

Four weeks after the lesion, the IA-lesioned NS had undergone substantial tissue atrophy accompanied by a marked dilatation of the lateral ventricle. The striatal GAD (FIG. 2a) and ChAT (not shown) levels remained low, although the specific activities (expressed per wet weight or μg protein) tended to be less reduced than the *total* activities at this time because of gradual tissue shrinkage.[4] In the grafted animals, the rostral NS, containing the striatal grafts, had on average three times the GAD activity of the group of animals that had only received lesions (FIG. 2). In the grafted group, specific GAD activity expressed per μg protein was not significantly different from the control value, but it was significantly below the mean control value both in terms of activity per mg wet weight and in terms of total activity for this structure. There were no graft-induced changes in the GP and SN at 3 weeks after the grafting (4 weeks after the lesion). Similar graft-induced changes in ChAT were seen at this time point in the NS.[4]

The final volume of the striatal graft tissue reached up to a maximum of 12 mm^3 in size at 20 weeks after the lesion and reduced the average IA-induced striatal atrophy from about 50-70% to about 30-40%, which was reflected in a twofold increase in striatal GAD (FIG. 2a) and ChAT activity (from 20-25% to 40-50% of normal total activity in the rostral NS).

It is noteworthy that the intrastriatal striatal grafts at 20 weeks after the lesion not only restored GAD and ChAT activity levels within the lesioned NS, but they were also capable of normalizing the depressed GAD activity in the adjacent GP region,[4] without affecting the SN region located at a greater distance from the implantation site.

Striatal Graft Connectivity

The morphological techniques currently available for assessing graft and host brain interconnections are based on visualization of various tracer substances, which are used regularly in neuroanatomy. The special condition of implanted cells into a host brain, however, emphasizes the necessity of graft-specific markers to effectively and safely visualize all direct connections between host brain and implanted cells. Various electrophysiological and brain metabolic techniques (see the results of the [^{14}C]2-D-deoxyglucose study, below) complement the morphological assessments of connectivity and may give more direct information about possible functional integration of the graft into the host brain. For the morphological study of graft-host interconnections, we have deposited wheat germ agglutinin-conjugated horseradish peroxidase (WGA-HRP) crystals inside fine glass capillaries into portions of the striatal grafts.[24] Visualization of possible retrogradely labeled host neurons and anterogradely labeled graft fibers was made according to the tetramethylbenzidine method of Mesulam.[25] In addition, we have processed some of the grafted brains for formaldehyde fluorescence histochemistry[26,27] in order to visualize possible dopamine-containing afferents to the striatal grafts from the host nigrostriatal pathway.[24]

HRP-labeled neurons were seen in the host brain in three of the five rats where the WGA-HRP deposit had been confined to the graft.[24] They were mainly found in SN, the spared portions of the host NS, and, to a lesser extent, in the thalamus. In addition, there was evidence of some weak labeling in the neocortex. Signs of anterograde labeling were detected in the host GP and SNr in one animal.

In the grafted rats, we generally found a substantial number (10-40) of retrogradely labeled cell bodies in SN ipsilateral to the WGA-HRP placement in the graft. The schematic overviews given in FIGURE 3 show the host NS, the grafted tissue (stippled), and the WGA-HRP deposit (black), as well as the total number of labeled neurons in SN and thalamus. Most labeled cell bodies were heavily labeled in a Golgi-like fashion. The labeling of SN neurons obtained from WGA-HRP deposits in the grafts was similar to that seen in the two control cases where the deposit had been made within the lesioned host NS (FIG. 3), although the number of labeled neurons tended to be somewhat larger in the control animals (range: 25-75) than in the grafted ones.

Indicated in FIGURE 3 are labeled thalamic neurons in a rat that had a large bilateral deposit of WGA-HRP, one in the grafted NS and one in the lesioned and shrunken contralateral host NS. Five labeled thalamic neurons were seen ipsilateral to the grafted NS, and 15 were found ipsilateral to the control injection. On both sides, the labeled neurons were scattered in the nuclei, normally giving rise to the thalamostriatal projection in the intact animal.[28–30]

In all grafted and control rats, some faintly HRP-labeled neurons were found in the deep layers of the frontoparietal cortex overlying the NS. This labeling, however, was faint in both the grafted and notably also in the control rats (with WGA-HRP deposits in the lesioned host NS). Since the exact number of labeled neurons was difficult to assess, they have not been plotted in FIGURE 3. In the striatum, labeled neurons were regularly found in the vicinity of the WGA-HRP deposit. In all grafted and control rats, some labeled neurons were found in the spared portions of the host NS, and in one case patches of labeled cell bodies, which were quite remote from the injection area, were found within the graft itself.

As the WGA-HRP tracer is transported both retrogradely and anterogradely, we also searched for terminal labeling in the primary NS efferent projection areas, the GP and SNr. In one of the WGA-HRP-implanted animals, we found indications for labeling of neuronal process in SNr, both on the side underlying the deposit in grafted NS as well as on the control side. The area of labeled neurons in SN pars compacta (SNc) and the area of labeled neuronal processes in SNr showed only partial overlap. Therefore, it seems likely that the SNr labeling represented terminal labeling of grafted NS efferents, instead of labeling of dendritic processes of retrogradely filled SNc neurons. This rather unexpected finding, however, requires confirmation by combined tracer techniques.

Labeling of axonal processes were also detected in the GP, adjacent to the grafted NS, as well as within the graft itself. Labeling was seen close to a heavily labeled bundle of fibers leaving the grafted NS and traversing spared portions of the host NS and GP. This fiber staining in the host GP may, therefore, represent either labeling of terminals or labeling of axons transversing the nucleus.[24]

In all grafted specimens processed for fluorescence histochemistry, dopamine-containing fibers were abundant within the striatal grafts. They formed distinct and partly interconnected patches, which were distributed throughout the graft tissue, although they were most abundant in the peripheral portions of the grafts (FIGS. 4a

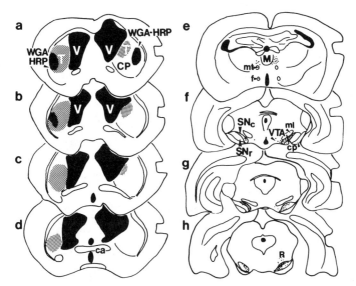

FIGURE 3. Camera lucida drawings of selected brain sections (from rostral to caudal) from a bilaterally lesioned and grafted rat. Drawings illustrate the grafted tissue (lightly stippled, labeled T) in caudate-putamen (CP) (sections **a-d**) as well as the site of the WGA-HRP deposits (black), one within the graft (left side) and one within the lesioned host CP (right side). The distribution of labeled cell bodies in thalamus and SN are indicated by dots. The total number of neurons found in the center median-parafascicular complex as well as in midline and interlaminar regions surrounding the dorsomedial nucleus (M) is indicated in **e**. Neurons in the SNc, SNr, ventral tegmental area (VTA), and retrorubral field (R) are shown in **f**, **g**, and **h**. The greatly dilated ventricles (V) are shown in solid black. ca: anterior commissure; cp: cerebral peduncle; f: fornix; ml: medial lemniscus; mt: mammillothalamic tract. (Data from reference 24).

& 4b). In many of these patches, the fiber density approached that seen in the normal NS. The areas between the fluorescent patches contained only scattered fluorescent fibers. A comparison with the adjacent cresyl violet-stained sections showed that neurons were equally abundant in areas of the graft with and without fluorescent dopamine-containing fiber patches, and the fiber patches did not appear to follow any obvious cytoarchitectonic boundaries within the grafts. The grafts were surrounded by the nonfluorescent bundles of myelinated host internal capsule fibers, which were packed along the periphery of the graft tissue (FIGS. 4a & 4b). In many places along the periphery of the grafts, the fluorescent fiber plexus in the atrophic host neuropil

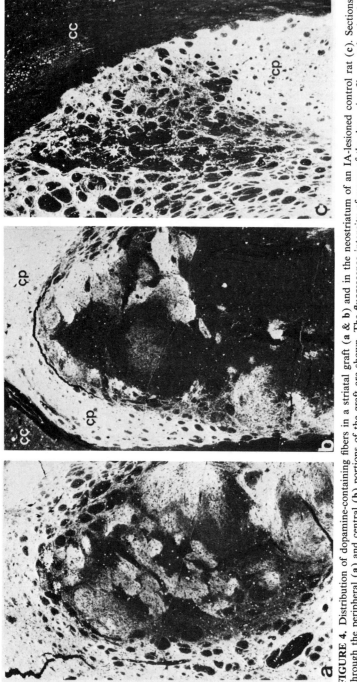

FIGURE 4. Distribution of dopamine-containing fibers in a striatal graft (**a** & **b**) and in the neostriatum of an IA-lesioned control rat (**c**). Sections through the peripheral (**a**) and central (**b**) portions of the graft are shown. The fluorescence intensity of many of the dopamine fiber patches in the graft is similar to that seen in the surrounding lesioned host caudate-putamen (cp). In **c**, the central zone of the IA lesion, which has a markedly reduced dopamine fluorescence, is marked by asterisks, and the peripheral zone, which had some minimal neuronal sparing, is marked cp. cc: corpus callosum. The sections in this figure were photographed with automated dark-field condenser scanner equipment, which was used courtesy of Mårtensson and Björklund, using a 4 × objective and 8 × ocular magnification. (Data from reference 24.)

was in direct continuity, across the graft-host border, with the fiber patches inside the graft, and, in favorable section planes, strands or bundles of fluorescent fibers could be traced across the graft-host border into the depth of the graft.

Fluorescence microscopy of the host SN revealed no major loss of fluorescent dopamine-containing neurons, neither in the grafted animals nor in the IA-lesioned control rats.

Graft Placement into Striatal Projection Areas

Although the theoretically most suitable graft location, in terms of neuronal replacement and reconnection, is homotopically into the damaged brain region, previous studies[1,31] have shown that dopamine- and cholinergic-rich fetal grafts are functionally more effective when implanted directly into or adjacent to their host efferent area (for example, the striatum or hippocampus). This is likely to be due to an easier access and establishment of efferent connections as well as direct transmitter diffusion into the target area. This possibility has also been tested for the striatal grafts, where we have placed the grafts into the main striatal target areas, the GP[5] (FIG. 1c) and the SNr (FIG. 5).[11] The functional consequences of grafting fetal striatal cells into the GP will be discussed below; it suffices to say here that the grafts reach a smaller size than in the IA-lesioned NS and that the general cellular and neurochemical organization already described for homotopic striatal grafts also appears to be maintained in those ectopic graft locations (FIGS. 1 & 5). Thus, a patchy and dense AChE staining was present over a rather even neuronal cell body distribution of the graft tissue (*cf.* GP in FIG. 1c). The compartmentalization of opiate (ME) and SP immunoreactivity was also apparent in the striatal grafts placed in the SNr (FIGS. 5a & 5c). A majority of the neurons studied could be stained with an antibody raised against GAD (FIG. 5a) (kindly donated by W. Oertel), which is consistent with the transmitter expression of the normal NS. There were also indications of SP reinnervation by the graft of the previously denervated SNr (FIG. 5c), a phenomenon not previously observed with homotopic graft placements into the NS. Abundant tyrosine hydroxylase-immunopositive fibers (presumably dopaminergic) could also be traced into the striatal transplant located in the SN.

Functional Aspects of Striatal IA Lesions and Striatal Neuronal Transplants as Assessed by Local Cerebral Metabolic and Behavioral Tests

The idea that damaged or lost transmitter systems could be "replaced" in a functionally meaningful way for the host-recipient brain has challenged the traditional concept of the brain as a structurally rigid network.[1,31–33] We, and others, have tested the hypothesis of "functional neuronal replacement" in the rats with striatal excitotoxic lesions[3–8,12] by physiological and behavioral tests, and found evidence that the fetal striatal transplants can integrate at least to some degree with the previously damaged host NS in a functionally effective manner.

In rats with a unilateral IA lesion of the NS,[3] we found, using measurements of local cerebral metabolism according to the [^{14}C]2-D-deoxyglucose method developed by Sokoloff *et al.,*[34] that the IA lesion caused a 60% reduction in glucose utilization

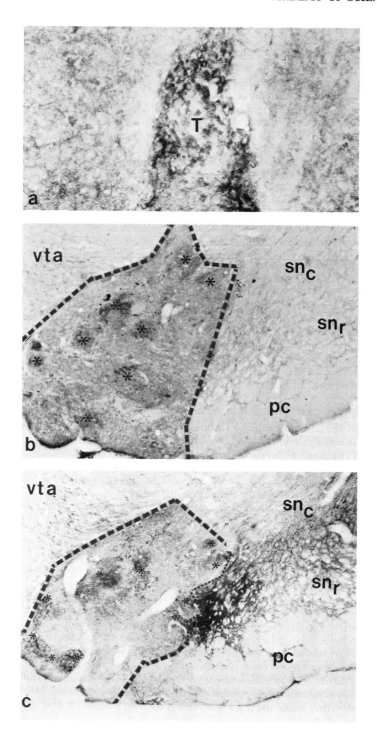

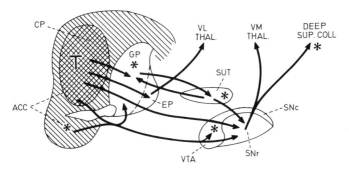

FIGURE 6. A diagram showing the principal arrangements of the major output pathways from the caudate-putamen and nucleus accumbens. Those primary and secondary targets that exhibited graft-induced reductions in [^{14}C]2-D-deoxyglucose utilization are marked by asterisks. ACC: nucleus accumbens; CP: caudate-putamen; EP: entopeduncular nucleus; GP: globus pallidus; SN: substantia nigra (c: compacta; r: reticulata); SUT: subthalamic nucleus; VL and VM Thal: ventrolateral and ventromedial thalamic nuclei, respectively; VTA: ventral tegmental area.

throughout the lesioned NS. Partially spared medial portions of the NS showed smaller reductions, and the NS tail appeared unaffected. In contrast to the ipsilateral decreases, the contralateral NS displayed increased mean glucose utilization values of between 19 and 28% over intact control levels in the different caudate regions measured. All major primary and secondary projection areas of the NS efferents (FIG. 6) showed significant uni- or bilateral increases in glucose use. The strongest increases were seen in the SNr (49% and 29% on the ipsi- and contralateral sides, respectively), in the GP (26% and 29%), in the subthalamic nucleus (18% and 19%), and in the deep superior colliculus (17% and 18%). Bilateral increases were also seen in several areas functionally associated with the extrapyramidal motor system, such as the ventral tegmental area, nucleus accumbens, sensorimotor cortex, and nucleus ruber, whereas other cortical and brain stem regions remained unaffected.

The striatal implant proper exhibited a significant glucose utilization of 69 ± 8% of the intact control neostriatum. The implant did not significantly increase glucose use in the surrounding, lesioned, or spared areas of the host caudate-putamen, although the contralateral increases in glucose use in animals with IA lesions alone were attenuated differently from those of the intact controls. The hypermetabolic responses in the primary and secondary striatal projection areas were normalized by the implant ipsilaterally in the GP and subthalamic nucleus and bilaterally in the deep superior

---

FIGURE 5. Striatal tissue transplants located in the substantia nigra region. (**a**) A photomicrograph of a section stained with an antibody directed against GAD. Heavy GAD cell and fiber staining is present in the transplant (T) (from the most dorsal portion of transplant; section adjacent to **b**). (**b**) Striatal transplant located in substantia nigra pars reticulata (snr) between the ventral tegmental area (vta) and substantia nigra pars compacta (snc) stained with an antibody reactive against ME. Opiate staining is present within the transplant (borders indicated by broken line), and patches of dense fiber staining are indicated by black stars. pc: cerebral peduncle. (**c**) Section of same transplant as in **b**, but stained with an antibody reactive against SP. Patches of dense fiber staining are indicated by black stars. A broken line indicates the transplant border; a thinner line, the border with SNr. Dense SP staining is present as a zone into the SNr, which was denervated of SP by the striatal IA lesion. Abbreviations as in **b**. Original magnifications for **a** and for **b** and **c**: ×512 and ×93, respectively; figure reduced to 66% of original size.

colliculi (FIG. 6). In the functionally associated areas, a significant transplant-induced effect was also seen in the ventral tegmental area and nucleus accumbens. Transplant-induced effects were not observed elsewhere in the brain.[3]

Following bilateral excitotoxic lesions of the anteromedial NS, the rats are known to develop not only locomotor hyperactivity but also substantial impairments in learning and memory.[13-15] Therefore, a critical test of the functional capacity of striatal transplants is whether they can affect performance in conditioned behaviors that are impaired by the lesion, as well as influencing nonconditioned spontaneous behaviors, such as locomotion. For this experiment,[5] rats received bilateral IA injections into the anteromedial NS. One week later, they received bilateral injections of a striatal cell suspension into the IA-lesioned anteromedial NS constituting the CP graft group (FIG. 1b). Another group of IA-lesioned rats received identical injections from the same striatal cell suspensions bilaterally into the principal NS projection area, the GP. These rats constituted the GP graft group (FIG. 1c). Lesioned rats without grafts belonged to the lesion-only group (FIG. 1a), and remaining rats served as unoperated controls.

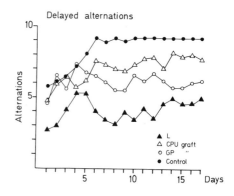

FIGURE 7. Four groups were tested in the delayed alternations paradigm using a delay of 30 ± 5 sec between trials. The average number of correct alternations for each group is plotted over time (see text). (Data from reference 5.)

Three months after the lesion and transplantation surgery, the rats were tested for their impairments in the acquisition of a spatial delayed alternation task and spatial position habits in a conventional elevated T-maze and for their locomotor hyperactivity in automated photocell cages. Operated animals were finally processed for quantitative morphometric analyses (see Summary and Discussion, below) of the IA lesions and the striatal grafts, using cresyl violet- and AChE-stained serial cryostat sections.

Although all control rats rapidly acquired the delayed alternation task, reaching criterion (27 correct choices in 30 trials over 3 days) in 7-12 days, none of the IA-lesioned rats reached criterion within 18 days of testing. Indeed, the mean performance of the lesioned group by the end of the test (between four and five correct alternations) was close to the random performance in the task (that is, five correct alternations) (FIG. 7). The IA-lesioned rats were significantly hyperactive in the overnight locomotor test, and this effect was further accentuated when the rats were tested under food deprivation. Under food deprivation, the lesioned rats were, on the average, about twice as active as the controls, although single individuals in the group were considerably more hyperactive.

Both graft groups were significantly improved in the acquisition of the delayed alternation task, as compared to the IA-lesioned rats, when tested 3 months after grafting (FIG. 7). The groups differed significantly in the number of correct choices ($F = 32.7$, $p < .001$), and Newman-Keuls tests indicated that each group differed from the others (control group > CP graft group > GP graft group > lesion-only group; all at least $p < .05$). Three of the eight rats in the CP graft group reached criterion (at days 13, 16, and 17), whereas the other rats in this group, although all close to this level of performance, did not reach the criterion level. By contrast, none of the rats in the GP graft group (that is, the rats with grafts placed in the GP region) reached criterion, and only three of the nine GP graft group rats reached above 21 of 30 correct alternations during the last 3 days of testing.

In the overnight spontaneous locomotor test, the lesion-induced hyperactivity was ameliorated in the CP graft group, both under the satiated and food-deprived conditions, which is consistent with previous studies.[3,6–8,12] The rats in the GP graft group did not differ from the controls that did not receive lesions in the satiated test but remained, on average, hyperactive in the food-deprived test.[5]

SUMMARY AND DISCUSSION

These studies of striatal transplants following an excitotoxic removal of the NS neurons can be summarized as follows:

1. Transplants of striatal primordia into the NS, GP, or SN form neural substrates with neurochemical, immunohistochemical, and receptor characteristics of adult or neonatal NS. Markers for GABA, ChAT, SP, ME, cholecystokinin, neuropeptide Y, and somatostatin, as well as muscarinic, opiate, and dopamine receptors, are distributed within the graft in neurochemically defined compartments.

2. Quantitative neurochemical analysis shows that with the present transplant procedure into the NS, total NS, GAD, and, to a similar degree, ChAT levels, which are reduced by about 80% after the IA lesion, are increased to 50-70% of control values as assessed 5 months after the lesion and grafting. In the NS-transplanted rats there is also a normalization of GAD levels in the previously denervated GP, but not to a significant degree in the SN.

3. Morphological assessment of striatal graft connectivity indicates that the NS graft has the capacity to establish normal efferent and afferent links with the host striatal circuitry, but it is not clear under what conditions such connections are a constant feature of the grafts. The presence of dense dopaminergic innervation in patch formations inside the graft as well as WGA-HRP retrogradely labeled neurons in the SNc can be taken as evidence for a link between the SNc and the NS graft. Variable findings of thalamic and cortical afferents together with tracer indications of efferent projections to the GP (and maybe SN) require further investigation.

4. Striatal grafts can be placed either homotopically into the IA-lesioned host striatum or ectopically into striatal target areas, that is, the GP and SN. The grafts develop similar cellular and neurochemical features in those different placements, but are notably of smaller size in the ectopic locations. Indications of SP reinnervation of the SNr with grafts placed in the SN, but not NS, point to the possibility of multiple graft placements in order to establish full target reinnervation.

5. Functional neuronal replacement is possible after IA lesions to the NS. First, studies of local cerebral metabolism show that glucose utilization is normalized in the ipsilateral GP and several other extrapyramidal areas associated with the NS, following striatal graft placement in the NS. Second, behavioral studies show that performance in nonconditioned (spontaneous locomotion) and conditioned behaviors (delayed al-

ternations) are within normal levels or improved in the grafted animals with grafts placed either into the IA-lesioned area of the NS or into the GP area, whereas the IA-lesioned animals are markedly impaired.

Functional recovery that occurs after transplantation probably involves a close interaction between striatal grafts and host brain in which IA lesions to the NS have been created. In a theory of striatal graft function, one may assume that the NS normally exerts a tonic inhibitory control over the principal primary output stations: the GP and SN (cf. FIG. 6). The basis for this is provided by the observations of markedly increased glucose utilization in these target regions after the IA lesion of the NS (see above) and by the observation that a majority of the striatal output neurons are GABA-ergic.[35] Also, the principal electrophysiological effects of NS stimulation in the pallidum and SN are inhibitory.[36] Then, if this is correct, it may be sufficient for the implanted striatal neurons to reinstate a relatively nonspecific tonic inhibitory action in the NS and the primary striatal target areas in order to account for the normalization of the hyperlocomotion and extrapyramidal hypermetabolic responses of rats with IA lesions of the NS. This view of the functional effects exerted by the striatal grafts is supported by the experimental findings of 1) normalization of the hypermetabolic response in the GP,[3] 2) a high GAD content[4] and GABA release capacity of the grafts (Isacson, unpublished results) as well as recovery of GAD activity in the denervated GP,[4] 3) preliminary evidence of the capacity for GP reinnervation,[24] and 4) a positive correlation between the proximity (distance) of the striatal grafts to the GP and the reduced behavioral hyperlocomotion.[5]

The NS functions are, however, quite complex, and the access and reinstated GABA-ergic inhibition by the striatal grafts are probably not the only factors to explain the functional effects seen in conditioned behaviors.[5] Thus, the improved performance in the delayed alternation test of grafted rats (compared to rats with IA lesions only (FIG. 7)) did not correlate with the proximity or the placement of the striatal grafts into the GP.[5] In fact, graft tissue located outside (compared to inside) the NS appeared to have less effect on the graft-induced recovery of this conditioned behavior. Instead, we found a significant correlation ($p < .01$) between striatal graft size within the NS and the performance in the delayed alternation test for individual grafted animals.[5] In contrast, the graft size factor in the NS did not correlate with reduced hyperlocomotion of the grafted animals.[5]

Regarding the interaction of all the afferent and efferent transmitters involved in the NS circuitry, the picture is even more complex. Some authors maintain that dopaminergic mechanisms are not involved in behavioral recovery such as that observed in hyperlocomotion.[7] They cite the absence of observable graft-induced effects following pharmacological dopamine potentiation and the relative absence of dopamine receptors in their striatal grafts. Their view, however, may be difficult to reconcile with several facts. First, under some conditions, obvious behavioral graft effects can also be found after pharmacological manipulation of the dopamine systems by haloperidol or amphetamine.[12,37,38] Second, the striatal grafts are clearly dopamine innervated, and show dopamine receptor binding in some preparations (FIG. 4).[9,11,24] In fact, additional experiments[38] have shown that the striatal grafts can reinstate behavioral functions such as paw reaching (coordinated movement control) in the rats with striatal IA-lesions, a task that normally requires a dopaminergic control over striatal function. In addition, in vivo measurements of local GABA release indicate a dopaminergic regulation of striatal grafts. Thus, it might be argued that a graft-mediated effect, for instance, on spontaneous locomotion behaviors by local GABA-ergic inhibition of the spared NS or adjacent GP modulated by dopamine both in the graft and in the nucleus accumbens, could account for some of the behavioral recovery seen in the rats with striatal implants into the excitotoxically lesioned striatum.

REFERENCES

1. BJÖRKLUND, A. & U. STENEVI. 1984. Annu. Rev. Neurosci. 7: 279-308.
2. SCHMIDT, R. H., A. BJÖRKLUND & U. STENEVI. 1981. Brain Res. 218: 347-356.
3. ISACSON, O., P. BRUNDIN, P. A. T. KELLY, F. H. GAGE & A. BJÖRKLUND. 1984. Nature 311: 458-460.
4. ISACSON, O., P. BRUNDIN, F. H. GAGE & A. BJÖRKLUND. 1985. Neuroscience 16: 799-817.
5. ISACSON, O., S. B. DUNNETT & A. BJÖRKLUND. 1986. Proc. Natl. Acad. Sci. USA 83: 2728-2732.
6. DECKEL, A. W., R. G. ROBINSON, J. R. COYLE & P. R. SANBERG. 1983. Eur. J. Pharmacol. 93: 287-288.
7. DECKEL, A. W., T. H. MORAN & R. G. ROBINSON. 1986. Brain Res. 363: 383-385.
8. DECKEL, A. W., T. H. MORAN, J. T. COYLE, P. R. SANBERG & R. G. ROBINSON. 1986. Brain Res. 365: 249-258.
9. MCGEER, P. L., H. KIMURA & E. G. MCGEER. 1984. *In* Neural Transplants: Development and Function. J. R. Sladek, Jr. & D. M. Gash, Eds. Raven Press. New York, NY.
10. MCALLISTER, J. P., II, P. D. WALKER, M. C. ZEMANICK, A. B. WEBER, L. I. KAPLAN & M. A. REYNOLDS. 1986. Dev. Brain Res. 23: 282-286.
11. ISACSON, O., D. DAWBARN, P. BRUNDIN, F. H. GAGE, P. C. EMSON & A. BJÖRKLUND. 1987. Neuroscience 22: in press.
12. SANBERG, P. R., M. A. HENAULT, S. H. HAGENMEYER-HOUSER, M. GIORDANO & K. H. RUSSELL. 1987. Ann. N.Y. Acad. Sci. This volume.
13. DIVAC, I. 1974. Physiol. Psychol. 2: 104-106.
14. DIVAC, I., H. MARKOWITSCH & M. PRITZEL. 1978. Brain Res. 32: 534-532.
15. DUNNETT, S. B. & S. D. IVERSEN. 1981. Behav. Brain Res. 2: 189-209.
16. BJÖRKLUND, A., U. STENEVI, R. H. SCHMIDT, S. B. DUNNETT & F. H. GAGE. 1983. Acta Physiol. Scand. Suppl. 522: 1-75.
17. CUELLO, A. C. & G. PAXINOS. 1978. Nature 271: 178-180.
18. KOHNO, J., S. SHIOSAKA, K. SHINODA, S. INAGAKI & S. TOHYAMA. 1984. Brain Res. 308: 309-317.
19. GRAYBIEL, A. M., C. W. RAGSDALE, E. S. YOUEOKA & R. P. ELDE. 1981. Neuroscience 6: 377-397.
20. NASHITO, M. A. & A. M. GRAYBIEL. 1985. J. Comp. Neurol. 237: 176-194.
21. ROTTER, A., N. J. M. BIRDSALL, A. S. V. BURGEN, P. M. FIELD, E. C. HULME & G. RAISMAN. 1979. Brain Res. Rev. 1: 141-165.
22. MOON EDLEY, S. & M. HERKENHAM. 1984. Brain Res. 305: 27-42.
23. VAN DER KOOY, D. 1984. Dev. Brain Res. 14: 300-303.
24. PRITZEL, M., O. ISACSON, P. BRUNDIN, L. WIKLUND & A. BJÖRKLUND. 1986. Exp. Brain Res. 65: 112-126.
25. MESULAM, M.-M. 1978. J. Histochem. Cytochem. 26: 106-117.
26. LOREN, I., A. BJÖRKLUND, B. FALCK & O. LINDVALL. 1980. J. Neurosci. Methods 2: 277-300.
27. BJÖRKLUND, A. 1983. *In* Handbook of Chemical Neuroanatomy. A. Björklund & T. Hökfelt, Eds. Vol. 1: 50-121. Elsevier. Amsterdam.
28. JONES, E. G. & R. Y. LEAVITT. 1974. J. Comp. Neurol. 154: 349-378.
29. NAUTA, H. J. W., M. B. PRITZ & R. J. LASEK. 1974. Brain Res. 67: 219-238.
30. VEENING, J. G., F. M. CORNELIUS & P. A. J. M. LIEVEN. 1980. Neuroscience 5: 1253-1268.
31. DUNNETT, S. B., A. BJÖRKLUND & U. STENEVI. 1983. Trends Neurosci. 6: 266-270.
32. FREED, W. J. 1983. Biol. Psychiatry 18: 1205-1267.
33. GAGE, F. H., A. BJÖRKLUND, U. STENEVI & S. B. DUNNETT. 1984. *In* Aging of the Brain. S. H. Gispen & J. Taber, Eds.: 125-137. Elsevier. Amsterdam.
34. SOKOLOFF, L. *et al.* 1977. J. Neurochem. 28: 897-916.
35. GRAYBIEL, A. M. & C. W. RAGSDALE. 1983. *In* Chemical Neuroanatomy. P. C. Emson, Ed.: 427-504. Raven Press. New York, NY.
36. KITAI, S. T. 1981. *In* Handbook of Physiology. V. Brooks, Ed.: 997-1015. Williams and Wilkins. Baltimore, MD.

37. ISACSON, O., P. BRUNDIN, F. H. GAGE & A. BJÖRKLUND. 1985. *In* Advances in Behavioral Biology. B. E. Will, P. Schmitt & J. C. Dalrymple-Alford, Eds. Vol. **28:** 519-535. Plenum. New York, NY.
38. DUNNETT, S. B., O. ISACSON, S. SIRINATHSINGHJI, D. J. CLARKE & A. BJÖRKLUND. 1987. Submitted for publication.

DISCUSSION OF THE PAPER

P. D. WALKER (*Temple University School of Medicine, Philadelphia, PA*): You saw dopamine patches with fluorescence histochemistry in the transplant, and yet you saw no change in dopamine content with your neurochemical studies. Was this simply an effect of graft placement or some other factor?

ISACSON: My first guess would be that it is a redistribution of fibers so the density of dopamine is the same in the grafted and the lesion animals, suggesting that the total network has been redistributed toward the graft. You can see that there was a slight tendency for increased total dopamine content in the grafted group. This tendency, however, was not significant. Many studies now support the view that there is a dopaminergic interaction within the striatal graft.

C. SOTELO (*INSERM U106, CMC Foch, Suresnes*): When you put the graft in the target area and you see that there is a functional recovery, how can you explain this recovery if it is not due to diffusion of neurotransmitter? You might think that the neurons are endocrine cells releasing things. Or, if you try to understand the brain by thinking of it as a kind of telephone system, and would see that neurons release things through specific pathways. Then it would be very difficult to understand that just by putting the graft in the target area you can have a functional recovery. It seems very difficult to understand how grafted neurons can have a nonmorphological function. The integration of the brain is the result of a very well balanced input-output organization.

ISACSON: When the grafts are placed homotopically into the striatum, they receive the afferent fibers of the host dopaminergic neurons, as well as input from the thalamus and most likely from the frontal cortex. I would like to emphasize that the behavior is *more* pronounced with the graft placement into the striatum compared to placement into the target areas (Isacson *et al.,* Proc. Natl. Acad. Sci. USA **83:** 2728-2732, 1986). As I mentioned previously, striatal grafts into the striatum appear to represent a condition where neuronal replacement is paralleled by a number of functional recoveries, and our morphological and neurochemical studies support the view that these recoveries depend on a balanced input and output organization.

SOTELO: Can you totally reconstruct the pathway and the secretory mechanism by putting the graft in the target area?

ISACSON: I think it is very probable that we can reconstruct the circuitry with graft placement homotypically, directly into the lesion area. This reconstruction is obviously less likely to occur with graft placement into the striatal target areas. I also think it is very probable that we can either circumvent the feedback mechanism or introduce a new feedback system similar to the one that normally operates. If this does occur, however, it will be a cruder operating system than the normal one.

SOTELO: You have the striatum as biological material, and you put in IA only to destroy neurons. Even if you always use the same parameters, I am sure that any one animal will always be a little different from any other, and that some cells will be spared. You can put your graft into the lesion site, but then spared cells could migrate. You could have a mixed population. If you want to convince neuroanatomists that you have a new secretory system, you need double labeling. You need to label the anatomical pathway with axonal flow systems, and, all the while, you must be convinced that the cells you are looking at are grafted cells.

ISACSON: Dr. McAllister can comment on that because he has already done a thymidine study, and his studies do not support your ideas.

J. P. MCALLISTER (*Temple University School of Medicine, Philadelphia, PA*): We labeled the donor tissue with tritiated thymidine 2 days before harvesting the tissue, and about 40% of the neurons within the transplant showed the label. They do not seem to migrate more than about 100 μ away from the transplants, so we are fairly convinced that the transplant contains primarily the donor cells. The host cells do not migrate into lesion site.

Could you comment on the types of neurons you think you are transplanting? We believe that in some of our transplants we are also getting some GP neurons. In some very preliminary studies, we have not been able to find any afferent or efferent connections with the host. We speculate that may be due to the fact that we are transplanting pallidal neurons with our striatal neurons, and that they are just hooking up to each other.

ISACSON: That is certainly a possibility. A striatal dissection, however, is definitely more precise than a mesencephalic or a raphe dissection, and would provide a fairly striatal-like population. The more rostral dissections give better results. If you were to select caudate that corresponded to caudate in man, you would get a more extensive reinnervation and, probably, efferent connections.

P. VOS (*University of Pennsylvania School of Medicine, Philadelphia, PA*): Given the D2 receptor work you have done in the dopamine afferent study, have you attempted in alternate sections to see if your afferents are lining up with your receptors?

ISACSON: Not in this preparation. It is not possible to combine dopamine histofluorescence with the D2 receptor preparation, but it is quite possible with the tyrosine hydroxylase stain.

VOS: Have you looked at benzodiazepine receptors?

ISACSON: No.

P. PASIK (*Mount Sinai School of Medicine, New York, NY*): You showed patches of cholinesterase, and you said that they coincided with the patches of dopamine reinnervation. This pattern is the exact opposite of the pattern you get in the normal cat: the so-called striatal cells are determined by cholinesterase and are just the negative image of the patches obtained by dopamine staining.

ISACSON: With the histofluorescence method, we have not made systematic comparisons with esterase staining, but the shape of the dopamine patches is very suggestive of corresponding to esterase-positive staining as well.

Receptor Characteristics and Behavioral Consequences of Kainic Acid Lesions and Fetal Transplants of the Striatum[a]

A. WALLACE DECKEL[b,c] AND ROBERT G. ROBINSON[c,d]

[c]*Department of Psychiatry and Behavioral Sciences*
and
[d]*Department of Neuroscience*
Johns Hopkins University School of Medicine
Baltimore, Maryland 21205

INTRODUCTION

Neural control of behavior is most often studied by creating lesions in, or "lesioning," the structure of interest, and then examining the behavioral consequences of such lesions. With the advent of the fetal brain transplantation methodology, a new method of examining neural control of behavior has become available. By combining a lesion of the structure of interest with "replacement" of the injured brain tissue, both the "negative" effects of the lesion and the "positive" effects of the transplant help to delineate the role of the brain region involved.

We have adopted such a strategy in studying the role of the striatum in the regulation of behavior by using excitotoxic lesions of the striatum, and implants of fetal striatum. The use of the transplants offer the hope that the behavioral role of the striatum will be better understood, and that the biological mechanisms by which the striatum influences behavior will become clearer.

GENERAL METHODOLOGY

Our methodology has been similar across the various experiments.[1-10] Kainic acid striatal lesions (0.8 μg/4 μl) are made bilaterally in the anterior-medial striatum in adult female Sprague-Dawley rats. Transplants are placed directly into the "lesioned"

[a]This work was supported by a grant from the Huntington's Disease Foundation of America.
[b]Present address: Department of Psychiatry, New Jersey Medical School, UMDNJ.

striatum, using a donor of gestational age E17-18. The transplants are stereotaxically implanted into the recipient striatum 7 days after the adult (host) striatum is lesioned, using nontrypsinized, aspirated injections of donor tissue. Volume of transplanted tissue is controlled, and has ranged from 2-3 mm³.

CHARACTERISTICS OF THE LESION

One early concern was that the kainate, despite the low doses used, would diffuse from the lesion site into other regions of the brain and cause extrastriatal damage.

TABLE 1. Cell Counts

Region of the Brain[a]	Cell Counts for Different Groups of Animals (mean ± SD)			One-way ANOVA[b]	
	Lesioned-and-transplanted	Lesioned	Controls	F	Significance
Striatum					
A 8920	15.8 ± 3.81	3.6 ± 1.9	27.7 ± 9.3	23.6 (2,15)	$p < .01$
A 8280	21.4 ± 6.8	4.7 ± 1.8	28.5 ± 5.5	36.5 (2,15)	$p < .01$
A 7890	18.3 ± 3.5	10.0 ± 5.5	23.8 ± 6.2	10.9 (2,15)	$p < .01$
Pyriform					
A 8280	50.5 ± 13.1	38.7 ± 17.4	52.2 ± 13.1	1.5 (2,15)	NS
Amygdala					
A 7020	16.1 ± 6.4	13.2 ± 3.4	21.2 ± 6.7	3.3 (2,15)	NS
Hippocampus					
A 3930	19.7 ± 0.93	22.4 ± 6.9	27.4 ± 4.7	3.3 (2,13)	NS
VMH					
A 4230	45.1 ± 5.4	39.2 ± 20.4	67.0 ± 33.9	1.9 (2,13)	NS

[a] The three regions of the brain are as defined in the atlas by Konig and Klippel.[11]
[b] The cell counts were compared for the three experimental groups in each region.

For this reason, cell counts within three regions of the striatum, as well as in the pyriform cortex, amygdala, hippocampus, and ventromedial nucleus of the hypothalamus (VMH), were done in control, kainic acid-lesioned, and lesioned-and-transplanted animals. The mean cell counts and standard deviations for each region of the brain are presented in TABLE 1. As can be seen, there were significant differences between groups for the three striatal regions after lesioning, but not for the pyriform cortex, amygdala, hippocampus, or VMH regions. Thus kainic acid does not appear to diffuse into widely diffuse regions of the neuraxis in the dosages employed, and does not cause obvious extrastriatal damage.

GENERAL ANATOMICAL CHARACTERISTICS OF THE TRANSPLANTS

Although all three regions of the kainic acid-lesioned striatum showed a significant decrease in the neuronal population in comparison to controls, the transplants grew robustly when placed into any of these regions of lesioned striatum. Ninety-two percent of the transplants evidenced excellent survival and growth when the host brains were sacrificed 5 months after transplantation.[1] The transplants grew 700-4900 μm in an anterior-posterior direction. Statistical analysis revealed the transplanted rats to have significantly more neurons than the lesioned-only group in regions A 8920 and A 8280, as defined by the atlas of Konig and Klippel,[11] but fewer neurons than controls in region A 8920. Occasional small patches of necrosis were seen in half of the transplants. When present, the necrosis appeared as small, oval, opaque crystalline patches that took the Nissl stain poorly, and were accompanied by occasional macrophages. Thus the transplants partially reversed the cell loss caused by the kainic acid lesions, and showed excellent survival overall.

More recently, comparisons of growth rates of fetal striatum transplanted into the intact (sham lesion) versus kainic acid-lesioned host brain were made in order to determine whether the neural environment significantly altered growth characteristics.[2,6] Transplants placed into the intact brain had only 72% of the mean cross-sectional area that transplants placed into the lesioned brain had, this despite the fact that an identical volume of transplant was made across groups. When mean cross-sectional striatal area (that is, host striatum plus transplant) was compared between transplanted and control brains, the lesioned-and-transplanted striatum had a *greater* cross-sectional area than controls (112%). Conversely, transplants placed into the nonlesioned brain had a *smaller* overall striatal area than controls.

Trophic factors exist in the lesioned brain,[12,13] and it is possible that such factors within the lesioned striatum accounted for the increased size of the transplants in the lesioned, as opposed to intact, brain. Alternatively, mechanical factors within the intact striatum could have limited the ability of the fetal striatum to expand and develop, and, through mechanisms similar to pressure atrophy, restrict development. In any case, fetal striatal transplants showed robust growth when placed within the previously lesioned host striatum, growing to a greater extent than when they were placed into the intact striatum.

RECEPTOR DEVELOPMENT

Dopamine Receptors

Dopamine (D2) receptor development was examined autoradiographically in transplants placed both into the intact as well as kainic acid-lesioned host brain striatum. The binding methodology is described elsewhere,[2] but included incubating coronal frozen sections (25 μm) of the anterior-medial striatum in a Tris buffer containing [^{3}H]spiperone (0.4 nM) and either haloperidol (0.4 μM, to block D2 receptor sites), cinancerin (0.3 μM, courteousy of Squibb Pharmaceutical, to block serotonin sites), or both. Striatal binding density was then calculated by computer densitometry (LOATS).

The transplants were clearly visible in the autoradiographs, appearing as a "cold" spot on the film with an optical density (OD) that was only slightly higher than that of the background (FIG. 1).

As TABLE 2 illustrates, the OD of transplants placed either into the intact brain or kainic acid-lesioned brain were similar, and significantly reduced from the OD of control striatum. D2 receptor density was also reduced in the lesioned-only striatum; nonetheless, there was significantly more D2 binding in the lesioned-only striatum than in the fetal striatal transplants placed into the lesioned brain. The OD of the surrounding host striatum appeared unchanged, or slightly higher from control striatum in the transplanted-only condition, possibly because of a "compaction" of the host striatum due to the additional mass of the transplant. Collectively, these results suggest that D2 receptors do not develop normally in striatal transplants, regardless of the neural environment they are placed into. The reasons for this remain unclear, and current work aimed at further exploring this phenomenon is underway.

β_1- and β_2-Adrenergic Receptors

To determine whether the failed development of the D2 receptors represented a catecholaminergic phenomenon, β_1 and β_2 receptor development was assessed autoradiographically. Briefly, slide-mounted tissue was incubated in 20 mM Tris containing 65 pM ^{125}I-labeled cyanopindolol.[5,14] Serial sections were incubated in the presence of either 1 μM L-propanolol, 70 nM β_1 antagonist ICI 89 406 or 50 mM β_2 antagonist ICI 118 551. Autoradiographs were analyzed by computerized densitometry (LOATS) to calculate densities of β_1, β_2, and total β receptors in the striatum under the different experiment conditions. The β_1 receptor density was significantly higher (mean OD: 0.164; SD: 0.027) than the β_2 receptor density (mean OD: 0.059; SD: 0.027). This was consistent with previous reports[14] describing the regional variation of β-adrenergic receptor density in the mammalian brain; β_1 density has been reported as being higher than β_2 in forebrain structures, and β_2 predominated within hindbrain areas. As shown in FIGURE 2, β-adrenergic OD within the transplanted striatum was virtually identical to that of surrounding host striatum. The β_1 OD reached 101%, with β_2 at 97%, of host striatum OD. As with the D2 binding, no differences were found between transplants placed into the intact, versus kainic acid-lesioned, host brains.

Although virtually no D2 receptors are found within the fetal striatal transplants, β-adrenergic receptor density reached control values. These results suggest that the failed D2 development did not reflect a more general failure of catecholaminergic receptor development, but rather points to a specific deficit of dopamine receptor development.

Cholinergic Receptor Binding

Cholinergic receptor binding was determined in the fetal striatum transplanted into intact (transplanted-only) as well as kainic acid-lesioned (lesioned-and-trans-

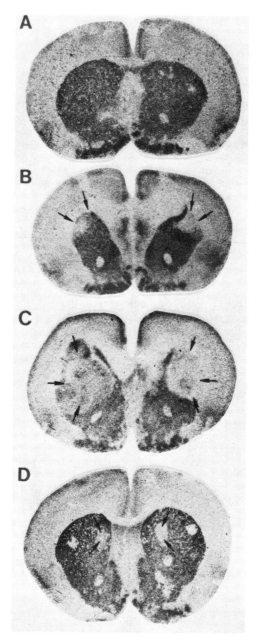

FIGURE 1. D2 autoradiography of brain sections. Each section is from a different group: (**A**) control; (**B**) lesioned-only (arrows point to the lesion); (**C**) lesioned-and-transplanted (arrows point to the striatal transplant); and (**D**) transplanted-only (striatal transplants in intact, that is, sham-lesioned, host striatum) (arrows point to the transplant).

planted) host striatum, with lesioned-only and sham-lesioned-sham-transplanted brains serving as controls. Brain slices (25 μm) were incubated either directly in 1 nM [^{3}H]N-methyl scopolamine ([^{3}H]NMS) (total binding), or underwent incubation in 1 nM [^{3}H]NMS + 10^{-4} carbechol or 1 nM [^{3}H]NMS plus 1 μM atropine, according to the methods of Wamsley et al.[15] Carbechol displaces high-affinity cholinergic receptor sites,[15] giving a measure of low-affinity receptor density. High-affinity sites were calculated by subtracting the OD of the carbechol condition from the total binding.

As TABLE 3 indicates, the OD of the total binding condition in the lesioned-only striatum (mean: 1.00; SD: 0.36) was significantly less than control striatum (mean: 1.26; SD: 0.14). OD of transplants placed either into intact brain (mean: 1.07; SD 0.20) or previously lesioned striatum (mean: 1.02; SD: 0.34) was significantly reduced from control values (FIG. 3).

TABLE 2. Dopaminergic Receptor Density

Group[a]	OD (mean ± SD)	Percentage of Control Striatum OD
Fetal Striatal Transplants		
TO	.040 ± .008	25
LT	.020 ± .004	16
Total Striatum[b]		
LO	.07 ± .05	43
LT	.05 ± .03	25
TO	.165 ± .040	114
CN	.145 ± .040	

[a] LO: lesioned-only; LT: lesioned-and-transplanted; TO: transplanted-only; CN: control.
[b] Host tissue and transplant tissue (region A 8280).

Compared to control striatum, high-affinity sites were significantly increased in the transplants, whereas the low-affinity cholinergic receptor sites were reduced in number (TABLE 3). Birdsall et al.[16] have argued that, of the classes of muscarinic agonist binding sites, the low-affinity receptors represent the functional (that is, channel-coupled) site, whereas the high-affinity site represents an uncoupled form of the receptor.[17] The current findings suggest that a shift from the low- to the high-affinity state occurs in the cholinergic receptors in fetal striatal transplants, regardless of the type of neural environment the tissue is placed into. The behavioral effects of this "shift," as well as the reduced density of low-affinity binding sites, remain unknown, but preliminary work (Deckel, unpublished results) suggested that the development of low-affinity receptors in the transplanted brains correlated significantly with the transplant-induced recovery.

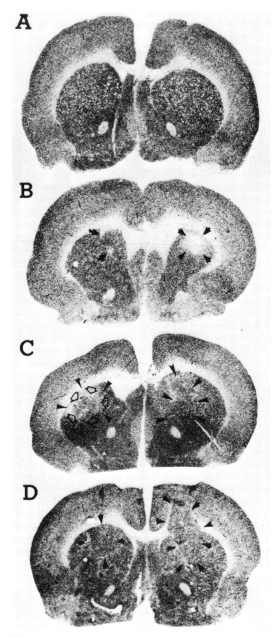

FIGURE 2. Total β-adrenergic receptor binding in brain sections. Each section is from a different group: (**A**) control; (**B**) lesioned-only (arrows point to the striatal lesion); (**C**) lesioned-and-transplanted (closed arrows point to the transplant; open arrows, to the lesion); and (**D**) transplanted-only (striatal transplants in intact host striatum) (arrows point to the transplant).

BEHAVIORAL MEASURES

Spontaneous Locomotor Activity

Following bilateral kainic acid lesions of the striatum, female rats showed an increase in spontaneous locomotion[1,2,4,6,7,9] that persisted for long periods of time after lesioning. When placed in a photocell chamber that calculated horizontal, vertical, and stereotypical movements (such as scratching, grooming, sniffing), the lesioned animals were hyperactive both as they became habituated to their surroundings, as well as during their active (night) period. Although male rats showed a decline in their hyperactivity for several weeks after lesioning,[18,19] the female rats continued to be hyperactive for the 9 months that we recorded their behavior (Deckel, unpublished results).

TABLE 3. Muscarinic Cholinergic Binding

Group[a]	Percentage of Control Striatum OD		
	Total Binding	High-affinity Binding	Low-affinity Binding
Fetal Striatal Transplants			
TO	85**	221*	70***
LT	81*	200*	71***
Total Striatum[b]			
LO	79*	147	82*
TO	90*	189	86***
LT	70***	137	70***

NOTE: *: $p < .05$; **: $p < .01$; ***: $p < .0005$.
[a] LO: lesioned-only; LT: lesioned-and-transplanted; TO: transplanted-only; CN: control.
[b] Host tissue and transplant tissue (region A 8280).

Transplants of E17-18 striatum into animals with bilateral kainic acid striatal lesions significantly remediated the lesion-induced hyperactivity. The lesioned-only animals were hyperactive over the 2 hr they were in the photocell chamber in horizontal and stereotypical movements. Specifically, the number of movements (FIG. 4A) and time spent moving (FIG. 4B) in the horizontal plane as well as the time spent moving in a stereotypical manner (FIG. 5) were all relatively increased over control values. The transplants reversed this hyperactivity, and led the lesioned animals to move similar to controls, and significantly less than the lesioned-only animals. Although the abnormality in horizontal activity was completely reversed (FIG. 4), the transplants affected stereotypical behavior in a complex manner in that they reduced the time the animals spent moving in a stereotypical manner (FIG. 5B), but increased the number of stereotypical movements (FIG. 5A). These results suggested that the transplants caused rapid, intermittent increases in stereotypic movements. This movement pattern was not seen in control or in lesioned-only animals.

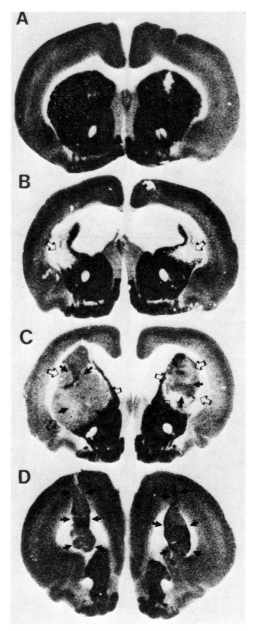

FIGURE 3. Autoradiography of total cholinergic receptor density in brain sections. Each section is from a different group: (**A**) control; (**B**) lesioned-only; (**C**) lesioned-and-transplanted; and (**D**) transplanted-only (striatal transplants in intact host striatum). Open arrows point to the lesioned striatum; closed arrows point to the transplant.

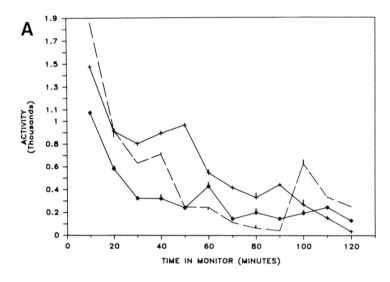

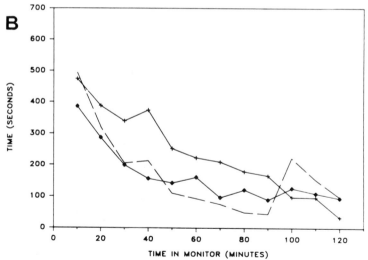

FIGURE 4. Locomotor activity in control (---), lesioned-only (+———+), and lesioned-and-transplanted (◆———◆) animals over the 2 hr they were placed in the animal activity monitor. (**A**) Horizontal activity. (**B**) Time spent moving in the horizontal plane.

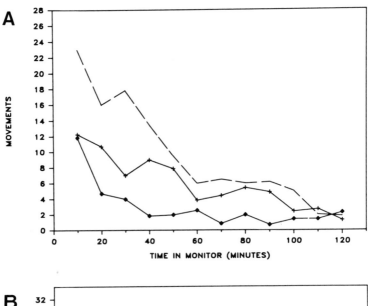

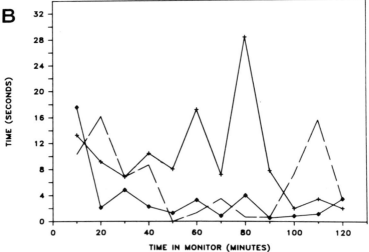

FIGURE 5. Locomotor activity in control (◆——◆), lesioned-only (+——+), and lesioned-and-transplanted (---) animals over the 2 hr they were placed in the animal activity monitor. (**A**) Number of stereotypical movements. (**B**) Time spent moving in the horizontal plane.

Drug-affected Locomotion

To assess the locomotor response to amphetamine injection, animals were placed in an open field, and horizontal activity and rearing behaviors were assessed. Specifically, animals were allowed to become habituated to the open field for 1 hr, and then were injected with amphetamine (1 mg/kg, i.p.). Horizontal activity and rearing behaviors were measured 0-5, 20-25, and 55-60 min following injection. A repeated measures design was utilized, with the animals (that is, the lesioned-only, lesioned-and-transplanted, and control animals) being placed in the field 2 weeks before surgery, and 2, 6, 10, and 14 weeks after surgery.

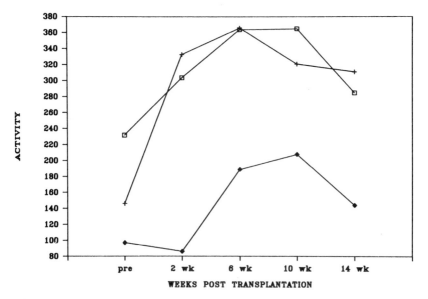

FIGURE 6. Locomotion in an open field 20-25 min after injection of amphetamine (1 mg/kg, i.p.). ◆: Controls; +: lesioned-only animals; and □: lesioned-and-transplanted animals.

Horizontal and vertical activities were measured during the 5-10 min after each amphetamine injection. No differences between groups were noted for any of the 5-10-min periods. The amphetamine did, however, cause a relative horizontal hyperactivity in the lesioned groups 20-25 and 55-60 min after injection (FIG. 6) that was not reversed by the transplants. There were no significant differences between groups at any time in their rearing behavior, nor was there evidence of a progressive motor deficit over the course of the experiment after the kainic acid lesions. Thus the transplanted animals, although apparently recovered on spontaneous locomotion, "reexpressed" the lesion-induced hyperactivity following amphetamine injection.

More recently, the effect of pre- and postsynaptic DA stimulation on the locomotor activity of rats was assessed.[2,6] In this experiment, four groups of animals were used: kainic acid lesioned-only, lesioned-and-transplanted, transplanted-only (that is, transplants into the sham-lesioned striatum), and control animals. Five months after trans-plantation, animals were run in an activity monitor for three drug trials, including a saline (1.0 ml/kg, i.p.), an amphetamine (1.0 mg/kg, i.p.), and an apomorphine (0.2 mg/kg, s.c.) condition; drugs were administered randomly to controls for drug order effect. Behavioral testing under the saline condition revealed that the lesioned-only group locomoted significantly further than did sham-operated controls on measures of horizontal activity (FIG. 7). Similarly, transplanted-only animals acted as if they had lesions of the striatum, showing a hyperactivity of similar magnitude to the lesioned-only group. Both control and lesioned-and-transplanted animals moved sig-nificantly shorter distances, and significantly slower, than the lesioned-only and trans-planted-only animals. Although the transplants normalized horizontal locomotor activity in the lesioned rats under the saline condition, they had no effect under the amphetamine or apomorphine trials. Both apomorphine and amphetamine caused lesioned animals to move significantly more often than controls, regardless of the presence of transplants.

Thus animals with kainic acid-induced lesions of the striatum showed a persistent daytime locomotor hyperactivity that, relative to controls, was accentuated after in-jection of amphetamine or apomorphine. Although the transplants normalized the locomotor changes seen under spontaneous ambulation, they had no effect on the amphetamine- or apomorphine-induced hyperactivity. Surprisingly, transplants of day E17-18 fetal striatum placed into the intact brain led to abnormalities in spontaneous locomotion similar to those seen in the lesioned group, but did not cause a hyperactivity in the amphetamine or apomorphine condition (FIG. 7).

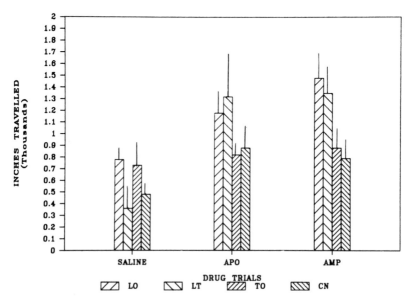

FIGURE 7. Locomotor response of lesioned-only (LO), lesioned-and-transplanted (LT), trans-planted-only (TO), and control (CN) animals after injection of saline (1 ml/kg, i.p.), apo-morphine (APO) (0.2 mg/kg, s.c.), and amphetamine (AMP) (1 mg/kg, i.p.).

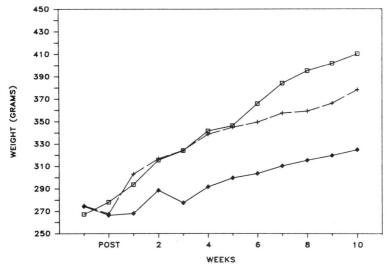

FIGURE 8. Weekly body weights for each of the 12 weeks after transplantation. ◆: Controls; +: lesioned-only animals; and □: lesioned-and-transplanted animals.

BODY WEIGHT EFFECTS

Past work examining the effects of striatal kainic acid lesions on body weight has been done in male rats.[20,21] The male rats with these lesions experienced a temporary adipsia and aphagia for several days after lesioning, eventually showing a gradual return of body weight to near control levels.[20,21]

When identical lesions were given to female rats, they demonstrated an adipsia and aphagia similar to those shown by the males, but subsequently showed an increase in body weight during the course of the experiment (FIG. 8).[10] The animals that received lesions followed by transplants of day E17-18 fetal striatum had body weights similar to animals of the lesioned-only group for the first 5 weeks after implantation, although they demonstrated a nonsignificant increase in their body weight 5 weeks after transplantation. There was no evidence that the transplants reversed the weight gain induced in female rats by the kainic acid striatal lesions.

The body weight increases in the lesioned-only and lesioned-and-transplanted animals appeared to be a partial result of increased food and water consumption. Lesioned-only, and lesioned-and-transplanted animals, consumed more food than controls over a 72-hr period (FIG. 9). In addition, both groups consumed more water than controls (FIG. 9), with the lesioned-and-transplanted animals drinking more than the lesioned-only animals, and lesioned-only animals consuming more water than controls. Thus the transplants not only failed to remediate the lesion-induced obesity, but either had no effect, or exaggerated the effect, on food and water consumption.

Although the increased food and water consumption in the lesioned-only and lesioned-and-transplanted groups would explain the body weight changes, we wondered whether changes in the metabolic rate of the lesioned animals existed that further

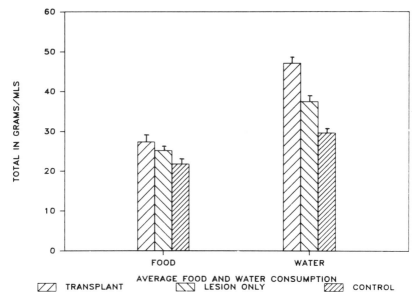

FIGURE 9. Three-day average of food and water consumption in control, lesioned-only, and lesioned-and-transplanted animals. Bars: SEM.

contributed to this phenomenon. To examine this on a preliminary basis, animals were deprived of food for a 24-hr period, and the amount of weight loss during the deprivation period and the amount of water consumption and food consumption following refeeding were all assessed. Surprisingly, control animals lost significantly more weight (25.3 g) than either the lesioned-only (16.8 g) or lesioned-and-transplanted (12.0 g) animals. As controls were less active than animals in the lesion groups, [1,4,7] these results suggested that the basal metabolic rates in the lesioned animals were reduced in comparison to controls. Food consumption during the 24 hr of refeeding also showed differences across groups, with lesioned-only animals consuming significantly more food (34.3 g) than the lesioned-and-transplanted animals (21.9 g); control consumption (27.1 g) was midway between the other two groups.

Collectively, these results suggested that the kainic acid striatal lesions caused an increase in body weight that is sex specific; only the female rats show this response, with male rats showing a decline in weight following identical lesions. The increase in body weight appeared to be a result both of the increased food and water consumption, as well as from the apparently decreased metabolic rate in the lesioned animals. The transplants had no effect on the body weight or on the feeding and drinking behaviors, but did influence the amount of food consumed during a period of refeeding. Taken together, these findings suggested a sex-specific striatal regulation of body weight that was not remediated by replacing the lost striatal tissue with fetal transplantation. Further work is underway to examine more carefully the biological variables that account for these effects.

PENTYLENETETRAZOL

Animals with kainic striatal lesions show intermittent grand mal seizures.[22] As a preliminary attempt to examine whether the transplants could reverse the seizure-induced effects of the lesion, a small group of lesioned-only, lesioned-and-transplanted, and control animals were given the convulsant pentylenetetrazol (PTZ) (70 mg/kg, s.c.) 14 weeks after transplantation. During the 20 min following injection of the PTZ, three measures were obtained, including latency to the first ictal response, latency to the first grand mal seizure, and total duration of the clonic phase of the grand mal seizure. There was a great deal of variation as to when the pre-ictal movements were seen in the lesioned-and-transplanted and control groups (FIG. 10), with the range extending from 63 to 668 sec in the former group, and 75 to 1155 sec in the latter group. Conversely, the range was narrower in the lesioned-only group, with all animals showing the first ictal response between 115 and 280 seconds. A similar pattern was found for latency to the first grad mal seizure. The lesioned-only group seized relatively quickly, and showed little variance as a group in response to the drug, whereas the lesioned-and-transplanted and control groups showed a wide range of response, with several animals not seizing for time periods well in excess of the most resistant lesioned-only animals. Finally, whereas all of the lesioned-only animals experienced a grand mal seizure following injection, only 50% of the lesioned-and-transplanted and 72% of the control animals seized during the 20 min following injection.

Although these results are preliminary and in need of replication, they suggest that the transplants may confer some protective effects against the lesion-induced seizures. The striatum is known to have GABA-ergic output neurons,[23] and the lesion-induced seizures may result from a disturbance of GABA-ergic processes.[24] It is possible that the transplants directly or indirectly modulate the GABA-ergic output

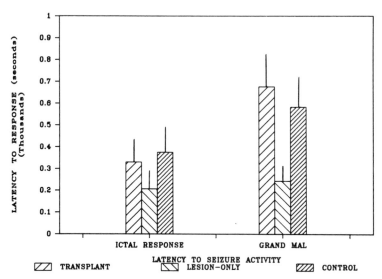

FIGURE 10. Latency to the first ictal response, and to the first grand mal seizure, after injection of 70 mg/kg PTZ in control, lesioned-only, and lesioned-and-transplanted animals.

system of the striatum, and in this manner reduce the seizure activity. There is some evidence to support this, as the transplants are known to increase GAD levels in the globus pallidus.[25] Further work will be required to more carefully evaluate this possibility.

T-MAZE (DELAYED REWARDED ALTERNATION)

Three groups of animals—1) lesioned only, rats with kainic acid striatal lesions; 2) implanted, rats with kainic acid striatal lesions and transplants of day E17-18 fetal striatum; and 3) control, rats with sham-lesions and sham transplants—were trained on a simple T-maze task where they were required to alternate visits to the sides of the T-maze in order to receive a food reward.[1] Rats were trained before surgery (21 trials/day) until they alternated 85% or more of the time for 3 consecutive days. Twelve weeks after implantation, and sham implantation, the animals were again run for 21 trials/day for 10 consecutive days without any pretraining.

Although there were no significant differences between groups on presurgery performance, 12 weeks after surgery the lesioned-only group alternated significantly fewer times than controls, as shown in FIGURE 11.

The implanted group performance level was midway between the lesioned-only group and control group levels. The average correct number of alternations in the control group exceeded the lesioned-only group in all 10 trials, and the implanted group in 9 of the 10 trials. Conversely, the implanted group showed significant recovery ($p < .05$) compared to the lesioned-only group, outperforming it in 9 out of 10 trials. Thus the transplants partially reversed the deficit in rewarded alternation caused by the lesion.

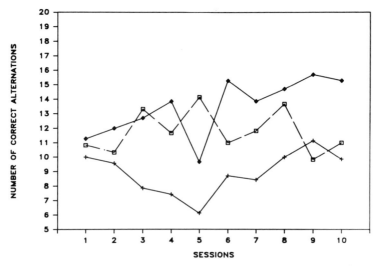

FIGURE 11. Number of correct alternations in the T-maze over the 10 sessions after surgery. ◆: Controls; +: lesioned-only animals; and □: lesioned-and-transplanted animals.

TABLE 4. Scores for Perserverance in Behavior before and after Surgery[a]

| Group | Score (mean ± SD) | | t | Significance |
	Before Surgery	After Surgery		
Implanted	10.3 ± 4.5	42.0 ± 38.1	1.99 (6df)	NS
Lesion-only	11.3 ± 5.5	57.3 ± 23.0	4.84 (7df)	$p < .01$
Control	16.3 ± 16.1	21.1 ± 39.8	0.27 (7df)	NS

[a] Scores were recorded in tests using the T-maze (delayed rewarded alternation) task.

Two different types of errors could be made by the lesioned-only group on the T-maze. First, the animals could have simply persevered in their behavior, for example, making one string of seven consecutive visits to the same side of the maze. Conversely, the animals could have "forgot" what side they had previously visited, in which case mistakes should not have occurred consecutively, but rather should have been distributed randomly throughout the trials. The number of consecutive mistakes made during training was used as a measure of perseverance. This measure was taken in training periods both before and after surgery for each rat. As shown in TABLE 4, measures of perseverance in the trials after surgery were higher than those in the trials before surgery for all groups: they were 408% higher for implanted rats (NS); 507% higher for lesioned-only rats ($p < .01$); and 130% higher for control rats (NS).

To assess whether the increased number of lesion-induced consecutive mistakes for each animal could simply be a function of increased mistakes, the number of consecutive mistakes was divided by the number of mistakes and multiplied by 100 to give the percentage of mistakes that were consecutive. For implanted rats, 42% of the mistakes were consecutive; for the lesioned-only rats, 50%; for the control rats, 21%. The remainder of the errors were attributed to "forgetting" by the animals.

In summary, transplants partially reversed the T-maze deficit caused by the lesion. Both quantitative (number of errors) as well as qualitative (type of error) aspects of the T-maze deficit were partially affected by the transplants.

SENSORIMOTOR NEUROLOGICAL EXAM

A brief sensorimotor neurological exam based on the test battery used by Dunnett et al.[26] was given to rats on a weekly basis over the 12 weeks following transplantation. The exam systematically examined five different types of neurological functioning, including 1) muscle tone, 2) orientation to vibrassae and olfactory stimulation, 3) response to blunt touch, 4) response to sharp touch, and 5) limb strength. Persistent and enduring deficits beginning after the kainic acid lesions were found in both the lesioned-only and implanted groups compared to controls. The implants had no effect on this behavioral deficit, as shown in FIGURE 12. At no time were the results for implanted animals statistically different from those for lesioned-only animals, nor were they similar to those for controls. Thus, on the sensorimotor neurological exam, there was no evidence of the ability of the transplant to modify the lesion-induced deficit.

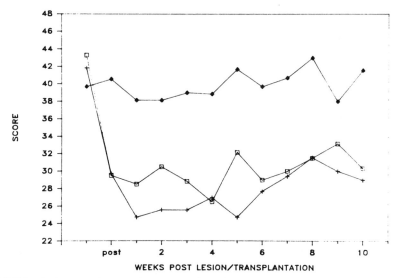

FIGURE 12. Score on the sensorimotor neurological exam over the 11 weeks after transplantation. ◆: Controls; +: lesioned-only animals; and □: lesioned-and-transplanted animals.

STRIATAL NEURONAL DENSITY AND RECOVERY

The recovery within the lesioned-and-transplanted group was only partial. Similarly, the transplants only partially reversed the neuronal cell loss caused by the striatal lesions. To better understand the relationship between cell counts and behavioral recovery, multiple regressions were used to examine whether neuronal cell density in regions A 8982, A 8280, and A 7890 of the striatum in control, lesioned-only, and lesioned-and-transplanted groups correlated with the behavioral measures.

Surprisingly, neuronal density in region A 8280 significantly correlated with six of the behavioral measures (TABLE 5). First, some locomotor activities, both under spontaneous as well as amphetamine-affected conditions, were inversely correlated with the cell counts. The fewer the cells in the striatum, the more hyperactive the animals were. Similar results were found on the T-maze, sensorimotor neurological exam, and response to pentylenetetrazol. The fewer the striatal cells, the more abnormal the behavior was.

These results suggest that quantitative aspects of the transplant methodology are important, and indicate that the extent of behavioral recovery seen after transplantation is likely to partially depend on the number of neurons transplanted.

DISCUSSION

The β_1- and β_2-adrenergic receptors develop in normal quantities in the fetal striatal transplants.[5] This indicates that the failure of the D2 receptors to "turn on" is not simply a catecholaminergic mechanism, but represents a specific failure of the DA system to develop. It is known that nigral afferents do not significantly penetrate transplanted striatum.[27] In normal development, the nigral afferents first start to release DA in the embryological striatum at gestational age day 14.[28] The first DA receptors are not detected, however, until several days later at day E18. It is possible that DA itself is required for the receptors to develop, and that the failed development of the D2 receptors in the transplants is secondary to the lack of penetration by nigrostriatal fibers of the host brain into the transplant.

Alternatively, it is conceivable that critical trophic factors known to foster D2 development are missing in the transplant. Specifically, cholecystokinin,[29] guanyl nucleotides,[30] estradiol,[31] and GM1[32] are all known to regulate DA receptor development. These, or other trophic factors, could be present in abnormal quantities in transplants; similarly, it is possible that these factors are generated during periods of neural development in other regions of the neuraxis, and diffuse to the striatum. Transplants of the fetal striatum in the adult brain could thus be without the benefit of these extrastriatal trophic factors, and thus account for some of the failed development.

The "shift" of the cholinergic receptor states from the low-affinity (that is, ion-channel-coupled, functional) state to the high-affinity (noncoupled) state found in the transplants is further suggestive of a cholinergic developmental abnormality. Other abnormalities in cholinergic systems within the transplant are found; acetylcholinesterase levels are decreased in nontrypsinized[9] and trypsinized[33] striatal transplants, and injection of cholinergic agonists/antagonists into lesioned animals disrupts the locomotor behavior of apparently recovered transplanted animals (Deckel, unpublished results). Guanyl nucleotides can experimentally interconvert the high-affinity cholinergic receptor state to a low-affinity one[34]; it is possible that these or other factors endogenous to the developing fetal brain are lacking, or reduced in amount, in the neural environment of the host adult brain. To what extent the reduced number of low-affinity sites in the transplants contributes to the incomplete reversal of the behavioral deficits remains unclear, but preliminary results suggest that the development of cholinergic receptor density correlates significantly with transplant-induced recovery (Deckel, unpublished results).

It is possible that the reduced OD of the total and low-affinity cholinergic receptor sites in the transplants is a function of the reduced neuronal density of the transplants. Low-affinity cholinergic OD reaches 70 and 71% of control values, respectively, when transplants are placed into intact, and lesioned, host striatum. The average neuronal density of the transplanted striatum was 57% (A 8920), 75% (A 8280), and 77% (A 7890) of control brain values; when cell counts were averaged across these three

TABLE 5. Correlations between Striatal Cell Counts in Region at A 8280 and Behavioral Outcomes

Behavior	R	R^2	F(df)	B	Significance
Locomotion					
Spontaneous	−.54	.29	6.44 (1,16)	−0.5	$p < .05$
Induced by amphetamine					
6 weeks after transplantation	−.48	.23	4.76 (1,16)	−5.6	$p < .05$
10 weeks after transplantation	−.50	.25	5.34 (1,16)	−5.5	$p < .05$
T-maze	−.70	.49	15.5 (1,16)	−0.7	$p < .001$
Sensorimotor neurological exam	−.57	.33	7.79 (1,16)	−0.6	$p < .01$
Latency[a]	−.64	.41	4.45 (2,13)	−28.0	$p < .05$

[a] Latency to the first ictal response after PTZ injection.

brain regions, the neuronal density reached 70% of control values. Thus the reduced OD of the cholinergic receptor density within the transplants could partially be a function of reduced cellularity within the transplants. This reduction of neuronal density of the transplants is important to consider not only when receptor density is being interpreted, but also when behavioral outcome studies are being analyzed. The neuronal density correlates with six of the behavioral measures reported here, suggesting that quantitative aspects of the transplantation methodology remain as an important variable to be considered in behaviorally oriented transplantation experiments.

To what extent remediation of the receptor abnormalities in the transplants would further normalize behavior following excitotoxic lesions remains unclear: The specific mechanisms by which the transplants remediate the behavioral deficits are unknown. A rich diversity of cell types are found within the transplants,[8,35] however, and GABA-ergic mechanisms may be involved in the recovery process. Glutamic acid decarboxylase levels are reinstated in the globus pallidus following ibotenic acid striatal lesions when fetal striatal transplants are placed into the lesioned area.[25] Pentylenetetrazol seizures, which may work via disruption of GABA-ergic systems,[24] are worsened by kainate lesions and partially remediated by the transplants. Thus GABA-ergic neurons, which are one of the major types of projection neurons in the normal striatum,[23] are likely to be contained within the transplants, and recovery may partially be a consequence of reestablishment of striatal GABA-ergic influence on its normal projection areas. Conversely, afferent connections to the transplant from the substantia nigra appear reduced, or lacking, within the transplant. Few monoamine-positive fibers are found to penetrate the transplant.[27] Similarly, few DA receptors are present within the transplant,[2,6] and the apparent remediation of locomotor deficits following kainic acid striatal lesions is reversed following injection of DA agonists.[2,6] Although little is known of the ability of cortical glutaminergic, thalamocortical, or other afferents to penetrate the transplants, it does appear as though nigrostriatal projections account for little, if any, of the observed recovery.

The use of fetal striatal transplants in neuroscience research is likely to lead to a better theoretical understanding of a number of different brain mechanisms. Although doubts remain, it is hoped that such transplants may serve as a clinical tool for the remediation of significant striatal pathology. Future work needs to be directed at elucidating (and remediating) the mechanisms that prevent the nigral afferents from penetrating the transplants; at examining the role that other afferent sources to the striatum may have in accounting for behavioral recovery; at more completely characterizing (and remediating) the intratransplant developmental abnormalities, such as the cholinergic and DA receptor abnormalities presented here; and at quantifying the number, and type, of outputs from the transplanted striatum to the host brain.

It is likely that interventions will need to be developed to improve the maturation and development of the transplant, and it is hoped that as these interventions are developed, the transplants will show successively greater ability to remediate the behavioral deficits resulting from striatal pathology.

ACKNOWLEDGMENTS

We thank Dr. Timothy Moran for his technical advice throughout the course of these experiments, Dr. Peter Whitehouse for assistance with the cholinergic receptor binding, and Albert W. Deckel, Sr. for reviewing the manuscript.

REFERENCES

1. DECKEL, A. W., T. H. MORAN, J. T. COYLE, P. R. SANBERG & R. G. ROBINSON. 1986. Anatomical predictors of behavioral recovery following fetal striatal transplants. Brain Res. 365: 249-258.
2. DECKEL, A. W., T. H. MORAN & R. G. ROBINSON. 1986. Behavioral recovery following kainic acid lesions and fetal implants of the striatum occurs independent of dopaminergic mechanisms. Brain Res. 363: 383-385.
3. DECKEL, A. W. & R. G. ROBINSON. 1986. Status marmoratus in fetal cortical transplants. Exp. Neurol. 91: 212-218.
4. DECKEL, A. W., R. G. ROBINSON, J. T. COYLE & P. R. SANBERG. 1983. Reversal of long-term locomotor abnormalities in the kainic acid model of Huntington's disease by day 18 fetal striatal implants. Eur. J. Pharmacol. 93: 287-288.
5. DECKEL, A. W., T. H. MORAN, K. SAAD & R. G. ROBINSON. 1986. β-Adrenergic receptor density in fetal striatal transplants. Eur. J. Pharmacol. In press.
6. DECKEL, A. W., T. H. MORAN & R. G. ROBINSON. 1985. Reversal of spontaneous locomotor hyperactivity following fetal transplants of the striatum occurs independent of dopamine mechanisms. Soc. Neurosci. Abstr. 11: 616.
7. DECKEL, A. W., R. G. ROBINSON & P. R. SANBERG. 1983. The ability of day 18 fetal striatal implants to reverse the long-term locomotor abnormalities in the kainic acid model of Huntington's disease. Soc. Neurosci. Abstr. 9: 860.
8. DEFIGLIA, M., L. SCHIFF & A. W. DECKEL. 1986. Synaptic organization of fetal striatal transplants in the normal and kainate-lesioned rat caudate nucleus. Soc. Neurosci. Abstr. 11: 365.
9. SANBERG, P. R., M. A. HENAULT & A. W. DECKEL. Locomotor hyperactivity: Effects of multiple striatal transplants in an animal model of Huntington's disease. 1986. Pharmacol. Bio. Behav. In press.
10. DECKEL, A. W., T. H. MORAN & R. G. ROBINSON. 1986. Striatal DA systems regulate body weight in female rats. Proc. Abstr. Annu. Meet. Eastern Psychiatry Assoc. 57: 72.
11. KONIG, J. F. R. & R. A. KLIPPEL. 1967. The Rat Brain. Huntington. New York, NY.
12. F. H. GAGE, A. BJÖRKLUND & U. STENEVI. 1984. Denervation releases a neuronal survival factor in adult rat hippocampus. Nature 308: 637-639.
13. NIETO-SAMPEDRO, M., S. R. WHITTEMORE, D. L. NEEDELS, J. LARSON & C. W. COTMAN. 1984. The survival of brain transplants is enhanced by extracts from injured brain. Proc. Natl. Acad. Sci. USA 81: 6250-6254.
14. RAINBOW, T. C., B. PARSONS & B. B. WOLFE. 1984. Quantitative autoradiography of β_1- and β_2-adrenergic receptors in rat brain. Proc. Natl. Acad. Sci. USA 81: 1585-1589.
15. WAMSLEY, J. K., M. A. ZARBIN, NIGEL, J. M. BIRDSALL & M. J. KUHAR. 1980. Muscarinic cholinergic receptors: Autoradiographic localization of high- and low-affinity agonist binding sites. Brain Res. 200: 1-12.
16. BIRDSALL, N. J. M., E. C. HULME & A. S. V. BURGEN. 1980. The character of the muscarinic receptors in different regions of the rat brain. Proc. R. Soc. London 207: 1-12.
17. BIRDSALL, N. J. M. & E. C. HULME. 1976. Biochemical studies on muscarinic acetylcholine receptors. J. Neurochem. 27: 7-16.
18. MASON, S. T., P. R. SANBERG & H. C. FIBIGER. 1978. Kainic acid lesions of the striatum dissociate amphetamine and apomorphine stereotype: Similarities to Huntington's chorea. Science 201: 352-355.
19. DIVAC, I., H. J. MARKOWITSCH & M. PRITZEL. 1978. Behavioral and anatomical consequences of small intrastriatal injections of kainic acid in the rat. Brain Res. 151: 523-532.
20. PETTIBONE, D. J., N. KAUFMAN, M. C. SCALLY, E. MEYER, I. ULUS & L. D. LYTLE. 1978. Striatal nondopaminergic neurons: Possible involvement in feeding and drinking behavior. Science 200: 1173-1175.
21. SANBERG, P. R. & H. C. FIBIGER. 1979. Body weight, feeding, and drinking behaviors in rats with kainic acid-induced lesions of striatal neurons. Exp. Neurol. 66: 444-466.
22. STONE, W. E. & M. J. JAVID. 1980. Effects of anticonvulsants and glutamate antagonists on the convulsant action of kainic acid. Arch. Int. Pharmacodyn. 243: 56-65.

23. KIM, J.-S., I. J. BAK, R. HASSLER & Y. OKADA. 1971. Role of γ-aminobutyric acid (GABA) in the extrapyramidal motor system. II. Some evidence for the existence of a type of GABA-rich strio-nigral neuron. Exp. Brain Res. 14: 95-104.

24. GAVISH, M., N. AVNIMELECH-GIGUS, J. FELDON & M. MYSLOBODSKY. 1985. Prenatal chlordiazepoxide effects on metrazol seizures and benzodiazepine receptor densities in adult albino rats. Life Sci. 36: 1693-1698.

25. ISACSON, O., P. BRUNDIN, P. A. T. KELLY, F. H. GAGE & A. BJÖRKLUND. 1984. Functional neuronal replacement by grafted striatal neurons in the ibotenic acid-lesioned rat striatum. Nature 311: 458-460.

26. DUNNETT, S. B., A. BJÖRKLUND, U. STENEVI & S. D. IVERSEN. 1981. Behavioral recovery following transplantation of substantia nigra in rats subjected to 6-OHDA lesions of the nigrostriatal pathway. I. Unilateral lesions. Brain Res. 215: 147-161.

27. SCHMIDT, R. H., A. BJÖRKLUND & U. STENEVI. 1981. Intracerebral grafting of dissociated CNS tissue suspensions: A new approach for neuronal transplantation to deep brain sites. Brain Res. 218: 347-356.

28. EDLEY, S. M. & M. HERKENHAM. 1984. Comparative development of striatal opiate receptors and dopamine revealed by autoradiography and histofluorescence. Brain Res. 305: 27-42.

29. A. DUMBRILLE-ROSS & P. SEEMAN. 1984. Dopamine receptor elevation by cholecystokinin. Peptides 5: 1207-1212.

30. CRESSE, I., T. B. UDSIN & S. H. SNYDER. 1979. Dopamine receptor binding regulated by guanine nucleotides. Mol. Pharmacol. 16: 69-76.

31. GORDAN, J. H. 1985. Estrogen modulation of striatal dopamine receptor sensitivity. Soc. Neurosci. Abstr. 15:

32. ALDINIO, C., G. VALENTI, G. E. SAVOINI, G. KIRSCHNER, L. F. AGNATI & G. TOFFANO. 1984. Monosialoganglioside internal ester stimulates the dopaminergic reinnervation of the striatum after unilateral hemitransection in rat. Int. J. Dev. Neurol. 2: 267-275.

33. WALKER, P., G. CHOVANES & J. MCALLISTER. 1986. Transplants of neostriatal primordia contain acetylcholinesterase-positive neurons. Am. Assoc. Anat. In press.

34. EHLERT, F. J., W. R. ROESKE & H. I. YAMAMURA. 1981. Muscarinic receptor: Regulation by guanine nucleotides, ions and N-ethylmaleimide. Fed. Proc. 40: 153-159.

35. MCALLISTER, J. P., P. D. WALKER, M. C. ZEMANICK, A. B. WEBER, L. I. KAPLAN & M. A. REYNOLDS. 1985. Morphology of embryonic neostriatal cell suspensions transplanted into adult neostriata. Brain Res. 23: 282-286.

DISCUSSION OF THE PAPER

S. B. DUNNETT (*University of Cambridge, England*): I would like to suggest that you can infer very little from a correlation in which you include both your control and lesion groups because they will provide two poles for scatter points. Whatever the transplant does down the middle, you will still get a significant correlation. Have you any behavioral measures correlated with neurobiological changes that apply just in these lesion and transplant groups?

DECKEL: Yes I do. But let me respond to your objection, which I have also heard from Dr. Isacson. I do not agree with it for a couple of reasons. Your data is sometimes extremely skewed in your lesion and transplant groups, both on the biological markers and on the behavioral outcomes. I do not know if in fact it was you who reviewed a recent paper of ours, but we included a few correlations because the referee insisted that we do so on just the lesion and transplant animals. We got this whopping correlation, but it did not mean anything because the data was so skewed: there was a flattening out of the biology and a flattening out of the behavior. It did not make a lot of sense.

Conceptually, it makes more sense to be able to divide the biology and the behavior and ask whether the two linked in any way. You have to make sure that you do not violate too many fundamental assumptions of regression analysis. But these are the same assumptions you may violate when you do regression analysis on the lesion and transplant animals alone. Your point is well taken, but I think you lose something doing the analysis in the way you suggest.

We have done the other analysis in some of the measures. The correlations generally give the same sort of pattern. There was not a tremendous amount of power because you lose significance when your numbers are reduced tremendously. With the cell counts, we have done the correlations with lesion-transplant animals and have found striking similarities between the cross-four groups as well as within the lesion-transplant group itself.

P. R. SANBERG (*Ohio University, Athens, OH*): My question concerns sex differences of the kind discussed in the paper by Dr. Stein, and whether these differences could account for the discrepancies between your data and our own. Unlike the female rats in your study, the male rats in our study maintained the same average speed and body weight and showed amphetamine recovery. Could this difference be due to sex differences? Have you tried any of the techniques mentioned by Dr. Stein? Have you, for example, tried correlations with the estrous cycle?

DECKEL: Yes. It is becoming clearer and clearer to us that female rat striatum is very different from male rat striatum in several respects. Sex differences could explain why your results and my results are somewhat different. We have done vaginal smears to see whether the animals were cycling or not, but we have not done the direct correlations between cycling and behavior. In fact the animals were cycling. We feel that some of the variants we have may be due to rats being in different phases of the estrous cycle. If anything, this tends to wash out our results as opposed to skewing them, but we do get some additional variants, as you mentioned. We have done some of these same things in male rats, and we hope to present the results soon.

O. ISACSON (*University of Lund, Sweden*): There is a positive correlation between your work, my work, and Dr. Sanberg's work, in that we all see significant recovery on a spontaneous behavior. I would like to look at motor activity and cognitive effects. But Dr. Sanberg and I see an almost completely dose-dependent compensation of both amphetamine and apomorphine in a rotational paradigm. This suggests the dopamine system may be involved. If you do not see a dopamine receptor density change that we see or an ingrowth that we see, you cannot infer that the dopamine system is not included; that is, correlations based on negative data alone are insufficient. And your correlations are also based on what might be expected: the greater the lesion the fewer the postsynaptic receptors and the greater the behavioral deficit.

So I wonder whether one might see different behavioral effects with different preparations?

DECKEL: Yes, you might expect different behavioral effects with different preparations, and differences in our preparations may account for many of the differences in our results.

We found a reduction in the D2 receptors that was more drastic than the reduction you found. Our reduction has been corrected for area, so you cannot attribute this difference in results to volumetric changes. You might wish to postulate that your recovery is occurring because of the dopaminergic systems, at least on the receptor side of things. Dopaminergic receptor systems are drastically reduced in our preparations, and this is one of the reasons, along with the behavioral data, why I tend to think there is nothing to point to the dopamine system in my preparation.

ISACSON: Even if you refute that as a possibility, you must think that the accumbens system is very well known for its dopaminergic input. You can change the nucleus accumbens system, which is dopaminergic, and get all these variable measures. So, even if the graft is acting by GABA-ergic inhibition, you could still have the dopamine system involved. You cannot exclude that one transmission system.

DECKEL: I would agree that we need to be cautious. I was delighted to see that Dr. Herman found the amphetamine-like effect that I found in the accumbens system. Particularly when a couple of other labs are not finding this effect in the striatum.

P. VOS (*University of Pennsylvania School of Medicine, Philadelphia, PA*): You discussed low-affinity and high-affinity muscarenic receptors. How different are the affinities?

DECKEL: They are very different. The low-affinity receptor sites are sevenfold or eightfold higher than the high-affinity receptor sites.

By the way I should acknowledge that this was done in the laboratory of Dr. Peter Whitehouse. I thank him for his help. I also want to thank Dr. Robert Robinson and Dr. Timothy Moran for their help.

VOS: Have you considered looking at muscarinic subtypes, specifically MI and MII, with, say, perenzapine?

DECKEL: Yes. That is in the future.

Embryonic Substantia Nigra Grafts

Factors Controlling Behavioral Efficacy and Reinnervation of the Host Striatum

WILLIAM J. FREED,[a] H. ELEANOR SPOOR,[a]
RENAUD DE BEAUREPAIRE,[a] JEFFREY A.
GREENBERG,[b] AND SAUL S. SCHWARZ[c]

[a]Preclinical Neurosciences Section
Neuropsychiatry Branch
National Institute of Mental Health
Saint Elizabeth's Hospital
Washington, DC

[b]Department of Neurosurgery
Georgetown University
Washington, DC

[c]Department of Neurosurgery
Naval Hospital
Bethesda, Maryland

INTRODUCTION

One of the primary goals of brain tissue transplantation is the development of methods to alleviate the effects of brain damage. Although most studies of brain tissue transplantation have thus far been restricted to animal models, the ultimate objective is to favorably influence the outcome of human neuropsychiatric disorders, such as Parkinson's disease. One of the major obstacles to the applicability of brain tissue transplantation, however, may be its limited efficacy.

Although brain tissue transplantation has now been applied to many experimental models, the first and most extensively studied system is the nigrostriatal dopamine system.[1-13] Loss of the dopamine-containing neurons of the substantia nigra (SN) and consequent degeneration of the nigrostriatal dopamine system has also been linked to the clinical syndrome of Parkinson's disease.[14] Two brain grafting techniques have been found to be capable of influencing the consequences of SN lesions in experimental models of Parkinson's disease: intracerebral adrenal medulla grafts, and embryonic SN grafts.[1-13] The two techniques appear to operate through different mechanisms: SN grafts produce dopamine-containing neurites that reinnervate the striatum. Adrenal medulla grafts, on the other hand, do not significantly reinnervate the striatum, but instead appear to act by secreting catecholamines and possibly other substances that enter into the host brain through diffusion.[1-6]

Both procedures can reduce the behavioral consequences of SN lesions, but neither procedure is completely effective. The efficacy of adrenal medulla grafts appears to be related to the degree of survival of the grafted tissues.[7,12,15] On the other hand, the limited efficacy of SN grafts is probably related to the limited degree to which neurites from SN grafts penetrate into the host striatum.[6,7,9,10] Axons and dendrites from SN grafts enter the striatum,[1-3,8-10] reduce denervation supersensitivity,[5] and form synaptic contacts with host neurons in parts of the striatum immediately adjacent to the grafts.[16,17] Even nearly 2 years after transplantation, however, the penetration of graft-derived neurites into the host striatum is limited to about 1.5 mm.[7] A hyperinnervation of SN grafts in the ventricle by catecholamine-containing neurites has also been noted,[1-3] suggesting that graft-derived neurites partially fail to enter the host brain (FIG. 1). In order to improve the performance of SN grafts we have, therefore, undertaken a series of experiments aimed at elucidating the factors that control reinnervation of the dopamine-denervated striatum by intraventricular SN grafts.

CHEMICAL SUBSTANCES

Ganglioside GM1

A number of recent studies have suggested that gangliosides, particularly ganglioside GM1, exert a stimulatory effect on the growth of dopaminergic neurites from the SN and on the survival of SN neurons after axotomy.[18-20] In vitro, ganglioside GM1 has been reported to stimulate neurite growth of several cell types.[21] We have therefore tested the effects of ganglioside GM1 on the innervation of the denervated striatum by neurites from SN grafts in the lateral ventricle.[22]

Animals with unilateral SN lesions received transplants of embryonic SN into the lateral ventricle as previously described. On the day of transplantation, and every subsequent day for 3 weeks, each animal received an injection of ganglioside GM1 10 mg/kg, ganglioside GM1 50 mg/kg, or vehicle. This injection schedule was adapted directly from reports of positive effects of ganglioside GM1 on the nigrostriatal system. At the end of the 3-week period, the animals were sacrificed and processed for fluorescence histochemistry,[23] and the growth of dopamine-containing neurites from the grafts into the caudate-putamen was quantified.

The depth of the catecholaminergic reinnervation of the host striatum was not significantly altered by ganglioside GM1 treatment. The depth of reinnervation (mean ± SEM) was 0.71 ± 0.09 mm in saline-treated animals, 0.79 ± 0.19 mm in animals receiving ganglioside GM1 10 mg/kg/day, and 0.52 ± 0.06 mm in animals receiving ganglioside GM1 50 mg/kg/day ($p = .35$, Kruskal-Wallis test). There is still a possibility that treatment with gangliosides over longer time periods would be effective. It is also possible, however, that gangliosides influence reactive fiber growth in vivo but not the extension of axonal processes by embryonic neurons.

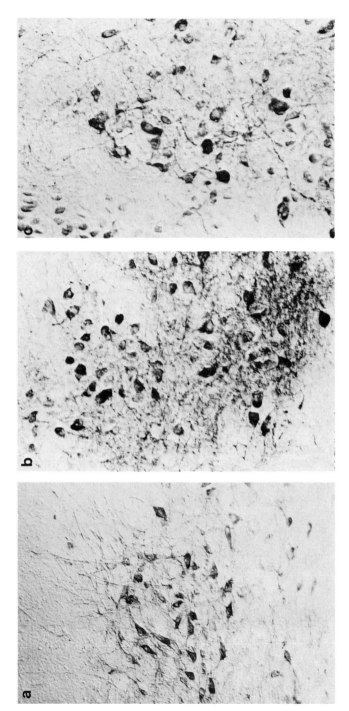

FIGURE 1. Comparison of neurons in normal SN and in SN transplanted to the lateral ventricle. Tyrosine hydroxylase immunocytochemistry, peroxidase-antiperoxidase method.[46] (**a**) Normal SN, Nomarski optics. (**b** & **c**) SN grafts in the lateral ventricle. Note the relative hyperinnervation of the grafted SN and random orientation of neurons as compared to **a**. Magnifications: ×280.

Haloperidol

Chronic haloperidol treatment stimulates dendritic sprouting in the SN.[24] Also, chronic haloperidol treatment can augment the supersensitivity of striatal dopamine receptors that is caused by SN lesions.[25] If the ingrowth of dopaminergic fibers into the denervated striatum depends on the properties of postsynaptic dopamine-receptor sites, augmenting dopaminergic supersensitivity by haloperidol treatment might increase fiber ingrowth.

Animals were given 0.01% haloperidol in 0.1% lactic acid in their drinking water beginning 3 days after SN lesions. Controls received 0.1% lactic acid vehicle. Two weeks later, the animals received SN grafts and were sacrificed after an additional 3 weeks, so that the total duration of haloperidol treatment was 5 weeks. Many of the haloperidol-treated rats did not survive this treatment because of aphagia and adipsia. Brains were processed for fluorescence histochemistry,[22,23] and depth of reinnervation was evaluated in every third 32-μ section.

Haloperidol treatment had no effect on the reinnervation of the striatum by SN grafts. The maximum depth of reinnervate was 0.67 ± 0.27 mm in vehicle-treated rats, and 0.63 ± 0.15 mm in haloperidol-treated animals ($p > .2$, Mann-Whitney test). The mean depth of reinnervation for the three sections in which the reinnervation was deepest was 0.63 ± 0.30 mm for vehicle-treated rats and 0.49 ± 0.12 mm for haloperidol-treated animals ($p > .2$). Thus, the properties of postsynaptic dopamine receptor sites are probably not a critical factor in the reinnervation of the striatum by SN grafts.

Estrogen

Estrogen stimulates the formation of synapses in the deafferented medial basal hypothalamus[27] and stimulates dendritic growth in birds.[26] Several effects of gonadal hormones, ovariectomy, and estrous cycles on dopaminergic neurons have been reported.[28] We therefore have tested the effects of chronic estrogen treatment on SN grafts.

Ovariectomized female rats received 5 μg of estradiol benzoate or peanut oil vehicle daily for 7 weeks before and 4 weeks after grafting. The reduction in apomorphine-induced rotation[29] in the animals treated with estrogen was $29 \pm 8\%$, as compared to $37 \pm 7\%$ for the animals treated with vehicle. This difference was not statistically significant ($T(14) = 0.71$, $p = .50$, two-tailed t test). Thus estrogen did not alter the reductions in apomorphine-induced rotational behavior that are produced by SN grafts.

HOST AGE

Several studies suggest that embryonic or immature brain tissue from the striatum contains factors that promote the survival and extension of neurites by developing SN neurons.[30-32] It is quite possible, therefore, that the absence of these substances in the mature brain accounts for the limitations of the ability of SN grafts to innervate the striatum. In order to investigate the ability of intraventricular SN grafts to innervate immature striatal target tissue, dual grafts of SN and striatum from gestational day 17 rat embryos were transplanted together into the lateral ventricles of animals with unilateral SN lesions.[33] The SN grafts were found to completely reinnervate the embryonic striatal grafts in preference to reinnervating the host brain. Little or no reinnervation of the host striatum was observed in animals with combined intraventricular SN and striatal grafts (FIG. 2). In control animals that received intraventricular SN grafts without a concomitant striatal graft, reinnervation of the host brain was invariably observed (FIG. 2).[33]

Thus the capacity of embryonic brain grafts to innervate embryonic striatum is not limited. When presented with a "choice" between an embryonic and a fully mature but denervated striatal target, grafted SN dopaminergic neurons exclusively innervate the grafted embryonic target, and do not produce the typical innervation of the dorsomedial striatum.

A means of exploiting the favorable neurite-promoting properties of embryonic target tissue was therefore sought. It is difficult to create a situation in a developmentally immature animal where a brain graft would be employed to ameliorate the effects of a lesion. An experiment was, therefore, performed in which the usual experimental paradigm was reversed, so that normal newborn rats received embryonic SN grafts or sciatic nerve control grafts on neonatal day 1, and subsequently received SN lesions.[34,35] Reinnervation of the striatum as well as catecholaminergic innervation of the septum was observed, although it was difficult to compare the degree of reinnervation with that observed in the mature hosts because of inconsistency of the positions of the grafts and areas of reinnervation. Behaviorally, however, these neonatally implanted grafts were highly effective. The incidence of aphagia and adipsia was markedly reduced in the animals with SN grafts, and the akinesia and rigidity were reduced as well. Animals with SN grafts were 3.7 times as active as control animals.[34] Most of the animals with SN grafts did not experience aphagia or become adipsic after the bilateral SN lesions were created, that is, after "lesioning." Furthermore, these animals maintained relatively normal eating, drinking, and body weight for at least 1 month after lesioning. Rigidity was also markedly reduced.[34,35]

Thus when SN grafts are implanted into neonatal animals, they successfully compete with the endogenous striatal dopaminergic innervation. Whether some of the reinnervation of the striatum produced by these neonatal grafts occurs after lesioning of the SN has not been entirely ruled out. Increased eating was, however, observed as early as 2 days after lesioning in the animals with SN grafts, suggesting that a major part of the reinnervation of the striatum produced by these grafts was already in place at the time of lesioning. It is clear, however, that the behavioral efficacy of SN grafts is markedly increased when implanted neonatally. Therefore neonatally implanted SN grafts protect animals from a subsequent SN lesion that produces severe debilitation in control rats.

CORTICAL LESIONS

Several studies suggest that competition between more than one system of neuronal fibers for a single terminal region can restrict the growth of either system, as compared to a comparable situation where only one fiber system is present.[36–38] When an em-

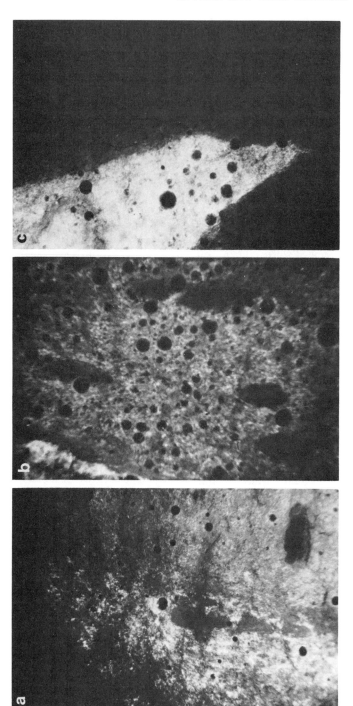

FIGURE 2. Pattern of reinnervation of host caudate-putamen and of caudate-putamen transplanted to the lateral ventricle. Glyoxylic acid-induced fluorescence histochemistry.[23] (**a**) SN graft and reinnervation of the host striatum. The graft is on the left side of the photograph and the host brain is on the right. (**b**) Reinnervation of the host caudate-putamen. Part of the graft can be seen in the upper left. (**c**) Innervation of embryonic striatum transplanted to the lateral ventricle by a co-grafted embryonic SN. Note that the embryonic striatal graft (upper left part of photograph) is densely innervated by catecholamine-containing neurites, whereas the host brain (right side of photograph) is not reinnervated. Magnifications for **a** and **c** and for **b**: ×180 and ×280, respectively.

bryonic SN graft is transplanted to the lateral ventricle, dopamine-containing neurites penetrate for short distances into the host striatum. In these experiments, the SN lesions are usually made long before the SN grafts are implanted. Thus there is ample opportunity for synaptic contacts formerly filled by the terminals of dopaminergic neurites to become filled by other competing axonal systems, either derived from interneurons or arising from major inputs to the striatum. One of the largest afferents to the striatum is the glutamate-containing corticostriatal pathway.[39-41] It was therefore hypothesized that perturbation of the circuitry of the striatum by lesioning of the overlying cerebral cortex would—either directly or indirectly—remove a competing innervation of the striatum and allow for an increased penetration of graft-derived neurites into the host brain.

On the other hand, it has been found that substances that promote the survival of neurons in tissue culture, as well as after transplantation to the brain, are secreted from injured brain tissue.[42-45] In any study involving brain injury, the possibility of stimulatory effects of the brain injury due to secretion of trophic substances should also be considered.

Animals received unilateral lesions of the SN by stereotaxic administration of 6-hydroxydopamine, and apomorphine-induced rotational behavior was measured for three testing sessions. An area of the dorsomedial frontal cortex was "lesioned" by aspiration under Chloropent anesthesia. Control animals received sham lesions. Apomorphine-induced rotational behavior was then measured for an additional two sessions. Ten days after the cortical lesions were created, each animal received an SN graft in the lateral ventricle as previously described.[2,3] Two weeks after the transplantation, measurements of rotational behavior began, and they continued for an additional three sessions. Three weeks after transplantation, each animal received Pargylene 75 mg/kg, and was sacrificed for fluorescence histochemistry as previously described.[22,23] Growth of dopaminergic neurites into the host striatum was assessed with a stage micrometer and eyepiece reticule as previously described.[22] Animals in which the graft was grossly displaced (for example, if the SN graft was located in the cortical lesion site) were eliminated. Approximately 50% of the cortex-lesioned rats were eliminated for this reason.

Because of the localized nature of the brain injury model that was employed, it was decided to evaluate the reinnervation of the striatum in four separate regions (FIG. 3), corresponding to the most dorsal fourth of the lateral ventricle (region a), the second and third most dorsal regions (b and c), and the most ventral fourth of the ventricle (d). In the most dorsal sector (a), mean dopaminergic neurite ingrowth was increased in animals with cortical lesions from 0.52 ± 0.14 mm to 0.78 ± 0.14 mm (each value a mean $\pm$ SEM, $T(13) = 4.71$, $p < .01$). In region b, there was a tendency toward increased neurite penetration in the cortex-lesioned animals, but this difference was not statistically significant ($p > .2$) (TABLE 1). There was no difference in sectors c and d (TABLE 1).

In several of the animals with cortical lesions the reinnervation of the caudate-putamen was found to closely follow the roof of the caudate-putamen, directly underneath the cortical lesion (FIG. 4). In some cases, the lateral extent of the reinnervation corresponded to the lateral extent of the cortical lesion (FIG. 4). In other animals, clumps of catecholamine-containing neurites were observed in parts of the caudate-putamen close to the cortical lesions.

In order to assess the possibility that the increased growth of dopaminergic neurites into region a was due to anatomical distortion of the striatum induced by the cortical lesions, selected sectors were counterstained with cresyl violet and subjected to gross anatomical measurements. There were no differences between the size of the caudate-putamen in the dorsoventral dimension and that in the mediolateral dimension. The

FIGURE 3. Method of division of the caudate-putamen into four dorsoventral regions for evaluation of the depth of reinnervation (for results, see TABLE 2).

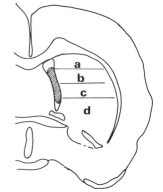

width of the right caudate-putamen was 3.46 ± 0.09 mm in controls and 3.50 ± 0.01 mm in lesioned animals. The dorsoventral size of the caudate-putamen was 5.18 ± 0.18 mm in controls and 5.41 ± 0.30 mm in lesioned rats. The area of the right caudate-putamen in coronal sections was also not altered (0.16 mm² for controls and 0.15 mm² for lesioned rats).

The possibility that the cortical lesions had resulted in a displacement of the grafts in a dorsal direction was also considered. The position of the center of each graft in the ventricle was determined using a scale of 0 to 100, 0 representing the ventral limit of the ventricle and 100 representing the dorsal limit of the lateral ventricle. The position of the dorsoventral center of each graft was determined according to this scale (FIG. 5). Grafts in control animals were located at 73%, that is, 73% of the distance to the dorsal end of the ventricle, whereas in cortex-lesioned rats the grafts were located at the 75% position. This difference was not statistically significant ($p > .2$).

The cortical lesions reduced rotational behavior substantially, before the implantation of SN grafts (FIG. 6). In animals with cortical lesions, SN grafts produced no additional decrease in rotational behavior. In the control group, which had received sham cortical lesions, the SN grafts produced a reduction in rotational behavior of approximately 35% (TABLE 2).

The cortical lesions were found to be relatively small, to be confined to the mediofrontal cortex, and to extend from approximately 1.0-1.5 mm lateral to the

TABLE 1. Depths of Catecholaminergic Reinnervation in Host Striatum

Region	Depth (mm)	
	Cortical Lesions	Sham Operations
a	.78 ± .14	.52 ± .14
b	.68 ± .14	.57 ± .17
c	.59 ± .08	.63 ± .12
d	.61 ± .14	.59 ± .12

NOTE: Each value represents a mean ± SEM.

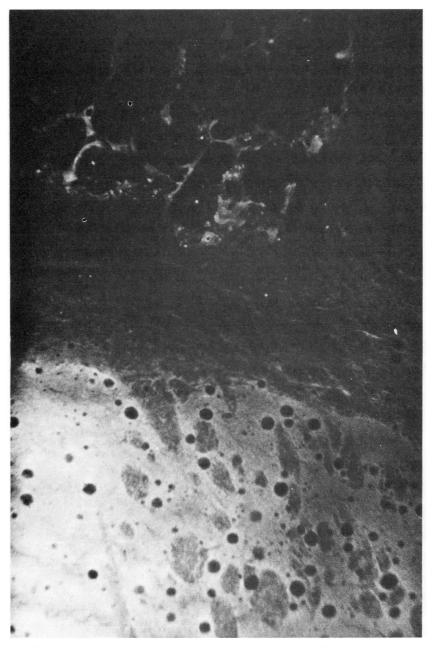

FIGURE 4. Reinnervation of the roof of the caudate-putamen by an SN graft in an animal that had received a cortical lesion 10 days before transplantation. Glyoxylic acid-induced fluorescence histochemistry. Magnification: ×130.

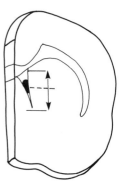

FIGURE 5. Illustration of the method of quantifying the position of the graft in the lateral ventricle. A 1-100 scale was created along the dorsoventral length of the lateral ventricle. The position of the center of the graft on this scale was determined for each animal. Mean values for control animals: 72.9 ± 3.1%; mean value for lesioned animals: 74.9 ± 3.1%.

midline to approximately 4.0-5.0 mm lateral to the midline (FIG. 7). There was some encroachment of the lesions into the white matter, but the striatum itself was not damaged in any of the animals. The lesions extended for considerable distances (on the order of 4 mm) in the rostrocaudal direction.

Therefore, injury to the overlying cerebral cortex has a stimulatory effect on the outgrowth of neurites from intraventricular SN grafts into the denervated striatum. Because of the localized nature of the increased neurite growth, it does not appear that this effect is due to the removal of a competing corticostriatal pathway. The topography of this pathway has been examined in rats in detail,[41] and lesions like those induced in the present study would be expected to remove the corticostriatal innervation from the medial striatum extending through all four regions, that is, a through d. Likewise, the primary effect would appear to involve the dopaminergic neurites, rather than the cell parenchyma, because the differences were only seen in the parts of the striatum physically closest to the lesion. An effect on the cell bodies of the grafted neurons would be expected to be manifest equally in all four regions.

Examination of published photographs of growth of dopaminergic neurites from cortical cavities suggests that reinnervation of the striatum using this procedure some-what exceeds that which occurs when similar grafts are implanted into the lateral ventricle.[8] The present study suggests that some of this difference could be due to

FIGURE 6. Effects of SN grafts on rotational behavior. The number of complete 360° contralateral rotations per hour induced by 0.1 mg/kg apomorphine·HCl was determined for each rat in the two groups of rats that were studied: after the first lesion (an SN lesion); after the second lesion (a sham lesion or a cortical lesion); and after implantation of an SN graft in the lateral ventricle. The mean values for the group that received sham lesions are indicated with triangles, and those for the group that received cortical lesions are indicated with circles. Data for the first 13 animals tested are shown here; data for all animals tested are shown in TABLE 2.

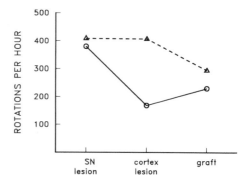

TABLE 2. Apomorphine-induced Rotational Behavior

	Number of Turns per Hour	
	Cortex-lesioned Group	Sham-lesioned Group
Before cortical lesions	346 ± 46	364 ± 49
After lesion or sham operation	177 ± 27	371 ± 60
After substantia nigra graft	194 ± 38	242 ± 56

NOTE: Each value represents a mean ± SEM.

direct effects of the lesions on dopaminergic neurites. It is also possible that the cortical lesions employed in these earlier studies[8] prevented SN grafts from causing reductions in apomorphine-induced rotational behavior. On the other hand, the cortical lesions were performed before SN lesioning in these earlier studies, and there are other procedural differences that preclude a direct comparison between the two studies.

DISCUSSION

In several studies of intraventricular SN grafts, it has been noted that dopaminergic neurites derived from these grafts almost always reinnervate the denervated host striatum, albeit to a limited extent.[1–3,8–10,16,17] Reinnervation of the septum is occasionally observed, but only when the dopaminergic neurons in the graft are located immediately adjacent to the septum and somewhat separated from the striatum by other parts of the graft that do not contain dopaminergic neurites (W. Freed, unpublished observations). Reinnervation of other structures that sometimes adjoin the grafted SN, such as the corpus callosum or hippocampus, has never been observed. Therefore, the dopamine-denervated striatum is a relatively favorable target for graft-derived dopaminergic neurites.

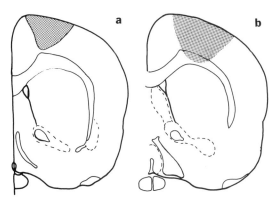

FIGURE 7. Representative cortical lesions. (a) Tracing representing a relatively small lesion. (b) Tracing representing a relatively large lesion, with some damage to the white matter.

On the other hand, the fully mature host striatum is not an entirely adequate target. Penetration of dopaminergic neurites into the host striatum is very limited, and complete reinnervation of the striatum is never observed. The efficacy of these grafts is not altered by chronic ganglioside GM1, haloperidol, or estrogen treatment.

Preliminary evidence suggests that the state of maturity of the host striatum is of prime importance in controlling reinnervation by SN grafts. Embryonic striatum placed in the lateral ventricle in combination with SN grafts is innervated in preference to the host striatum, and the effects of SN grafts are much more pronounced when these grafts are transplanted into immature brains. Thorough investigation of the molecular mechanisms that control innervation of immature striatal neurons by dopaminergic neurites will therefore become important for the ultimate success of SN grafts.

It also appears to be possible to augment the growth of SN-graft-derived dopaminergic neurites by local injury to the brain. Of course, it is unlikely that brain injury per se could be employed to enhance the function of SN grafts if and when these grafts are applied clinically. Nevertheless, this provides a clue that may ultimately lead to other techniques that may be employed to augment the performance of SN grafts. Perhaps, for example, brain-injury-induced neuronotrophic factor could be administered locally to enhance the performance of SN grafts. A means of inducing the production of such factors without actual injury to the brain may be found. Or, it is possible that a very minor local brain injury would provide a significant stimulation of growth. As yet, however, the mechanisms through which brain injury and target cell immaturity enhance the growth of dopaminergic neurites are unclear. The possibility that the two effects are related is intriguing. For example, brain injury might induce nearby neurons to adopt some of the properties of immature neurons responsible for the attraction of dopaminergic neurites. Or, alternatively, brain-injury-induced neuronotrophic factor(s) may be similar or identical to substances produced by immature striatal neurons that attract a dopaminergic innervation. Further study of these possibilities is likely to yield data that will not only be useful in enhancing the function of SN grafts, but that may also be useful in developing an understanding of mechanisms of growth and plasticity of dopaminergic systems.

REFERENCES

1. PERLOW, M. J., W. J. FREED, B. J. HOFFER, A. SEIGER, L. OLSON & R. J. WYATT. 1979. Brain grafts reduce motor abnormalities produced by destruction of the nigrostriatal dopamine system. Science **204:** 643-647.
2. FREED, W. J., M. J. PERLOW, F. KAROUM, A. SEIGER, L. OLSON, B. J. HOFFER & R. J. WYATT. 1980. Restoration of dopaminergic function by grafting of fetal rat substantia nigra to the caudate nucleus: Long-term behavioral, biochemical, and histochemical studies. Ann. Neurol. **8:** 510-519.
3. FREED, W. J. 1983. Functional brain tissue transplantation: Reversal of lesion-induced rotation by intraventricular substantia nigra and adrenal medulla grafts, with a note on intracranial retinal grafts. Biol. Psychiatry **18:** 1205-1267.
4. FREED, W. J., J. M. MORIHISA, E. SPOOR, B. J. HOFFER, L. OLSON, A. SEIGER & R. J. WYATT. 1981. Transplanted adrenal chromaffin cells in rat brain reduce lesion-induced rotational behavior. Nature **292:** 351-352.
5. FREED, W. J., G. N. KO, D. L. NEIHOFF, M. J. KUHAR, B. J. HOFFER, L. OLSON, H. E. CANNON-SPOOR, J. M. MORIHISA & R. J. WYATT. 1983. Normalization of spiroperidol binding in the denervated rat striatum by homologous grafts of substantia nigra. Science **222:** 937-939.

6. FREED, W. J., L. DE MEDINACELI & R. J. WYATT. 1985. Promoting functional plasticity in the damaged nervous system. Science **227:** 1544-1552.
7. FREED, W. J., H. E. CANNON-SPOOR & E. KRAUTHAMER. 1985. Factors influencing the efficacy of adrenal medulla and embryonic substantia nigra grafts. *In* Neural Grafting in the Mammalian CNS. A. Björklund & U. Stenevi, Eds.: 491-504. Elsevier. Amsterdam.
8. BJÖRKLUND, A., S. B. DUNNETT, U. STENEVI, M. E. LEWIS & S. D. IVERSEN. 1980. Reinnervation of the denervated striatum by substantia nigra transplants: Functional consequences as revealed by pharmacological and sensorimotor testing. Brain Res. **199:** 307-333.
9. DUNNETT, S. B., A. BJÖRKLUND, R. H. SCHMIDT, U. STENEVI & S. D. IVERSEN. 1983. Intracerebral grafting of neuronal cell suspensions. IV. Behavioral recovery in rats with unilateral 6-OHDA lesions following implantation of nigral cell suspensions in different forebrain sites. Acta Physiol. Scand. Suppl. **522:** 29-37.
10. DUNNETT, S. B., A. BJÖRKLUND & U. STENEVI. 1983. Dopamine-rich transplants in experimental parkinsonism. Trends Neurosci. **6:** 266-270.
11. GASH, D. M., T. J. COLLIER & J. R. SLADEK, JR. 1985. Neural transplantation: A review of recent developments and potential applications to the aged brain. Neurobiol. Aging **6:** 131-150.
12. STROMBERG, I., M. HERRERA-MARSCHITZ, U. UNGERSTEDT, T. EBENDAL & L. OLSON. 1985. Chronic implants of chromaffin tissue into the dopamine-denervated striatum: Effects of NGF on graft survival, fiber growth, and rotational behavior. Exp. Brain Res. **60:** 335-349.
13. GAGE, F. H., U. STENEVI, T. CALSTEDT, G. FOSTER, A. BJÖRKLUND & A. J. AGUAYO. 1985. Anatomical and functional consequences of grafting mesencephalic neurons into a peripheral nerve "bridge" connected to the denervated striatum. Exp. Brain Res. **60:** 584-589.
14. BERNHEIMER, H., W. BIRKMAYER, O. HORNYKIEWICZ, K. JELLINGER & K. SEITELBERGER. 1973. Brain dopamine and the syndrome of Parkinson and Huntington: Clinical, morphological, and neurochemical correlations. J. Neurol. Sci. **20:** 415-455.
15. FREED, W. J., H. E. CANNON-SPOOR & E. KRAUTHAMER. 1986. Intrastriatal adrenal medulla grafts from young and aging donors: Long-term survival and behavioral effects. J. Neurosurg. **65:** 664-670.
16. FREUND, T. F., J. P. BOLAN, A. BJÖRKLUND, U. STENEVI, S. B. DUNNETT, J. F. POWELL & A. D. SMITH. 1985. Efferent synaptic connections of grafted dopaminergic neurons reinnervating the host neostriatum: A tyrosine hydroxylase immunocytochemical study. J. Neurosci. **5:** 603-616.
17. MAHALIK, T. J., T. E. FINGER, I. STROMBERG & L. OLSON. 1985. Substantia nigra transplants into denervated striatum of the rat: Ultrastructure of graft and host connections. J. Comp. Neurol. **240:** 60-70.
18. TOFFANO, G., G. SAVOINI, F. MORONI, G. LOMBARDI, L. CALZA & L. F. AGNATI. 1983. GM1 ganglioside stimulates the regeneration of dopaminergic neurons in the central nervous system. Brain Res. **261:** 163-166.
19. TOFFANO, G., G. E. SAVOINI, F. MORONI, G. LOMBARDI, L. CALZA & L. F. AGNATI. 1984. Chronic GM1 ganglioside treatment reduces dopamine cell body degeneration in the substantia nigra after unilateral hemitransection in rat. Brain Res. **296:** 233-239.
20. SABEL, B. A., G. L. DUNBAR, W. M. BUTLER & D. G. STEIN. 1985. GM1 gangliosides stimulate neuronal reorganization and reduce rotational asymmetry after hemitransections of the nigrostriatal pathway. Exp. Brain Res. **60:** 27-37.
21. LEDEEN, R. W. 1984. Biology of gangliosides: Neutriogenic and neurotrophic properties. J. Neurosci. Res. **12:** 147-159.
22. FREED, W. J. 1984. Ganglioside GM1 does not stimulate reinnervation of the striatum by substantia nigra grafts. Brain Res. Bull. **14:** 91-95.
23. DE LA TORRE, J. C. 1980. An improved approach to histofluorescence using the SPG method for tissue monoamines. J. Neurosci. Methods **3:** 1-5.
24. BENES, F. M., P. A. PASKEVICH & V. B. DOMESICK. 1983. Haloperidol-induced plasticity of axon terminals in rat substantia nigra. Science **221:** 969-971.
25. RECHES, A., R. H. WAGNER, V. JACKSON, E. YABLONSKAYA-ALTER & S. FAHN. 1983.

Dopamine receptors in the denervated striatum: Further supersensitivity by chronic haloperidol treatment. Brain Res. **275:** 183-185.

26. MATSUMOTO, A. & Y. ARAI. 1979. Synaptogenic effect of estrogen on the hypothalamic arcuate nucleus of the adult female rat. Cell Tissue Res. **198:** 427-433.

27. DEVOOGD, T. & F. NOTTEBOHM. 1981. Gonadal hormones induce dendritic growth in the adult avian brain. Science **214:** 202-204.

28. ROBINSON, T. E., D. M. CAMP, D. S. JACKNOW & J. B. BECKER. 1982. Sex differences and estrous-cycle-dependent variation in rotational behavior elicited by electrical stimulation of the mesostriatal dopamine system. Behav. Brain Res. **6:** 273-287.

29. UNGERSTEDT, U. 1971. Postsynaptic supersensitivity after 6-hydroxydopamine-induced degeneration of the nigrostriatal dopamine system. Acta Physiol. Scand. Suppl. **367:** 69-93.

30. HEMMENDINGER, L. M., B. B. GARBER, P. C. HOFFMAN & A. HELLER. 1981. Target neuron-specific process formation by embryonic mesencephalic dopamine neurons *in vitro.* Proc. Natl. Acad. Sci. USA **78:** 1264-1268.

31. PROCHIANTZ, A., U. DIPORZIO, A. BERGER & J. GLOWINSKI. 1979. *In vitro* maturation of mesencephalic dopaminergic neurons from mouse embryos is enhanced in the presence of their striatal target cells. Proc. Natl. Acad. Sci. USA **76:** 5387-5391.

32. DENIS-DONINI, S., J. GLOWINSKI & A. PROCHIANTZ. 1983. Specific influences of striatal target neurons on the *in vitro* outgrowth of mesencephalic dopaminergic neurites: A morphological quantitative study. J. Neurosci. **3:** 2292-2299.

33. DE BEAUREPAIRE, R. & W. J. FREED. 1987. Embryonic substantia nigra grafts innervate embryonic striatal co-grafts in preference to mature host striatum. Exp. Neurol. **95:** 448-454.

34. SCHWARZ, S. S. & W. J. FREED. 1987. Brain tissue transplantation in neonatal rats prevents a lesion-induced syndrome of adipsia, aphagia, and akinesia. Exp. Brain Res. **65:** 449-454.

35. SCHNEIDER, G. E. 1973. Early lesions of superior colliculus: Factors affecting the formation of abnormal retinal projections. Brain Behav. Evol. **8:** 73-109.

36. SCHWARZ, S. S. & W. J. FREED. 1987. Neonatally transplanted brain tissue protects the adult rat from a lesion-induced syndrome of adipsia, aphagia, and akinesia. Ann. N.Y. Acad. Sci. This volume.

37. LEONG, S. K. & R. D. LUND. 1973. Anomalous bilateral corticofugal pathways in albino rats after neonatal lesions. Brain Res. **62:** 218-221.

38. OLSON, L., A. SEIGER & M. ALUND. 1978. Locus ceruleus fiber growth *in oculo* induced by trigeminotomy. Med. Biol. **56:** 23-27.

39. GOLDMAN, P. S. & W. J. N. NAUTA. 1977. An intricately patterned prefronto-caudate projection in the rhesus monkeys. J. Comp. Neurol. **171:** 369-386.

40. MCGEER, P. L., E. G. MCGEER, U. SCHERER & K. SINGH. 1977. A glutamatergic corticostriatal path? Brain Res. **128:** 369-373.

41. WEBSTER, K. E. 1961. Corticostriatal interrelations in the albino rat. J. Anatomy (London) **95:** 532-545.

42. NIETO-SAMPEDRO, M., E. LEWIS, C. COTMAN, M. MANTHORPE, S. SKAPER, G. BARBIN, F. LONGO & S. VARON. 1982. Brain injury causes a time-dependent increase in neuronotrophic activity at the lesion site. Science **217:** 860-861.

43. NIETO-SAMPEDRO, M., M. MANTHORPE, G. BARBIN, S. VARON & C. W. COTMAN. 1983. Injury-induced neuronotrophic activity in adult rat brain: Correlation with survival of delayed implants in the wound cavity. J. Neurosci. **3:** 2219-2229.

44. GAGE, F. H., A. BJÖRKLUND & U. STENEVI. 1984. Denervation releases a neuronal survival factor in adult rat hippocampus. Nature **308:** 637-639.

45. COLLINS, F. & K. A. CRUTCHER. 1985. Neurotrophic activity in the adult rat hippocampal formation: Regional distribution and increase after septal lesion. J. Neurosci. **5:** 2809-2814.

46. STERNBERG, L. A. 1979. Immunocytochemistry. 2nd edit. John Wiley & Sons. New York, NY.

DISCUSSION OF THE PAPER

S. C. McLOON (*University of Minnesota, Minneapolis, MN*): Did you alter the position of the lesion in the cortex to a more caudal position, or even to the other side, and see if it had an effect?

FREED: We did not alter the position of the lesions. Actually, the lesions extended anteriorly in a rostral-caudal direction for a fairly long distance. In most cases, they were in the same anterior-posterior position as the graft.

M. NIETO-SAMPEDRO (*University of California, Irvine, CA*): Did you place any of your transplants in the injured cavity?

FREED: By accident we did.

NIETO-SAMPEDRO: Do they survive and grow? Do they innervate? Do they grow along the corpus collosum to innervate the opposite cortex?

FREED: Yes. When they are in the cortical cavity they often reinnervate the same part of the striatum as they do when they are in the ventricle.

NIETO-SAMPEDRO: We found there is a very strong local effect. These things are not very diffusable. They are highest just adjacent to the injury. You found an increase in innervation and survival for dopamine neurons?

FREED: I do not know about survival, only about the innervation. We do not have any counts of cells. But we did see that wherever the grafts were displaced they still reinnervated that same dorsal part of the caudate putamen. In some cases, they were in a tear in the roof of the ventricle lodged in the corpus collosum or in the cortical lesion site, but, wherever they happen to be, they often seem to reinnervate that same dorsal part of the roof of the caudate putamen.

P. R. SANBERG (*Ohio University, Athens, OH*): When you do the cortical graft, you think that the reason you might have more innervation in the dorsal area is because this is an area that is innervated by the cortical-striatal pathway. Perhaps you are getting degeneration there.

FREED: We did an experiment that was designed so we could test both possibilities. We removed the cortical striatal reinnervation, thus either removing the competing fibers or getting the trophic effect. The cortical striatal reinnervation would be expected to extend through all four quadrants, although in the quadrants c and d it would be relatively medial. It would not extend to the lateral parts of quadrants c and d, but it would go through all four quadrants. One of the things we concluded is it is not a competition. The pattern of change looks more like a trophic effect from the lesion.

S. B. DUNNETT (*University of Cambridge, England*): We have done a number of similar experiments with grafts into such a cortical cavity. Your data on the cavity stimulating outgrowth is really interesting. Two aspects, however, are slightly discrepant with my experience. First, when we have cavities that do not penetrate the corpus collosum, there is a sheet of intact fibers. When we put a graft into a cavity there is very little penetration across the fiber bundles of the corpus collosum. Consequently, there is very little reinnervation of the striatum. This seems to differ with what you were saying about your cavity never actually exposing the caudate.

FREED: Right. In animals in which the graft was accidentally placed into the cavity, we did see some reinnervation of the dorsal striatum. I am not sure that the fibers went through the corpus collosum, and I am not sure how they got into the caudate. They may have gone through the wound that we made when we made the graft. I cannot conclude much from the animals in which the grafts were placed into the cortical cavity because those grafts were in all sorts of different places. In some grafts, however, there were neurons extending more medially toward the ventricle or in a mixed position. In some of the grafts that were located entirely within the cortical cavity, there was still reinnervation of the dorsal striatum. I do not know by what route the reinnervation reached the striatum.

DUNNETT: The second point I am interested in concerns the slide that you showed in the beginning of those experiments. The slide suggested there was a decline in rotation following cortical cavity alone. I routinely test rotation after lesion and then after cavity and have found that the trend, if anything, is in the opposite direction. The rotation gets stronger after the lesion or after the cavity even before the graft is implanted.

FREED: We do not know whether the decrease may recover, but these lesions are probably somewhat larger than the lesions you make. Do you also make your cavities before you make the substantia nigra lesions?

DUNNETT: Yes, sometimes together, but usually it is the lesion first and the cavity a week or two after that, and then the grafting several weeks after the cavity.

FREED: That is similar to what we do. I really do not know what accounts for the difference. It may just be the size of the lesions.

J. R. SLADEK, JR. (*University of Rochester School of Medicine, Rochester, NY*): When you look at fluorescent sections through the microscope, do you actually see a connection between the dopaminergic cells and what you are referring to as reinnervation of the striatum, or are you assuming that any fluorescence in the striatum must be attributable to the dopamine cells?

FREED: You usually can trace it. The idea was to put the grafts in the ventricle. In these cases, it was possible to trace the fibers. Occasionally we will have an animal in which the original denervation is incomplete, and there will be some residual fluorescence in the ventral parts of the striatum in those animals that we do not use. But, in virtually all the animals we do use, the denervation is complete. You can actually trace the fibers.

SLADEK: Do they actually work through the ventricular ependyma to gain access to the target?

FREED: In many cases the ependyma is damaged. In our recent experiments the ependyma is more damaged than in our early experiments. We make the graft sufficiently lateral that the ependyma is nicked a little bit. If we look closely, we usually see the fibers entering through breaks in the ependyma. I am not sure, however, that they always enter that way.

SLADEK: Are you using the Falck-Hillarp technique?

FREED: No, the glyoxylic acid technique.

V. SINALI (*Institute of Neurology, Milan, Italy*): Did you ever compare the efferents of the medulla to those of the substantia nigra?

FREED: Not in this situation. In fact, the adrenal medulla grafts do not really reinnervate the striatum at all, so I do not know how applicable that would be in this situation.

Summary

S. FAHN (*Columbia University, New York, NY*): I will keep my remarks fairly brief, and, instead of summarizing all the contributions made in this session, I will make some general remarks about some clinical aspects of brain grafting techniques. As a clinical neurologist, perhaps I have the prerogative to do so.

It really is an exciting area when coming from the outside and not being involved. When I attend a conference like this, I can see that progress is being made, and I realize that before long more clinical applications will be taking place—probably in countries outside of Sweden—in addition to what is already happening and what will happen in Sweden.

The possibility of transplanting tissues to correct neurological deficits was first recognized for patients with dopamine deficiency syndromes and parkinsonism. Our first speaker today, Dr. Brundin, mentioned that the clinical relevance of transplanting dopamine-containing cells into striatum soon became quite obvious. In fact, the clinical aspects of treating patients with parkinsonism with L-DOPA and the fact that these patients can respond tends to support the concept that dopamine in the striatum probably functions much like a neurohormone functions. It bathes the tissue with a transmitter, and you do not need one-to-one cell contact to get that type of motor function.

In a sense, just as L-DOPA can be used clinically, so can one then conceive of transplanting a source of dopamine in the striatum. The progress that we see in the rodent models and in primates, and that we hope to eventually see in humans, gives real credence to this. Progress such as enhancing the effect of these transplants makes them more potent. Different hosts in cross-species types of experiments using cyclosporin A really show that scientists are thinking about how they can be used eventually for human work.

A few years ago, we would not have considered that there would be much promise for grafting techniques in diseases that have a specific point-to-point deficit where cell-to-cell contact is needed for the functioning of the tissues. Therefore, it comes somewhat as a surprise to see results of striatal tissue transplants into diseased striatum.

We know clinically that there are a number of diseases that involve the striatum as their primary target. Huntington's disease is the leading one, but other, less frequent diseases say such as chorea acanthocytosis also have striatal degeneration. There are a number of multisystem atrophies in which the patients have disease resembling parkinsonism, such as progressive supranuclear palsy and striatonigral degenerations. These patients do not respond to L-DOPA therapy, partly because the striatum is also involved. The receptors are gone, and then giving L-DOPA does not really help much.

Can striatal transplants be effective in diseases that directly involve the striatum? We have heard today some very promising remarks in two of the papers, and it looks like some locomotor functions can improve after this. One would like to see better models than the rodent models for striatal lesions, however. The clinical picture that one sees in humans includes either choreic movements or clumsiness of motor performance; or the dopamine system is also involved, with some Parkinson-like effect that does not respond to L-DOPA. Therefore, one would like to see a more sophisticated animal model than what the rodents would show with striatal lesions. Perhaps work on models with higher animals such as the primate offer a reasonable approach to look at this type of transplantation system.

I wonder why a transplant into diseased striatum would work better than the striatal tissue itself would work in this diseased striatum. Does one not need one-to-one cell contact if the transplant is to do its job? Does one not need to find the target organs? It was a bit of a surprise to see the rodent model respond in a behavioral locomotion pattern, and, of course, it would be interesting to determine whether the primate would respond the same way. Should one go for the target side of the striatum? Should one look in the pallidum and in the reticulata as transplantation sites? It may not be as easy with striatum as it is with the dopamine nigrostriatal system in which the dopamine acts like a hormone, as I mentioned. Nevertheless, we would not have predicted even 10 years ago that we would be talking about transplant work at all. We could not have foreseen using transplants in animals, much less in treating human disease. So I am very encouraged to see this kind of progress: it is really very heartening.

Transplantation Techniques and the Survival of Adrenal Medulla Autografts in the Primate Brain

JOHN M. MORIHISA

Department of Psychiatry
Georgetown University School of Medicine
and
Psychiatry Service
Veterans Administration Medical Center
Washington, DC

RICHARD K. NAKAMURA, WILLIAM J. FREED,
MORTIMER MISHKIN, AND RICHARD J. WYATT

National Institute of Mental Health
Washington, DC

INTRODUCTION

Development of effective therapeutic approaches to central nervous system disorders has been constrained by the limited potential of the brain to repair itself. Thus, the possibility that dysfunctional systems in the human brain might be repaired by replacement with grafted tissue has encouraged a number of experimental approaches and strategies.[1-5] Based on the finding that Parkinson's disease most consistently involves pathologic changes in the substantia nigra, the main source of dopaminergic innervation to the striatum,[6-7] a rat rotational model[8-11] involving this system has been used to investigate the possibility of using dopamine-containing grafts in an experimental therapeutic approach to this disorder. Indeed, it has been demonstrated that either fetal substantia nigra or adrenal medulla tissue, which are biological sources of dopamine, transplanted into the rat brain can reduce rotational behavior caused by experimental deprivation of dopaminergic innervation.[2,12-14] Moreover, it has been shown that fetal substantia nigra can reverse experimentally induced abnormalities of postsynaptic dopaminergic binding sites.[15]

In this paper we discuss our extension of investigations in the rat to a preliminary study in the nonhuman primate.[16]

METHODS

Seven fully mature male rhesus macaques (*Macaca mulatta*) were studied. Each animal received a unilateral neurotoxic lesion of the substantia nigra with 6-hydroxy-dopamine. After at least 2 months, each animal received an implant of either fetal substantia nigra (animals A1 and A2) or adrenal medulla tissue (animals A3 through A7). All operations were performed aseptically with the animals under deep pento-barbital anesthesia. Three or more months later, each animal was killed and the brain of each animal studied with fluorescence histochemistry.

Neurotoxic Lesions

X-ray-corrected stereotaxic coordinates were derived for the location of the sub-stantia nigra.[17] A 2-cm trephine was used to make an opening in the skull. After a 22-gauge needle was introduced through an incision in the dura and lowered into the substantia nigra, 4 μg/μl (in 4 ml of lactated Ringer's solution) of 6-hydroxydopamine was injected into multiple sites dispersed in a three-dimensional pattern designed to encompass the entire substantia nigra.

Tissue Implantation

At least 2 months after the creation of the neurotoxic lesions, animals A1 and A2 received a second operation in which the embryonic tissue was implanted. A 2 cm $\times$ 2 cm bone flap was opened over the left cerebral cortex. Embryonic substantia nigra divided into pieces approximately 0.25 mm^3, in a Ringer's solution, were drawn up into a 22-gauge needle. In this approach, stereotaxic coordinates were corrected using X-rays of the skull,[17] and these corrected coordinates were used when lowering the needle into the head of the caudate. For each implantation site, the needle con-tained an average of six pieces of tissue per injection in a volume of approximately 10 to 20 μl.

Animals A3 through A7 received autografts of their adrenal medulla, which was removed through a posterolateral retroperitoneal approach. The adrenal medulla was carefully separated from the cortex because adrenal corticosteroids limit the trans-formation of chromaffin cells from the endocrine phenotype to a neuronal pheno-type.[18,19] The adrenal medulla was divided into pieces with volumes of approximately 0.25 mm^3 and drawn up into a 22-gauge needle with an average of 5 to 10 pieces of tissue per injection in a volume of approximately 10 to 20 μl.

Animal A3 received stereotaxic implantation of adrenal medulla tissue in a manner similar to that used for animals A1 and A2. In animals A4 through A7, direct visualization of the caudate was used in order to improve the reliability of anatomic placement. The left hemisphere was cut with a diamond saw to create a 5 cm $\times$ 2 cm bone flap that extended over the midline. The midline was then exposed by reflecting a dural flap hinged on the saggital sinus. The corpus callosum at the level of the head of the caudate nucleus was exposed by sacrificing a few anastomotic veins and then gently retracting the left hemisphere. With the aid of a surgical microscope, a rectangular window was cut (less than 1 mm $\times$ 1 cm) in the anterior body of the corpus callosum. The corpus callosum was approximately 35-mm long. We entered approximately 15 mm from the anterior end and angled the window to the left until we entered the lateral ventricle. The opening was then enlarged to approximately 1 cm in length, with the final window starting approximately 10 mm from the anterior end of the corpus callosum. This window provided a clear view of the left caudate nucleus on the lateral wall of the ventricle. The 22-gauge needle was inserted into the body of the caudate and the adrenal medulla tissue injected.

Fluorescence Histochemistry

Falck-Hillarp fluorescence histochemistry[20] was used to study the brains from animals A1 and A2. Animals A3 through A7 were perfused with a magnesium paraformaldehyde solution[21] and studied, according to the method described by de la Torre,[22] using catecholamine fluorescence induced by glyoxylic acid.

RESULTS

The fluorescence histochemistry demonstrated that the dopaminergic denervation of the caudate nucleus was essentially complete in all animals. Graft tissue was easily identifiable by the presence of specific catecholamine fluorescence. No catecholamine-containing graft tissue, however, was detected in the two animals that received the fetal substantia nigra implants. In contrast, all five animals implanted with adrenal medulla tissue did demonstrate at least some catecholamine histofluorescence in the tissue grafts (TABLE 1). Although some parts of the grafts appeared fused with the parenchyma of the brain, there was no evidence of axonal reinnervation of the caudate. The graft sites all demonstrated catecholamine diffusion, but most fluorescent cells retained the typical morphology of an adrenal chromaffin cell.

DISCUSSION

These findings indicate that peripheral tissue autografts can survive intraparenchymal implantation into the central nervous system of the nonhuman primate, and that these grafts appear to retain the potential as a biological source of catecholamines. The number of surviving cells, however, is limited, and there was no evidence of reinnervation of host. Although no fetal substantia nigra grafts survived, it should be pointed out that only two animals were used, and these animals were studied before we adopted the approach of directly visualizing the implantation site.

Nevertheless, even with the successful adrenal grafts, the limited yield presents a problem for therapeutic application because the human striatum is approximately 250 times larger than the rat striatum; furthermore, it is clear that a large number of grafts would be required to completely reinnervate the striatum.[23] Although residual surviving substantia nigra neurons in Parkinson's disease patients, as well as advances in our understanding of the topographic specialization of the striatum, should significantly reduce the number needed, it is still likely that multiple graft sites will be required. A direct visualization approach provides a flexibility and anatomic reliability that will be useful in our experimental investigation.

A technique in which computed tomography and stereotaxis were combined, and in which tissue to be implanted was surrounded by a steel spiral holder,[24] to ensure the accurate placement of adrenal medullary tissue has been reported for two patients with Parkinson's disease.[25] To decrease the likelihood of producing further damage to the central nervous system, the steel spiral holder may be abandoned in the future.[25] If so, easily verifiable anatomic placement in the caudate might be achieved in experimental models by other means, that is, through direct visualization.

Specifically, if implantation in many sites distributed throughout the caudate is required, direct visualization may offer an advantage over multiple stereotaxic inser-

TABLE 1. Central Nervous System Grafts (*Macaca mulatta*)

Animal	Surgical Approach	Months between Graft and Sacrifice	Fluorescence Technique	Number of Graft Sites Found	Catecholamine Fluorescence Cell Count
A1	Stereotaxic	3	Falck–Hillarp	None	None
A2	Stereotaxic	3	Falck–Hillarp	None	None
A3	Stereotaxic	5	de la Torre	2	< 10
A4	Direct visualization	3	de la Torre	2	< 10
A5	Direct visualization	8	de la Torre	2	190
A6	Direct visualization	5	de la Torre	5	310
A7	Direct visualization	5	de la Torre	4	630

tions through the cortical hemispheres. Indeed, multiple stereotaxic placement raises the possibility of undetected bleeding into the ventricular system with its potential for morbidity. Direct visualization allows the surgeon greater assurance that bleeding has been controlled before closing.

Although it is too early to assess the clinical efficacy of these experimental approaches, any possibility that this strategy may evolve into a reasonable therapeutic modality requires the testing and refinement of a variety of surgical techniques. The stereotaxic approach has been applied in human cases,[25] but this does not preclude the value and importance of pursuing animal models with which we may further define and elaborate the multiple parameters that determine tissue graft survival as well as optimal therapeutic efficacy. Thus, the object here is not to indicate which approach is superior, but to emphasize the importance of exploring the feasibility of several approaches in order to maximize the likelihood that we will be able to eventually delineate an optimal therapeutic approach.

ACKNOWLEDGMENTS

We thank Luis de Medinaceli for carrying out the adrenalectomies, Lars Olson and Ake Seiger (supported by grants 04X-03185 and 14P-5867 from the Swedish Medical Research Council and by the Magnus Bervalls Stiftelse) for the fluorescence histochemistry of the two substantia nigra grafts, Eleanor Krauthamer for the histologic preparation of the central nervous system tissue, and Jere Phillips for the veterinary support of this project.

REFERENCES

1. BJÖRKLUND, A., R. H. SCHMIDT & U. STENEVI. 1980. Functional reinnervation of the neostriatum in the adult rat by use of intraparenchymal grafting of dissociated cell suspensions from the substantia nigra. Cell Tissue Res. **212:** 39-45.

2. BJÖRKLUND, A., S. B. DUNNETT, U. STENEVI, M. E. LEWIS & S. D. IVERSEN. 1980. Reinnervation of the denervated striatum by substantia nigra transplants: Functional consequences as revealed by pharmacological and sensorimotor testing. Brain Res. **199:** 307-333.

3. GASH, D., J. R. SLADEK & C. D. SLADEK. 1980. Functional development of grafted vasopressin neurons. Science **210:** 1367-1369.

4. LEWIS, E. R. & C. W. COTMAN. 1982. Mechanisms of septal lamination in the developing hippocampus analyzed by outgrowth of fibers from septal implants. II. Absence of guidance by degenerative debris. J. Neurosci. **2:** 66-77.

5. LUND, R. D. & A. R. HARVEY. 1981. Transplantation of tectal tissue in rats. I. Organization of transports and pattern of distribution of host afferents within them. J. Comp. Neurol. **201:** 191-209.

6. FALLON, J. H. & R. Y. MOORE. 1978. Catecholamine innervation of the basal forebrain. IV. Topography of the dopamine projection to the basal forebrain and the neostriatum. J. Comp. Neurol. **180:** 545-580.

7. SZABO, J. 1980. Organization of ascending striatal afferents in monkey. J. Comp. Neurol. **189:** 307-321.

8. ANDEN, N. E. 1975. Animal models of brain dopamine function. *In* Advances in Parkinsonism. W. Birkmayer & O. Hornykiewicz, Eds.: 169-177. Hoffman-LaRoche. Basel.

9. UNGERSTEDT, U. 1971. Postsynaptic supersensitivity after 6-hydroxydopamine-induced degeneration of the nigrostriatal dopamine system. Acta Physiol. Scand. **367:** 69-93.

10. UNGERSTEDT, U. 1976. 6-Hydroxydopamine-induced degeneration of the nigrostriatal dopamine pathway: The turning syndrome. Pharmacol. Ther. Behav. **2:** 37-40.

11. MORIHISA, J. M. & S. D. GLICK. 1977. Morphine-induced rotation in rats and mice: Species differences, persistence of withdrawal-induced rotation and antagonism by naloxone. Brain Res. **123:** 180-187.

12. FREED, W. J., M. J. PERLOW, F. KAROUM, A. SEIGER, L. OLSON, B. J. HOFFER & R. J. WYATT. 1980. Restoration of dopaminergic function by grafting of fetal rat substantia nigra to the caudate nucleus: Long-term behavioral, biochemical and histochemical studies. Ann. Neurol. **8:** 510-519.

13. FREED, W. J., J. M. MORIHISA, H. E. SPOOR, B. J. HOFFER, L. OLSON, A. SEIGER & R. J. WYATT. 1981. Transplanted adrenal chromaffin cells in rat brain reduce lesion-induced rotational behavior. Nature (London) **292:** 351-352.

14. FREED, W. J., F. KAROUM, H. E. SPOOR, L. OLSON, J. M. MORIHISA & R. J. WYATT. 1983. Catecholamine content of intracerebral adrenal medulla grafts. Brain Res. **269:** 184-189.

15. FREED, W. J., G. N. KO, D. L. NIEHOFF, M. J. KUHAR, B. J. HOFFER, L. OLSON, H. E. CANNON-SPOOR, J. M. MORIHISA & R. J. WYATT. 1983. Normalization of spiroperidol

binding in the denervated rat striatum by homologous grafts of substantia nigra. Science **222:** 937-939.

16. MORIHISA, J. M., R. K. NAKAMURA, W. J. FREED, M. MISHKIN & R. J. WYATT. 1984. Adrenal medulla grafts survive and exhibit catecholamine-specific fluorescence in the primate brain. Exp. Neurol. **84:** 643-653.

17. AGGLETON, J. P. & R. E. PASSINGHAM. 1981. Stereotaxic surgery under X-ray guidance in the rhesus monkey, with special reference to the amygdala. Exp. Brain. Res. **44:** 271-276.

18. TISCHLER, A. S. & L. A. GREENE. 1980. Phenotypic plasticity of pheochromocytoma and normal adrenal medullary cells. In Histochemistry and Cell Biology of Autonomic Neurons, SIF Cells, and Paraneurons. O. Eranko, S. Soinila & H. Paivarinta, Eds. Advances in Biochemical Pharmacology. Vol. **4:** 61-88. Raven Press. New York, NY.

19. UNISCKER, K., B. RIEFFERT & W. ZIEGLER. 1980. Effects of cell culture conditions, nerve growth factor, dexamethasone, and cyclic AMP on adrenal chromaffin cells in vitro. In Histochemistry and Cell Biology of Autonomic Neurons, SIF Cells, and Paraneurons. O. Eranko, S. Soinila & H. Paivarinta, Eds. Advances in Biochemical Pharmacology. Vol. **4:** 51-59. Raven Press. New York, NY.

20. FALCK, B., N. A. HILLARP, G. THIEME & A. TORP. 1962. Fluorescence of catecholamines and related compounds condensed with formaldehyde. J. Histochem. Cytochem. **10:** 348-354.

21. LOREN, I., A. BJÖRKLUND, O. LINDVALL & R. H. SCHMIDT. 1982. Improved catecholamine histofluorescence in the developing brain based on the magnesium and aluminum (ALFA) perfusion techniques: Methodology and anatomical observation. Brain Res. Bull. **9:** 11-26.

22. DE LA TORRE, J. C. 1980. An improved approach to histofluorescence using the SPG method for tissue monoamines. J. Neurosci. Methods **3:** 1-5.

23. WYATT, R. J., J. M. MORIHISA, R. K. NAKAMURA & W. J. FREED. 1986. Transplanting tissue into the brain for function: Use in a model for Parkinson's disease. In Neuropeptides in Neurologic and Psychiatric Disease. J. B. Martin & J. D. Barchas, Eds.: 199-208. Raven Press. New York, NY.

24. LEKSELL, L. & B. JERNBERG. 1980. Stereotaxis and tomography: A technical note. Acta Neurochir. **52:** 1-7.

25. BACKLUND, E.-O., P. O. GRANBERG, B. HAMBERGER, E. KNUTSSON, A. MARTENSSON, G. SEDVALL, A. SEIGER & L. OLSON. Transplantation of adrenal medullary tissue to striatum in parkinsonism. J. Neurosurg. **62:** 169-173.

DISCUSSION OF THE PAPER

QUESTIONER: Did you see any behavioral changes or look for behavioral changes with these transplants? Could you tell us the age of the substantia nigra graft?

MORIHISA: The fetal grafts were 59 and 71 days. We did see behavioral changes, and we did make attempts to measure them and develop neurological examinations for the primates. I was unimpressed, however, with our ability to really distinguish the normal healing process from actual changes that could be related to the graft. In the course of the study, we had some animals that received lesions but did not receive a graft for a very long time. To my dismay, these animals also improved significantly following surgery over many months. So at this point, with this particular approach, I did not feel that there were any behavioral findings that we could confidently report. I have heard more encouraging findings from some other approaches.

J. R. SLADEK, JR. (*University of Rochester Medical School, Rochester, NY*): I noticed on the two substantia nigra grafts that you attempted Falck-Hillarp histochemistry and on the others that you used other approaches. Falck-Hillarp histochemistry is more involved than the other techniques. Is it more difficult to get the same intensity of fluorescence that you would get with a glyoxylic acid preparation. It is possible in those two first animals that you simply did not have a technique that was adequate for the visualization?

MORIHISA: Dr. Lars Olson and Dr. Åke Seiger performed the Falck-Hillarp study. For obvious reasons, it is hard to transport material across the ocean. We sent material from two animals by airplane. I know the substantia nigra implants in these animals did not have any histofluorescence, and perhaps Dr. Olson can talk about the histofluorescence in the rest of the brain.

OLSON: Many things could have gone wrong. Fluorescence in the rest of the brain was in bad condition in those two animals. I think the trip over the ocean was bad for them.

MORIHISA: We thought they did not survive travel in good condition. And that is one of the reasons we developed our own histofluorescence capability using the glyoxylic acid technique.

P. PASIK (*Mount Sinai School of Medicine, New York, NY*): In the direct approach you put some weight in terms of the success of the survival. Does this apply essentially to the caudate? Implantation in primates may become more successful when the putamen and the caudate are reinnervated.

MORIHISA: Yes, I agree, and I would suggest that there is an additional technical concern. The issue was raised that the stereotaxic approach carries with it a lower morbidity. We would, however, raise one technical issue, which is that if one needs many implants into the striatum to achieve a good therapeutic result, the multiple stereotaxic punches might lead to more morbidity than a single direct visualization where we could make multiple implantations. Nevertheless, it is most likely that as we gain new insights into the topographic distribution of the key dysfunctional neural elements in Parkinson's disease, we will be better able to develop effective experimental therapeutic approaches.

Thus, our final point would be that we see this work as an experimental approach and not one to be considered as an alternative therapeutic approach but rather one to experiment with to try to elaborate the neuroscientific principles important to transplant survival and growth as well as therapeutic efficacy.

An *in Vivo* and *in Vitro* Assessment of Differentiated Neuroblastoma Cells as a Source of Donor Tissue for Transplantation[a]

JEFFREY H. KORDOWER,[b,c] MARY F. D. NOTTER,
HERMES H. YEH, AND DON M. GASH

Department of Neurobiology and Anatomy
University of Rochester School of Medicine
Rochester, New York 14642

INTRODUCTION

It is now well established that the central nervous system is receptive toward the implantation of cells derived from donors of the same species. Indeed, not only do these cells survive, they are capable of ameliorating motoric, cognitive, or endocrine deficits produced through acute lesions, congenital defects, or the aging process.[1,2] Most transplantation studies have employed fetal or embryonic anlage as donor material. After transplantation, such tissues have been demonstrated to project toward host targets[3] and to establish synapses[4] in a pattern as would be expected of their normal disposition *in situ*. Host neurons can project to grafted cells as well,[4] suggesting that functional interactions between host and graft may develop. Indeed, in certain cases, specific graft-host interactions appear obligatory for the restoration of lesion-induced deficits.[5]

The success of fetal neural transplants in rodents has led to the suggestion that neural implants might serve a clinical role in treating neurodegenerative disorders. This suggestion raises a number of issues and concerns, not the least of which being the source of donor tissue. In light of the ethical questions surrounding the use of fetal cells for human transplantation, the identification of alternative, nonfetal sources of donor material could be extremely valuable. Indeed, nonfetal cells survive transplantation for extended periods of time and, in some cases, can restore behavioral dysfunctions. Grafts of adrenal medullary tissue into the lateral ventricle[6] or caudoputamen[7] attenuate apomorphine-induced motor asymmetry in rats in which

[a] This work was supported by ADRDA 86-063 (J.H.K.), BRSG 2 507RR05404-23 (H.H.Y.), NS19711 (M.F.D.N.), and NIH1S109 (D.M.G.).

[b] A recipient of the John Douglas French Foundation Fellowship for the Study of Alzheimer's Disease.

[c] Address for correspondence: Department of Neurobiology and Anatomy, Box 603, University of Rochester School of Medicine and Dentistry, Rochester, New York 14642.

unilateral nigrostriatal lesions have been created. Adrenal medullary grafts have also been attempted in Parkinson's patients.[8] Vigorous regeneration of adult superior cervical ganglion is also seen after transplantation into the fourth ventricle of intact rats.[9] This paper details studies conducted by our research group evaluating the potential of differentiated neuroblastoma cells as a novel source of cells for use as donor tissue for transplantation.

WHY NEUROBLASTOMA CELLS?

Neuroblastoma cells provide unique features that make them an advantageous donor material for certain types of transplantation studies. Whereas some cell lines produce a number of neurotransmitters, others produce a single transmitter or peptide. For example, Seeger and colleagues[10] have characterized two tumor cell lines derived from the bone marrow of a metastatic cancer. One of them, the LA-N-1, is an adrenergic cell line containing dopamine, norepinephrine, and epinephrine. The other, the LA-N-2, consists of tumor cells that appear to be almost purely cholinergic as demonstrated by biochemical assays for choline acetyltransferase (ChAT).

Most transplant studies employ dissections of fetal tissue microdissected from specific regions of the central nervous system. These dissections contain both the cell types desired and additional cell groups from surrounding regions. Having a cell line that produces a single neurotransmitter allows for greater specificity in assessing structure-function relationships or treating transmitter-specific neurodegenerative disorders. It would also seem plausible that there are a limited number of cells that can be transplanted without compromising the host. It might prove advantageous to have all of the grafted cells contain the desired neurotransmitter or neuromodulator. Additionally, some neuroblastoma cell lines contain trophic factors. Clones of the C1300 cell line contain and secrete nerve growth factor[11] and thus may promote their own survival and integration within the host.

Furthermore, undifferentiated cells are, in a sense, immortal. Their ability for continuous continual mitosis means that they represent a virtual inexhaustible supply of donor cells. They can be stored frozen or maintained in culture for years, adding great flexibility for transplantation experiments.

Undifferentiated, mitotic neuroblastoma cells have been employed in two transplant studies reported by other laboratories. PC12 cells, an adrenergic cell line, was transplanted into the striatum of rats in which unilateral nigrostriatal lesions were created. In one study,[12] transplants into the striatum reduced apomorphine-induced rotation. However, no cells survived beyond 2 weeks after transplantation. Jaeger[13] transplanted PC12 cells into 4-, 10-, and 12-day-old rat pups. For up to 2 months, tyrosine hydroxylase-immunoreactive cells were demonstrated to have survived and proliferated.

If neuroblastoma cells are to be a practical source of donor material, they need to be transformed from their natural tumorous state. This can be accomplished by treating the cells with one or more of the known differentiating agents. For a number of reasons, differentiating the cells in culture makes them a better candidate for transplantation. After this treatment *in vitro*, the cells can be rendered permanently amitotic. Although their genotype remains unaltered, their phenotype takes on features characteristic of normal mature neurons. Following differentiation, the cells can extend long processes from the perikarya.[14] Ultrastructural analyses reveal that these processes possess organelles similar to neurosecretory vesicles.[11] Like neurons, these cells can release neurotransmitter in response to electrical or chemical stimulation.[15]

Dependent upon the specific cell line, differentiation often increases the level of neurotransmitter within cells. In certain clones of the well-studied C1300 mouse cell line, differentiation with cAMP treatment significantly increases the levels of acetyl-cholinesterase (AChE), ChAT, tyrosine hydroxylase, and dopamine β-hydroxylase.[11]

The electrical properties of differentiated clones of C1300 neuroblastoma cells have also been extensively studied. Intracellular recordings demonstrate resting potentials similar to those seen in nerve cells.[16] These cells are capable of generating action potentials that are dependent upon sodium and calcium ionic fluxes.[11]

It would appear that neuroblastoma cells, once they are differentiated, have two qualities that may allow them to be well integrated and regulated by the host. After differentiation, the cell surface undergoes significant changes. C1300 cells treated with bromodeoxyuridine (BRDU) or dibutyryl cAMP produce new low molecular weight cell surface glycopeptides.[11] Differentiation of a neuro 2a subclone induces cell surface gangliosides that bind tetanus toxin.[17] Such cell surface characteristics are similar to those of differentiated neurons, and it is the cell surface characteristics that, in part, determine the interactions between nerve cells. Additionally, receptors for neurotransmitters and neuropeptides have been identified on neuroblastoma cells.[11] After differentiation, the number of receptors can increase[11] and can be modified in a manner similar to that used for cells found in the central nervous system. Repeated cholinergic agonist administration results in a decreased number of muscarinic receptors both in the brain[18] and on N1E-115 neuroblastoma cells,[19] effects that are reversed after removal of the agonist. It is suggested that these binding sites have properties similar to those seen in the central nervous system because differentiated neuroblastoma cells have many "neuronal-like" characteristics and because areas of membrane contact specializations with "synaptic-like" vesicles are seen in structurally apposed differentiated neuroblastoma cells in vitro.[11]

CRITERIA FOR DETERMINING A NEUROBLASTOMA CELL LINE SUITABLE FOR TRANSPLANTATION

With respect to neuroblastoma cells, we propose the following basic criteria for determining their suitability for transplantation: 1) the grafted cells must survive in a differentiated state for extended periods of time; 2) the grafted cells should become well integrated within the host; 3) the grafted cells should not produce an inflammatory response; 4) the grafted cells must be able to moderate behavioral deficits; 5) criteria 1-4 must be demonstrated in nonhuman primates. The following is a review of the experiments carried out to date by our laboratory group aimed at assessing the extent to which differentiated neuroblastoma cells fulfill these criteria.

PREPARATION OF DIFFERENTIATED NEUROBLASTOMAS FOR TRANSPLANTATION

Each neuroblastoma cell line has unique characteristics; hence different cell lines are maintained, treated, and differentiated in different ways. In the first series of experiments, C1300 and LA-N-2 cells were employed. The C1300 neuroblastoma cells (clone NB41A3) are derived from the parent cell line that originated spontaneously from the spinal cord region of the mouse and is believed to be of sympathetic origin.[11] It was adapted to tissue culture systems by Augusti-Tocco and Sato.[20] This cell line contains both catecholaminergic and cholinergic markers.[11] In addition, it produces high levels of gangliosides.[11] The LA-N-2 cells were characterized by Seeger and colleagues.[10] These cells are of human origin and also have been demonstrated to contain the enzymatic markers indicative of acetylcholine-containing cells. For the present study, C1300 cells were obtained from the American Type Culture Collection. The LA-N-2 cells were generously donated by Dr. Seeger.

FIGURE 1 is a schematic representation of how these cells are maintained and treated until the time of transplantation. Before their use, they are stored frozen at $-140°$ C in liquid nitrogen. At a desired time, they are thawed and grown in either Falcon flasks containing Ham's F-12 medium (C1300 cells) or in a stoppered flask with Leibovit's medium (LA-N-2 cells). Both of these media are supplemented with 15% heat-inactivated fetal calf serum, gentamycin (50 μg/ml), and fungizone (2.5 μg/ml). Once a significant number of cells has grown, they are labeled with [^{3}H]thymidine (3-5 μCi/ml). This allows the cells to be visualized after transplantation with autoradiography. The [^{3}H]thymidine is left in the media for a time period equal to the doubling time of the cell (24 hr for the C1300; 56 hr for the LA-N-2). For differentiation, the cells are incubated with mitomycin C (0.5 μg/ml) followed 6 hr later by 10^{-5} M BRDU. The cells remain in this solution for 2-4 days (the actual length of time is determined by whether processes can be visualized by an inverted light microscope). Mitomycin C/BRDU was chosen as the differentiating agent because pilot studies have demonstrated superior cell survival after transplantation as compared to prostaglandin E1/cAMP treatment.[21] BRDU prevents mitosis by incorporating a false uracil into the replicating DNA.[22] After differentiation, the cells are removed from the culture dish by trypsin and counted by a hemocytometer. The cell suspension is centrifuged, the supernatant is decanted, and the resulting pellet is resuspended in a phosphate-buffered saline (PBS) solution containing 1% fetal calf serum at a dilution of approximately 10 000 cells/μl. The viability of the cells is assessed before the transplantation by trypan blue dye exclusion with an average viability of about 93% (the minimum acceptable viability is 85%). The cells were kept on ice until transplantation.

IMMUNOCYTOCHEMICAL STAINING FOR ChAT IN NEUROBLASTOMA CELLS

Even though it has been established by others that both C1300 and LA-N-2 cells contain significant levels of ChAT,[10,11] it was important to substantiate the cholinergic nature of these cells for two reasons: first, to make sure that the multiple generations produced in our laboratories did not induce any mutations that would alter the expression of cholinergic markers; second, since neuroblastoma cells are sensitive to environmental conditions, ChAT staining verified that the procedures outlined above did not alter the neurochemical phenotype of the cell.

Two sets of C1300 and LA-N-2 cell were placed on coverslips. One set was differentiated with mitomycin C/BRDU treatment whereas the other set served as a control. The cells were otherwise maintained and treated as before except that

[³H]thymidine treatment was omitted. The medium was gently decanted and washed (2 × 5 min with PBS). The cells were then fixed with 4% paraformaldehyde-1% glutaraldehyde for 1.5 hr. Immunocytochemical staining for ChAT was carried out via the peroxidase-antiperoxidase method[22] according to established procedures (Immunonuclear) except for the following: 1) a 0.5% triton prewash was employed in lieu of the recommended 0.4% prewash; 2) the primary antibody was diluted 1:50; 3) and the initial 10 min application of 0.05% diaminobenzadine was omitted. A substitution of PBS for the primary antibody served as a control.

FIGURE 2 illustrates the results. C1300 and LA-N-2 cells demonstrated positive ChAT immunoreactivity in both the differentiated and undifferentiated state. Control

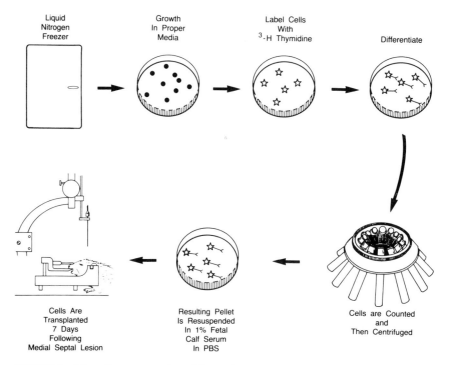

FIGURE 1. Schematic representation of the methods we used to prepare differentiated neuroblastoma cells for intracerebral transplantation.

incubated cells failed to display any immunoreactivity. There was no apparent difference in the intensity of staining between the two conditions. For both cell lines, there was some heterogeneity in staining. Most of the cells displayed immunoreactivity; some cells did not (see arrow in FIG. 2A). These data are consistent with the published reports that these cell lines contain the synthesizing enzyme for acetylcholine, and suggest that this property is unchanged by differentiation with mitomycin C/BRDU treatment. FIGURE 2 also illustrates the altered morphology of these cells after differentiation. The undifferentiated C1300 cells (FIG. 2A) are round with minimal processes emanating from their cell bodies. This is in sharp contrast to the long multiple neurites extending from the perikarya after mitomycin C/BRDU treatment (FIG. 2B).

DEMONSTRATION OF FUNCTIONAL SYNAPSES *IN VITRO* BY DIFFERENTIATED NEUROBLASTOMA CELLS

As an initial strategy aimed at assessing the viability of differentiated neuroblastoma cells for transplantation, it is helpful to examine their physiological properties *in vitro* and compare these findings to well-established characteristics of neurons in culture systems. Since acetylcholine is the neurotransmitter at the neuromuscular junction, the putative release of acetylcholine from the LA-N-2 neuroblastoma cells after differentiation was determined in a co-culture system with muscle cells by an electrophysiological analysis.

Procedure

The methods for the preparation and maintenance of striated muscle cell cultures as well as for the electrophysiological assay have been described in detail elsewhere.[24,25]

LA-N-2-Muscle Co-culture

Primary muscle cultures were prepared by fusion of myoblasts derived from hindlimbs of newborn rat pups treated briefly with trypsin, mechanically dissociated, and grown in 35-mm tissue culture dishes. The cultures were exposed to cytosine arabinoside (1 μM) from day 2 to day 4 to select for nondividing cells. Between 3 and 5 days in culture, myoblasts fused into myotubes that were 200-400 μm in length. LA-N-2 cells were seeded into plastic petri dishes, differentiated with mitomycin C/BRDU, as described earlier, again dissociated with mild trypsin, and added (1 $\times$ 10^5 cells/plate) to 5-6-day-old muscle cultures.

Electrophysiological Assay

The co-cultures were placed in a chamber on a stage of an inverted microscope with Hoffman modulation optics and examined throughout the experiment. The temperature was maintained at 34 $\pm$ 1° C (pH 7.4). Glass micropipets (tip resistance: 40-70 MΩ) filled with 3 M KCl were used to record intracellularly from muscle cells. The electrophysiological activity was displayed on-line on an oscilloscope and penwriter.

Our strategy of monitoring acetylcholine release from LA-N-2 cells was prompted

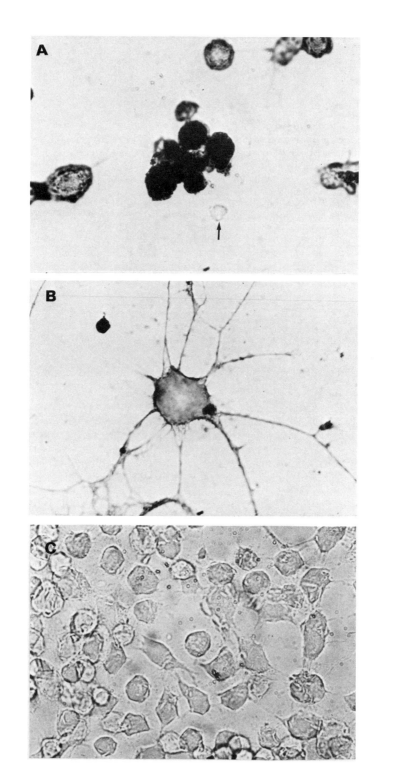

by previously reported studies of synaptic function in culture using a similar co-culture system consisting of retinal and muscle cells.[24-27] In such a co-culture, cholinergic retinal neurons formed functional synapses with muscle cells. Similarly, in the present study, muscle cells innervated by differentiated LA-N-2 cells were detected by recording spontaneous depolarizing synaptic potentials. Only those muscle cells with stable membrane potentials of at least -45 mV were used. Muscle cells are useful as postsynaptic targets because their membranes have areas with a high density of cholinergic receptors and because their physiological response to acetylcholine has been extensively studied both *in vivo* and in culture. In addition, their relatively large size permits prolonged, stable intracellular recording for the physiological monitoring of acetylcholine release from LA-N-2 cells.

Results

Under our co-culture conditions, LA-N-2 cells could innervate muscle cells sampled electrophysiologically as early as 3 hr after co-culture. Between 3 and 5 hr after co-culture, $77.0 \pm 4.3\%$ (mean $\pm$ SEM; three experiments) of the muscle cells sampled exhibited spontaneous depolarizing potentials. Typically, the muscle cell responses lasted 10 msec and were variable in amplitude and frequency. The incidence of innervated muscle cells remained relatively unaltered over the first 4 days of co-culture. In all cases in which synaptic potentials were detected, one or more LA-N-2 cells could be localized adjacent to, or on, the muscle cells being sampled (FIG. 3A). In FIGURE 3B, the penwriter records of muscle cells in co-culture show a muscle cell that was innervated (top record) and one that was not innervated (bottom record). Muscle cells that have not been innervated, as those that have been cultured alone, do not display activity, which may be confused with synaptic potentials.

The results of our electrophysiological experiments indicate that differentiated LA-N-2 cells are synaptically competent, releasing acetylcholine under our co-culture conditions. The strategy of using striated muscle cells as a postsynaptic target will permit a sensitive bioassay for monitoring transmitter output from LA-N-2 cell lines, and other cultured cell lines, and for investigating factors that may regulate their activities. Whether the presence of functional synapses formed by LA-N-2 cells in co-culture, as first demonstrated electrophysiologically here, is correlated with morphological signs of synaptic investment remains to be demonstrated at the ultrastructural level.

FIGURE 2. ChAT-positive immunoreactivity in (A) undifferentiated C1300 cells and (B) a C1300 cell differentiated with mitomycin C/BRDU. This is in contrast to the lack of immunoreactivity in control incubated undifferentiated C1300 cells (C). Original magnifications: $\times 1000$; figure reduced to 54% of original size.

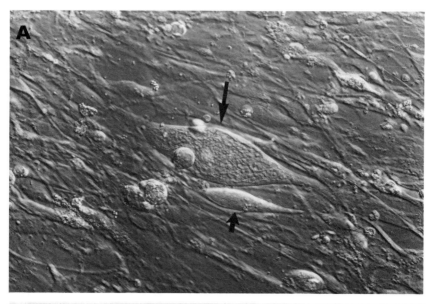

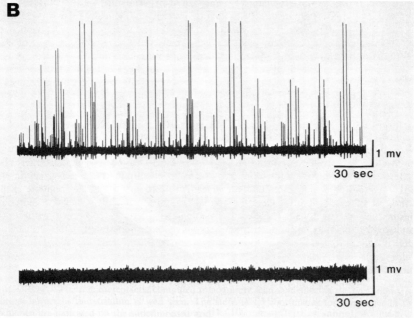

FIGURE 3. (A) Hoffman modulation optics image of a differentiated LA-N-2 cell (short arrow) in apposition to a muscle cell (long arrow) in a co-culture system. (B) The topmost penwriter record illustrates the action potentials recorded from muscle co-cultured with, and in apposition to, a differentiated LA-N-2 cell; the bottommost record illustrates the lack of electrical potentials in the absence of LA-N-2 cells.

MORPHOLOGICAL COMPARISON OF UNDIFFERENTIATED AND DIFFERENTIATED NEUROBLASTOMA CELLS AFTER INTRAHIPPOCAMPAL TRANSPLANTATION

Procedure

Four groups of rats were used in this experiment. All groups received electrolytic lesions of the posterodorsal medial septum in order to remove cholinergic afferents to the hippocampus. Seven days later, they received transplants of neuroblastoma cells into the dorsal hippocampus. Both the lesion and the period of time between surgeries were employed because both have been demonstrated to enhance graft survival, which is presumably due to the release of endogenous trophic factors.[28,29] Group 1 received a transplant of undifferentiated, unlabeled C1300 cells. Group 2 received a similar transplant of C1300 cells that were labeled with [³H]thymidine and differentiated with mitomycin C/BRDU treatment as described earlier. Groups 3 and 4 were treated in an identical fashion as groups 1 and 2, respectively, except that LA-N-2 cells were transplanted in lieu of the C1300 cells. All cells were stereotaxically implanted into two sites of the dorsal hippocampus, one each in the medial and lateral aspects at the level of the tuberal and mammillary regions of the hypothalamus, respectively. Transplants were made in a 1-μl volume through a 31-gauge internal cannula (Plastic Products) connected to a 5-μl Hamilton syringe by PE-20 tubing. There were approximately 20 000 cells/μl. All rats were sacrificed 7 days later. Frozen sections (40 μ thick) were cut on a sliding knife microtome. Sections from rats that received undifferentiated cell transplants were processed for cell body visualization with cresyl violet. Similar sections from rats that received transplants of differentiated cells were processed for Nissl staining and autoradiography.

Results

There is a clear distinction in morphology between transplants of undifferentiated and differentiated cells for the LA-N-2 and C1300 cell lines. Both types of cells flourish in the central nervous system. As is often seen *in vitro,* however, both types do not migrate significantly in the undifferentiated state. Rather, the mass of cells within the host appears attributable to their *in vivo* cell division. When undifferentiated LA-N-2 cells are transplanted, they can encompass much of the entire dorsal hippocampus. A similar finding is seen with the C1300 cells (FIG. 4A). These cells have obliterated much of the dorsal aspect of the pyramidal cell layer of the hippocampal formation. Additionally, both cell types are found in association with host vasculature. It is not uncommon to find five to seven layers of grafted cells completely surrounding a single blood vessel. Both the LA-N-2 and C1300 cells appear to remain mitotic without differentiation because numerous cells display nuclei with tumorous features, such as an alignment of mitotic spindles characteristic of late anaphase mitosis. These cells are heterogeneous in their morphology and are easily distinguishable from host cells in the hippocampus. In contrast, transplanted differentiated neuroblastoma cells integrated so well into the parenchyma of the host that they were not identifiable with routine Nissl staining. Autoradiography revealed that numerous LA-N-2 and C1300

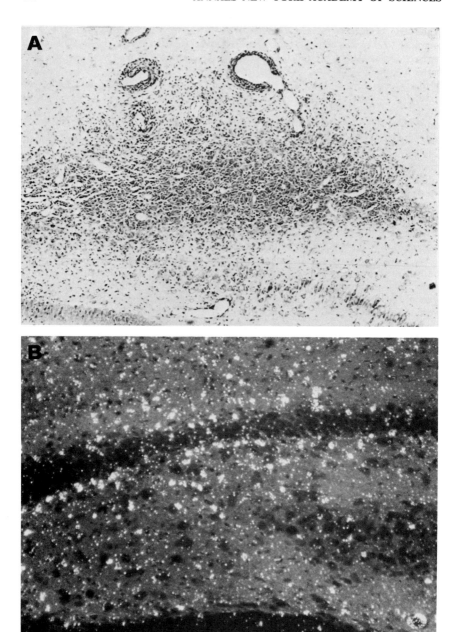

FIGURE 4. (A) Nissl stain of undifferentiated C1300 neuroblastoma cells transplanted into the hippocampus 7 days before sacrifice. (B) Dark-field image of the large number of autoradiographically labeled neuroblastoma cells that were differentiated with mitomycin C/BRDU and then transplanted into the hippocampus 7 days before sacrifice. Original magnifications for **A** and **B**: ×100 and ×200, respectively; figure reduced to 70% of original size.

(FIG. 4B) cells survive transplantation throughout the host hippocampus. These cells migrated well away from the injection site and, unlike their undifferentiated counterparts, migrated away from each other. There did not appear to be any obvious regional pattern of survival, with many labeled cells surviving in all of the classical CA fields of the hippocampus. Also, there was no evidence of any cells reverting to a tumorous state, nor any indication of an inflammatory response. Some cells were seen around blood vessels, but the pattern was qualitatively different from that of the undifferentiated cells. Instead of completely surrounding the blood vessels, often four to five cells could be seen in a restricted region of the perivascular space.

TIME COURSE OF SURVIVAL OF INTRAHIPPOCAMPAL GRAFTS OF DIFFERENTIATED NEUROBLASTOMA CELLS

Procedure

In this pilot study, two groups of rats received either LA-N-2 or C1300 cells and were differentiated and labeled as described earlier. As in the third experiment, they were then transplanted bilaterally into the hippocampus of rats that had received medial septal lesions 7 days earlier. Groups of rats were then sacrificed 7, 30, or 120 days later, and 40-μ-thick sections through the hippocampus were processed for autoradiography. Two additional groups received identical transplants of LA-N-2 or C1300 cells that were rendered nonviable by 1) a 1-hr incubation *in vitro* with 1% sodium azide or by 2) trypsinization followed by resuspension in PBS with 10% dimethysulfoxide for 1 hr. Ninety-nine percent of these cells were nonviable as determined by trypan blue exclusion, and they served as a control for any positive autoradiographic labeling that might have been within the hippocampus, due to the presence of nonviable cells, or the incorporation of the label by scavenger cells. These rats were sacrificed 30 days later and were also processed for autoradiography.

Results

Both cell types showed a similar survival 7 days after the transplantation. Numerous ARG-labeled cells were observed in parenchyma of the host hippocampus (FIG. 5). Additionally, many cells were seen around blood vessels and below the hippocampus in the cerebrospinal fluid. These cells appeared attached to the ventral surface of the hippocampus by an extracellular matrix (FIG. 6). Fewer cells were labeled 30 and 120 days after transplantation, although a considerable number of each cell type remained. Additionally, the pattern of distribution between the cell groups took on a different appearance. Most C1300 cells were discerned primarily within the parenchyma of the host (FIG. 5), and were often intermingled with perikarya intrinsic to the hippocampus. In contrast, few LA-N-2 cells were found in the parenchyma. Rather, cells survived predominantly around blood vessels and in the ventricular space just ventral to the hippocampus. Rats that received the nonviable cell grafts did not display [^{3}H]thymidine labeling. An inflammatory response was not evident in any group.

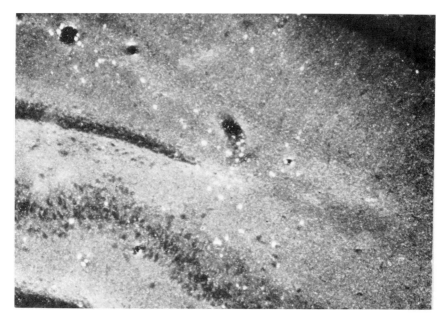

FIGURE 5. Dark-field image of differentiated C1300 neuroblastoma cells visualized with autoradiography surviving within the parenchyma of the hippocampus for 120 days after transplantation. Original magnification: ×100; figure reduced to 70% of original size.

TRANSPLANTS INTO NONHUMAN PRIMATES

The nonhuman primate is the species of choice for evaluating any treatment that has the potential for clinical use.[30] Since monkeys have a brain structure that is similar to man, their use in delineating an optimal donor tissue may be critical.

Procedure

Four African Green (*Cercopithicus aethiops*) monkeys received fornix transections. An additional monkey underwent a sham surgical procedure. Twenty days later, all monkeys received intrahippocampal transplants of the acetylcholine-containing, human-derived, IMR-32 neuroblastoma cells.[31] These cells were labeled with [³H]thymidine and differentiated with either prostaglandin E_1/cAMP ($N = 3$) or mitomycin C/BRDU ($N = 2$). Animals were sacrificed 51-270 days after transplantation. Brains were perfused and processed for ARG and AChE histochemically.

Results

ARG-labeled cells were found in four monkeys. Some neuroblastoma cells were seen around blood vessels and within the host parenchyma. Like the human-derived LA-N-2 cells, a large number of IMR-32 cells were seen outside the hippocampus in the lateral ventricle (FIG. 6). About 90% of these cells stained positively for AChE and appeared attached to the parenchyma by neuritic protuberances. AChE-containing grafted cells were also seen along the needle tract. Not all of the ARG-labeled cells were AChE positive.

DISCUSSION

The present series of experiments were carried out as initial steps in determining whether differentiated neuroblastoma cells are a practical source of donor material for transplantation. This determination is to be made with respect to the five criteria outlined previously. It has been demonstrated that both human- and rodent-derived neuroblastoma cells, once differentiated, survive transplantation into the denervated host without reverting to a tumorous state. Indeed, whereas undifferentiated neuroblastoma cells continue to proliferate within the host, cells survive in large numbers

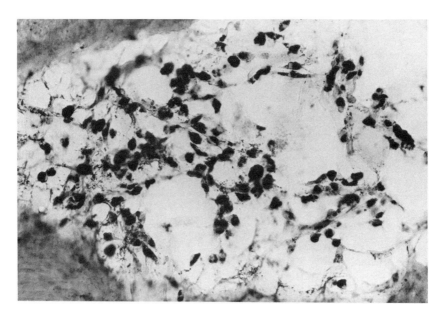

FIGURE 6. Differentiated IMR-32 neuroblastoma cells staining for AChE and surviving for 9 months in the ventricular space below the hippocampus in the African Green (*Cercopithicus aethiops*) nonhuman primate. Original magnification: ×200; figure reduced to 67% of original size.

up to 4 months in the rat and 9 months in the monkey after mitomycin C/BRDU treatment and continue to display a nontumorous phenotype in every animal examined. Like fetal neuron transplants, these cells integrate well within the host, and the brain as an "immunologically privileged site" appears to protect the grafted cells from a significant inflammatory response. Rejection may be further prevented because many neuroblastoma cell lines display only a weak expression for the major human transplantation antigens.[32]

Additionally, these cells appear to function in vitro like normal neural crest-derived neurons. In co-cultures of differentiated cholinergic LA-N-2 cells and muscle cells, synaptic potentials can be detected in the postsynaptic muscle cells, consistent with the presence of functional LA-N-2-muscle synapses as has been reported for certain cholinergic neurons co-cultured with muscle cells.[24-27] Moreover, recent data have demonstrated that intrahippocampal transplantation of LA-N-2 or C1300 cells can attenuate the cognitive dysfunction induced after medial septal lesions.[33]

Although the cell lines tested exhibited positive ChAT immunoreactivity in vitro, we are cautioned by our finding that they did not do so in the rat after transplantation. This apparent discrepancy may be due to environmental factors in vivo and in culture, due to factors specific for the cell lines tested, or due to the species of the host. In fact, we have been able to visualize AChE-positive cells after transplantation of IMR-32 cells into nonhuman primates. Since this cell line is of human origin, it is possible that factors within the nonhuman primate may aid in the expression of the cholinergic phenotype. These findings highlight the necessity of testing different types of neuroblastoma lines and of ultimately choosing the one that is best suited for a particular condition. It is possible that transplanting only a cell line will not be an optimal source of donor material. Indeed, a homogeneous source of cells such as cultured cell lines may not necessarily be best for transplantation because the role of glia in transplanted suspensions or tissue blocks of fetal cells is still unclear.

The data presented clearly prompt further investigation into the possibility of cultured cell lines, such as differentiated neuroblastoma cells, as donor material for transplantation. Differentiated neuroblastoma cells exhibit many neuron-like properties, such as those of altered cell surface proteins, including receptors. These are factors that would appear to be prerequisites for integration into the mammalian central nervous system. Similarly, our electrophysiological data indicate that they can take on some fundamental functional characteristics as well. Taken together, these findings suggest that cultured lines, such as differentiated neuroblastoma cells, may be a viable and practical source of donor cells for transplantation.

ACKNOWLEDGMENTS

We wish to thank Kim Gesell for typing the manuscript, Dorothy Herrera for photographic assistance, and B. Ferbal and V. MacKay for technical assistance.

REFERENCES

1. BJÖRKLUND, A. & U. STENEVI, EDS. 1985. Neural Grafting in the Mammalian CNS. Fernstrom Foundation Series. Vol. 5. Elsevier. Amsterdam.

2. SLADEK, J. R., JR. & D. M. GASH, EDS. 1984. Neural Transplants: Development and Function. Plenum. New York, NY.
3. LUND, R. D. & S. D. HAUSCHKA. 1976. Science **193:** 582-584.
4. MAHALIK, T. J., T. C. FINGER, I. STROMBERG & L. OLSON. 1985. J. Comp. Neurol. **240:** 60-70.
5. MARCIANO, F. F. & D. M. GASH. 1986. Brain Res. **370:** 338-342.
6. FREED, W. J., J. M. MORIHISA, E. SPOOR, B. J. HOFFER, L. OLSON, Å. SEIGER & R. J. WYATT. 1981. Nature **292:** 351-352.
7. FREED, W. J., J. J. PERLOW, F. KAROUM, Å. SEIGER, L. OLSON, B. J. HOFFER & R. J. WYATT. 1979. Ann. Neurol. **8:** 510-519.
8. BACKLUND, E.-O., L. OLSON, Å. SEIGER & O. LINDVALL. 1987. Ann. N.Y. Acad. Sci. This volume.
9. ROSENSTEIN, J. M. & M. W. BRIGHTMAN. 1984. *In* Neural Transplants: Development and Function. J. R. Sladek, Jr. & D. M. Gash, Eds.: 423-443. Plenum. New York, NY.
10. SEEGER, R. C., S. A. RAYNER, A. BANERJEE, H. CHUNG, W. E. LANG, H. B. NEUSTEIN & W. F. BENEDICT. 1977. Cancer Res. **37:** 1364-1367.
11. BOTTENSTEIN, J. E. 1981. *In* Functionally Differentiated Cell Lines. G. H. Saton, Ed. Alan R. Liss. New York, NY.
12. HEFTI, F., J. HARTIKKA & M. SCHLUMPF. 1985. Brain Res. **348:** 283-288.
13. JAEGER, C. A. 1985. Exp. Brain Res. **59:** 615-624.
14. PRASAD, K. N. 1975. Biol. Rev. **50:** 125-268.
15. NELSON, P. G., J. H. PEACOCK, T. AMANO & J. MINNA. 1970. J. Cell. Physiol. **77:** 337-352.
16. SCHUBERT, D., A. J. HARRIS, S. HEINEMANN, Y. KIDOKORO, J. PATRICK & J. H. STEIN-BACH. *In* Tissue Culture of the Nervous System. G. Sato, Ed.: 55-86. Plenum. New York, NY.
17. NOTTER, M. F. D. & J. F. LEARY. 1986. Dev. Brain Res. In press.
18. COSTA, L. G., B. W. SCHWAB & S. D. MURPHY. 1982. Biochem. Pharmacol. **91:** 3407-3413.
19. FEIGENBAUM, P. & E. E. EL-FAKAHANY. 1985. J. Pharmacol. Exp. Ther. **233:** 134-140.
20. AUGUSTI-TOCCO, A. & G. SATO. 1969. Proc. Natl. Acad. Sci. USA **64:** 311-315.
21. KORDOWER, J. H., M. F. D. NOTTER & D. M. GASH. 1984. Soc. Neurosci. Abstr. **10:** 981.
22. BISCHOFF, R. & H. HOLTZER. 1970. J. Cell Biol. **44:** 134-150.
23. STERNBERGER, L. A. 1985. Immunocytochemistry. 2nd edit. Prentice Hall. New York, NY.
24. PURO, D. G., B.-A. BATTELLE & K. E. HANSMANN. 1982. Dev. Biol. **91:** 138-148.
25. YEH, H. H., B.-A. BATTELLE & D. G. PURO. 1984. Dev. Brain Res. **10:** 63-72.
26. PURO, D. G. & H. H. YEH. 1983. J. Neurosci. Res. **10:** 241-250.
27. YEH, H. H., B.-A. BATTELLE & D. G. PURO. 1984. Neuroscience **13:** 901-909.
28. COTMAN, C. W. 1984. *In* Neural Transplants: Development and Function. J. R. Sladek, Jr. & D. M. Gash, Eds.: 305-324. Plenum. New York, NY.
29. GAGE, F. H. & A. BJÖRKLUND. 1986. Neuroscience **17:** 89-98.
30. KORDOWER, J. H. & D. M. GASH. Integrative Psychiatry. In press.
31. TUMILOWITZ, J. J., W. W. NICHOLS, J. J. CHOLON & A. E. CREENE. 1970. Cancer Res. **30:** 2110-2118.
32. LAMPSON, L. A., C. A. FISHER & J. P. WHELAN. 1983. J. Immunol. **130:** 2471-2478.
33. KORDOWER, J. H., M. F. D. NOTTER & D. M. GASH. 1987. Brain Res. In press.

DISCUSSION OF THE PAPER

QUESTIONER: I think the idea of using a cancer cell therapeutically is ironic but nice. During the last couple of days we have heard a lot about undifferentiated nonneuronal cells migrating. You said that the cells migrated into ventricles and that you thought that this was part of the procedure. Have you looked to see whether these cells were in a mitotic state? Did they migrate from the zone of transplantation? This, of course, would not be desirable.

GASH: We find them within several millimeters of the implantation site. My impression is that they diffuse out at the time of implantation. They are injected as a cell suspension. We do not see extensive migration though the needle tracks we follow down, but whenever these cells get into the ventricular system, they can be carried by diffusion.

D. G. STEIN (*Clark University, Worcester, MA*): I have two questions: one on the cells and one on the behavior. First, even though your cells are amitotic, have you thought about injecting cultured neurons to see if they migrate and accumulate in blood vessels? This could still indicate a significant difference between neurons and these other cells.

Second, I notice that it was a 30-sec interval that was the second most difficult interval. It appeared to me that all of the groups that were treated or untreated performed the same even though they were somewhat different from the normal intact controls. Could you comment on why they all came together even though one of the groups was not treated and still performed as well as the others?

GASH: We have followed Garth Thomas's paradigm for behavioral analysis on this, and Jeffrey Kordower and I have worked closely with Garth. He has found that rats with septal lesions can, with training, show recovery. In fact, the animals that we tested at the 30-sec delay interval had the experience of training in the tests conducted at the 0- and 10-sec time intervals (days 1 and 2 of testing). The most pronounced deficits we saw were on the first day of testing.

We have not looked at neuronal migration. We have not looked at transplants of fetal cholinergic neurons. The neuronal migration I would have to talk about would be from our hypothalamic transplants, in which we do see migration out of the grafts of vasopressin neurons and for short distances. The tendency for IMR-32 cells to congregate around blood vessels may be a different property than you find in normal neurons, but I suspect it is going to vary from cell line to cell line.

QUESTIONER: What is the pharmacology of your muscle cell co-cultures?

GASH: The studies with co-cultures were done with Hermes-Jeh. Our technique was developed to look at newborn rat myoblasts that have been cultured and have formed myotubules. This technique has been used to look at retinal cell myotubule interactions and also cholinergic neurons innervating myotubules.

P. PASIK (*Mount Sinai School of Medicine, New York, NY*): What is the longest survival time for neurons that you have transplanted within the primate brain?

GASH: The longest survival has been 9 months in the African Green monkey brain. We transplanted about 80 000 cells in each of four sites per animal. The greatest number of cells we have seen surviving in one site this long after transplantation was several hundred.

Biochemical and Behavioral Correction of MPTP Parkinson-like Syndrome by Fetal Cell Transplantation[a]

ROY A. E. BAKAY[b]

Department of Surgery
Emory University
Yerkes Regional Primate Research Center
and
Veterans Administration Medical Center
Atlanta, Georgia

DANIEL L. BARROW,[c] MASSIMO S. FIANDACA,[c]
P. MICHAEL IUVONE,[d] ARTHUR SCHIFF,[e]
AND DELWOOD C. COLLINS[f]

Departments of [c]Surgery, [d]Pharmacology,
[e]Neurology, and [f]Medicine
Emory University
Atlanta, Georgia

INTRODUCTION

Although it has been known throughout this century that transplanted nervous tissue could survive in the host, it was not until the demonstration that grafted neurons could actually function in their new environment and affect the behavior of their recipients that neurotransplantation received wide attention, and began to be studied in a number of neurobiological research centers.[1] The first reports of behaviorally functioning neurotransplants were from studies conducted in rats with experimental damage to the mesostriatal dopamine system.[2,3] Not only were the biochemical and

[a] This project was funded by the American Parkinson's Disease Association. Support was also received from Emory University; the Yerkes Regional Primate Research Center; the Veterans Administration; and the National Institutes of Health, through Core Grant RR-00-165 and Grant ROI-NS17524 (to P. M. I.).

[b] Address for correspondence and reprint requests: The Emory Clinic, 1365 Clifton Road, N.E., Atlanta, Georgia 30322.

623

behavioral abnormalities corrected, but the transplanted dopaminergic cells actually gave rise to fibers that reinnervated the neostriatum of the host. These and other studies suggested that dopaminergic neurons might be capable of surviving transplantation in primates and have clinical application to patients with Parkinson's disease. What was lacking at that time was an acceptable primate model for parkinsonism. The demonstration of selective neurotoxicity of 1-methyl-4-phenyl-1,2,3,6-tetrahydropyridine (MPTP) to dopaminergic cells of the substantia nigra in human[4] and in nonhuman primates[5,6] has led to the development of a primate model that is clinically, biochemically, and neuropathologically similar to idiopathic parkinsonism. Combining these two important neurobiological areas of investigation, we attempted to investigate whether MPTP-induced parkinsonism in nonhuman primates could be reversed by fetal mesencephalic transplantation.

The first step in designing the experiment was to draw upon the experience derived from transplantation in the rat. One of the keys to success appears to be the transplantation of the fetal tissue at the "critical" interval of maturation. The critical time for fetal transplantation has been serially examined and found to be that stage of gestation just before the final mitosis and final migration of the stem cell for that particular area of brain. Fortunately, the embryology of the rhesus monkey has been evaluated, and the final mitosis for those cells destined to become dopaminergic in the ventral mesencephalon shown to occur between the 35th and 42nd day.[7] Fetal tissue transplantation failures at older gestational ages seem to confirm that transplantation should be performed during this interval, or within this "window," to be successful. The second key to success in fetal transplantation is the technique used to place the tissue in the host. Intraventricular and intracerebral solid grafts, although quite successful in the rat, appeared to represent undesirable methods for grafting in primates. The stereotactic placement of fetal cell suspensions is much more attractive. This is especially true considering that the sprouting from the graft extends a distance of only several millimeters and that the primate brain is 100 to 200 times larger than that of the rodent, suggesting that multiple graft sites would be required.

Our study of fetal mesencephalic transplantation in the treatment of the MPTP model of parkinsonism began in 1984. The preliminary results of the first two transplanted animals were reported at the World Society for Stereotactic and Functional Neurosurgery in Toronto, in 1985.[8] At that time, only two animals had been studied. Since then, we have performed additional transplantations and have gained experience with the MPTP model of parkinsonism. The data and insight accumulated to date form the substance of this report.

MATERIALS AND METHODS

MPTP Preparation

Nine rhesus monkeys (*Macaca mulatta*) aged 2-16 years and weighing 3-11 kg were used for this initial study. The monkeys were adapted to life in individual primate cages, without restraints, in heated and humidified quarters on a 12-hr light/dark cycle (light cycle: 0700-1900). The animals received food and water *ad libitum*. Eight monkeys received at least 0.33 mg MPTP/kg/day i.v. over five separate injection days, as recommended by Burns *et al.*[5] The total doses required to make these animals permanently symptomatic varied from 11 mg of MPTP over 6 weeks to 68 mg of MPTP over 37 weeks. This represents a total dose range of 2.7-21.9 mg/kg, with most animals requiring 4-7 mg/kg. Once the acute behavioral effects (abnormal movements and alterations in motor behavior and posture) of the drug therapy subsided, usually over a period of a few days to several weeks, the animals received further i.v. injections of MPTP (usually at 1-2 mg/day). To ensure the persistence of behavior resembling that which would be seen in Parkinson's disease, that is, Parkinson-like behavior, the clinical behavior and the level of activity of the monkeys were followed for at least 2 months after the final dose of MPTP. Nontransplanted animals with the Parkinson-like syndrome served as controls to assure that spontaneous recovery did not occur after 2 months. If, in a given animal, there was significant improvement during this 2-month interval, the animal received more MPTP and was observed until the deficits were pronounced and stable for 2 months.

During the acute phase of treatment, most of the animals displayed serious Parkinson-like behavior that occasionally affected their eating, drinking, and grooming behavior. Extremely symptomatic animals were given oral Sinemet (Merck, Sharpe & Dohme) in suspensions that provided approximately 100 mg of L-3,4-dihydroxy-phenylalanine (L-DOPA), every 4-6 hr. As previously described by Burns et al.,[5] 30 min after the dose of Sinemet the behavior and movement of the animals were markedly improved. The animals were gradually weaned off the Sinemet so that the chronic effects of the MPTP could be monitored. Two of the animals could not be weaned from the Sinemet without developing severe rigidity and akinesia. These animals were maintained on Sinemet for at least 2 months after their last dose of MPTP, at which time they were sacrificed for neuroanatomical studies. Three of the symptomatic animals have undergone transplantation. An additional animal, not having received intravenous MPTP, received two separate mesencephalic tissue injections from two different fetuses, into multiple subcortical locations. This animal never displayed a movement disorder and served as an immunological and surgical control.

Behavioral Analysis

Spontaneous caged behavior was recorded on videotape with a Canon videocassette recorder. Six-hour taping sessions were conducted during the same part of the day for each animal. Animal behavior was evaluated by an observer having experience with typical rhesus behavior but unaware of the treatment schedule of any of the animals. Each 6-hr videotape was subdivided into 15-sec time intervals, during which the dominant animal behavior and position were recorded. *Behavior* was either stationary or active. *Position* was either "up" (where both feet of the animal were off the bottom of the cage) or "down" (where the animal had one or both feet touching the bottom of the cage). *Crossover* was defined as a movement from the up to down position, or vice versa; *stationary behavior,* as a combination of time spent sitting, eating, pruning, or in a perched position, not involving skilled or complex whole body movements; *sitting,* as a time when the animal maintained a position with knees flexed, whether or not the buttocks rested on the bottom of the cage; *eating,* as any type of stationary eating, drinking, or chewing activity in any position; *pruning,* as any type of cleaning, grooming, or self-examination behavior, in any position; *perched,* as having all four limbs off the floor of the cage, holding onto the bars, without movement; *active behavior,* as a combination of time spent in acrobatic, circling, and other types of activity involving complex movements or whole body movements; *acrobatic behavior,* as any type of physical activity requiring complex motor movement, such as jumping, somersaults; *circling,* as any type of circular walking behavior where the animal returned to the point of origin within a short period of time; *other,* as any type of active or complex behavior not defined by the previous two definitions of active behavior. Many other behavioral parameters were observed. These were difficult to quantitate, but were readily visible on the videotapes (such as rapidity of movements, aggressive behavior, and facial expression). Clinical evaluation of behavior was made with regard to the degree of hyperkinesia, rigidity, flexed posture, and tremor. Each sign of Parkinson-like behavior was assigned a grade from normal to severe on a 0-4 scale.

Biochemical Analysis

Biochemical studies were carried out on cerebrospinal fluid (CSF) obtained from the monkeys via cisterna magna taps. Two methods of analysis were used: a radioenzymatic assay[9] and a high-pressure liquid chromatography (HPLC) technique.[10] The radioenzymatic method determined CSF concentrations of dopamine and L-DOPA. An HPLC method was used for determining CSF concentrations of two dopamine metabolites, homovanillic acid (HVA) and 3,4-dihydroxyphenylacetic acid (DOPAC), as well as the serotonin metabolite 5-hydroxyindole acetic acid (5-HIAA). In addition, punch biopsies were obtained from unperfused caudate nuclei of untreated and MPTP-treated monkeys for tyrosine hydroxylase (TH) activity determination.[11] Similar tissue was obtained by surgical resection of the right caudate nucleus from two of the transplanted animals (designated ROZ and RMZ) prior to perfusion. This was achieved under general anesthesia by a transcallosal exposure of the head of the caudate, through the right lateral ventricle. The tissue was immediately frozen in freon and placed on dry ice for catecholamine histofluorescence utilizing the glyoxylic acid method of de la Torre,[12] and TH assay. The animal was then given a lethal dose of pentobarbital and transcardially perfused with 10% formalin for histological evaluation.

Transplantation Technique

Fetal age is determined by a timed-breeding program that is routinely carried out at the Yerkes Regional Primate Research Center. Pregnant female monkeys have palpable uterine changes at about 30 days gestation. Since the breeding time is approximately 36-48 hr, there may be a 1-2-day error in estimated gestational age (EGA). Fetuses are obtained via cesarean section, with the mother under general anesthesia. Fetal crown-to-rump (CR) length is measured, and microsurgical dissection of the integument from the fetal central nervous system is performed allowing clean resection of the ventral mesencephalon. Ventral mesencephalic tissue then undergoes incubation for enzymatic dispersion with a 0.01% trypsin-pancreatin solution, followed by mechanical dispersion of mesencephalic cells using flamed-pipet techniques as described by Brundin *et al.*[13] The last fetus to be transplanted used a modified technique with the addition of DNase to the standard trypsin-pancreatin solution.

The first fetus, used to transplant ROZ and RSY, had an EGA of 35 days and a CR length of 15 mm. A final volume of 1 ml was made up of the mesencephalic cell suspension, having a cell count of 1900 cells/μl. Trypan blue was used to stain nonviable cells, and approximately 60% were found to be viable, making the viable cell count 1140 cells/μl. A total of three stereotactically placed injections of 10-15 μl each were made in each of six graft tracts in ROZ (three in each caudate). An additional 10-15 μl of this suspension was injected into each of four subcortical tracts in RSY.

The second fetus, used to transplant RMZ and RSY had an EGA of 37 days and a CR length of 16 mm. A final volume of 500 μl of suspension, having a cell count of 1700 cells/μl, was used for transplantation. Trypan blue staining again determined that 60% of the cells were viable (1020 cells/μl). The same procedure, volume per injection, and number of injections were carried out in RMZ and RSY as has just been described for ROZ.

The final fetus's mesencephalic tissue was transplanted only into Z352. Its EGA was 36 days, and its CR length was 16 mm. A final volume of 300 μl of mesencephalic cell suspension was used for transplantation. Three injections of 10 μl were carried out in each of nine striatal tracts (five on the left and four on the right). Cell counts had been determined as 723 cells/10 μl with 90% viability (650 viable cells/10 μl) using the modified dispersion technique.

RESULTS

Behavior after MPTP Treatment

Behavior that was videotaped before treatment with MPTP was quite characteristic for normal rhesus monkeys, although showing some variation in the quantity of specific behaviors among the different monkeys. The animals exhibited the various types of stationary and active behaviors described previously. The animals displayed marked differences from baseline behavior after MPTP therapy. The effects were seen after a single i.v. injection in some animals, and they were seen in all animals following two or three doses of MPTP (0.33 mg/kg) over several days. The abnormalities increased in severity after each successive dose. The onset of symptoms occurred within 5-10 min of drug administration and initially lasted up to 1 hr. After five consecutive doses, some of the motor deficits persisted for varying periods of time but resolved to near baseline over the ensuing weeks. All animals required repeated doses of MPTP with large interanimal variability in the total dosage required to obtain a stable Parkinson-like syndrome (range: 2.7-21.9 mg/kg). Most animals required 4-7 mg/kg for the development of a stable syndrome.

The major quantitative behavioral change was that the total time spent sitting was markedly increased in all of the chronic Parkinson-like animals. All animals were quite hypokinetic and rigid after the MPTP treatments. The animals all walked with a flexed posture, had little facial expression, and showed increased drooling and difficulty swallowing their food. Some showed marked difficulty in feeding themselves. These acute changes either resolved completely, prompting further MPTP dosing, or persisted in varying degrees. Postural tremor occurred in only one animal that was moderately affected by the MPTP, and lasted only 2 weeks. Episodes of freezing were seen in all severely affected monkeys. Despite variability of drug dosages and clinical response, stable Parkinson-like animals were produced (TABLE 1). Markedly symptomatic animals responded well to initial doses of oral Sinemet, with a nearly normal return of function. Prolonged replacement therapy (1-2 months) with routine doses of Sinemet caused various complications in two animals, similar to those previously described in humans with Parkinson's disease receiving chronic L-DOPA replacement therapy (that is, the on-off phenomenon, end-of-dose hypokinesia and rigidity, and L-DOPA insensitivity). Short drug holidays in these animals, with veterinary support for alimentation, allowed the drug to be reinstated with some success. An example of a complex unsuccessful response to drug therapy is shown in FIGURE 1 and TABLE 2.

Anatomical studies were carried out in normal monkeys as well as in three MPTP-treated, chronically Parkinson-like monkeys. Unperfused tissue subjected to the de la Torre catecholamine fluorescence method[12] showed fluorescent cell bodies in the untreated substantia nigra (FIG. 2), as well as fluorescent cell processes in the striatum (FIG. 3). MPTP-treated animals displayed little or no specific fluorescence in their substantia nigra (FIG. 4), especially in the region of the pars compacta. Fluorescent

TABLE 1. Clinical Evaluation of a Rhesus Monkey before and after MPTP Administration in Animal Z352[a]

Clinical Sign	Before MPTP	After MPTP		
		Immediately	1 Month[b]	8 Months[b]
Hypokinesia	0	3	3	3
Rigidity	0	3	3	3
Flexed posture	0	3	3	3
Tremor	0	0	0	0

[a] The clinical findings are graded as follows: 0: normal; 1: mild; 2: moderate; 3: severe; 4: severe on medication.
[b] Without medication.

cell processes were not seen in the striatum of an MPTP-treated animal (FIG. 5). Perfused tissue underwent normal histologic staining and routine microscopy. The untreated animals displayed a normal complement of cells in the substantia nigra and striatum. MPTP-treated monkeys displayed marked neuronal loss in the substantia nigra, especially the pars compacta. The striatum showed no light microscopic evidence of nerve cell degeneration or gliosis. Perfused tissue also underwent special staining for examination by transmission electron microscopy (TEM). Of interest, the MPTP-treated monkeys exhibited degenerating axon terminals in the striatum by TEM that were not seen in untreated monkeys.

Biochemistry after MPTP Treatment

The results on CSF levels of dopamine and L-DOPA obtained with a radioenzymatic assay[9] have proven to be quite variable, possibly because of cross-reaction

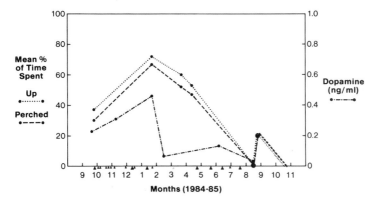

FIGURE 1. Behavior and biochemical performance of RLZ.

with compounds other than dopamine and L-DOPA. The average dopamine concentration in the cisternal CSF of untreated animals was 124 ± 132 pg/ml ($N = 13$). The average L-DOPA concentration in cisternal CSF was 866 ± 467 pg/ml ($N = 13$). Dopamine and L-DOPA levels in CSF 1 month after the last dose of MPTP were decreased to 22 ± 12 pg/ml ($N = 6$) and 600 ± 432 pg/ml ($N = 6$), respectively. Animals with a chronic Parkinson-like syndrome had dopamine and L-DOPA levels in their CSF of 76 ± 99 pg/ml ($N = 4$) and 612 ± 462 pg/ml ($N = 4$), respectively. CSF analysis via the HPLC method disclosed the following untreated control levels ($N = 3$): HVA: 258 ± 20 ng/ml; DOPAC: 4.57 ± 0.19 ng/ml; and 5-HIAA: 72.8 ± 2.4 ng/ml. The CSF of MPTP-treated animals 1 month after their last dose of the drug showed the following dopamine metabolite levels ($N = 4$): HVA: 67 ± 11 ng/ml; DOPAC: 2.43 ± 0.22 ng/ml; and 5-HIAA: 68.8 ± 12 ng/ml. The HVA and DOPAC levels after MPTP treatment differed significantly ($p < .01$) from the control values, showing drops in concentration of 75% and 32%, respectively. The CSF 5-HIAA levels in MPTP-treated animals did not differ from

TABLE 2. Analysis of Videotaped Home Cage Activity of Animal RLZ before and after MPTP Administration and after Subsequent L-DOPA Therapy

| | | Immediately | After L-DOPA | |
| | | | --- | --- |
Activity	Before MPTP	after MPTP	1 Month	2 Months
Up in cage [a]	22 ± 9	0	12 ± 6	0
	(6-45)		(0-60)	
Active behavior[a]	2 ± 2	1 ± 1	2 ± 1	0
	(0-10)	(0-4)	(0-7)	
Crossover[b]	33 ± 12	0	1 ± 1	0
	(11-58)		(0-2)	

[a] Mean number of minutes per hour with standard deviation and range ($N = 12$).
[b] Mean number of crossovers per hour from top to bottom of cage with standard deviation and range ($N = 12$).

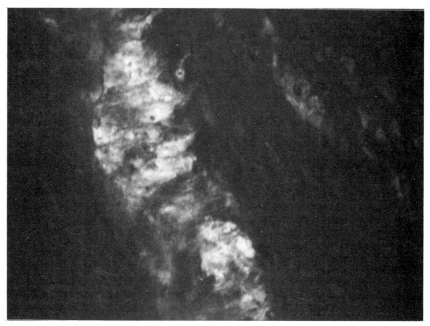

FIGURE 2. This photomicrograph of normal rhesus monkey substantia nigra demonstrates the catecholamine-fluorescent cells in the pars compacta.

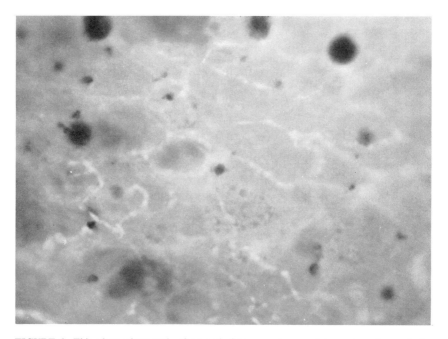

FIGURE 3. This photomicrograph of normal rhesus monkey caudate nucleus demonstrates catecholamine-fluorescent fiber processes interspersed among nonfluorescent neurons.

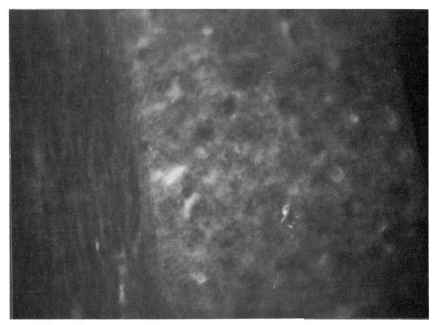

FIGURE 4. This photomicrograph of the substantia nigra of an MPTP-treated rhesus monkey with Parkinson-like behavior demonstrates the paucity of catecholamine-fluorescent cells in the pars compacta.

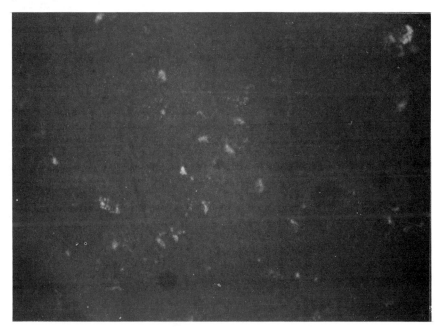

FIGURE 5. This photomicrograph of the caudate nucleus of an MPTP-treated rhesus monkey with Parkinson-like behavior demonstrates the relative lack of catecholamine-fluorescent processes. The small spots represent lipofuchsin.

those in controls. TH activity in the caudate nuclei of MPTP-treated monkeys was greatly reduced (control: 4.9 pmol/min·mg protein, $N = 2$; MPTP: 0.32 pmol/min·mg protein, $N = 2$).

Behavior after Transplantation

After the transplantation procedure, all three monkeys that displayed Parkinson-like behavior showed functional improvement. The amount of time that one of these animals (ROZ) spent "up," along with the number of crossovers, increased following transplantation. The mean percentage of time spent in active behavior after transplantation was only slightly elevated compared to the level seen after MPTP treatment, and did not reach the level seen before MPTP treatment (TABLE 3). The other monkey that showed early Parkinson-like behavior (RMZ) also showed changes in the fraction of time spent sitting after transplantation, such that the stationary activity of the animal was essentially brought back toward the baseline. Active behavior and the number of crossovers showed little change from the levels seen in this animal after MPTP treatment such that the changes that were seen after transplantation are difficult to interpret (TABLE 3). Both ROZ and RMZ, after receiving their intrastriatal grafts, showed marked improvement in their overall body tone, in the overall quickness of their movements, in their ability to feed themselves, and in their ability to swallow food and secretions. Improvement in these behaviors was initially noted during the first month after transplantation in both animals (TABLE 4). The animals were observed for a total of 2 months after transplantation before being sacrificed for anatomical analysis. The monkey with chronic Parkinson-like behavior (Z352) has shown

TABLE 3. Analysis of Videotaped Home Cage Activity of Two Rhesus Monkeys before and after MPTP Administration and after Fetal Mesencephalic Tissue Transplantation

Animal	Activity	Before MPTP	After MPTP	After Transplantation	
				1 Month	2 Months
ROZ	Up in cage[a]	13.8 ± 10	12.3 ± 10	33 ± 16	34 ± 16
		(0-30)	(0-25)	(8-57)	(6-55)
	Active behavior[a]	20 ± 21	2 ± 4	4 ± 4	6 ± 3
		(0-58)	(0-12)	(0-16)	(1-12)
	Crossover[b]	22 ± 16	12 ± 8	19 ± 9	19 ± 7
		(0-46)	(0-23)	(9-40)	(7-29)
RMZ	Up in cage[a]	13 ± 5	18 ± 7	24 ± 10	30 ± 12
		(4-20)	(4-26)	(1-32)	(10-56)
	Active behavior[a]	28 ± 10	19 ± 6	24 ± 8	22 ± 14
		(11-44)	(5-28)	(7-38)	(2-46)
	Crossover[b]	41 ± 11	38 ± 10	35 ± 12	35 ± 10
		(22-55)	(15-52)	(6-49)	(22-58)

[a] Mean number of minutes per hour with standard deviation and range ($N = 12$).

[b] Mean number of crossovers per hour from top to bottom of cage with standard deviation and range ($N = 12$).

TABLE 4. Clinical Evaluation of Three Rhesus Monkeys before and after MPTP Administration and after Fetal Mesencephalic Tissue Transplantation[a]

| Animal | Clinical Sign | Before MPTP | After MPTP | After Transplantation | |
				1 Month	2 Months
ROZ	Hypokinesia	0	3	2	1
	Rigidity	0	2	1	1
	Flexed posture	0	2	1	1
	Tremor	0	0	0	0
RMZ	Hypokinesia	0	2	2	1
	Rigidity	0	2	1	0
	Flexed posture	0	2	1	0
	Tremor	0	1[b]	0	0
Z352	Hypokinesia	0	3	2	2
	Rigidity	0	3	3	2
	Flexed posture	0	3	3	3
	Tremor	0	0	0	0

[a] The clinical findings are graded as follows: 0: normal; 1: mild; 2: moderate; 3: severe; 4: severe on medication.
[b] For 2 weeks.

much less initial improvement (TABLE 4) but continues to be monitored and is still improving.

The surgical control animal (RSY) received a total of two separate sets of subcortical transplants, 1 month apart, from two different fetuses. RSYs behavior before and after each surgical procedure did not change from baseline and showed no behavioral changes from normal after a 13-month follow-up. This animal is being evaluated for any chronic immunologic reactions.

Anatomical studies have been completed only on our first two animals with Parkinson-like behavior that received transplants. Routine histologic sections showed that the substantia nigra of these transplanted animals had cell losses similar to those seen in our control MPTP animals. The caudate nuclei of ROZ and RMZ showed catecholamine fluorescent cells in the regions of the tracts of the stereotactic implants (FIG. 6). Some fluorescent cells had migrated away from the tracts, into the substance of the caudate nucleus. A rich network of catecholaminergic fibers extending from these catecholaminergic cells was also observed. No specific cell counts were carried out on these sections, but approximately 50-100 cells/tract were observed. Since a total of six tracts were present in each animal, we are postulating the presence of, at most, 300-600 viable catecholamine-producing cells in each of these animals, 2 months after transplantation.

Biochemistry after Transplantation

After transplantation, CSF biochemical analysis again included determinations of dopamine and L-DOPA via the radioenzymatic method, since analysis by HPLC was not available on the first two animals that received transplants (TABLE 5). When

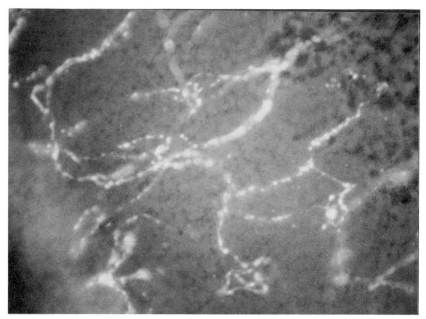

FIGURE 6. A fetal mesencephalic transplant tract is located on the left of this catecholamine fluorescence photomicrograph. Note the fluorescent fibers that extend into the adjacent host caudate.

comparing the data from these animals to the data from our other animals with chronic Parkinson-like behavior (dopamine and L-DOPA levels of 76 ± 99 pg/ml ($N = 4$) and 612 ± 462 pg/ml ($N = 4$), respectively), we see that the L-DOPA levels for RMZ and ROZ after MPTP treatment are much lower than those for the other animals, but within the large standard error. After transplantation, ROZ and RMZ show increases in CSF L-DOPA both at 1 month and 2 months (FIG. 7).

The activity of TH was determined in punch biopsies taken from the caudate

TABLE 5. CSF Biochemical Analysis after Transplantation

| | Dopamine Level (pg/ml) | | L-DOPA Level (pg/ml) | |
	ROZ	RMZ	ROZ	RMZ
Before MPTP treatment	380	242	710	640
After MPTP treatment[a]			160	170
After transplantation				
1 month after	75	55	240	180
2 months after	122	84	780	840

[a] CSF dopamine levels after MPTP treatment are not available because of technical difficulties with the assay.

nucleus of an MPTP-treated monkey that had received transplants. The caudate TH activity far from the grafts was similar to that previously determined in MPTP-treated animals. Regions closer to the graft showed intermediate levels of TH activity; in areas immediately surrounding the transplanted cells, however, the measured activity was 3.9 pmol/min·mg protein (normal control: 4.9 pmol/min·mg protein ($N = 2$)).

DISCUSSION

Although this study includes only a few animals, we believe that our results suggest answers to several questions. First of all, we were able to show that animals treated with MPTP do develop a Parkinson-like syndrome and that the MPTP-treated primate will be a good animal model to study transplant plasticity in the central nervous system. There was a marked variation in the amount of MPTP that was necessary to

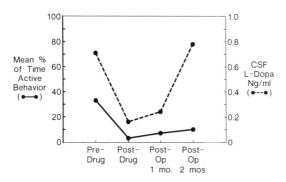

FIGURE 7. Behavioral and biochemical performance of ROZ.

induce the stable Parkinson-like syndrome, but, with careful titration, monkeys with unquestionable Parkinson-like behavior could be produced. Furthermore, these animals could remain functional enough to feed and care for themselves without the need of medications. So far, we cannot adequately explain the reason why these animals show such a large variation in the amount of MPTP necessary to produce a chronic Parkinson-like state. One possible mechanism that we are currently exploring is the age of the animal in relation to nigrostriatal susceptibility to MPTP. Burns *et al.*[14] and Langston (personal communication, 1985) have proposed that age progressively decreases the total dopaminergic cell population in both humans and rhesus monkeys. With normal aging, there is a dropout of nigral dopaminergic cells. It has been postulated that less of a toxic insult to the nigral dopaminergic cell population would be necessary in an older animal compared to a younger animal because the older animal has already lost an age-dependent portion of the nigrostriatal system. Whatever the mechanism, this new model of parkinsonism and the new techniques for tissue transplantation provide useful tools in attempts to replace lost physiologic function in primates.

Parkinsonism is an outstanding model system for transplantation investigations because there is but a single major neurotransmitter deficit resulting from the loss of a single discrete population of cells whose axons terminate predominantly on a single target. Furthermore, the neurotransmitter influence is generally one of "permissiveness" on the target organ rather than one providing specific informational input.

Fetal mesencephalic transplantation has the theoretical advantage that the precise neurons that are required for reversal of the neurological deficit can be integrated into the host. Mesencephalic transplants have demonstrated spontaneously active neurons that fire at rates indistinguishable from those of normal nigral neurons.[15,16] The transplanted neurons have also demonstrated the ability to sustain intracranial self-stimulation, suggesting that the transplanted neurons, under certain circumstances, convey specific, temporally organized information axonally to the reinnervated striatum.[17,18] A major disadvantage of utilizing fetal neural transplants is the difficulty in acquiring this tissue should such therapy ever be applied to the human situation. The legal[19] and moral[20,21] debates have already started. Other disadvantages of these heterotopic allografts are the risk of immunologic rejection and the potential initiation of an autoimmune encephalopathy.

The question that begs to be answered is whether these techniques can significantly improve the behavioral deficit of human parkinsonism. The answer is complex because not only must the transplant survive and continue to function, but it must do so without immunological injury to the host. Although biochemical and anatomical data are essential to guide the development of these transplantation techniques, ultimately, only the behavioral improvement matters. Therefore, a successful transplantation must be defined as one in which the graft becomes anatomically integrated within the host and in which persistent, clinically significant behavioral improvement results.

Unquestionably, we have been able to demonstrate the anatomical integration of fetal mesencephalic cells into the caudate nucleus of the host. These cells have definitely altered the biochemical milieu, and the result has been behavioral improvement. We have performed immunologic evaluations in animals that have shown such improvement, and these evaluations, to date, have not demonstrated any evidence of antibody formation by lymphocytotoxic cross-match reactions in the serum of the host. Furthermore, no inflammatory cell response around the graft site has been detected in the two animals in which this has been investigated. The control animal, which received two different allograft tissues (documented to be allografts by rhesus monkey tissue typing), demonstrated no immunologic response in the CSF or serum following either set of subcortical injections, which were made approximately 1 month apart. This absence of immune reaction occurred even though one of the parents was the same for both fetuses. Similarly, no evidence of an immune encephalopathy has been demonstrable in the CSF by immunoglobulin G electrophoresis or myelin basic protein determinations. Despite this "success," the key element that is missing is persistence. The transplants must continue to promote behavioral improvements over the natural life of the animal in order to be truly successful. Long-term studies are required in order to answer the question of whether effective and immunologically safe transplantation can be performed in primates.

The degree to which the behavioral abnormalities can be reversed appears to be quite different in the initial two animals and the subsequent third animal that displayed Parkinson-like behavior (this may be due to a number of parameters, such as severity of symptoms, duration of symptoms, number of cells transplanted, age of the animals). The questions raised by this discrepancy can only be answered by further studies, and the answers to these questions may lie in factors that are not apparent at this time.

CONCLUSIONS

Intensive basic science research is being performed in the area of neural tissue transplantation to determine if such techniques are suitable for application to the human condition. Parkinsonism is an excellent disease in which to study the potential usefulness of this technology. Human studies at this time are extremely premature, and the only means by which future human benefit can be predicted is through a firm research foundation through development of transplantation techniques in nonhuman primates. This paper helps confirm that fetal tissue can be used to reverse the neurologic deficits of parkinsonism in primates. But, like all papers of any substance, it raises more questions than it answers: What is the optimal tissue for transplantation? Where are the optimal target sites for graft placement? What adjuvant therapy may be required for enhancing graft success? What is the potential for immunological complications from allografts? All of these questions require answers before a human study may begin. The most important question to be answered, however, is whether severe deficits can be improved and remain improved over the long term. We believe that the long-term demonstration of successful reversal of a nonhuman primate Parkinson-like syndrome by transplantation techniques should precede any human investigations.

ACKNOWLEDGMENTS

We wish to thank the outstanding staff at the Yerkes Regional Primate Research Center for their support, which proved indispensible to the execution of this project. We also wish to thank Joyce Klemm and Mary Alice Smith for their technical assistance.

REFERENCES

1. BJÖRKLUND, A. & U. STENEVI. 1985. Intracerebral neural grafting: A historical perspective. *In* Neural Grafting in the Mammalian CNS. A. Björklund & U. Stenevi, Eds.: 3-14. Elsevier. Amsterdam.
2. BJÖRKLUND, A. & U. STENEVI. 1979. Reconstruction of the nigrostriatal pathway by intracerebral nigral transplants. Brain Res. **177:** 555-560.
3. PERLOW, M. J., W. J. FREED, B. J. HOFFER, O. SEIGER, L. OLSON & R. J. WYATT. 1979. Brain grafts reduce motor abnormalities produced by destruction of the nigrostriatal dopamine system. Science **204:** 643-647.
4. DAVIS, G. C., A. C. WILLIAMS, S. P. MARKEY, M. H. ELBERT, E. D. CAINE, C. M. REICHERT & J. J. KOPIN. 1979. Chronic parkinsonism secondary to intravenous injection of meperidine analogues. Psychiatr. Res. **1:** 249-254.
5. BURNS, R. S., C. C. CHIUEH, S. P. MARKEY, M. H. ELBERT, D. M. JACOBOWITZ & J. J. KOPIN. 1983. A primate model of parkinsonism-selective destruction of dopaminergic neurons in the pars compacta of the substantia nigra by N-methyl-4-phenyl-1,2,3,6-tetrahydropyridine. Proc. Natl. Acad. Sci. USA **80:** 4546-4550.
6. LANGSTON, J. W., L. S. FORNO, C. S. REBERT & I. IRWIN. 1984. Selective nigral toxicity after systemic administration of 1-methyl-4-phenyl-1,2,3,6-tetrahydropyridine (MPTP) in the squirrel monkey. Brain Res. **292:** 390-394.

7. LEVITT, P. & P. RAKIC. 1982. The time of genesis, embryonic origin and differentiation of the brain stem monoamine neurons in the rhesus monkey. Dev. Brain Res. **4**: 35-37.
8. BAKAY, R. A. E., M. S. FIANDACA, D. L. BARROW, A. SCHIFF & D. C. COLLINS. 1985. Preliminary report on the use of fetal neural tissue transplantation to correct NMPTP-induced primate model of parkinsonism. Presented at the Ninth Meeting of the World Society for Stereotactic and Functional Neurosurgery. Toronto.
9. PEULER, J. D. & G. A. JOHNSON. 1977. Simultaneous single isotope radioenzymatic assay of plasma norepinephrine, epinephrine and dopamine. Life Sci. **21**: 625-635.
10. MENA, M. A., E. G. AGUADO & J. G. DE YEBENES. 1984. Monoamine metabolites in human cerebrospinal fluid: HPLC/ED method. Acta Neurol. Scand. **69**: 218-225.
11. IUVONE, P. M. 1984. Calcium, ATP and magnesium activate soluble tyrosine hydroxylase from rat striatum. J. Neurochem. **43**: 1359-1368.
12. DE LA TORRE, J. C. 1980. An improved approach to histofluorescence using an SPG method for tissue monoamines. J. Neurosci. Methods. **3**: 1-5.
13. BRUNDIN, P., O. ISACSON, F. H. GAGE, U. STENEVI & A. BJÖRKLUND. 1985. Intracerebral grafts of neuronal cell suspensions. *In* Neural Grafting in the Mammalian CNS. A. Björklund & U. Stenevi, Eds.: 51-59. Elsevier. Amsterdam.
14. BURNS, R. S., S. P. MORKEY, J. M. PHILLIPS & C. C. CHIUEH. 1984. The neurotoxicity of 1-methyl-4-phenyl-1,2,3,6-tetrahydropyridine in monkey and man. Can. J. Neurol. Sci. **11**: 166-168.
15. WUERTHELE, S. M., W. J. FREED, L. OLSON, J. MORIHISA, L. SPOOR, R. J. WYATT & B. J. HOFFER. 1981. Effect of dopamine agonists and antagonists on the electrical activity of substantia nigra neurons transplanted into the lateral ventricle of the rat. Exp. Brain Res. **44**: 1-10.
16. HOFFER, B., G. ROSE, G. GERHARDT, I. STROMBERG & L. OLSON. 1985. Demonstration of monoamine release from transplant-reinnervated caudate nucleus by *in vivo* electrochemical detection. *In* Neural Grafting in the Mammalian CNS. A. Björklund & U. Stenevi, Eds.: 437-447. Elsevier. Amsterdam.
17. DUNNETT, S. B., P. J. FRAY, A. BJÖRKLUND, U. STENEVI & S. D. IVERSON. 1981. Self-stimulation from substantia nigra transplants reinnervating the 6-OHDA-lesioned neostriatum of rats. Neurosci. Lett. (Suppl.) **7**: 532.
18. FRAY, P. J., S. B. DUNNETT, S. D. IVERSON, A. BJÖRKLUND & U. STENEVI. 1982. Nigral transplants reinnervating the dopamine-depleted neostriatum can sustain intracranial self-stimulation. Science **219**: 416-419.
19. CARNAHAN, W. A. 1984. Legal implications of the use of embryonic cells for transplants. Appl. Neurophysiol. **47**: 69-72.
20. MURPHY, P. J. 1984. Moral perspectives in the use of embryonic cell transplantation for correction of nervous system disorders. Appl. Neurophysiol. **47**: 65-68.
21. NEVILLE, R. C. 1984. Ethics in medical donations. Appl. Neurophysiol. **47**: 73-76.

DISCUSSION OF THE PAPER

D. M. GASH (*University of Rochester School of Medicine, Rochester, NY*): Several groups have looked at MPTP toxicity. Our group has reported that there is a spontaneous recovery, as you have also indicated. What was the number of control animals, and did any of them show spontaneous recovery?

BAKAY: We had four animals that we considered controls in that they got nothing—in other words, no MPTP. They were just normal animals. We injected MPTP in a total of nine animals, three of which received a transplant. So six of these nine animals did receive a transplant. We make our animals Parkinson-like by a series of small injections of MPTP over time. We allow a recovery time of a couple of weeks, evaluate the animals in terms of their CSF markers, and evaluate behavioral performance on a clinical basis. After the recovery period, we begin another series of injections. This series may last 12 to 36 weeks, so that once the series is completed we have not found spontaneous recovery. During the series you will find some degree of recovery.

GASH: I know that Langston's reported recovery is as long as 3 months or longer following the last dose, so there is a question of how much of the endogenous system can recover. How long do you wait before you decide the animals are not recovering?

BAKAY: Once we have got the animal to maintain itself on a certain behavioral level and a 70% diminution in the DOPAC levels in the CSF, we will wait 2 months before transplanting. For one of them, we waited 8 months and saw no change. The two animals we transplanted earlier were the most successful. Again, does it relate to some sort of spontaneous recovery, or does it relate to the fact that maybe these animals are less severely involved? Maybe there is a critical interval during which you can transplant. All these questions are critical, and but I do not have the answers to them.

E. A. DEBLER (*Nathan S. Klein Institute, New York, NY*): The doses of MPTP you gave, what size were they?

BAKAY: We started off with 0.33 milligrams per kilogram for 5 days. I think Burns recommended this. We subsequently dropped down to lower doses because we were afraid of overdosing some of the animals. In fact we did. Some animals were so severely involved that we had to give them medications.

J. D. ELSWORTH (*Yale University School of Medicine, New Haven, CT*): What was the technique you used to measure the CSF L-DOPA values?

BAKAY: The dopamine and the L-DOPA were measured by an RIA assay. In addition, our pharmacologist, Dr. Iuvone, provided HPLC data. He also performed the TH analysis that on the tissue.

ELSWORTH: The slide showed CSF L-DOPA. Are you saying that the RIA gave an accumulative L-DOPA and dopamine value?

BAKAY: Right.

ELSWORTH: So it is not specifically measuring either one of those compounds.

BAKAY: Right. We have not been happy with the RIA assay because it seems to be quite variable. We have gone back to using almost exclusively the HPLC data.

P. PASIK (*Mount Sinai School of Medicine, New York, NY*): How old were the donor fetuses? You mentioned something about embryonic day 38 or 42. What basis did you use to select that?

BAKAY: From the readings in the literature, from the rat information, we knew that the critical time is just before the last mitosis. The critical time for the rat is certain age, and that for the monkey is very different. From the literature Rakic has published, we knew that mitosis in monkeys occurs between the 35th day and the 42nd day, and so we decided to implant grafts during this interval. We also knew about the work done by Drs. Freed and Morihisa. Their work showed that animals that are older do not appear to have success in their transplants, so we decided we would use the 35-42-day interval.

Certainly, the fetal cells we have taken out do fluoresce.

PASIK: Then you essentially extrapolated from the rat data.

BAKAY: Correct.

J. R. SLADEK, JR. (*University of Rochester School of Medicine, Rochester, NY*): The slide you showed us of the normal "nonlesioned" *Macaca* had fascicles of the occular motor complex exiting the brain. This must mean that you showed us an area of the ventral tegmental area as well as possibly nigra. As Doug Boudin pointed out at the Neuroscience Meetings, and as we and lots of others have seen, that area is somewhat spared after MPTP with respect to dopamine content. Indeed, because the fibers of the nigral striatal pathway pass through the ventral tegmental area and are swollen, this area has one of the higher contents of dopamine. Yet, even though you used low doses of MPTP to make sure your animals were easy to maintain, your second slide showed absolutely no fluorescence in this area. It is somewhat paradoxical that you do not see any fluorescence at all.

BAKAY: We did see some fluorescent cells. I took an area that was reasonably represented. If you look very carefully at the low-power view, you will see there was an area that was fluorescent. Under high power, there was a cell there that fluoresced. We used the third nerve as a landmark only in the first slide. The second slide is from an area more laterally where the SNc is closer to the peduncle.

SLADEK: But if it does have that area, that really should be quite contrary to what you showed. And again, in the first slide of the nigral implant, where you showed that cluster of cells, there appears to be a large myelinated bundle. I am curious as to what this is. Clearly, in the caudate, we would not expect to see it.

BAKAY: I am not sure what you are referring to. Are you talking about the tract of the fetal transplantation itself?

SLADEK: No. You showed material in which there was a cluster of very bright cells, and of course the neuropil was very bright also. There was this large bundle that looked almost like a myelinated bundle. My first impression was like a case of dé jà vu. It looked like the nigral area, but of course this is not what you intended to show. Still, I would like to know where this bundle was in the caudate.

BAKAY: One of the pictures was very close to the ventricle, and the other part was closer to the internal capsule.

SLADEK: Where were your placements with respect to the capsule and the ventricle?

BAKAY: They were very close. We tried to make a diagonal between the two. We injected all along the line where the maximum diameter of caudate-putamen was and tried to inject straight across it. We made a series of injections—each one along the way so that the entire tract would be filled with cells. We took a diagonal approach across the widest angle. In some areas, it was much closer to the ventricle than others; in others, it was much closer to the internal capsule.

Reversal of Parkinsonism by Fetal Nerve Cell Transplants in Primate Brain[a]

J. R. SLADEK, JR.,[b] T. J. COLLIER,[c] AND
S. N. HABER[d]

Department of Neurobiology and Anatomy
University of Rochester School of Medicine
Rochester, New York 14642

A. Y. DEUTCH,[e] J. D. ELSWORTH,[e] R. H. ROTH,[e,f]
AND D. E. REDMOND, JR.[e,f,g]

[e]*Department of Pharmacology*
and
[f]*Department of Psychiatry*
Yale University School of Medicine
New Haven, Connecticut 06510

INTRODUCTION

Parkinson's disease is an age-related, neurodegenerative disorder that afflicts close to 500 000 people in the United States alone. This progressive disease results in hypokinesia, episodes of freezing, tremor, difficulty in initiating movement, and other signs. Although the etiology is unclear, a marked loss of dopaminergic input to the striatum from the substantia nigra is known to be a constant feature of the disease. Replacement pharmacotherapy with the dopamine (DA) precurser, 3,4-dihydroxy-phenylalanine (L-DOPA), is somewhat effective in treating the disorder, but usually does not provide lasting reversal of the associated motor disorders.[1]

[a]This work was supported by Grants AG 00847, NS 15816, MH 14092, MH 25642, and MH 14276. It also received core support from the St. Kitts Biomedical Research Foundation, the Axion Research Foundation, and the University of Rochester.

[b]Address for correspondence: University of Rochester School of Medicine and Dentistry, 601 Elmwood Avenue, Rochester, New York 14642.

[c]An Alzheimer's Disease and Related Disorders Association Faculty Scholar.

[d]Supported by RSCDA K04-NS 01071.

[g]Supported by RSCDA K05-DA 00075 and K05-MH 00643.

A strikingly close animal model of this disease has been produced in monkeys by the administration of the neurotoxin N-methyl-4-phenyl-1,2,3,6-tetrahydropyridine (MPTP). In several species of primates, including human upon accidental exposure, the parkinsonian deficits have been long lasting and in part improved by L-DOPA therapy.[2] MPTP induces a significant loss of nigrostriatal DA neurons as measured biochemically and morphologically.[3] Thus, parallels between MPTP-induced and naturally occurring parkinsonism make the former a particularly useful model for assessing the therapeutic value of neural grafts in the treatment of parkinsonism.

A great deal is known about the usefulness of grafts of fetal DA-containing neurons to improve lesion-induced motor abnormalities in rats.[4,5] Dopaminergic neuronal grafts from fetal rat brain survive, grow, and functionally integrate into host adult brain. These interrelated phenomena are seen even in the absence of immunosuppressant drug administration. Grafts of adrenal chromaffin cells, which are known to produce DA as an essential precursor to their releasable product, epinephrine, also can improve these motor abnormalities in rats, but to a lesser extent than grafts of fetal neurons.[6] The first attempts at therapeutic grafting in humans suffering from parkinsonism have utilized the adrenal chromaffin cells of the patients as donor tissue and have not resulted in any significant or lasting improvements in motor deficits.[7] Although the reasons for this consistent lack of improvement in the first human autograft recipients are unknown, it is clear that any potential utilization of therapeutic attempts with fetal neurons as donor tissue should be preceded by thorough examination of transplantation procedures and results, both short and long term, in nonhuman primates in order to address essential questions about the safety and effectiveness of this procedure. The present study was designed as an initial exploration of fetal neuron survival, growth, and function after transplantation into monkey brain.

METHODS

Five adult male African Green monkeys (*Cercopithecus aethiops sabaeus*) from the St. Kitts colony were treated with MPTP (0.30-0.40 mg/kg, four to five times over 5 days) as part of a baseline study to determine the effective dosages, extent of nigrostriatal damage, behavioral similarity to parkinsonism, and neurochemical correlates of the disease as reported elsewhere.[3,8] Six untreated monkeys served as controls. Nine additional monkeys were treated with MPTP, three for use as transplant recipients and five as nontransplanted controls. MPTP doseages were 0.25-0.40 mg/kg administered six times over 5 days for controls and 0.40 mg/kg for the intended transplant recipients. Over 30 different behavioral observations and ratings were made before and after MPTP treatment and for a period of 10 weeks after transplantation. Biochemical measures of the DA metabolite, homovanillic acid (HVA), were made at comparable time courses from cisternal taps of cerebrospinal fluid (CSF).

Transplantation of fetal substantia nigra (SN) was performed according to protocols established in nonhuman primates. Solid grafts of SN from a single late gestational fetal African Green monkey were transplanted simultaneously and bilaterally into multiple sites (that is, three penetrations in each striatum with three drops/penetration for a total of 18 solid grafts) into the striata of two adult hosts, which were designated S092 and S054. A third monkey (S114) served as a control and received early gestational SN bilaterally, into the overlying cingulate cortex as well as hypothalamic DA neurons in the left striatum and noradrenergic neurons from the locus ceruleus and subceruleus in the right striatum. After transplantation, animals were monitored for up to 10 weeks. Host brains were perfused for immunohisto-chemical analysis for demonstration of the DA synthetic enzyme, tyrosine hydroxylase (TH), using primary antiserum (Eugene Tech, Allendale, NJ) according to a standard protocol.[9]

RESULTS

General Observations

The multiple cannula tracks and associated graft tissue were seen easily in his-tological sections in each implanted monkey (FIGS. 1, 2 & 5). In S092, these bilaterally placed tracks were seen to penetrate the cerebral cortex, corpus callosum, and caudate nucleus. With dark-field illumination, the tracks refracted light differently than host tissue; this difference aided identification of graft tissue. In most instances, the tracks were filled with neural tissue either from the host brain or from the grafts (FIGS. 3, 4 & 5). With the latter, grafted tissue generally appeared more lightly stained than the surrounding host neuropil; this difference aided the identification of TH-stained fibers and cells within the grafts.

Monkey S092

Large numbers of TH-positive neurons were seen within the striata, bilaterally, in this monkey (FIGS. 1 & 2). Most of these neurons were located in the caudate nucleus, although some were seen in the putamen also. Many were clustered deep within the head of the caudate nucleus near the cannula tracks. These neurons were relatively small and showed multiple branched processes. Some were simpler in shape with only one or two visible processes in each 50-μm-thick section. The neuritic processes branched freely throughout the neuropil of the host. Initial quantitative estimates of cell numbers indicate approximately 60 000 TH-positive cells present in both striata in S092.

Monkey S054

Cells stained for TH, comparable to those seen in S092, were also seen in this monkey. These cells numbered on the order of 15 000 in the combined striata and, as in the previous animal, were seen in clusters. Additionally, numerous larger, more multipolar neurons were identified in and near the cannula tracks (FIG. 3). These neurons gave rise to a rich plexus of beaded processes that branched freely throughout the host neuropil. The cannula tracks were filled with transplanted tissue that stained more lightly than the surrounding host neuropil (FIG. 3). This tissue, which was seen

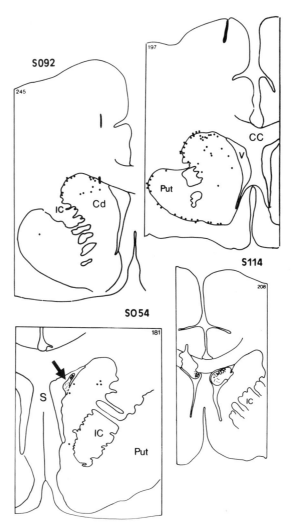

FIGURE 1. This composite diagram illustrates two coronal levels through S092 and one each for S054 and S114. TH-positive cells and fibers appear as large and small dots, respectively. The thick vertical dark lines in S092 represent cannula tracks. Numerous TH-containing neurons are seen in the caudate nucleus (Cd) and putamen (Put), especially at rostral levels as illustrated. These neurons also occur in clusters near the cannula tracks. Similar TH-positive neurons were seen in S054, but to a lesser extent. Additionally, this monkey showed growth of grafted tissue from the cannula tracks into the adjacent lateral ventricle (arrow). TH-positive neurons and fibers were seen in these ventricular grafts. In S114, ventricular grafts were even more prominent and contained dense clusters of TH neurons and fiber networks. CC: corpus callosum; IC: internal capsule; S: septum; V: lateral ventricle.

deep within the head of the caudate nucleus, contained numerous beaded fibers and TH-positive neurons. Grafted tissue extended from the caudate nucleus into the adjacent lateral ventricle, where it expanded in a feather-like array (FIG. 4). Expansion in size of the fetal tissue was apparent because of the increased width of the grafted tissue in comparison to the width of the cannula tracks. Cells within the grafts appeared to give rise to extensive TH-positive networks that consisted of delicate fibers continuous with the TH perikarya within the grafts (FIG. 4).

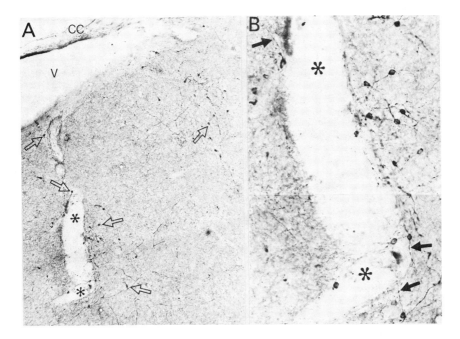

FIGURE 2. (A) A cannula track (asterisks) and clusters of TH-positive neurons (open arrows) are seen in S092. The corpus callosum (CC) and lateral ventricle (V) are noted for orientation. (B) A portion of the field is enlarged to better visualize the densely stained neurons and their beaded processes (solid arrows). Original magnifications for A and B: ×100 and ×250, respectively; figure reduced to 63% of original size.

Monkey S114

There were several unique features of the transplanted areas in this monkey. TH-positive neurons, in contrast to those in S092 and S054, were not seen in the neuropil of the host striata in spite of the transplantation of dopaminergic and noradrenergic neurons in this region. Large pieces of grafted tissue, however, were identified in each host target site. They were seen within the caudate nucleus, lateral ventricle, corpus callosum, and overlying cingulate cortex (FIG. 5). This tissue was considerably greater in size in comparison to that seen in S054; this latter tissue also showed growth into the lateral ventricles. Moreover, each piece of grafted tissue was characterized by an organotypic appearance of TH-positive neurons and fibers. Thus, the graft of hypothalamic DA neurons into the left striatum revealed a large piece of grafted tissue filled with smaller unipolar-to-bipolar neurons reminiscent of hypothalamic DA cells

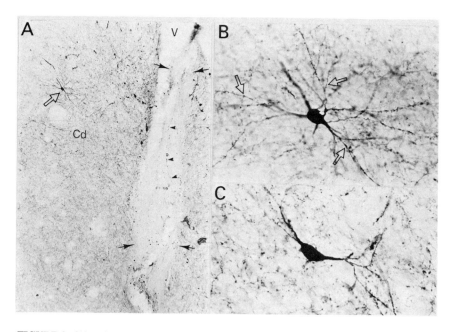

FIGURE 3. (A) A fetal graft (outlined by arrows) is seen in the caudate nucleus (Cd) of S054. It was continuous dorsally with graft tissue that extended into the lateral ventricle (V) as illustrated in FIGURE 4. A TH-stained fiber (arrowheads) is located within the grafted tissue. A relatively large TH-stained neuron (open arrow) is seen near the graft. This multipolar neuron is seen to advantage in B where its beaded processes (open arrows) are evident. Another example of a branched, TH-positive neuron found in the caudate nucleus of S054 is seen in C. Original magnifications for A and for B and C: ×200 and ×700, respectively; figure reduced to 58% of original size.

(FIG. 6). Similarly, the grafts of the dorsal pons into the right caudate nucleus showed clusters of two types of neurons: a dense collection of medium-sized bi- and multipolar neurons and a much less dense cluster of larger, more multipolar neurons, resembling the nuclei locus ceruleus and subceruleus, respectively (FIGS. 7 & 8). Grafts in SN into the cerebral cortex consisted of dense collections of medium-sized, multipolar neurons of uniform size and shape (FIG. 9).

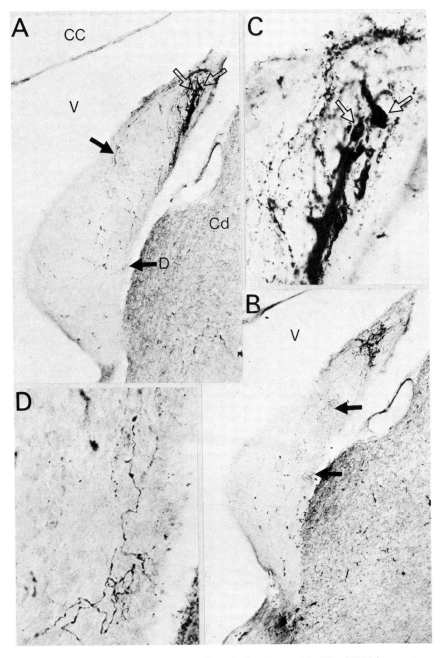

FIGURE 4. An extension of grafted tissue into the lateral ventricle (V) of S054 is seen at an interval of 150 μm in **A** and **B**. The graft contains TH-positive neurons (open arrows) and fibers (closed arrows), which are seen to advantage in **C** and **D**, respectively. CC: corpus callosum: Cd: caudate nucleus; V: lateral ventricle. Original magnifications for **A** and **B** and for **C** and **D**: ×65 and ×340, respectively; figure reduced to 82% of original size.

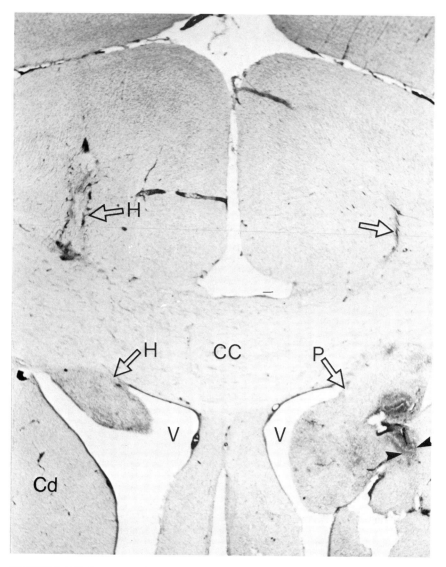

FIGURE 5. This low-power photomicrograph shows the tissue taken from fetal hypothalamus (H) and pons (P) 10 weeks after grafting into S114. A portion of the cannula track (open arrow) on the right side is visible dorsal to the corpus callosum (CC) in this Nissl-stained section. The pontine graft appears to invade the caudate nucleus (Cd) at this level (arrowheads) whereas part of the hypothalamic graft is seen in the cingulate cortex immediately dorsal to the corpus callosum on the left side. Each graft has a large component in the lateral ventricle (V). Original magnification: ×6; enlarged to 105% of original size.

Behavioral and Neurochemical Correlates

Before transplantation, all three monkeys showed signs consistent with the putative damage from MPTP to the nigrostriatal system. These parkinsonian signs included bradykinesia, motor freezing, difficulty with initiating movement, and both resting and postural tremors. That the nigrostriatal system was damaged by this treatment was confirmed by measurement of the CSF concentration of HVA and by subsequent analysis of the nigrostriatal system with TH staining. After transplantation, S092 and S054 showed significant declines in the parkinsonian signs. The motor recovery was greatest in S092, which showed skilled motor coordination, no difficulty in initiating movement, and an absence of postural and resting tremor. This improvement was noted as early as 1-2 days after transplantation surgery. This animal showed a consistently improved parkinsonian score over the duration of the recovery period. Freezing episodes were not apparent. Monkey S054 also showed an improvement after grafting. His motor abnormalities and severe tremor disappeared for 1-2 days and gradually returned during the next several days. Improvement again was seen within 18 and 70 days after surgery with the severity and frequency of tremor diminished. Monkey S114 appeared to improve briefly after surgery, but showed a decline consistent with that of MPTP-treated monkeys that did not receive fetal grafts. This animal was aided by hand-feeding, regular passive exercise, and assistance in altering body position during the entire postsurgical period.

HVA levels in CSF increased in both monkeys that showed functional recovery. In S092 this level rose to 89% of baseline; in S054 it rose to 40% of baseline by 69 days after transplantation surgery (FIG. 10). HVA was not elevated in S114, rather it was depressed, comparable to levels seen in nontransplanted monkeys that received MPTP over a comparable time period.

DISCUSSION

The present results support the therapeutic use of neural transplantation in neurodegenerative disorders, particularly in Parkinson's disease, which is characterized in part by a specific decline of an identified transmitter system. Clearly, the disease is based on a more complex etiology than a loss of only dopaminergic nigrostriatal neurons. Nevertheless, the reversal of parkinsonian signs after transplantation of fetal SN into a primate species closely related to human represents an essential, preliminary next step in the exploration of this question. If this procedure is to become an effective therapeutic strategy in treating parkinsonism, a number of questions raised by this study need to be addressed in nonhuman primates to ensure maximum efficacy and safety as discussed below.

Both monkeys bearing parkinsonian signs that received grafts of fetal SN into the striatum showed an improvement in the mean parkinsonian summary score up to the time of brain removal. The degree of functional recovery in each monkey appeared to correspond closely with both the levels of HVA detected in the CSF and the number of TH-positive neurons found in the implanted striata. This correspondence between cell survival and functional reversal raises an important question about the minimum number of DA neurons required for amelioration of the parkinsonian signs. It has been estimated that about 250 000 DA neurons exist in the SN of the adult old world

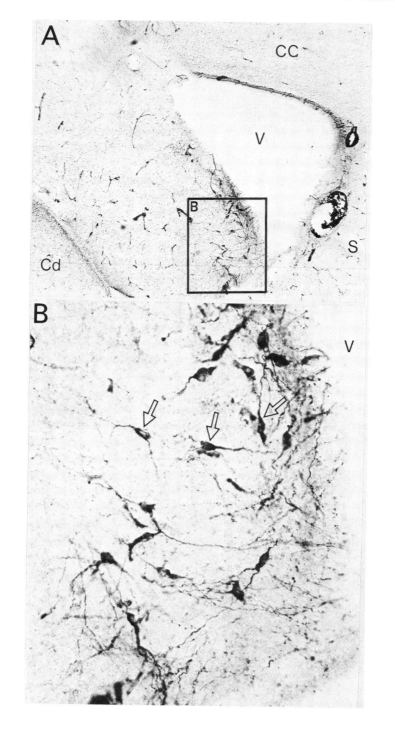

monkey[10] and that 500 000 exist in human. In rodent models of neurological dysfunction associated with either DA or vasopressin deficiencies, improvement in function is seen when only a small percentage (10-20%) of transmitter-specific neurons survive grafting. Moreover, parkinsonian signs are not usually manifested in humans until approximately 80% of the DA neurons of the SN are destroyed. This implies a reserve capacity of the nigrostriatal system, that is, that the DA-mediated behavioral status can be sustained by a small percentage of the neurons of the system even during probable progressive cell loss, which might occur naturally. Thus, it is likely that a relatively small percentage of DA neurons transplanted into the striatum can supply sufficient DA for functional improvement. Accordingly, the estimated 15 000 TH neurons seen in S054 would be sufficient to improve the motor deficits induced by MPTP. That a more rapid response after grafting was seen in S092 is probably related to the greater availability of DA as approximately 60 000 TH neurons were seen after grafting in this monkey. It is perhaps noteworthy that many of the TH-positive neurons in the graft recipient that showed the smaller number of grafted neurons exhibited more elaborate neuritic branching. This may be due to the greater potential availability of synaptic sites in the host striatum. Integration at the synaptic level has been reported after transplantation of fetal SN in the 6-hydroxydopamine-depleted rodent striatum[11] and is likely to occur in primates as well.

Numerous TH-positive neurons were seen through the head of the caudate nucleus and to a lesser extent in the putamen in S092 and S054. Because these neurons were found at a distance of several millimeters from the nearest cannula track, at least two possibilities are raised to explain this phenomenon. Neurons can be induced to shift their transmitter phenotype *in vitro*.[12] Although unreported in the rodent transplant literature, it is not possible to eliminate from consideration that a shift occurred in transmitter expression by a population of noncatecholaminergic neurons of the host brain after the introduction of adult brain. There is no evidence from prior graft experiments in rodents to support this concept, however. A second explanation is that neuronal migration of grafted fetal neurons occurred. Two observations are of interest in this regard. A great number of TH-positive neurons were found several millimeters rostral to the most rostral cannula tracks whereas fewer neurons were seen at levels caudal to the most caudal placements. This rostrally oriented gradient could be accounted for if migrating neuroblasts utilize existing axonal pathways as guidance cues, particularly if existent nigrostriatal axons of the host brain that course in a caudal-to-rostral direction serve as directional avenues. Thus, a situation somewhat analogous to that proposed for the guidance of migrating neuroblasts might also occur in host, adult brain. The second observation of interest in this regard is the marked accumulation of TH neurons seen at the borders of the striatum, especially rostrally. Their accumulation at the junction of the head of the caudate nucleus and the overlying corpus callosum and at the rostral pole of the striatum could be consistent with neuroblast migration that was arrested upon reaching the limits of the appropriate target. This would require a highly ordered level of donor-target specificity. Such

---

FIGURE 6. The hypothalamic graft in S114 reveals large numbers of TH-positive neurons (arrows) seen to advantage in **B** wherein the area enclosed in the rectangle is enlarged. Numerous, bipolar neurons display a size, shape, and neuritic arbor reminiscent of dopaminergic neurons from the hypothalamus. CC: corpus callosum; Cd: caudate nucleus; S: septum; V: lateral ventricle. Original magnifications for **A** and **B**: ×70 and ×350, respectively; figure reduced to 85% of original size.

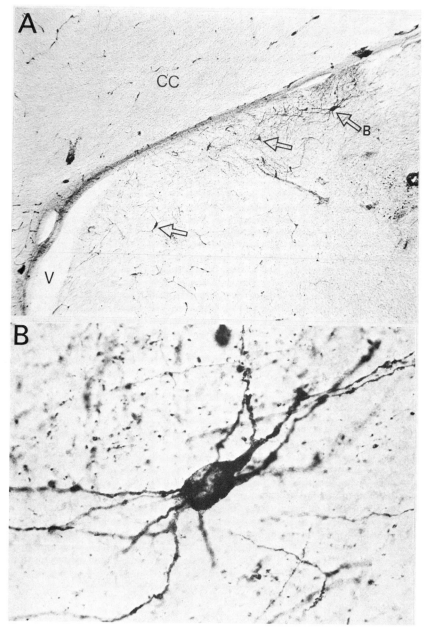

FIGURE 7. Relatively large, TH-positive neurons (open arrows) taken from the region of the nucleus subceruleus and locus ceruleus are found in a large graft (of which only a small portion is illustrated) located primarily in the lateral ventricle (V) in S114. The morphology of these neurons is comparable to that of noradrenergic subceruleal neurons. These neurons are enlarged in **B**. CC: corpus callosum. Original magnifications for **A** and **B**: ×75 and ×720, respectively; figure reduced to 87% of original size.

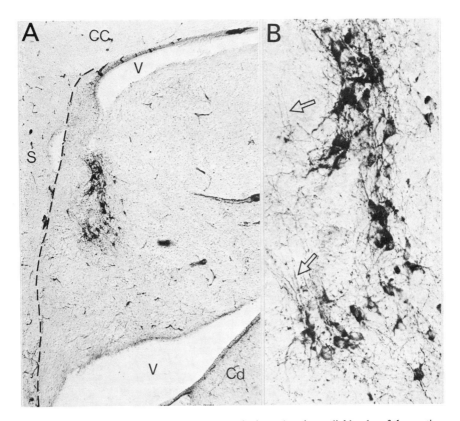

FIGURE 8. A cluster of densely packed neurons is situated at the medial border of the pontine graft in S114. The border between the graft and septum (S) is marked by a dashed line. The morphological appearance and arrangement of these cells resembles noradrenergic neurons of the locus ceruleus in primates. The rich branching patterns of processes (open arrows) of these grafted neurons are evident in **B**. CC: corpus callosum; Cd: caudate nucleus; V: lateral ventricle. Original magnifications for **A** and **B**: ×70 and ×285, respectively; figure reduced to 80% of original size.

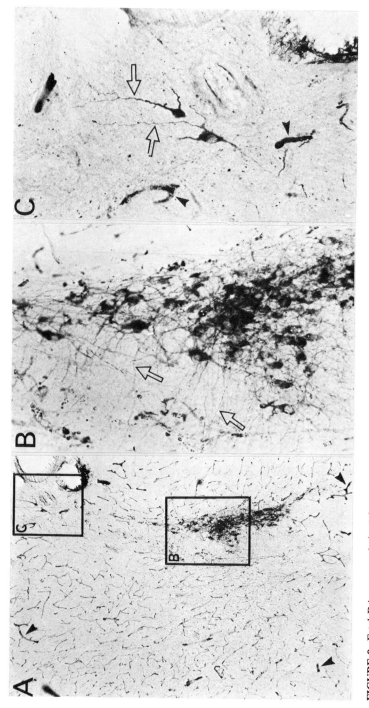

FIGURE 9. Fetal DA neurons derived from the mesencephalon are depicted after grafting into the cerebral cortex in S114. The regions of the graft outlined by the rectangles are enlarged in **B** and **C** to better illustrate the nigral appearance of the cells and their processes (open arrows). The graft and host neuropil are replete with blood vessels (arrowheads) that appear darkly stained because of endogenous peroxidase. Original magnifications for **A** and for **B** and **C**: ×50 and ×200, respectively; figure reduced to 90% of original size.

specificity is supported by the apparent lack of migration of the nigral grafts placed into the cingulate cortex of S114. Although these donor neurons were derived from a fetus of early gestational age, and presumably were relatively more migratory, they showed no evidence of migration into surrounding cerebral cortex. Rather, they appeared organotypic with clusters of densely packed DA neurons and associated neurities.

Functional recovery was not seen in S114 in spite of the presence of multiple grafts, each of which revealed extensive survival and growth of catecholaminergic neurons. Hypothalamic DA neurons placed into the lateral ventricle and caudate apparently were insufficient in either number or DA release to promote recovery. The

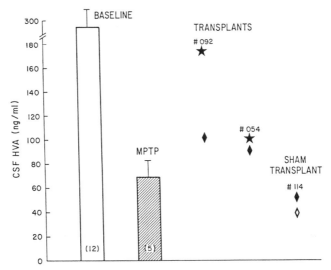

FIGURE 10. Effect of MPTP treatment and fetal neuron transplantation on cisternal CSF HVA concentration measured by gas chromatography-mass spectrometry. The stippled bar shows the reduction in CSF HVA content 1 month after MPTP administration compared with the baseline level (open bar). Three monkeys (S092, S054, and S114) received grafts 1 month after MPTP treatment. The closed diamonds show CSF HVA concentration at approximately 18 days after the transplant procedure. The starred values indicate the value 69 days after the grafts of fetal neurons in S092 and S054. Monkey S114 had an additional CSF sample drawn immediately before the transplant operation (open diamond). This monkey died before 69 days.

latter explanation is favored because the lack of any elevation in CSF HVA levels in this animal suggests a lack of release or metabolism or both of DA from this graft. On the other hand, a slight increase in the norepinephrine metabolite, 3-methoxy-4-hydroxyphenylglycol, was seen in this animal, suggestive of release of this closely related transmitter by the grafted locus ceruleus. These observations may be useful in judging the potential value of non-nigral donor tissue for transplantation, for example, if DA-prone neuroblastoma cells or adrenergic adrenal chromaffin cells were used as a source of DA and norepinephrine. If future experiments in monkeys continue to support this preliminary finding of a lack of improvement after grafting of these nonnigral sources of catecholamines, then it is probable that these sources will be considered unsuitable for functional grafting. Coupled with the lack of success of alternate cell types to reverse parkinsonism in the first human transplant recipients[7] and other behavioral deficits in monkeys receiving surgical lesions,[13] fetal neurons derived from the SN appear to offer the best opportunity for successful grafting in primates.

ACKNOWLEDGMENTS

The authors are appreciative of the competent assistance of Brian Daley, Pat Zambito, Dottie Herrera, Jeanine Schu, the staff of the St. Kitts Biomedical Research Foundation, and a group of dedicated Summer Fellows including Daniel R. Feikin, Joseph T. Fenerty, Paul N. Foster, Lori Kaplowitz, Valerae Lewis, and Lawrence M. Salzer for the care and treatment of monkeys and the assistance with neural grafting procedures.

REFERENCES

1. FAHN, S. & D. B. CALNE. 1978. Considerations in the management of parkinsonism. Neurology 28: 5-7.
2. BURNS, R. S., C. C. CHIUEH, S. P. MARKEY, M. H. EBERT, D. M. JACOBOWITZ & I. J. KOPIN. 1983. A primate model of parkinsonism: Selective destruction of dopaminergic neurons in the pars compacta of the substantia nigra by N-methyl-4-phenyl-1,2,3,6-tetrahydropyridine. Proc. Natl. Acad. Sci. USA 80: 4546-4550.
3. ELSWORTH, J. D., A. Y. DEUTCH, D. E. REDMOND, JR., J. R. SLADEK, JR. & R. H. ROTH. 1987. Neurons within primate substantia nigra differ in susceptibility to 1-methyl-4-phenyl-1,2,3,6-tetrahydropyridine toxicity. Life Sci. 410: 193-202.
4. FREED, W. J., G. N. KO, D. L. NIEHOFF, M. J. KUHAR, B. J. HOFFER, L. OLSON, H. E. CANNON-SPOOR, J. M. MORIHISA & R. J. WYATT. 1983. Normalization of spiroperidol binding in the denervated rat striatum by homologous grafts of substantia nigra. Science 222: 937-939.
5. SCHMIDT, R. H., M. INGVAR, O. LINDVALL, U. STENEVI & A. BJÖRKLUND. 1982. Functional activity of substantia nigra grafts reinnervating the striatum: Neurotransmitter metabolism and [^{14}C]2-deoxy-D-glucose autoradiography. J. Neurochem. 38: 737-748.
6. FREED, W. J., J. M. MORIHISA, E. SPOOR, B. J. HOFFER, L. OLSON, A. SEIGER & R. J. WYATT. 1981. Transplanted adrenal chromaffin cells in rat brain reduce lesion-induced rotational behavior. Nature 292: 351-352.
7. BACKLUND, E.-O., P.-O. GRANBERG, B. HAMBERGER, G. SEDVALL, A. SEIGER & L. OLSON. 1985. Transplantation of adrenal medullary tissue to striatum in parkinsonism. In Neural Grafting in the Mammalian CNS. A. Björklund & U. Stenevi, Eds.: 551-556. Elsevier. Amsterdam.
8. REDMOND, D. E., J. R. SLADEK, JR., R. H. ROTH, T. J. COLLIER, J. D. ELSWORTH, A. Y. DEUTCH & S. HABER. 1986. Fetal neuronal grafts in monkeys given methylphenyl-tetrahydropyridine. Lancet i: 1125-1127.
9. HABER, S. N. & W. J. H. NAUTA. 1983. Ramifications of the globus pallidus in the rat as indicated by patterns of immunohistochemistry. Neuroscience 9: 245-260.
10. BOWDEN, D. M., M. F. DUBACH, R. SNYDER, S. ASKARI & D. C. GERMAN. 1985. Three-dimensional computer analysis of MPTP-induced aminergic cell loss in the monkey. Soc. Neurosci. Abstr. 11: 166.
11. MAHALIK, T. J., T. E. FINGER, I. STROMBERG & L. OLSON. 1985. Substantia nigra

transplants into denervated striatum of the rat: Ultrastructure of graft and host interconnections. J. Comp. Neurol. **240:** 60-70.

12. PATTERSON, P. H. & L. L. Y. CHUN. 1974. The influence of non-neuronal cells on catecholamine and acetylcholine synthesis and accumulation in cultures of dissociated sympathetic neurons. Proc. Natl. Acad. Sci. USA **71:** 3607-3610.
13. GASH, D. M., M. F. D. NOTTER, L. B. DICK, A. L. KRAUS, S. H. OKAWARA, S. W. WECHKIN & R. J. JOYNT. 1985. Cholinergic neurons transplanted into the neocortex and hippocampus of primates: Studies on African Green monkeys. *In* Neural Grafting in the Mammalian CNS. A. Björklund & U. Stenevi, Eds.: 595-603. Elsevier. Amsterdam.

DISCUSSION OF THE PAPER

M. J. PERLOW: (*University of Illinois, Chicago, IL*): That was a terrific presentation. I would like to ask about the SN graft that you had in the cortex. This graft had a an unusual morphological appearance: it showed no sprouting. In the MPTP animal, does the cortex show a loss of DA? And, if it does, why did the graft fail to sprout? Is there any explanation of the nature of its varicosities, why it is different in that different position of the brain as compared to the graft in the caudate?

SLADEK: This is a very important question. If there is a decrease in synaptic density in the cortex, would that not have been enough to induce the DA cells from the nigral grafts to innervate them? I think we have seen a number of studies that support the specificity of the right cell and the right part of the brain. I could only suggest that what is being retained in the fetal graft and in the adult damaged host is the point-to-point specificity between an appropriate target and an appropriate piece of transplanted tissue. My interpretation is that the inappropriate tissue did not send axons out beyond the limits of the transplanted cell.

The extent to which mesolimbic DA fibers are damaged by MPTP, however, is much less than that for nigral striatal DA fibers. This is because the medially placed ventral tegmental area A10 neurons are quite stable in these and other preparations.

Toward a Transplantation Therapy in Parkinson's Disease

A Progress Report from Continuing Clinical Experiments

ERIK-OLOF BACKLUND,[a] LARS OLSON,[b]
ÅKE SEIGER,[b] AND OLLE LINDVALL[c]

[a]Department of Neurosurgery
University of Bergen School of Medicine
N-5021 Haukeland Hospital
Bergen, Norway

[b]Department of Histology
Karolinska Institute
S-104 01 Stockholm, Sweden

[c]Department of Neurology
University Hospital
S-221 85 Lund, Sweden

INTRODUCTION

An experience widely known among clinicians seeing patients with Parkinson's disease is that in spite of ambitious therapy many patients eventually become seriously disabled. The introduction of a medical therapy utilizing L-DOPA and direct dopamine agonists has dramatically changed the conditions for many patients, insofar as quality of life is concerned. This medical therapy, however, does not influence the progressive and serious nature of the disease.

Surgery has long been used to ameliorate symptoms in parkinsonism. It was found empirically that a stereotactic lesion in the pallido-campo-thalamic connections gave relief from contralateral tremor. To some extent, rigidity can also be diminished by such surgery. Today, stereotactic thalamotomy is a routine procedure in patients with tremor as the predominant symptom. In this procedure, a lesion of a size up to approximately 80 mm³ is made in the ventrolateral thalamus, most often in the nucleus ventrointermedius. The surgical risks are fairly low, and, for many tremor patients, thalamotomy produces a significant and permanent improvement.[1] Unfortunately, a bilateral thalamic lesion will significantly increase the risks for neurological deficits and is considered contraindicated by most neurosurgeons. Thalamotomy is thus most often performed as a unilateral procedure, on the side contralateral to the most affected side of the body.

Hypo- or akinesia, often the most disabling symptom, remained a therapeutic problem until the introduction of L-DOPA. L-DOPA, however, in its turn proved to pose a number of problems. Many patients and doctors are now familiar with such troublesome factors as drug resistance, so-called on-off phenomena, and side effects (such as hyperkinesias and psychiatric symptoms, which are due to relative over-dosage). The need for new therapeutic approaches in parkinsonism has become obvious, especially for patients that are hypokinetic or rigid or both.

The main objectives of this review are to describe how we selected patients, to describe the methods we used, and to present summarized patient histories for the four patients that received transplants of autologous adrenal medullary tissue to the striatum (for further details, see Backlund *et al.*[2] and Lindvall *et al.*[3]).

RATIONALE

The papers in this volume give the theoretical and experimental basis for our clinical study (see also Olson *et al.*[4]). Some of the findings that suggest transplants in humans may be effective, however, should be specified: 1) Transplanted chromaffin cells are able to transform themselves toward a neuron-like cell type[5] and to innervate brain tissues.[6] 2) The pathological motor behavior in animals in which lesions are induced with 6-hydroxydopamine can be partly counteracted by transplantation of adrenal medullary tissue to the striatum.[7,8] 3) Adult material can be used for such grafting.[5] Furthermore, human trials could benefit from improved surgical procedures, which have resulted from the recent marriage of sophisticated imaging techniques and established stereotactic surgical procedures.

A neurosurgeon familiar with thalamotomy as a tremor-alleviating operation would understand the results of the animal studies to suggest there was a possibility of designing an operation that would alleviate not only tremor, but hypokinesia and rigidity as well. The possibility of using the improved surgical procedures would also be evident. It was the hope of realizing such possibilities that led to the original proposal for the present clinical study. In 1979, the author of this paper (E. B.) suggested that autologous adrenal medulla or sympathetic ganglion tissue could be transplanted to the striatum in a few selected patients with Parkinson's disease that were at the Karolinska Hospital. An application for approval of a patient project was submitted to the local ethical committee and, after some further animal experiments were performed, approval was given early in 1981. One year later, the first operation was performed.

Hypothetically, the ideal therapeutic approach in Parkinson's disease would be to counteract the furtive degeneration of the nigrostriatal system. This, however, would require a thorough knowledge of the pathogenetic mechanisms, which are largely unknown at present. The second-best approach would involve an attempt to substitute the deficient transmitter-producing cells by transplantation. Such an attempt was made in the present study. With this second approach, it may not be necessary to reestablish the structural neuronal interplay in detail: a mere enhancement of transmitter concentration in the depleted area, by providing a new cellular source of catecholamines, seems to be sufficient to influence motor function. This is supported by results from recent animal experiments.[9]

SELECTION OF PATIENTS

From the clinician's point of view, parkinsonism can often be characterized as being either of the "tremor type" or of the "rigidity-hypokinesia type" when the individual patient is considered. As mentioned above, thalamotomy is rewarding for a patient of the tremor type, whereas L-DOPA may give only moderate tremor relief. On the other hand, treatment with dopamine agonists and particularly with L-DOPA gives the best results in a patient of the rigidity-hypokinesia type. The latter characteristics would therefore best qualify a patient for transplantation, if he also has proven to respond to dopaminergic medication. This was taken into account when the selection criteria were formulated (TABLE 1). These criteria were used to select the four patients that have been operated on thus far.

TABLE 1. Selection Criteria

A patient suitable for transplantation should:
1. Be under 60 years of age
2. Not suffer from dementia
3. Have Parkinson's disease of the rigidity-hypokinesia type
4. Have suboptimal response from L-DOPA and bromocriptine
5. Have bilateral adrenal glands appear on computed tomography scans
6. Have given his or her informed consent to transplantation

METHODS

In the first two patients, the degree of disability was assessed by standard neurological examinations and a self-scoring system. Every 2 hr, seven times a day, the patient estimated symptoms of parkinsonism on a scale of 0 to 3, with 0 corresponding to the absence of symptoms and 3 to maximal symptoms. Dyskinesia symptoms were scored similarly. The total for either daily score could thus vary between 0 and 21.

For the two most recent patients, the clinical assessment protocol was more extensive, aiming at a more objective quantification of the symptomatology. Because of this, the patients were in the hospital for 1 month before and for 3 months after the operation. They had their usual medication except for two short drug-free periods, the first of which began about 1 week before and the second of which began immediately after the operation. The clinical assessment of the motor performance was carried out two or three times daily, and recordings of the behaviors listed below were made.

1. Rigidity: Evaluations were made using a scoring system on passive joint movements with the patient relaxed in supine position: 0: absent; 1: slight; 2: moderate, 3: severe. Major joints in all four extremities and the neck were examined.

2. Tremor: Tremor was recorded as being either present or absent.

3. Successive Movements: The time needed for tapping the knee alternately with the palm and dorsum of the hand 20 times was recorded.

4. Finger Dexterity: The time needed for tapping the thumb with the forefinger

and then with each finger in rapid succession, eventually coming back to the forefinger, 10 times, was recorded.

5. Fist Clenches: The time needed to carry out 20 fist clenches with each hand was recorded.

6. Foot Tapping: The patient tapped the floor with the ball of the foot as rapidly as possible, using the heel as a fulcrum. The time needed for 20 taps was recorded.

7. Gait: The number of steps and the time needed to walk 7 m, turn around, and walk back were recorded.

On-off phenomena were assessed by the patients themselves, who kept a daily log of the number and duration of on-off periods. These self-evaluations were verified independently by a trained observer. In addition to the clinical assessment, the test battery designed to evaluate the effects of the transplantation included computed tomography scans, sensory- and movement-evoked potentials, quantitative electro-encephalogram recordings, measurements of regional cerebral blood flow and mono-amine metabolites in the cerebrospinal fluid, positron emission tomography using a dopamine receptor ligand, and psychiatric and psychological examinations.

The operation was commenced under local anesthesia. By means of a standard computed-tomography-guided stereotactic technique,[10] coordinates were determined for target points in the head of the right caudate nucleus or in the putamen. For the former, the brain coordinates for a single implantation site (patient 1) were 10 mm from the midline, 10 mm anterior to the anterior commissure, and 10 mm above the horizontal intercommissural plane. In patient 2, an additional implantation was made 3 mm more anteriorly. In the putamen (patients 3 and 4), two targets were used: the first was 20 mm from the midline, 5 mm anterior to the anterior commissure, and 5 mm above the intercommissural plane (FIG. 1). The second target in the putamen was located in the same horizontal plane, but at the level of the anterior commissure in the anterioposterior direction. Furthermore, it was 25 mm from the midline. The targets were chosen in the central area of these two nuclei.

During the same operation, now continued with the patient under general anes-thesia, approximately two-thirds of the left adrenal gland (patients 1 and 2) or the entire gland (patients 3 and 4) was removed via a standard extraperitoneal approach. Fragments of medullary tissue were carefully dissected free from the adrenal cortex under rigorous sterility and using microsurgical techniques. This was done in cold saline solution, mixed with serum from the patient. The tissue pieces were trimmed to a size of approximately 1 mm^3 each, and a 16-19-mm-high column consisting of such pieces was loaded into a specially designed cannula. One graft in each patient was arranged in a small steel spiral holder, which was used as a radiographic marker, should emergency X-ray localization and destruction of the grafted tissue have become necessary. On postoperative day 1, the position of the spiral was checked by X-ray (FIG. 2).

PATIENT HISTORIES

Patient 1

This 55-year-old man had an 8-year history of Parkinson's disease with a rapid deterioration during the last year. In spite of optimal medication, he was very hy-pokinetic and rigid and had pronounced on-off phenomena. The operation was per-

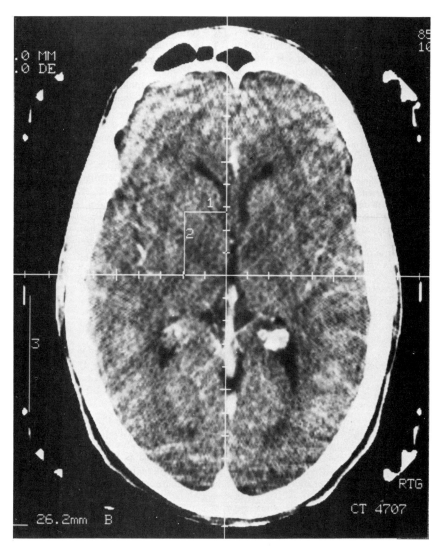

FIGURE 1. Patient 3: Stereotactic computed tomography scan made during the operation. The lateral border of the striatum is well seen. The stereotactic coordinates for the target in the putamen are indicated on the superimposed grid.

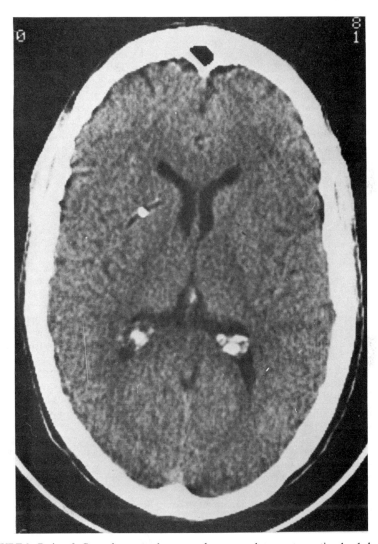

FIGURE 2. Patient 3: Control computed tomography scan made on postoperative day 1 showing the steel spiral (giving minor artifacts) in the predetermined target position (see FIG. 1). The brain parenchyma in the area of the operation has a normal appearance.

formed in March 1982. Approximately 15 pieces of chromaffin tissue, each with a volume of 1-2 mm^3, were placed in the steel spiral holder, which was then introduced into the caudate target.

The operation was uneventful, and the patient woke up promptly. All medication had been withdrawn 10 days preoperatively. Before the operation, the patient was bedridden, was totally dependent, and could only move his arms slightly. The immediate postoperative condition seemed unchanged. One day later, he was mobilized in a wheelchair. His arms were then found to be less rigid than before the operation, and this slight improvement lasted approximately 1 week. He then gradually reverted to a condition similar to the preoperative one.

This patient has now been followed, and no further deterioration has been noted. Some minor adjustments of his drug therapy have been made, but his medication at present does not differ significantly from that of the immediate postoperative period. His unchanged condition during the 4 years after the operation contrasts to his deterioration during the year before the operation.

Patient 2

This 46-year-old woman had a 5-year history of Parkinson's disease with rigidity and, gradually, severe hypokinesia. She had pronounced on-off phenomena. There was a striking contrast between her fairly satisfactory condition during the on phases and her severe disability during the off phases. An attempt to reduce her medication before the operation seriously incapacitated the patient, and it was necessary to perform the operation without preoperative dose reduction.

The operation was performed in May 1983. A larger amount of adrenal medullary tissue was used, and was deposited at two sites in the head of the caudate nucleus, using the steel spiral for only one of the sites. With the exception of one L-DOPA dose given 1 hr after the operation, no medication was given for 4 days. During postoperative days 1 and 2, the patient was observed to move both arms more freely, with less rigidity than before the operation. She gradually regained her preoperative rigidity, and it was considered necessary to reinstate the drug therapy on postoperative day 4. Three days later, hypokinesias and on-off effects were again seen.

Two weeks after the operation, the patient had slight psychiatric symptoms of paranoic character. Simultaneously, her hyperkinesias were also more pronounced. It was reasoned that these symptoms might have indicated overdosage, that is, that they might have been caused by the additive effects of the transplant and the L-DOPA medication. When the latter was lowered, the patient had no more psychiatric symptoms and returned to her preoperative state, except for a persistent slight improvement of motor function in her arms, as indicated by repeated ADL testing. For about half a year it was possible to keep her on a lower L-DOPA dosage than before the operation. Later, it became necessary to gradually increase the dose again.

At a follow-up 2½ years later, she was somewhat more disabled than before the operation. She could no longer profit functionally from the on periods to the same degree as was possible before the operation. On the other hand, her dependence in general was about the same. Her main problem was gait impairment, and she preferred to use a wheelchair instead of walking supported by two persons.

Patient 3

This 46-year-old man had a 14-year history of Parkinson's disease. He benefitted considerably from L-DOPA treatment during the first 6 years of his disease, but then disabling on-off phenomena appeared. During the off periods, he had general hypokinesia, which was most pronounced in his left arm and leg, where he also had marked rigidity. During the on periods, he could walk and move his arms rather normally, but, most often, he had hyperkinesias in his head and trunk.

The operation was performed in March 1985. Two transplants were inserted into the right putamen. The steel spiral was used for the anterior transplant.

The medication was withdrawn just before the operation. After the operation, the patient spontaneously displayed improved motor performance with his left arm and leg as compared to his status both during the preoperative off periods and during the short drug-free interval before the transplantation. This improvement seemed to last 2-3 days after the operation. The medication was reinstated on postoperative day 3.

About 4 hr after the operation, the patient had a reduction of muscle rigidity in his left arm, as compared to preoperative off phases, whereas no obvious effect on muscle tone was observed in his right arm. On postoperative day 1, the rigidity reduction was less pronounced bilaterally, mainly in his left arm, and, on postoperative day 2, the rigidity in all extremities was similar to that registered before the operation, during the drug-free test period.

Acute effects of the transplantation were also recorded in arm and hand function tests, as exemplified by the results from the first clenching test (FIG. 3). On day 2 of the drug-free interval before the transplantation, the time to perform all these tests was much prolonged on the left side, whereas smaller changes were observed on the right side. When the tests were performed on day 2 of drug-free interval after the transplantation, that is, 42 hr after drug withdrawal, the performance was clearly better. In good agreement with the patient's own report, the time to perform the tests was much reduced on the left side, whereas the effects of the transplantation were smaller on the right side. On postoperative day 2, the results of the tests approached those recorded before the operation, although there seemed to be some minor improvement on the left side.

Interestingly, the on periods after the operation were significantly longer than those before the operation (FIG. 4). This improvement lasted for about 2 months, but then the patient returned to his preoperative state, that is, spending about 50% of his time in the on phase. At a follow-up 6 months after the operation, the patient considered his general condition to be similar to that before the operation. This was in good agreement with the results from the clinical examinations, which indicated that there were no or only slight differences between measures of motor performance before and those after the operation.

No signs of brain damage were found by repeated neurological examinations during the follow-up period, and the operation did not influence the results from either the psychological tests or the psychiatric examinations.

Patient 4

This 63-year-old man, who had Parkinson's disease since 1975, responded well to L-DOPA treatment during the first 5 years of his disease. Later, however, severe on-

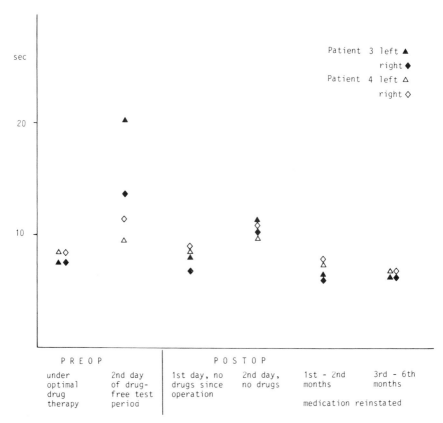

FIGURE 3. Patients 3 and 4: Motor performance in the arms as exemplified by the fist clenching test. In patient 3, on day 2 of the preoperative drug-free interval, the time to perform all arm and hand function tests (including fist clenching) was much prolonged, particularly on the left side. When the tests were repeated on day 2 of the drug-free interval after the operation (that is, on postoperative day 1), the performance was much improved on the left side, whereas smaller changes were observed on the right side. On the next day, the time to perform the tests was prolonged, but there still seemed to be some minor improvement, particularly on the left side, as compared to the performance before the operation. In patient 4, the fist clenching test suggested some minor acute improvement after transplantation, but this was not supported by the results from the other arm and hand function tests. In both patients, the test results 3-6 months after the transplantation seemed to be slightly better than those before the transplantation; however, these improvements were not clinically significant.

off phenomena appeared. As in patient 3, there were difficulties in improving his condition by changing the medication. During off phases, his body balance was impaired and his gait seriously disturbed. He walked with typical "freezing" and propulsion. For short periods during on phases, he could have a practically normal motor performance, but, during the rest of the time, he suffered from disturbing hyperkinesia in his head, trunk, and extremities.

The operation was performed in March 1985. The transplantation procedure was identical with that used for patient 3. Surprisingly, within a few minutes after the insertion of the transplants into the putamen, signs of peripheral vasoconstriction appeared. There was a transient rise in blood pressure, and the patient's hands and feet were white and cold. He was kept on a ventilator overnight. Chest X-rays showed signs of incipient pulmonary edema, and the patient was given diuretics. The condition normalized gradually, and, during the morning hours of the following day, he was extubated and found to have normal respiration.

When the patient was examined about 8 hr after the operation, there seemed to be a slight reduction of muscle rigidity in his left arm as compared to that during the off phases before the operation. On postoperative days 1 and 2, the rigidity increased, particularly on the right side. No significant differences compared to the preoperative rigidity scores were observed. In this patient, the motor performance tests showed less clear-cut changes. Although the results in the fist clenching test seemed to suggest some minor improvement (FIG. 3), this was not supported by the finger dexterity test.

During the first postoperative days, without medication, the patient said he walked more easily and had better balance than during the preoperative drug-free periods. After reinstatement of medication, he found himself able to walk in the mornings, even *before* the first daily L-DOPA dose, which had been impossible for at least half a year before the operation. This period of improvement lasted for about 2 months, and then his condition became the same as it was before the operation. In contrast to patient 3, this patient did not experience an increase of time spent in on periods. Three to 6 months after the operation, the results in all the motor performance tests were slightly better than they were before the operation. These minor changes should be interpreted cautiously, however, since the general state of the patient, as well as his own report, indicated his condition to be approximately the same as it was before the operation. Routine neurological examinations performed several times after the operation showed no pathological changes.

DISCUSSION

Any interpretation of the postoperative courses in these four patients has to be tentative. There are, however, some common features in all four cases, suggesting that

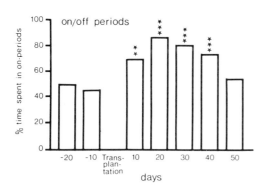

FIGURE 4. Before the operation, patient 3 spent approximately 50% of his time in on periods. During the first 50 postoperative days, with a maximum around postoperative day 20, the time spent in on periods was significantly increased (**: $p < .01$; ***: $p < .001$) compared to preoperative values.

the operation temporarily reduced the pathological motor symptoms. It remains to be definitely established that this effect is due to a release of catecholamines from the implanted tissue; however, the similarities in duration and degree of functional effects seen after the operation in the present study, as compared to numerous animal experiments using adult adrenal medulla grafts, suggest this to be the case. This is further supported by the results obtained with auditory-evoked and readiness potentials in patients 3 and 4, which indicate an increased catecholaminergic activity'in the basal ganglia after transplantation.[3]

It is important, though, to remember that symptoms of parkinsonism may vary spontaneously from time to time, such as after changes in the treatment program. Furthermore, it could be argued that the mechanical lesion created by inserting the cannula into the striatum, small as this lesion is, could influence the motor symptoms of the patient the way a thalamic lesion influences tremor. This seems unlikely, however, as a limited lesion of the striatum is not known to influence the motor system in man. In capsulotomy, for example (a psychosurgical operation), the fairly extensive stereotactic lesion created in the anterior limb of the internal capsule encroaches significantly upon both the caudate and the putamen. No influence upon the motor system has been registered in patients treated with capsulotomy.[11] On the other hand, lesions in the human brain, even discrete lesions, may initiate functional and structural changes of varying and partly obscure character.[12]

New techniques are now emerging that may allow the local effects of implanted transmitter-characterized cell populations to be monitored directly. Thus, in the future, it may be possible to study various neurotransmitters in the vicinity of the transplant, using a dialysis probe.[13] This technique has been elegantly used in recent animal experiments.[14]

The brief and limited response in our patients after the transplantation seems to indicate a limited survival of the graft. Thus, in the next series, we plan to infuse growth-promoting substances, such as nerve growth factor (NGF), into the recipient area. Recent studies in rats[8,9] have shown that administration of NGF to the adrenal medullary implant leads to better cell survival as well as more pronounced and more lasting functional effects. The most efficient way yet found to administer NGF involves continuous infusion via an intracerebral dialysis probe during the first weeks after grafting. It would be within acceptable surgical risks to have such a probe installed in situ in a patient's brain for at least 1 week. An implantable micropump for long-term NGF delivery is probably an even better alternative. Improved graft survival could then be expected, leading to a more efficient and more lasting reduction of the parkinsonian symptoms.

When transplants from the central nervous system are used in animal experiments, the use of a cell suspension is more versatile than grafting solid pieces of tissue. The use of suspensions was not possible in this project because, given the available techniques, the human adrenal medulla does not seem suitable for dissociation. New techniques, however, will be tried. The future may also offer better alternatives in the form of transplants derived from established cell lines with specific neurohumoral characteristics. Interesting animal experiments were reported recently.[15]

The stereotactic technique gives the neurosurgeon wide opportunities to perform precise operations at a very low risk in any region of the human brain. As a rule, such operations are performed under local anesthesia only. Local anesthesia, however, has not yet been utilized in the present project. Recent observations in rats indicate that fetal nerve cells can be stored for several days before transplantation.[16] If this is also the case for adult human adrenal medulla cells, the graft could be taken in a separate operation, before the introduction of the transplant into the brain, and the transplantation could then be performed without general anesthesia. If local anesthesia could be used, a more refined transplantation procedure would be possible because preoperative electrophysiological and biochemical exploration of the target regions could be conducted with the patient awake.

Furthermore, our attention is also directed toward the possible use of substantia nigra neurons from aborted human fetuses. Although the serious ethical implications of such a strategy need further clarification, recent experimental data give clear indications that at least the immunological problems in human transplantations can be mastered. Fetal dopamine neurons have been successfully grafted from mouse[17] and from aborted human fetuses[17-19] to the adult rat brain after administration of the immunosuppressive drug cyclosporin A. In our opinion, it seems necessary at this time to continue the present study. Autologous adrenal medulla grafts, however, should be introduced using an improved technique, and tentative studies using human fetal dopamine neurons should be started. Such innovations may provide directives for the development of a transplantation therapy in Parkinson's disease.

When the present project was initiated, an essentially new therapeutic principle was founded. Compared to many other degenerative diseases in the human central nervous system, Parkinson's disease is a condition extensively studied and now partly understood, making it a challenging domain for clinical application of results from frontier research in experimental neurobiology. The experiences from the present study indicate that neurosurgery is approaching exciting new therapeutic fields.

REFERENCES

1. TASKER, R. R., J. SIQUEIRA, P. HAWRYLYSHYN & L. W. ORGAN. 1983. Appl. Neurophysiol. **46:** 68-83.
2. BACKLUND, E.-O., P. O. GRANBERG, B. HAMBERGER, E. KNUTSSON, A. MÅRTENSSON, G. SEDVALL, Å. SEIGER & L. OLSON. 1985. J. Neurosurg. **62:** 169-173.
3. LINDVALL, O., E.-O. BACKLUND, L. FARDE, G. SEDVALL, R. FREEDMAN, B. HOFFER, Å. SEIGER & L. OLSON. 1987. Ann. Neurol. In press.
4. OLSON, L., E.-O. BACKLUND, G. GERHARDT, B. HOFFER, O. LINDVALL, G. ROSE, Å. SEIGER & I. STRÖMBERG. 1986. *In* Advances in Neurology. M. D. Yahr & K. J. Bergmann, Eds. Vol. **45:** 85-94. Raven Press. New York, NY.
5. OLSON, L. 1970. Histochemie **22:** 1-7.
6. OLSON, L., Å. SEIGER, R. FREEDMAN & B. HOFFER. 1980. Exp. Neurol. **70:** 414-426.
7. OLSON, L., E.-O. BACKLUND, G. SEDVALL, M. HERRERA-MARSCHITZ, U. UNGERSTEDT, I. STRÖMBERG, B. HOFFER & Å. SEIGER. 1984. *In* Catecholamines, Part C. Neuropharmacology and Central Nervous System: Therapeutic Aspects. E. Usdin, A. Carlsson, A. Dahlström, J. Engel, Eds.: 195-201. Alan R. Liss. New York, NY.
8. STRÖMBERG, I., M. HERRERA-MARSCHITZ, U. UNGERSTEDT, T. EBENDAL & L. OLSON. 1985. Exp. Brain Res. **60:** 335-349.
9. STRÖMBERG, I., T. EBENDAL, Å. SEIGER & L. OLSON. 1985. Cell Tissue Res. **241:** 241-249.
10. LEKSELL, L. & B. JERNBERG. 1980. Acta Neurochir. **52:** 1-7.
11. LEKSELL, L. & E.-O. BACKLUND. 1979. *In* Modern Concepts in Psychiatric Surgery. E. R. Hitchcock, H. T. Ballantine & B. A. Meyerson, Eds.: 213-216. Elsevier/North-Holland. Amsterdam.
12. GESCHWIND, N. 1985. Ann. N. Y. Acad. Sci. **457:** 1-12.
13. UNGERSTEDT, U. 1984. *In* Measurement of Neurotransmitter Release *in Vivo.* C. A. Marsden, Ed.: 81-105. John Wiley & Sons. London.
14. ZETTERSTRÖM, T., P. BRUNDIN, F. H. GAGE, T. SHARP, O. ISACSON, S. B. DUNNETT, U. UNGERSTEDT & A. BJÖRKLUND. 1986. Brain Res. **362:** 344-349.
15. HEFTI, F., J. HARTIKKA & M. SCHLUMPF. 1985. Brain Res. **348:** 283-288.

16. GAGE, F. H., P. BRUNDIN, O. ISACSON & A. BJÖRKLUND. 1985. Neurosci. Lett. **60:** 133-137.
17. BRUNDIN, P., R. E. STRECKER, O. LINDVALL, O. ISACSON, O. G. NILSSON, G. BARBIN, A. PROCHIANTZ, C. FORNI, A. NIEOULLON, H. WILDNER, F. H. GAGE & A. BJÖRKLUND. 1987. Ann. N. Y. Acad. Sci. This volume.
18. OLSON, L., I. STRÖMBERG, M. BYGDEMAN, A. C. GRANHOLM, B. HOFFER, R. FREEDMAN & Å. SEIGER. 1987. Exp. Brain Res. In press.
19. STRÖMBERG, I., M. BYGDEMAN, M. GOLDSTEIN, Å. SEIGER & L. OLSON. 1986. Neurosci. Lett. **71:** 271-276.

DISCUSSION OF THE PAPER

C. SOTELO (*INSERM U106, CMC Foch, Suresnes*): Having been a nerve biologist for 25 years, I would rather do experiments in animals than in humans. But the question I want to address is a very simple one. Dr. Rosenstein, Dr. Pappas, and Dr. Jaeger tell us that when they inject chromaffin cells in the brain, the first thing they do is change the vascular bed. They then have fenestrated capillaries. Could the change in the blood-brain barrier explain all the positive results you observed at 2 months because peripheral monoamines can go to the striatum of these patients?

LINDVALL: The problem is that there are many ways to explain these data with the changes at 2 months. One explanation is that it is just a matter of the drug withdrawal in connection with the operation or some entirely unspecific effect. It could be an effect of the transplant, but this is something that we do not know. We assume that the transplant itself cannot give the patient enough relief during the 2 months after transplantation, but it could be that these patients have lost the capacity to buffer the very big oscillations in L-DOPA concentrations in the blood. Normally, when the L-DOPA is taken up in the brain and dopamine is released, the L-DOPA is converted to dopamine by other neurons and by vessels, inducing on-off phenomena. But with a transplant, perhaps L-DOPA and amines are taken up by the transplant and are then released slowly to help to prolong the off periods.

SOTELO: I was in contact with some neurologists when I was working with experimental models for epilepsy. All essential epilepsia that had been operated in Santan in Paris had the common denominator of outreaching of the blood-brain barrier. You say that your transplants are not harmful to the patients, but are you sure that they do not develop epilepsia?

LINDVALL: We followed these patients with computed tomography scans every day during the week after the operation and saw no sign of any barrier change. We also followed the patients with frontal electroencephalogram recordings. We still saw no change.

BACKLUND: Furthermore, we have an enormous wealth of knowledge concerning this specific question in materials of thalamotomy. The frequency of EEG pathology and seizure disorders after thalamotomy is so small that no neurosurgeon would consider it a contraindication for thalamotomy, and thalamotomy is an operation of about the same magnitude as this one.

QUESTIONER: You referred to patients P1 and P2. Have patients P3 and P4 been done?

LINDVALL: Yes.

QUESTIONER: The medulla grafts that you are injecting contain manyfold greater content of epinephrine and norepinephrine than dopamine. Is it known what these two other catecholamines do in animal models with Parkinson's disease in terms of affecting their symptoms in any way?

OLSON: In the animal experiment, it seems very clear that it is the transplant itself that causes the relief, and there is a good correlation between the number of surviving cells and the amount of reduction of rotational behavior, for instance. If you add nerve growth factor you get a larger graft with more fiber outgrowth and much better results. I do not think that there is a permanent disturbance of the blood-brain barrier.

The patient could theoretically make more L-DOPA available, but that passes the blood-brain barrier anyway. And, in answer to the question about the various catecholamines after grafting, we very carefully separate the adrenal medulla from the adrenal cortex. Therefore, the chromaffin cells will not be able to make adrenalin any more because this is dependent upon high local steroid concentrations. After a while, they will only make noradrenalin and larger amounts of dopamine than they usually do. We think that the beneficial effect is caused by a mixture of these two catecholamines. Noradrenalin and adrenalin, for that matter, also work, but they are much less potent on dopamine receptors. The acute effects of implanting chromaffin tissue in rats on rotational behavior is caused by a massive release of adrenalin and noradrenalin that can be completely blocked by dopamine receptor blocking drugs.

QUESTIONER: Do you have convincing evidence of survival of these cells in long-term PET scans?

LINDVALL: Not in the human experiments. We have not analyzed all the data yet. In the PET scan experiment that Dr. Backlund mentioned, we had the idea that maybe one could see receptor sensitivity changes due to the transplantation. Therefore, we have used a dopamine receptor ligand with the PET scan that is available in Sweden. The data are not ready yet, but we have not seen any changes. So this is a problem of course. We have performed an analysis of the cerebrospinal fluid, and, in the first two patients that were operated in the caudate nucleus, there seemed to be some changes that could indicate survival of the graft. But the interesting changes are the functional effects. One should be very cautious when attributing these changes to the graft. But there is a striking similarity between these changes and the changes in rodents that can be attributed to the graft.

M. J. PERLOW (*University of Illinois, Chicago, IL*): You present results where the patient has some subjective feelings that his symptoms get better as a result of this procedure. The patient subsequently becomes worse. You ascribe the beneficial result to catecholamine release. I do not find any evidence in your paper that there was any catecholamine release, and I wonder how you could come to that conclusion. Could you tell me why you say catecholamines are released from these transplanted neurons? There are a number of other reasons why patients or the patients you have could get better.

One possibility, which you mentioned, is the drug holiday. Also, we know that Parkinson patients, as they showed in the monkey, have a large emotional response to getting better. It is conceivable that your patients felt better during the period of time you examined them—that they were more alert and responded better emotionally. Another possibility is that the catecholamine cells do in fact live in the brain and that the patients get better as a result of these catecholamine transplants. There are other compounds in the catecholamine cells besides the catecholamines. These cells contain all sorts of different enkephalins and medullary proteins. These proteins could be the cause of the amelioration of the symptoms.

Researchers in France—I am not sure of their names—analyzed autopsy material from patients that had Parkinson's disease and found a reduction in Met-enkephalin in several areas of the brain, including the putamen, where there was a rather large decrease. If these catecholamine cells do in fact live, which I think still remains to be seen, the amelioration of the effects may not be due to the catecholamines themselves but perhaps to the enkephalins and the other peptides.

LINDVALL: What we are sure of now of the four implantations in putamen and caudate nucleus is that we cannot find any harmful effects of the transplantation. If there are any changes, they are only minor ones and do not last long. For the patients, the present transplantation procedure is of very little value. I think a more interesting way to look at the data would be to draw similarities to the animal experiments. The patients were admitted to the neurological clinic a month before transplantation so that they could be examined repeatedly many times before transplantation. Unilateral changes are very difficult to attribute to the expectations of the patient.

PERLOW: It is hard to say. The same kind of experimental criteria we use for experiments on animals should be applied to humans. Such a rigorous approach may be appropriate for patients with Parkinson's disease simply because the disease is so devastating.

LINDVALL: I agree.

PERLOW: But I think for the long term for the greater number of Parkinson patients who exist all over the world, that you should apply these rigid criteria.

LINDVALL: You misunderstand me if you think that I disagree with this because I very much agree. The results with adrenal medulla in humans—from the patient's point of view—are quite negative. But then one should very carefully consider whether there could be some positive data. I did not mention the neurophysiological data with readiness potentials and sensory evoked potentials that were performed by Robert Freedman in Denver, but they also seem to indicate that there is an increased catecholaminergic transmission in the basal ganglia on the site of the transplantation. This increase, however, subsides after 1 or 2 weeks; that is, the increase is maximal 2 days after the transplantation.

A. W. DECKEL (*Johns Hopkins University School of Medicine, Baltimore, MD*): Do you still use the metal cannula in your patients?

LINDVALL: You mean the small spiral?

DECKEL: Yes.

LINDVALL: From the beginning we wanted to have a marker in case an emergency extraction of the transplant would be necessary. But in the last two patients we have used it in one of the targets and only the cells in the other target.

DECKEL: Has there been basic work done to see what the effects of the metal cannula are on the development of the graft? One could imagine that all sorts of parameters are altered. Also, a few years ago Dr. Freed offered to try some of your methods in monkeys here in the States. Has anyone taken him up on his offer?

OLSON: I can answer about the metal cannula. It is not actually a cannula. It is a loosely wound steel spiral that carries the grafts. The spiral carrying the 15 to 20 pieces of graft material is placed at the first implantation site only. A spiral is not needed to locate the second site because its position can be defined with respect to the spiral at the first site. We have done some animal experiments implanting the same type of metal spiral into rat brain. We were looking for a gliosis and such possible chronic changes. There was surprisingly little gliosis caused. But I agree that it is probably less satisfactory to leave this spiral in the brain, although I understand that neurosurgeons quite often leave little metal pieces in the human brain.

J. M. GORELL (*Henry Ford Hospital, Detroit, MI*): Have you and your group measured cerebrospinal fluid levels of homovanillic acid and of other metabolites of other catecholamines, both before and after transplantation? If not, it would be a very good thing to do. Also, is there any way of trying, in a clinical situation, to see whether rejection is a continuous process?

LINDVALL: We have performed an analysis of the cerebrospinal fluid on these patients, but we do not have the data. There is no rejection of these adrenal grafts because they were taken from the patients themselves.

Summary

P. PASIK (*Mount Sinai School of Medicine, New York, NY*): This session included six fascinating papers on the application of neural grafting in primates. They covered a rather wide range of basic subjects: the variety of subjects covered already points to the multiplicity of problems encountered with such procedures.

Two of the papers dealt mostly with technical aspects. Dr. Morihisa demonstrated a higher yield of grafted tissue by using a direct visualization of the site of the implant in the host brain. It is possible that some of his findings are related to the results of several of the reports that were given in the first two sessions, as well as to the report given by Dr. Freed, who showed that the degree of neurite development from substantia nigra tissue grafted into the caudate nucleus was greater in animals which had additional cortical injury. As repeatedly shown at this meeting, there must be a variety of factors produced at the site of brain injury which promotes the survival of grafted neurons. We are seeing now that this applies to the primate brain as well. The other technical paper, this one by Dr. Backlund, gave a detailed account of the neurosurgical procedure for adrenal autografts into the striatum of Parkinson's disease patients.

Two papers, one of which was delivered by Dr. Bakay and the other by Dr. Sladek, addressed the issue of amelioration of symptoms by nigral grafts into the striatum of rhesus or cercopithecus monkeys, the symptoms of parkinsonism having been produced by MPTP intoxication. They both coincided in reporting behavioral and biochemical improvement with some morphologic evidence of so-called graft integration into the host brain. One of the important variables in this type of study—a variable that has only been touched upon and perhaps should be emphasized—is the fetal age of the implant. It has been clear from several presentations at this symposium that the optimal age in the rat is about the 15th embryonic day. The equivalent in primates is not known. This information is badly needed although it appears from Dr. Sladek's data that it may not be so critical as initially thought. In fact, the salutatory effect was obtained with fetal material of both E49 and E182 in African Green monkeys. It should be recalled that gestational ages vary greatly among the nonhuman primates used in these experiments. It is roughly 165 days for the rhesus but 195 for the African Green. It is possible that the more recent primate model of parkinsonism, that is, MPTP-intoxicated marmosets, as it was going to be reported in this session by Dr. Jenner, may have not only the advantage of lower cost but also of a briefer gestation, which is about 140 days.

The integration of the graft into the host brain is one of the most critical issues. Nothing is known; hard data is completely lacking in primates. We have seen beautiful anatomical demonstrations, particularly by Dr. Sladek, but the actual connectivity at the synaptic level is missing. Even if one assumes that some of the findings in the rat can be extrapolated, that data is limited, with rare exceptions as demonstrated yesterday by Dr. Sotelo in the cerebellum and Dr. Gibson in the hypothalamus, to the output of the grafted neurons which apparently enter into synaptic partnership with the appropriate target cells. A most intriguing problem is that of newly formed inputs onto the grafted cells. In other words, what kinds of circuits are established not only with the target elements but also with the afferents onto the grafted cells? An obvious requirement is adequate knowledge of the circuitry present in the involved structures of the normal brain, and although much has been advanced in the understanding of the synaptology of, for instance, the basal ganglia system, we are only starting to unravel some of its complexities. A case in point is given by the nigrostriatal and strionigral relationships. Although the dopaminergic (DA) projection from the substantia nigra pars compacta to striatum is unquestionable, it is not clear which striatal cells are receiving this input. It is also known that neurons of the substantia nigra pars reticulata (SNr), which are probably GABA-ergic, also innervate the striatum, and that these cells must be present in the nigral graft as well. Finally, an output from the striatum reaches the SNr, and this output is predominantly GABA-ergic. We have recently demonstrated the presence of GABA-immunoreactive terminals in the monkey SNr, presynaptic to both similarly labeled dendrites and to unlabeled dendrites, and suggested that this connectivity could be the basis for the disinhibition of DA neurons elicited by striatal stimulation. In the case of the graft, both DA and GABA neurons from the SN are placed in a striatal environment which in turn contains both GABA-ergic efferent cells and GABA-ergic interneurons. We can speculate that the possibilities of reproducing the normal circuitry are all there. The DA neuron may contact GABA striatal cells, in turn synapsing on other GABA neurons of the graft, in turn contacting other GABA neurons of the DA cells. The question is how to go about finding this out. We are fortunate at this point to have the methodology available to explore these questions. It involves the electron microscopy of tissues processed with double-labeling immunocytochemistry. Our electron micrographs from caudate nucleus treated in this fashion show axonal boutons labeled for tyrosine hydroxylase with peroxidase–antiperoxidase complex, presynaptic to a neuronal soma labeled for Leu-enkephalin with ferritin particles. Therefore it demonstrates a direct connection of a DA terminal with a Leu-enkephalin neuron. It would be highly desirable to examine graft and host tissue with this technique.

Attempts to improve symptoms due to deficiency in other systems are also being made, and we had in this session Dr. Gash's presentation offering a promising result with the use of neuroblastoma cells which apparently can manufacture acetylcholine. It is striking that two of his cell lines were of rodent origin. The use of such cell lines opens the possibility of using xenografts in future studies of this system and other systems. Such situations bring into consideration what may become an important ethical issue for the future, namely the implantation of rat brain cells into the human brain.

Finally, the most thought-provoking paper was by Dr. Lindvall. In this paper the general approach of brain grafts has been taken to the human level. Although the multipotentiality of neural crest derivatives is an established fact, it is still surprising that adult adrenal tissue may transform into DA-producing cells if that indeed is the basis for the transient improvement of parkinsonian patients when fragments of their own adrenals are implanted into the striatum. Although the results are rather disappointing, they represent a first attempt at this type of human experimentation, which brings again a whole slew of ethical issues, impractical to be discussed in this forum.

Final Discussion

A. BJÖRKLUND (*University of Lund, Sweden*): This panel discussion is designed to focus on this afternoon's session. We have asked three associated scientists, Dr. Wyatt, Dr. Redmond, and Dr. Olson, to also participate in this discussion. Each has been asked to make a brief statement or comment on issues that they think would be relevant to discuss further, something that has to be clarified, or something that may have been neglected.

After these brief remarks we'll widen the discussion to include questions that may be related to difficulties in this field, interpretational problems, or other fundamental issues.

I would like to see that we don't get sidetracked by minor technical details such as how to send a brain from Europe to America without losing the fluorescence.

L. OLSON (*Karolinska Institute, Stockholm, Sweden*): I thought I'd first make some general remarks on the "my graft is bigger than your graft" problem. An instructive example involves grafting to an area other than the brain, namely, the anterior chamber of the eye. The advantage of this technique is that you can study development of isolated areas and it is easy to follow growth of individual grafts. In a spinal cord graft after a couple of months *in oculo,* for example, if such grafts are taken from fetuses at different embryonic stages a plot can be made of the growth rate.

We have found that there is a very sharp decrease in the growth potential in the volume of the graft from what you would expect with grafts from older fetuses. You can also compare growth potentials for grafts taken from different areas of the brain, but it is very important to keep in mind, especially when comparing grafts described in different studies, that the state of development of a graft will affect its potential for growth. It is equally important to keep in mind the age of the recipient.

A locus ceruleus from a rat grafted to the eye chamber illustrates that some areas do not grow as much as other areas, but they do differentiate well in aged animals. (I'm not referring now to studies of aging.) Cortex grafts in animals 1½ months old, which are barely adults, will grow better than those in 7½-month-old animals. This is important to bear in mind when you compare studies.

The final point I want to make refers to the eye chamber; it is also important where you graft the tissue piece. We have an eye that carried a single graft of cortex cerebrum, and a similar piece of embryonic fetal cortex cerebrum was grafted into another eye that already carried a mature locus ceruleus graft and was placed in contact with that. This greatly enhanced the volume increase in growth and development of the cortex cerebrum graft; it was much bigger and more normally organized and more normal electrophysiologically than the first graft. So, in comparing sizes, it is important to exactly compare where the grafts are placed.

D. E. REDMOND (*Yale University, New Haven, CT*): I have been asked to comment about the possibility of applying transplant techniques to clinical problems. Parkinson's disease, for example, is an important clinical problem that may lend itself to the first ethical experimentation in this area. This is because, first, Parkinson's disease is an age-related disease so that many of its victims are already quite advanced in years. Treatment, although ameliorative, does not prevent the progression of the disease and is inadequate even when it's working. Consequently, there are good ethical reasons for exploring alternative therapy. Second, Parkinson's disease seems to be caused to some extent by structural deterioration of the brain; it does not seem to be the kind of disorder that would be easily dealt with by replacement, medication, and other kinds of treatment.

I would like to mention the importance of the MPTP [1-methyl-4-phenyl-1,2,3,6-tetrahydropyridine] model which may have changed the speed with which investigators will eventually progress to human studies. At the time the Swedish group began their clinical studies the MPTP model was not really well demonstrated. Now, however, something very similar to Parkinson's disease can be induced in monkeys and so it is possible for a number of different kinds of techniques to be studied which will provide a great deal of information before further clinical experiments are undertaken.

R. J. WYATT (*National Institutes of Health, Washington, DC*): I would first like to make a few comments about the ethical issues that are raised by our work. The first involves putting foreign tissues into the brain and the second refers to the use of material from aborted fetuses. With respect to the introduction of foreign material we have never felt that this is a major issue. Pig heart valves are used in cardiac surgery, so we even go across species. Very little issue is taken with such use as long as we are trying to make the body whole, or to cure disease, or to make a patient more comfortable. Ethical problems do arise, however, when we start thinking about going beyond the boundaries of our species for transplantation into the brain.

The use of fetal tissue is governed by state law, in most cases, under the Uniform Anatomical Gift Act, recommended by the National Conference of Commissioners on Uniform State Laws. This act allows the use of fetal tissue for research purposes provided that one parent grants permission and the other does not object, and that the tissue is not taken from a live fetus. I think most people would also agree that the decision to have an abortion must be independent of the need for a graft. This does not dispose of the ethical issues, but the guidelines are in place and they are being used.

I would now like to raise some technical issues. For example, what is the optimal size of the graft? We are not referring to the use of dispersed cells, for, of course, there is no size issue there. And with respect to the lump or whole-tissue grafts, most investigators have come to the conclusion that your graft cannot be much larger than one cubic millimeter. With respect to how divergent the tissue can be, we know that tissue can be grown across species, particularly with immunologic suppression, and we can probably go across histocompatability lines within the same species.

Can there be a tissue bank? That possibility was originally looked into by Mark Perlow, who succeeded in using cultured adrenal cells for grafts several years ago.

Scale can be a problem if you want to disperse transplant material throughout a large volume of brain tissue. Dispersing half-cubic-millimeter grafts into the 40-cubic-millimeter striatum of a rat would be much easier, for example, than dispersing half-cubic-millimeter grafts into a human striatum, which has a volume of about 10 000 cubic millimeters, if one considers the caudate and putamen.

A potential problem becomes apparent when we consider how many grafts would be required to evenly distribute transplant tissues throughout the parkinsonian striatum. More than 3000 grafts would be needed. In any event, a large number of grafts would be needed to effect a successful long-term change in parkinsonian patients.

Because going through the cortex is the easiest if not the preferred way to reach the cortex, I would like to ask the neurosurgeons the following question: What is the maximum number of punctures that can be made in the cortex without worrying about doing damage to the human?

I'd like to encourage Dr. Björklund not to give up on the adrenal. We were able to place adrenal medulla grafts into the cortex of a monkey simply by dipping them in with a forceps; 6 weeks later we found that literally tens of thousands of cells were surviving without any evidence of rejection. We have also had success transplanting material from the adrenal medulla into the monkey caudate: we found substantial numbers of grafted cells surviving after transplants were performed. Adrenal medulla cells may well become as useful as fetal cells, at least for the Parkinson's model. The reasons why we're having greater success now than we did 7 or 8 years ago when we first started using grafts in monkeys is unclear, except that probably relates as much to experience as anything else. There is a potential for success just by continuing to try to develop ways of "gentling in" the tissue.

J. R. SLADEK, JR. (*University of Rochester School of Medicine, Rochester, NY*): I'll respond to Dr. Wyatt's question about the numbers of grafts, although I would caution that our results are still quite preliminary and that the numbers of animals are quite small. Even with as few as three implants per site we are either getting a massive induction in primate brain of some endogenous cell type that is shifting its transmitter phenotype to accommodate the need for dopamine or alternately we are getting a pretty extensive migration of cells from the implant site toward the rostrum of the caudate nucleus, a migration guided perhaps by the remaining axons. That may offer some optimism that neurosurgically in humans we wouldn't need to place that extensive a number of grafts.

BJÖRKLUND: I would like to comment on the numbers of grafts. The number of nigral neurons that normally innervate the striatum in the rat is roughly about 10 000, while about half a million innervate the striatum of the human, a size disparity of 50. Thus we need 50 times more neurons to cover the human striatum then we would need in the rat striatum.

Now the minimum number of cells that produce measurable effects in the rat is on the order of 100 to 250 cells, which would be between 5000 and 7500 cells in the human. Dr. Sladek's experiments had cell counts of more than 50 000, well above the expected minimum. Is that compatible with the reported functional effects? Would fewer cells have sufficed to produce measurable effects? And if so, how many? We cannot be sure because the estimated minimum does not take into account biological differences that might accompany scaling up. Scaling up is more than just adding numbers, it's also biology. When scaling up from a small structure to a large structure one may also impose biological problems which may not be simple; for example, the distance over which neurons would have to grow in order to reach the target may be absolutely limited and that may not be scaled up just because we're working with a larger brain. If so, then size will remain a problem.

SLADEK: One additional advantage in using fetal nerve tissue as opposed to adrenal chromaffin cells with respect to numbers is that during development the brain loses numbers of cells in particular loci. Consequently, it is entirely likely that by using fetal cells we're actually implanting 50 to 100 percent more of the nigral cells than would exist in the adult brain if ontogeny requires a certain pruning effect due to an overproduction of dopamine cells. This might favor the use of the fetus.

T. FREEMAN (*New York University Medical Center, New York, NY*): I would like to discuss a few volumetric constraints about upgrading to the phylogenetic order and how these constraints relate to transplantation and the source of tissue for transplantation. As Harmon and Carpenter showed in 1953, and as Dr. Wyatt just pointed out, the human striatum is more than one and a half orders of magnitude larger than the rat striatum. This difference in scale, as it relates to sources of transplantation, may not be as depressing as was thought from a neurosurgical point of view. It's unlikely that 1500 grafts will be necessary.

Steven Dunnett and Professor Björklund have shown that somatotopic symptoms may be treated by transplantation to particular areas of the striatum. PET scans could help determine which regions of the striatum should receive transplants by determining which regions are losing dopamine; it may not be necessary to transplant into every region of the human striatum. Furthermore, the descending pathways that Dr. Coonsall described in the monkey go primarily to the putamen. Symptoms of Parkinson's disease could be treated by completely saturating that particular region. It's unlikely that the volume of tissue necessary for transplantation would be as great as that anticipated in the worst-case scenario.

Dr. Bakay's experiment has shown that the outgrowth from transplants from a higher phylogenetic order are unfortunately of a short distance. One would hope that that could be improved upon, given that cells assume the morphology of the species that they come from. But until then, it will be necessary to have a large number of grafts close together.

So in terms of the source of tissue it is likely that a larger number of cells than are available right now will be necessary. But Professor Sladek's finding that the amount needed may not be as great as we thought is quite exciting, for it may be possible to get more tissue.

Human fetal tissue should not be used as a source for work with humans, however, until it can be shown that a sufficient volume of tissue can be removed from one fetus for a clinically significant transplantation in the volume of a striatum necessary for human clinical improvement.

REDMOND: I'd like to underscore that point with respect to the MPTP model. One of the things that happens with MPTP treatment is that you can produce tremendous depletions in both dopamine content and dopamine cell numbers without producing any apparent functional change in the animal. This indicates the functional reserve that neurons are capable of, and there's no reason to think that transplanted dopamine neurons wouldn't also have a similar capacity to increase their biological function.

BJÖRKLUND: I would like to ask about the MPTP model. How problematic is the recovery of action in the MPTP model and how unpredictable is it? Is it possible to master the model to the extent that one can get and maintain predictable long-range impairments? And can such impairments be obtained without having very sick animals—animals that may be very difficult or even ethically problematic to keep in research?

D. M. GASH (*University of Rochester School of Medicine, Rochester, NY*): Those who are working with MPTP find that there is a dose dependency such that you can get animals with various degrees of impairment. The approach we're taking is to have animals that slowly develop Parkinson's disease from MPTP treatment and that can take care of themselves. This is essentially equivalent to the early stages of the disease that one sees clinically.

In terms of recovery of function I would refer you to other groups, such as Bill Langston's group, which is working with squirrel monkeys, I believe. They have seen spontaneous recovery as late as 3 months after the last dose of MPTP was given. As scientists we have to remember that we have to run the right control experiments, which means that in trials with transplants in monkeys we have to have control groups large enough to do statistically rigorous analysis between the transplant recipients and the control animals. We also have to be patient since the time course in primates is much longer than that in rodents. We have to allow time for the disease symptoms to develop. We have to show that the impairments are stable. We then have to use the right control groups in order to show that transplants may be effective and compare our results with those obtained with other forms of therapy, such as L-dopa.

R. A. E. BAKAY (*Emory University, Atlanta, GA*): We have used a number of MPTP animals and have had extensive discussions with the NIH and Dr. Langston. If a series of standard doses of MPTP is given to an animal, about 10 percent will begin to recover spontaneously. It behooves one to wait for at least 2 months and possibly 3 months before transplantation; we even waited 8 months in one animal.

You can get a very stable animal using MPTP if you are very careful and titrate your doses. Changes are occurring in the animal even as it is being dosed. You have to be very patient: we have sometimes dosed our animals for as long as 36 weeks before making sure that it was, in fact, a parkinsonian animal. The MPTP model is an outstanding one, although there may be better ways to give it than intravenously. Some researchers at the NIH are directly injecting MPTP into the substantia nigra to obtain lesions. They have even found a circling model produced by unilateral lesion. The effectiveness of this will have to be determined by further investigation.

P. PASIK (*Mount Sinai School of Medicine, New York, NY*): My comment is rather heretical. At this meeting we have heard how useful the MPTP model is in helping us evaluate transplantation as a possible technique in humans. But beyond that the MPTP model may serve a more important purpose in elucidating both pharmacologic manipulation as well as the disease process itself, thereby possibly rendering transplantation unnecessary. Studies by others and ourselves have shown, for instance, that monoamine oxidase inhibitors, particularly of the B type, like diprenyl, completely protect the monkey from the MPTP effect.

So it may be shown that we can somehow arrest the actual chronic process of the disease by protecting the few survivor neurons by giving monoamine oxidase inhibitors. By so doing we would risk less in alleviating such a terrible condition by drugs rather than by using transplantation.

GASH: We've heard that there are three possible approaches to using transplants for alleviating Parkinson's disease, but it's still too early to say which might be the most successful. Fetal tissue has the longest track record and adrenal medullary grafts transplanted in rodents may be effective. The third approach, which may also be effective, is the use of cultured cell lines. It's too soon to make a commitment to any one approach.

I would also like to agree with Dr. Redmond: we have a good animal model in the MPTP-treated primate and we had best spend time evaluating these three approaches in animals before more clinical experiments are done.

BAKAY: I agree that each of these three means by which tissue can be implanted shows promise, but needs to be investigated extensively.

Dr. Gash's work with cultured cell lines is outstanding and I would certainly encourage him in it. However, I am concerned that even if 1 percent of those cells were not "turned off" they could grow into a tumor over time. Since we're talking in terms of primates—whose survival time is 20 to 30 years in monkeys.—you may not see any changes for a couple of years.

The method using material from the adrenal gland has the greatest potential. Some of the things that Dr. Freed has shown are encouraging, although some of the older glands don't work as well in terms of reversing deficits; perhaps they need to be cultured with other factors such as nerve growth factor before implantation. With respect to fetal tissue my personal view is that as long as society feels that abortions are legal there is no ethical difference between using that aborted tissue than there is in using an organ from a person who has died in a motor vehicle accident. It isn't just neuroscientists who are going to have a problem with the use of fetal tissue because researchers in a number of other areas of biology are going to be interested in its use as well.

M. DEL CERRO (*University of Rochester School of Medicine, Rochester, NY*): A comment was made that no one had presented material on eye chamber transplants, but I would like to note that my colleagues and I did display a poster on this subject at this conference. Some of our results are relevant to the problem of how donor age may complicate comparisons of graft sizes. Good transplant material may be obtained from a donor within a certain interval, and this interval depends on the system. Our work with the eye chamber and ventricular transplants shows that, for the retina at least, the window of time is incredibly wide—good growth can be obtained from embryonic day 13 to postnatal day 3.

The problem of determining the best age for using retinal transplants applies to other systems as well. And researchers besides ourselves work with mixtures of cells taken from donors of different ages. So, one of our concerns is found in the question: what is the best age for survival of a given cell population within a mixture?

OLSON: We already have some idea of the way these transplants might work. It has been shown convincingly at the electron microscopic level that transplanted fetal dopamine neurons form synapses with host caudate neurons. We also know from electrophysiological studies that identified dopamine cells in the grafts are spontaneously electrically active. Consequently, all the prerequisites are there for these cells to put out dopamine.

Adrenal grafts probably work because of diffusion of catecholamines, and they work in a way similar to the way L-dopa therapy does. Also, we have tried to implant dialysis fibers chronically into striatum of rats and then simply infuse L-dopa or dopamine, which is, of course, a perfect treatment for the symptoms in the rat.

PASIK: Dr. Olson, when I referred to working out the microcircuitry of these implants I was referring essentially to primates. I don't know of any studies that you have shown which permit extrapolating from rodent to primate. I don't know to what extent that's valid in this particular case.

M. SEGAL (*Weizmann Institute, Rehovot, Israel*): The strategy of what kind of cells to use and what kind of implantation to try depends on your basic assumption of what a transplant is doing. If the transplant can work in the first day after transplantation as Dr. Sladek has shown, you don't need any synapses. Dr. Gash has shown that you just have to introduce some cells there and they will produce acetylcholine. Synapses are not needed, and you don't need to wait a long time. Perhaps the best strategy would to be to design a cell that would produce a lot of dopamine. Or perhaps you could just place a slow-release capsule that contained dopamine and that would solve all the biological problems and moral issues. You could place in the striatum some kind of device that would release dopamine over a period of years.

C. SOTELO (*Inserm U106, CMC Foch, Suresnes, France*): I think that it's time to issue a warning. As a biologist I believe that tissue transplantation is a wonderful tool. We have a lot of things to learn, and we are grateful to those who have begun to develop this technique. But I would ask the neurosurgeons to call a bit of a moratorium on clinical experiments in humans and to wait to learn what's happened with the monkeys to see whether transplantation is the best way to treat some MPTP Parkinson's disease. Don't forget that the most important thing in Parkinson's disease is to understand the etiology of this disease. As Alain Prochiantz has said, if this disease is caused by a virus or if it is an autoimmune disease, the fact that you change neurons doesn't stop the process. Even if the neurons you implant are beautiful, even if they are capable of producing all types of catecholamines, and even if they integrate morphologically, they will still probably be killed by the disease, which continues to be degenerative and progressive.

Consequently, we need to wait at least several years in order to be sure that transplantation is the best and the most appropriate way to treat patients who do not respond to L-dopa.

OLSON: I agree in principle that this is true now that the MPTP model exists. I wanted to comment upon the death of the neurons. We know that they die very slowly. So, if the disease process goes on and captures the new neurons, there is no reason to believe that they will die faster than the old ones so the procedure could still be beneficial; isn't that so?

SOTELO: To have a hypothesis you must have an idea of what has happened. Did the disease start very early or very late in human life? Some disease is slow, but there is a progressive Parkinson's disease that evolves quickly. We don't have any idea about the physiology; how you can be sure that the embryonic cells or the chromaffin cells grafted in the brain will not die in 3 or 4 years? If these patients have a progressive disease, we estimate 4 to 5 years as the average survival time. Human beings today in the occidental countries live for about 70 years, so for as long as 30 years you should know what's happened with the cells you have transplanted.

WYATT: I agree that we should do the studies and develop techniques in monkeys before going on to humans. I disagree with you, Dr. Sotelo, about this last point, though. If you could "buy" a patient 4 years of life it would be worth it—I don't see that there's any question about that. So once we have the technique worked out in monkeys, neurosurgeons can apply it in humans. I think it ought to be tried. If it doesn't work, it doesn't work. If a patient gets 4 more years, fine; if he gets 10 years that's magnificent.

P. BRUNDIN (*University of Lund, Sweden*): I'd like to offer a brief analogy: Diabetic patients with renal problems get transplants and sometimes those kidneys get affected by the disease. But those patients are helped a great deal by transplantation. Even though they can survive on dialysis for some time, these patients like the renal grafts a lot more.

J. M. MORIHISA (*Veterans Administration Medical Center, Washington, DC*): The last issue points up an essential dichotomy between developing a therapeutic modality which will help lessen suffering and the elucidation of basic neuroscientific principles. Thus, as we try to decide which techniques are most useful and effective, we must also remember that one of the greatest prizes in this adventure may be in a better understanding of the disease process, which may then in turn lead to an unexpected new approach to treatment of Parkinson's disease. I would say do not concentrate on possible new approaches in terms of eliminating one or the other, but pursue all of them in their many forms to try and elucidate the underlying principles that make them work.

G. D. PAPPAS (*University of Illinois, Chicago, IL*): We're mixing up some concepts here. Transplantation is not the answer for anything; transplantation is a tool that basic neuroanatomists and cell biologists should use, but transplants don't do anything for us. They delay understanding what goes wrong. The problems we have are fundamentally not ethical problems; rather, they're problems of intellectual and basic research.

Certainly there is a place for kidney transplants right now, but this procedure does not answer the questions in renal disease. We're overlooking the fact that this is patch-up technology. Just as artificial lungs were not the answer to the problem of polio, transplants are not going to be the answer to anything in the long run. While transplantation is an important tool in rodent research and in research in cellular interactions, we should remember that it is a halfway technology. Let's not confuse technology and basic research.

R. M. LINDSAY (*Sandoz Institute for Medical Research, London, England*): We're here discussing perhaps four human experiments and one or two hundred experiments in monkey experiments when most of us have carried out perhaps ten million experiments in rats. So perhaps we could discuss some of the cellular and molecular findings of the rat experiments, how these may lead ultimately to not having to use transplants at all, and how our understanding may be enhanced of how degenerative diseases occur.

PAPPAS: No one here is against preventive therapy; certainly everyone agrees that the best way to treat a disease is to prevent it. But in reality these diseases occur, and we are focussing on one particular approach that might improve the quality of life for individuals with neurodegenerative diseases. At the same time we are interested in basic science. But we don't want to get so theoretical about the approach that we forget the reality that people have Parkinson's disease now and will probably continue to develop Parkinson's disease or other neurodegenerative diseases in the future.

Our ultimate goal is to improve the quality of life for these persons. No one is against preventing diseases, but if they develop let's look at the most practical way of treating them.

BAKAY: These experiments in rats are a basic science tool and as such are absolutely essential. My work was certainly not in isolation, Dr. Pappas; I used all of your work. But this technology must also be viewed in terms of what it can do for people. While controls in both Dr. Sladek's and in my work are needed, I don't think that the controls of a placebo operation are appropriate.

The bypass study did not have a placebo group. No surgery was done without a connection being made: the control group was a medically treated group, and we should remember that. If we're ever going to show that the transplant is an effective mode of therapy, it must do better than the available medical treatment—that's essentially the bottom line. The same thing is true in cardiology: you have to show that a cardiac operation gives better results than can be gotten with medical therapy. Certainly pumping drugs in is a good idea; however, the problem is not in getting the drugs there, the problem is that in a progressive disease the receptors become supersensitive, which creates a problem later on. We are very interested in what will occur later on: our work is preliminary and 5 years from now I may have to take it all back.

PAPPAS: No debate. Of course you have to treat victims of polio with mechanical machines—we're not heartless about these things. But let's understand what really counts here—the importance of basic biomedical research. I reiterate: we have to have technology, but the problem is only going to be solved by basic research. We have to continue the other work, but we must understand the difference between technology and fundamental research.

E. C. AZMITIA (*New York University, New York, NY*): We know so little at this point that to close any door is unwise. If there are patients who are not responding to drug treatment and who do consent to undergo experimentation, then it probably should be done. If the monkey MPTP model is working, then we should all work to increase research on primates. There's a danger in this country that research in nonhuman primates is on the decline. The work presented at this session on primate research demonstrates that we need to increase our efforts in this direction. We should start to set up the facilities and the guidelines for primate work. We should try to persuade the general public that we need this support to attack some of these critical issues.

I would like to emphasize that when we do approach these problems we should remember that we're addressing them as scientists. It would probably be a very good education for all of us to reread Claude Bernard's book on experimentation and to review the theories behind it. When we propose a new theory we are responsible to try and *disprove* rather than prove it. When we design our experiments, we should be heavy on the control side. We should use and analyze our material double-blind. Maybe we should go so far as to have controls within some of our human patients by not putting in the grafts. It sounds cruel, but I think that these are the kinds of things we have to do to be very rigorous. Our findings should not raise false expectations for other patients. A patient may feel that by receiving a graft he's going to get better. So controls may be necessary in the same way that you divide your drug treatment groups into placebo and experimental groups. For this kind of experimental surgical procedure it might be wise to have those kinds of controls in order to see whether we just raised expectations or whether the procedure of placing the cannula into the brain can have beneficial effects. We must be more rigorous with ourselves. If in Dr. Sladek's experiments, in which he had three animals, two of those animals had been controls and one had been the experimental subject, the results, as elegant as they were, would have been even more convincing. We can't forget that we are scientists, and while it's nice to be the first to prove our own theories correct, science progresses by *disproving* theories. Don't forget the controls, for they are necessary for this type of work.

O. LINDVALL (*University of Lund, Sweden*): A short comment about controls: for our experiment it would have been of great value to have some kind of control so we could attribute changes to catecholamine release. But I want to make it clear that the major findings in the human trials with adrenal medulla have been negative thus far—they have shown that we cannot help the patient with this approach as it is done today. Although we haven't seen any negative effect, we must tell our patients that we don't have a transplantation therapy at present, and at the moment I think it would be unethical to do any sham procedures. On the other hand, if we had seen spectacular changes, then we would have considered doing sham procedures.

AZMITIA: In testing an experimental drug is it ethical to give the drug to half of the population while giving a placebo to the other half?

I don't understand how in experimental testing you can say it's unethical to have a control. You can say that it doesn't make sense or that it's not economic, but I don't see how you can say it's not ethical.

OLSON: First, in a sense we do have a motivational control and that is because we did unilateral implantations on one side and there was no way the patient would figure out on which way to be better because they didn't realize about the crossed projections from the caudate. The acute beneficial effects were contralateral to the implantation, which is strong evidence that it was related to the surgery and probably even to release of catecholamines, although that is not proven.

So in a sense we have controls. You might question whether or not it was right to do these first experiments, but imagine the following: imagine that they worked much better than they did, except that in two patients it didn't work and afterwards we had to say to them, "Sorry, but you were the controls." That would be a very tough situation.

AZMITIA: Imagine if all four did improve dramatically and it was due simply to implanting the cannula. . . .

REDMOND: There's no argument that animal experiments should be done with adequate controls. That's just one of the reasons to try and encourage additional animal experiments because all different kinds of control groups need to be set up. We have treated 19 monkeys with MPTP and we used a whole variety of control animals for every different part of the procedure. As far as the human clinical trials are concerned, there are some ethical problems that make it more difficult to determine exactly when and how to control for procedures. Many things can be done in animals that cannot ethically be done in humans.

WYATT: The issue of human controls is extremely important. It is instructive to look at the case with coronary bypass surgery. This was done by eager surgeons for years with no change in mortality rate and only some benefit in morbidity. Now it's clear that for certain conditions it works and other conditions it doesn't.

E.-O. BACKLUND (*University of Bergen, Norway*): I appreciate all these comments and welcome controversy. We had a parallel example among neurosurgeons a number of years ago when it was argued within the context of so-called psychosurgery whether one should also perform sham operations in treating epilepsy. But the negative attitudes to such thoughts were overwhelming. And you can't, of course, compare sham operations with placebos.

S. FAHN (*Columbia University, New York, NY*): Although Parkinson's disease is a degenerative and progressive one that doesn't spontaneously lessen in the long run, there are many examples of transient remission. One example is the phenomenon known as paradoxical kinesia, in which the patient suddenly gets better and the patient with Parkinson's disease is the first one out of the burning building. Or, you throw a ball quickly to a patient who couldn't move and all of a sudden he's moving and catching the ball before it hits him. This is a well known phenomenon; obviously these patients are not paralyzed and when the circuitry is activated, these persons can move their limbs.

Similar things have been seen after surgical procedures that have been performed for other reasons—not in the type of operation we're describing here. A transient improvement will occur after surgery, even without medication just for a couple of days and then the condition reverts to baseline. The same thing occurs with electroshock therapy: there have been a number of examples in patients with Parkinson's disease who have had electroshock therapy for depression. Some of these patients had remission of parkinsonian symptoms for several weeks afterwards. Performance became close to normal, but after a period of time their conditions also reverted to baseline. So, even in a disease like Parkinson's, which is degenerative, there are transient periods of remission that must be taken into account.

I don't know why the patients in Sweden got better for a short period of time after the operation; maybe it was related to the operation and maybe not. The fact that those patients didn't get better provides a control group of sorts for other experiments. We know that the actual transplantations of some of these tissues were failures. So, just by transplanting something or inserting a probe into the striatum is itself not going to be beneficial. These operations, then, are almost like sham operations for the next type of procedure, which may be the implantation of fetal tissue.

We should always bear in mind the natural biology of Parkinson's disease. The question of whether it is ethical to do sham operations should remain controversial; we shouldn't close the door on the possibility. Other surgeons may think that sham operations are not so unethical. Certainly the external carotid-internal carotid procedures were done for patients with cerebrovascular disease for years. Only when the double-blind study was finally done was it shown to be worthless. Yet people thought they might have gotten better from it just because there were open trials.

So we must still keep all the proper controls in place. It always amazes me how careful basic laboratory scientists are to have controls in animal experiments, but once they start working on patients, the controls disappear out the window and we're left with bad treatments for years. The history of medicine is replete with accounts of leech treatments and the like that were used before scientists or doctors began using controlled approaches to treatment and testing. We must be even more careful because of the seriousness of this surgical procedure and the potential harm that can be done to some of these patients.

FREEMAN: The primary dictum for surgeons and clinicians is "first do no harm." A placebo is a harmless control while neurosurgery is not. Consequently some other form of comparison is mandatory.

SLADEK: If you ask 400 000 or 500 000 parkinsonian patients in this country alone whether they would be willing to undergo an operation that might prevent the progression of disease or lessen some of the motor deficits, they will invariably say yes. If you ask a leukemia patient whether he or she would like a bone marrow transplant again I think the answer would be yes. Eight years ago I informed my mother that she would require two heart valves from a pig to stay alive. She was a bit skeptical, but I'm delighted to say that as a result she's alive and delightful at 75 years of age. So the point is that while such surgical intervention is not going to cure the disease, it is capable of doing such good that it would be irresponsible not to pursue this approach.

LINDSAY: I must take exception to Dr. Sladek's remark that the availability of human guinea pigs wanting to have an experiment done on them is a reason for doing an experiment. I think that we as scientists must decide whether a treatment has some real possibility of success rather than decide to do it simply because there are 500 000 people willing to try it out simply because they don't know what the answer will be.

During the period several years ago in Britain when interferon was popular there was the sudden hope that interferon was going to solve everything. The amount of public debate and the amount of agony it caused to people who thought there was a cure around the corner certainly outweighed any of the results.

SLADEK: I must respond to your inference about my remarks. I did not mean to imply that we should make human guinea pigs out of a population of depressed and debilitated parkinsonian patients. I completely agree with what my colleague Dr. Redmond has said about the need for primate research and I think that we are years away from operations in humans. I encourage our very courageous colleagues from Scandinavia to continue their work. I would like to see them move in the direction of fetal nerve cells because I believe that it is much easier to expect a fetal nerve cell to behave like a neuron than it is for some other cell type to do so. But I do not want to leave the wrong impression that we should be ready to move this work on until we really know the long-term effects of fetal grafting. If you recall from earlier evidence I showed, the early gestational grafts were enormous. They may be growing in an unchecked or unregulated manner and, indeed, perhaps an obstruction from those grafts would worsen the situation and kill the patient. But on the other hand, when I recall so many unhappy parkinsonian patients depressed at facing a progressive disease that will probably kill them in 10 years, I don't want to see us stand still either.

PASIK: I'm beginning to become a little bit disturbed because I thought that some kind of consensus was developing, but apparently there is no consensus at all. I thought that we were moving toward the idea of having obtained a relatively good model of parkinsonism, not Parkinson's disease, mind you, but a model in an animal that shows parkinsonian signs. Then I thought that we were going toward experimentation with that particular model. When we have a method absolutely beyond doubt and when that method—be it transplantation or something else—is able to alleviate or cure the disease in the animal, then and only then will we dare touch another human being.

I'd like to recount an anecdote related to Dr. Azmitia's remark about a patient requesting surgery. When I was a resident in neurology I presented a case in which the patient started with sciatica, which caused him intractable pain. Eventually a laminectomy was performed, and later, because the patient still had pain, a chordotomy was carried out. Further procedures were done which had the effect of chopping his nervous system up to the point where he was like a zombie.

I asked him, "How do you feel?" "Bad," he answered. So I asked, "Do you still have the pain?" "Yes." "Would you like another operation?" "Yes," he said again. That's my point.

BRUNDIN: Unfortunately this debate has become polarized between neurobiologists and clinicians. I suggest that the clinicians should go to a laboratory and look down a microscope and the neurobiologist should go to a neurological clinic and look at a patient.

Serotonin Metabolism in Raphe Neurons Transplanted into Rat Hippocampus

S. B. AUERBACH,[a,b] F. C. ZHOU,[c] B. L. JACOBS,[d]
AND E. C. AZMITIA[c]

[b]Rutgers University
Piscataway, New Jersey 08854

[c]New York University
New York, New York 10003

[d]Princeton University
Princeton, New Jersey 08544

Fetal raphe cells transplanted into adult rat brain survive and form functional synaptic connections,[1] but little is known about metabolism and release of serotonin (5-HT) from transplanted neurons. Serotonergic neurons are autoactive and thus, even in the absence of presynaptic input, may release 5-HT. As indices of neuronal activity, rates of 5-HT synthesis and catabolism were measured before and after neurotoxin lesions of the serotonergic innervation of the hippocampus in adult rats and after transplantation of fetal raphe tissue into the 5-HT-denervated hippocampus.

For bilateral lesions of the serotonergic innervation of the hippocampus, male rats (280-350 g) received desmethylimipramine (10 mg/kg, i.p.) and then were injected with 5,7-dihydroxytryptamine (5,7-DHT) into the dorsal and medial raphe nuclei (coordinates relative to the midsagittal line at lambda: 0.0 mm L, 0.2 mm A, and 6.8-7.8 mm V). Two weeks after these lesions, rats were given a unilateral injection of minced tissue from the raphe area of day 15 rat fetuses. Hippocampal coordinates were 1.0-5.0 mm L, 4.5 mm A, and 3.7 mm V. One month after transplantation, rats were used in studies of 5-HT metabolism.

The rate of 5-HT synthesis was estimated by the accumulation of 5-hydroxytryptophan (5-HTP) 1 hr after injecting rats with m-hydroxybenzylhydrazine (100 mg/kg, i.p.). The metabolites and 5-HT were analyzed by high-performance liquid chromatography.[2,3] The normal value for 5-HTP accumulation in the hippocampus was 0.23 ± 0.02 ng/mg wet wt (mean $\pm$ SEM), as shown in TABLE 1. The 5,7-DHT lesion reduced 5-HTP accumulation to 65% of the normal value. In contrast, 5-HTP accumulation in hippocampus that had received a lesion and raphe transplants was significantly increased, to 65% above normal. TABLE 1 also shows that the 5,7-DHT lesion reduced 5-HT and 5-hydroxyindoleacetic acid (5-HIAA) levels to about 50% of normal, and raphe transplants restored the 5-HT level to 138% and the 5-HIAA level to 118% of normal. Catabolism of 5-HT was estimated by the increase in the

[a]Address for correspondence: Rutgers University, Department of Biological Sciences, Box 1059, Piscataway, New Jersey 08854.

TABLE 1. Monoamine Content in Hippocampus 60 Min after Decarboxylase Inhibition

| | Monoamine Content (ng/mg wet wt) | | |
Group	5-HT	5-HIAA	5-HTP
Normal rats	0.34 ± 0.03	0.22 ± 0.02	0.23 ± 0.02
Rats with raphe lesions	0.16 ± 0.03[a]	0.11 ± 0.02[a]	0.15 ± 0.03[a]
Rats with transplants	0.47 ± 0.11[b]	0.26 ± 0.05[b]	0.38 ± 0.09[b]

NOTE: Each value is a mean ± SEM. Each group included 10 rats.
[a] Significantly different from corresponding values for normals ($p \leq .001$).
[b] Significantly different from corresponding values for rats with raphe lesions ($p \leq .001$).

5-HIAA level after injection with probenecid (200 mg/kg, i.p.). As calculated from the values shown in TABLE 2, the normal conversion rate of 5-HT to 5-HIAA is 0.18 ng/mg wet wt/hr. The rate is reduced to 88% of normal by the 5,7-DHT lesion. Although raphe transplants in this group of rats restored the 5-HT level to 121% and the 5-HIAA level to 117% of normal, 5-HIAA accumulation was not significantly greater in hippocampus that had received transplants than it was in hippocampus that had received lesions. These results suggest that the turnover of 5-HT is elevated in nerve terminals that survive the 5,7-DHT lesion. Thus the ratio of 5-HTP to 5-HT is 0.94 for the 5-HT-depleted hippocampus and 0.68 for the normal hippocampus. Similarly, the normal ratio of 5-HIAA accumulation to 5-HT is 0.54, and it is increased to 1.08 for the partially 5-HT-depleted hippocampus. The raphe transplants restored these estimates of turnover to lower, more normal levels.

Acute stress (scrambled footshock, 30 min) did not affect 5-HIAA accumulation as calculated from data shown in TABLE 2, but was associated with a 17% depletion

TABLE 2. Monoamine Content in Hippocampus 30 Min after Probenecid Administration

| | | | Monoamine Content (ng/mg wet wt) | |
Group	Probenecid	Shock	5-HT	5-HIAA
Normal rats	0	0	0.33 ± 0.01	0.24 ± 0.01
	+	0	0.36 ± 0.01	0.33 ± 0.01
	+	+	0.30 ± 0.01[a]	0.34 ± 0.01
Rats with raphe lesions	0	0	0.13 ± 0.03[b]	0.08 ± 0.02[b]
	+	0	0.16 ± 0.02[b]	0.15 ± 0.03[b]
	+	+	0.17 ± 0.03[b]	0.15 ± 0.02[b]
Rats with transplants	0	0	0.40 ± 0.02[c]	0.28 ± 0.03[c]
	+	0	0.37 ± 0.02[c]	0.34 ± 0.02[c]
	+	+	0.34 ± 0.03[c]	0.30 ± 0.03[c]

NOTE: Each value is a mean ± SEM. The normal groups included four rats; the groups with lesions and the groups with transplants included five rats.
[a] Significantly different from corresponding value for nonshocked, normal rats ($p \leq .01$).
[b] Significantly different from corresponding value for normal rats ($p \leq .001$).
[c] Significantly different from corresponding value for rats with raphe lesions ($p \leq .001$).

of 5-HT from normal hippocampus. Footshock stress did not significantly affect the 5-HT level in the hippocampus with lesions or in the hippocampus with raphe transplants.

In conclusion, these results show that 5-HT metabolism occurs in raphe tissue when transplanted into the 5-HT-denervated hippocampus, consistent with the possibility that 5-HT is released from the transplanted neurons. The data also suggest that partial denervation accelerates 5-HT turnover in surviving nerve terminals, but that serotonergic neuronal activity is relatively unresponsive to modulation by acute stress.

REFERENCES

1. AZMITIA, E. C. & P. M. WHITAKER. 1983. Neurosci. Lett. **38:** 145-150.
2. AUERBACH, S. B., F. C. ZHOU, B. L. JACOBS & E. C. AZMITIA. 1985. Neurosci. Lett. **61:** 147-152.
3. AUERBACH, S. B. & P. LIPTON. 1985. J. Neurochem. **44:** 1116-1130.

Transplants Modify the Response of Immature Neurons to Damage[a]

BARBARA S. BREGMAN

Department of Anatomy
University of Maryland School of Medicine
Baltimore, Maryland 21201

Although descending serotonergic axons can regenerate after chemical lesions in adult animals, they show little regrowth after mechanical lesions. It has been suggested that after mechanical lesion, the local environment at the lesion site prevents the regrowth of these axons. In newborn animals, the serotonergic axons show no regrowth after either chemical or mechanical lesions. Axotomy by either method in the newborn animal results in the death of the raphe-spinal neurons. We have recently demonstrated that in newborn rats, transplants of fetal spinal cord tissue to lesion-sustaining spinal cord prevents the retrograde cell death of immature axotomized rubrospinal neurons.[1] After spinal cord lesions sustained neonatally, even late-developing, uninjured axons are unable to grow through the site of a lesion, but can take an aberrant route through adjacent undamaged spinal cord tissue. The current experiments were designed to determine 1) whether transplants of fetal spinal cord tissue to lesion-sustaining spinal cord in newborn rats prevent the retrograde cell death of immature axotomized raphe-spinal neurons; 2) whether these transplants provide a terrain that supports the growth of serotonergic axons across the site of the neonatal lesion; and 3) whether the axons that cross the transplant are late-growing axons, regenerating axons, or both.

Spinal cord transections were made at T6 in newborn rat pups. Transplants of spinal cord tissue from fetuses 12-14 days in gestation (E12-14) were placed into the lesion site in half of the animals. Peroxidase-antiperoxidase immunocytochemical techniques were used to examine the serotonergic input to the transplant and to the host spinal cord caudal to the transplant. Retrograde double-labeling techniques with fluorescent tracers were used to determine whether late-growing or regrowing neurons contribute to this innervation.

At E12-14, the spinal cord does not contain any serotonergic innervation. At birth, serotonergic fibers can be identified at all levels of the spinal cord, but the pattern of innervation remains immature until 14 days after birth. Immunocytochemical analysis of the transplant from 1 month to 1 year survival reveals a moderate to dense serotonergic innervation throughout the transplant. No serotonin-immunoreactive cell bodies are present within the transplants. Neonatal transection (without transplant) abolishes the serotonergic innervation of the spinal cord caudal to the lesion within 7 days after transection. In animals with transplants, however, serotonergic axons are identified both within the transplant and within the host spinal cord

[a] This work was supported by Grant NS19259 from the National Institutes of Health and by Grant 5-448 from the March of Dimes.

caudal to the transection. In the host spinal cord caudal to the transplant, fascicles of serotonergic fibers are often located in an ectopic position, but, despite their abnormal position within the white matter, the serotonergic fibers innervate normal targets within the gray matter, for example, the intermediolateral cell column. Growth is not limited to spinal cord segments immediately adjacent to the lesion and transplant; serotonergic fibers are present throughout the host cord as far as the lumbar enlargement. Analysis of the nucleus raphe magnus indicates that the transplants prevent the retrograde cell death of immature axotomized raphe-spinal neurons. Thus, late-developing or regrowing serotonergic axons are able to cross the site of a neonatal spinal cord transection by growing through the transplant and to innervate the host spinal cord caudal to the lesion. Preliminary double-labeling experiments indicate that both late-growing and regenerating neurons contribute to this innervation.

REFERENCES

1. BREGMAN, B. S. & P. J. REIER. 1986. Neural tissue transplants rescue axotomized rubrospinal cells from retrograde death. J. Comp. Neurol. 244: 86-95.

Transplanting Strips of Immature Retinal Tissue and Suspensions of Dissociated Retinal Cells into Normal and Extensively Damaged Eyes[a]

M. DEL CERRO, D. M. GASH, M. F. D. NOTTER,
G. N. RAO, S. J. WIEGAND, L. Q. JIANG, AND
C. DEL CERRO

*University of Rochester Medical School
Rochester, New York 14642*

As a continuation of our previous work on intravitreal retinal transplants in the rat,[1-3] we present here an overview of new studies in which the developing retina was transplanted into normal and extensively damaged adult eyes.

MATERIALS AND METHODS

Embryonic (postconceptual days 13-18) and perinatal rats of the Long-Evans strain served as donors. The transplant consisted of either a strip of neural retina, approximately 1 mm^3 in volume, or 2 μl of a suspension of enzymatically dissociated neural retinal cells in culture medium, at a concentration of 60-600 × 10^3 cells/μl. The hosts were young adult males of either Long-Evans or Lewis strain. In some experimental series, the host retina had been previously damaged by continuous light exposure to decimate photoreceptor cells, or by intraocular injection of kainic acid to destroy ganglion cells and amacrine cells. Donor cells were labeled with Fast Blue, [³H]thymidine, or both. Survival times ranged from 0 to 120 posttransplantation days.

RESULTS

Successful transplants result in a mass of retinal tissue developing on the host retina or anterior chamber (FIG. 1), and the cells forming this mass carry the label

[a] This work was supported by Grant EY 05262 from the National Eye Institute and by the Rochester Eye Bank.

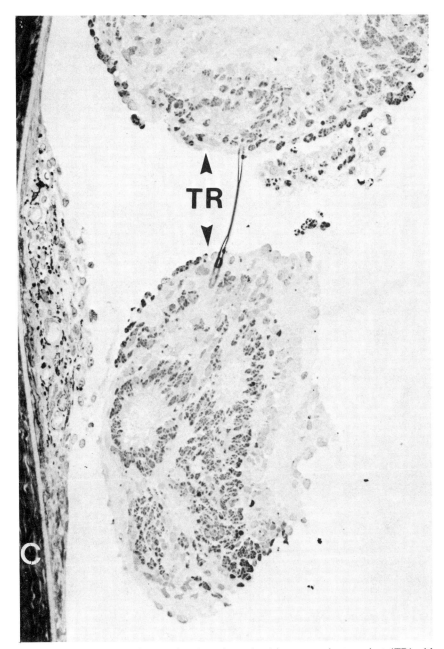

FIGURE 1. A thin layer of connective tissue (arrowheads) connects the transplant (TR) with the host cornea (C). A Long-Evans rat (embryonic day 14) was the donor; a Lewis rat was the host. Survival: 26 days. Original magnification: ×325; enlarged to 123% of original size.

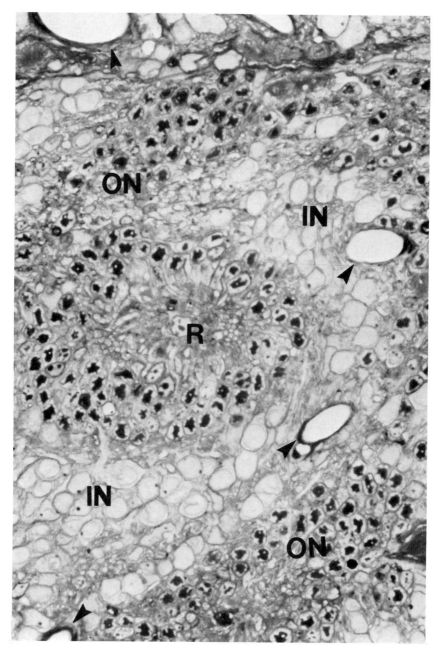

FIGURE 2. Light micrograph showing an instance of rosette (R) formation and dysplasia of outer nuclear (ON) layer cells in the inner nuclear (IN) layer. Numerous vessels are present in the field (arrowheads). A Long-Evans rat (embryonic day 14) was the donor; another Long-Evans rat was the host. Survival: 30 days. Original magnifications: ×750; enlarged to 123% of original size.

identifying them as donor cells. Light and electron microscopical examination of the transplants show differentiation of the nuclear and plexiform layers, which are populated by the expected neuronal and glial types. Differentiation includes the appearance of numerous rod cells, and a few cones. Rosettes often form within the transplant (FIG. 2). The lumina of these rosettes are limited by an outer limiting membrane and are filled by cilia-bearing inner segments, and by contorted outer segments. Some macrophages loaded with cytoplasmic debris, apparently from the outer segments, are also a constant feature within the rosettes. As the transplants grow on the host retina and become progressively vascularized, the layers of the transplant blend with those of the host retina. Synapses of both the conventional and ribbon types are found within the plexiform layers of the transplant. Successful grafts occurred in eyes with normal as well as in eyes with extensively damaged retinas. Neither clinical nor histological indications of immune-mediated rejection occurred in these series, even though the transplants involved outbred donors and included hosts of a different strain.

DISCUSSION

These experiments confirm the viability of intraocular retinal transplants. In particular, the results indicate the following: 1) It is possible to successfully transplant embryonic and perinatal rat retinas to the eyes of adult hosts of the same, or even of a different strain. 2) Transplant growth takes place in contact with normal, but, more significantly, in contact with extensively damaged retinas. 3) Intraocular retinal transplants fulfill the basic requirements to be considered as tools for possible neuronal replacement and reconstruction of damaged circuits in the adult retina.

REFERENCES

1. DEL CERRO, M., D. M. GASH, G. N. RAO, M. F. NOTTER, S. J. WIEGAND & M. GUPTA. 1985. Intraocular retinal transplants. Invest. Ophthalmol. Vis. Sci. **26:** 1182-1185.
2. DEL CERRO, M., D. M. GASH, G. N. RAO, M. F. NOTTER, S. J. WIEGAND & C. DEL CERRO. 1985. Retinal transplants into the anterior chamber and vitreal cavity of adult rats. Invest. Ophthalmol. Vis. Sci. Abstr. **26:** 336.
3. DEL CERRO, M., D. M. GASH, G. N. RAO, M. F. NOTTER, S. J. WIEGAND & C. DEL CERRO. 1985. Retinal transplants into normal and extensively damaged adult retinas. Soc. Neurosci. Abstr. **11:** 15.

Effects of Transplanting Rabbit Substantia Nigra into the Striatum of Rats with Experimental Hemiparkinsonism

JERZY DYMECKI, ANGNIESZKA JEDRZEJEWSKA,
MACIEJ POLTORAK, OLGIERD PUCILOWSKI,
ANDRZEJ BIDZINSKI, AND WALDEMAR WOSKO

Department of Neuropathology
Department of Pharmacology and Neurophysiology
and
Department of Biochemistry
Psychoneurological Institute
Warsaw, Poland

Most of the reports on the survival and effects of cross-species intracerebral grafts concern mouse-to-rat transplantations. We did not find in the literature any reports concerning rabbit-to-rat intracerebral transplantations.

The aim of our study was to evaluate the effects of transplanting rabbit substantia nigra (SN) into the brains of rats with experimentally induced hemiparkinsonism. Ventral mesencephalon, containing the SN, was removed from gestational day 21 rabbit embryos and transplanted into the striatal region or into the lateral ventricle of each of 90 adult albino Wistar rats. A unilateral lesion was created in the SN of each rat by injecting 6-hydroxydopamine; the transplant was then placed ipsilateral to the lesion. No immunosuppressive treatment was applied. In a control group, sham transplantations were performed by introducing a needle without injecting any material.

Before and 2, 4, and 6 weeks after transplantation, apomorphine-induced rotational behavior was tested. Survival of the grafts was evaluated using histological and histofluorescence methods. The Heubrich and Denzer technique was used to perform biochemical analyses to determine the dopamine content in isolated·right and left sides of the striatum.

A significant decrease in the number of rotations (to 46% of the number of rotations before transplantation) was observed in the experimental group 2 weeks after transplantation. The decrease was still pronounced after 4 weeks (57%). By 6 weeks after transplantation, rotational behavior had returned to 64% of baseline levels (TABLE 1). Animals with sham transplantations showed a moderate increase in the number of rotations.

Histological and histofluorescence examination, performed 2 weeks after transplantation, showed survival of about 50% of the grafts. After 4 weeks, however, about 70%, and after 6 weeks, almost 90% of the grafts demonstrated signs of rejection.

696

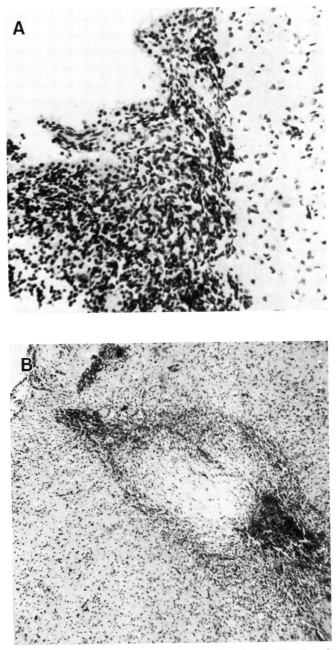

FIGURE 1. (**A**) Intraventricular graft 1 week after transplantation. Proliferation of blastic cells and lymphocytes in the area of the graft, which is closely connected to the striatum. (**B**) Intraparenchymal graft 2 weeks after transplantation. Necrosis in the central part of the graft, surrounded by a rich lymphocytic reaction.

TABLE 1. Rotational Behavior Induced by Apomorphine in Animals with SN Lesions before and after Transplantation of Rabbit SN

	Number of Rotations during 5-min Test (mean ± SEM)	Percentage of Baseline Rotation
Before transplantation[a]	28 ± 3	100
After transplantation		
2 weeks	13 ± 3[b]	46
4 weeks	16 ± 2[b]	57
6 weeks	18 ± 3[b]	64

[a] Two weeks after SN lesion.
[b] $p < .05$ as compared to rotations before transplantation.

The percentage of grafts surviving was higher when they were located in the lateral ventricle (FIG. 1A). In the area of grafts, particularly in the intraparenchymal ones, a rich lymphocytic reaction was observed (FIG. 1B). This reaction increased until 2 weeks had passed since the transplantation, and then gradually decreased.

The biochemical evaluation of dopamine content in the striatum was only performed in those animals that showed a decrease in rotation after transplantation. No significant differences, however, were observed after transplantation as compared with the dopamine content after the lesion alone.

It is concluded that heterologous rabbit-to-rat SN grafts survive for short periods of time and reduce apomorphine-induced rotational behavior until rejection occurs. The intraventricular localization of grafts increases the probability of survival. The presence of a lymphocytic reaction, which accompanies both intraventricular and intraparenchymal grafts, indicates that immunological mechanisms are involved in graft rejection.

Cross-species Grafts of Embryonic Rabbit Mesencephalic Tissue Survive and Cause Behavioral Recovery in the Presence of Chronic Immunosuppression

THOMAS B. FREEMAN,[a] LESLIE BRANDEIS,[b] JOHN PEARSON,[b] AND EUGENE S. FLAMM[a]

[a]*Department of Neurosurgery*
and
[b]*Department of Pathology*
New York University Medical Center
New York, New York 10016

A new model of xenogeneic neural grafting is described. Embryonic rabbit ventral mesencephalic tissue from outbred E14-17 rabbits was transplanted into Sprague-Dawley rat striatum in which lesions had been created with 6-hydroxydopamine (6-OHDA) (TABLE 1).

Optimal survival and function was seen in animals receiving suspension grafts from E14-15 donors. E14 mesencephalic tissue remained over 80% viable in basic medium at room temperature for at least 7 hr. Furthermore, about 10% of cells seen in smears of E14 ventral mesencephalon were tyrosine hydroxylase positive.

Chronic immunosuppression with cyclosporin A significantly improved survival of grafted dopaminergic neurons (chi-square test: df $= 1$; $\chi^2 = 0.05$). No animal that received grafts in the absence of immunosuppression demonstrated more than 16 surviving dopaminergic neurons, whereas immunosuppressed recipients had up to 3754 viable cells. The survival of transplants, however, was highly variable; only 8 of 14 immunosuppressed animals that received transplants showed evidence of surviving dopaminergic cells. At least one graft from each of the four rabbit donors survived.

Amphetamine-induced rotational activity was also significantly improved in the grafted-immunosuppressed group when compared to both the immunosuppressed (Wilcoxon test: $p < .02$) and nonimmunosuppressed control groups (Wilcoxon test: $p < .001$).

The outgrowth pattern of dopaminergic axonal terminal densities from grafts resembled the normal distribution of nigrostriatal projections (FIG. 1). Tyrosine hydroxylase staining stopped abruptly at the interface between striatum and corpus callosum. Likewise, ectopically placed dopaminergic cells in the cortex did not demonstrate axonal outgrowth. Therefore, rabbit dopaminergic cell outgrowth depends in part upon specific signals from the target region of the rat host that are functional across widely divergent species.

Three animals demonstrated behavioral recovery in the absence of more than 16 surviving grafted dopaminergic cells (two had no surviving dopaminergic cells). The striatum surrounding these graft regions showed an increase in dopaminergic terminal densities and axonal regions surrounding the graft for a distance of 1-3 mm. It is possible that some factor from these grafts induced a behaviorally significant neural reorganization of the remaining host striatal dopaminergic axons. If true, the specific stimulatory factor or restricted cell population that induced axonal sprouting or biochemical maturation cannot be determined from this experiment. Such a trophic factor, however, if present, would also be effective across species.

TABLE 1. Materials and Methods

Hosts	Outbred female Sprague-Dawley rats, 180-200 g at the start of the experiment.
Lesions	Unilateral 6-OHDA lesion of the right nigrostriatal pathway.[1]
Behavioral testing	Methamphetamine (5 mg/kg, i.p.)-induced rotation model of dopamine deficiency.[2]
Donor tissue	Embryonic mesencephalic tissue from outbred New Zealand White rabbits.
Donor gestational age	E14-17, where E0 is the day of conception.[a]
Method of transplantation	Stereotactic injection of suspension transplant.[4]
Coordinates of injection	Two microliters of suspension was injection into two locations in the dorsal striatum (L = 2.5 mm, AP = 2.0 mm rostral to bregma, and V = 3.5 and 4.5 mm below dura; incisor bar at 5.0 mm above the intraaural line).
Histology	Tyrosine hydroxalase immunocytochemistry performed 9 weeks after transplantation.
Method of immunosuppression	Chronic administration of cyclosporin A (10 mg/kg/day, i.p.) beginning 1 day before transplantation (N = 14).

Control animals	1. Animals that had lesions and did not recieve grafts (N = 14).
	   a. Controls receiving daily vehicle injections (N = 10).
	   b. Controls receiving daily cyclosporin A injections (N = 4).
	2. Animals that had lesions and received grafts but no immunosuppression (N = 7); injection of vehicle was given daily.

[a] These dates correspond to the period of mesencephalic dopaminergic cell proliferation, terminal differentiation, and migration[3] in the rabbit. In rodents, this period in ontogeny coincides with optimal survival of neural grafts.[4]

Because of the potential use of neural grafting techniques in the treatment of Parkinson's disease,[5] it is necessary to develop a source of tissue that is appropriately integrated into the host and of sufficient quantity to graft into the striatum of man (which is $2\frac{1}{2}$ orders of magnitude larger than the striatum of rats).[6] Xenogeneic grafts from animals that breed in litters may provide a source of tissue that will meet these criteria.

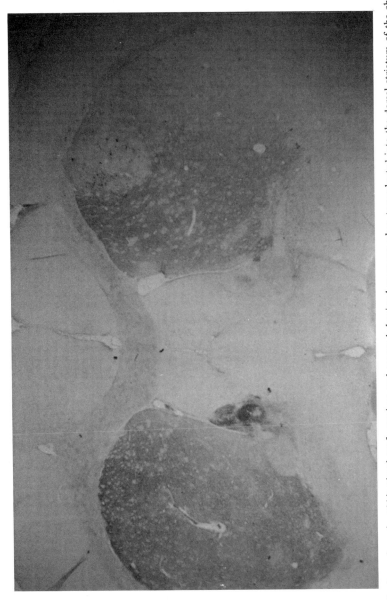

FIGURE 1. An embryonic rabbit nigral graft survives and causes behavioral recovery when transplanted into the dorsal striatum of the chronically immunosuppressed rat. Axonal extensions from embryonic rabbit grafts grow into appropriate target regions of the rat striatum. Dopaminergic cell outgrowth depends upon signals from the target region of the host that are functional across widely divergent species.

REFERENCES

1. MARSHALL, J. F. & U. UNGERSTEDT. 1977. Eur. J. Pharmacol. **41:** 361-367.
2. DUNNETT, S. B., A. BJÖRKLUND & R. H. SCHMIDT. 1983. Acta Physiol. Scand. Suppl. **522:** 29-37.
3. TENNYSON, V. M. & C. MYTILINEOU. 1973. J. Comp. Neurol. **149:** 233-258.
4. BJÖRKLUND, A., U. STENEVI & R. H. SCHMIDT. 1983. Acta Physiol. Scand. Suppl. **522:** 1-8.
5. PERLOW, M. J., W. J. FREED & B. J. HOFFER. 1979. Science **204:** 643-647.
6. HARMAN, P. J. & M. B. CARPENTER. 1950. J. Comp. Neurol. **93:** 125-138.

Myelin Basic Protein Expression after Cortical Transplants into Shiverer Brain

E. FRIEDMAN, G. NILAVER, P. W. CARMEL,
AND N. LATOV

Departments of Neurological Surgery and Neurology
Columbia University
New York, New York 10032

Mutant mice with neurological deficits are useful models for studying the development and proliferation of oligodendrocytes and the formation of myelin. The autosomal recessive mutant shiverer has a gene deletion resulting in the virtual lack of myelin basic protein (MBP).[1] Antibodies to MBP stain normal mouse myelin but fail to stain shiverer brain, providing a means to distinguish host from graft. Cortex from fetal and neonatal timed pregnant CD-1 mice was employed as a source of oligodendrocyte precursors. Fragments of frontal cortex, in Dulbecco's medium, were implanted stereotactically in the lateral ventricle of anesthetized adult shiverers. Host brains were examined immunohistochemically with polyclonal antibodies to MBP at 2–7 weeks after implantation. Immunostaining for axonal sprouting and glial proliferation was performed as well, on paraffin sections.

Donor oligodendrocytes were found to proliferate and mature, and MBP immunoreactivity was noted in the shiverer host as early as 28 days after implantation. The new MBP reactivity was not only seen in the graft, but to a greater degree detected in adjacent major commissures (corpus callosum), following the host tracts, and crossing over into the contralateral hemisphere (FIG. 1). Noncontiguous myelination was evident in distant septal nuclei. The highest density of MBP staining occurred with the youngest fetal tissue (15–16 day gestation). There was no evidence of graft necrosis or rejection despite the strain difference and intraventricular graft placement. Glial fibrillary acidic protein[2] revealed minimal gliotic reaction. Staining for neurofilament protein[3] (an axonal marker) paralleled the MBP immunoreactivity, suggesting that CD-1 axons penetrate the host and may be the guidewires along which transplanted oligodendrocytes gain access to the host brain.

Implantation of fetal grafts into mutant mice provides an elegant *in vivo* system for studying oligodendrocyte function in the setting of dysmyelination, and for pursuing new strategies to treat demyelinating diseases.

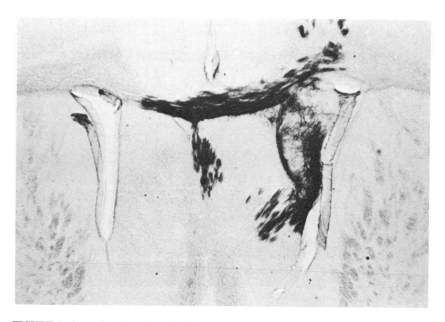

FIGURE 1. Coronal section through shiverer brain. The section was 100 μm thick, and was cut on a vibratome. MBP staining extends from the graft, seen within the lateral ventricle, into the deep septal region, and crosses to the contralateral hemisphere via the host corpus callosum. Original magnification: ×30; reduced to 68% of original size.

REFERENCES

1. BARBARESE, E., M. L. NIELSON & J. H. CARLSON. 1984. J. Neurochem. **40:** 1680-1686.
2. LATOV, N., G. NILAVER, E. A. ZIMMERMAN, W. G. JOHNSON, A. J. SILVERMAN, R. DEFENDINI & L. COTE. 1979. Dev. Biol. **72:** 381-384.
3. TAPSCOTT, S. J., G. S. BENNETT, Y. TOYAMA, F. KLEINBART & H. HOLTZER. 1981. Dev. Biol. **86:** 40-54.

Transplanted Raphe Neurons Reverse Sleep Deficits Induced by Neonatal Administration of 5,7-Dihydroxytryptamine

G. GANDOLFO,[a] A. McRAE-DEGUEURCE,[b] L. GLIN,[a]
AND C. GOTTESMANN[a]

[a]Laboratoire de Psychophysiologie
Faculté des Sciences et Techniques
Nice, France

[b]Institut National de la Santé
et de la Recherche Médicale Unité 259
Bordeaux, France

It has been shown that serotonin (5-HT) plays a role in initiating and maintaining paradoxical sleep.[1] We extended this finding by demonstrating that 5-HT neurons can reverse the paradoxical sleep deficit induced by neonatal administration of 5,7-dihydroxytryptamine (5,7-DHT). Neonatal male Wistar rats (4 days old) received an intracisternal injection of 5,7-DHT (100 μg). An age-matched sham group received a vehicle injection. Three months later, when the adaptations to the loss of the 5-HT system were well formed, the animals were implanted with cortical, hippocampal, electromyographic, and electrooculographic electrodes for sleep-waking cycle study. Seven behavioral stages were defined, and each stage was graded using an automatic sleep-waking scoring system: 1) attentive or active waking with theta activity in the dorsal hippocampus; 2) waking without theta; 3) cortical slow waves, first stage of sleep; 4) cortical spindles as sleep deepens; 5) intermediate stage characterized by spindles and theta activity; 6) paradoxical sleep without eye movement; 7) eye movement periods of paradoxical sleep. The electrophysiological recordings established that total paradoxical sleep level was decreased from 10.5 to 6.4% ($p < .01$) whereas the slow wave stage, which corresponds to light sleep, was increased from 21.9 to 28.7% ($p < .01$) in the 5,7-DHT-treated rats when compared to the sham group. The other stage levels were not significantly modified.

The 5,7-DHT-treated rats then received injections of a suspension containing dissociated 5-HT neurons taken in 16-day-old embryos in the cisterna magna. One month later, sleep-waking recordings were again performed. The total level of paradoxical sleep increased to 9.6% ($p < .01$) whereas the light sleep decreased to 25.3%. Thus paradoxical sleep and light sleep were restored to nearly normal levels whereas the other stages were not modified. Immunocytochemical observations revealed 1) the disappearance or a massive decrease of 5-HT-immunoreactive neurons in the dorsal and medial raphe nuclei and 2) numerous transplanted neurons with processes in the tissue surrounding the fourth ventricle.

This transplant paradigm employed in conjunction with this sleep model provides a powerful tool to selectively investigate neurobiochemical correlates to sleep-waking states. In fact, the results presented here could be related to a perturbation of thermoregulation induced by the 5-HT denervation of the anterior hypothalamus.[3] Indeed, hypothermia induces a decrease of paradoxical sleep.[4] This hypothesis will be verified by raphe cell transplants in the anterior hypothalamus of neonatal 5,7-DHT-treated rats.

REFERENCES

1. SALLANON, M., F. PETITJEAN, C. BUDA, M. JANIN & M. JOUVET. 1983. Mise en jeu de structures hypothalamiques dans les mécanismes indolaminergiques du sommeil paradoxal. C. R. Acad. Sci. Paris 297: 531-534.
2. GLIN, L., G. GANDOLFO, G. LACOSTE, M. RODI & C. GOTTESMANN. 1985. Sleep-waking analysis on microcomputer in the rat. In Sleep 1984. W. P. Koella, E. Rüther & H. Schulz, Eds.: 455-457. Gustav Fischer Verlag. Stuttgart.
3. MYERS, R. D. 1978. Hypothalamic action of 5-hydroxytryptamine neurotoxins: Feeding, drinking and body temperature. Ann. N.Y. Acad. Sci. 305: 556-575.
4. SAKAGUCHI, S., S. F. GLOTZBACH & H. C. HELLER. 1979. Influence of hypothalamic and ambient temperatures on sleep in Kangaroo rats. Am. J. Physiol. 237: R80-R88.

Brain Transplantation in the Study of Host Regulation of Susceptibility to Experimental Allergic Encephalomyelitis[a]

DAN GOLDOWITZ, FRED D. LUBLIN,
AND ROBERT L. KNOBLER

Departments of Anatomy and Neurology
Jefferson Medical College
Thomas Jefferson University
Philadelphia, Pennsylvania 19107

Experimental allergic encephalomyelitis (EAE) is an organ-specific cell-mediated immune disorder of the central nervous system (CNS), and is induced by immunization with CNS antigens in adjuvants.[1] EAE has served as an animal model of the human demyelinating disease multiple sclerosis. There are genetic differences in susceptibility to the development of EAE among strains within a given species.[2] Although previous studies have shown that EAE is an immune-mediated disease, using inbred strains of mice that differ in their susceptibility to EAE, there also is a restriction to its development that is independent of the effector arm of the immune system.[3] This restriction may be located at the level of the CNS.

In order to study the cellular and molecular basis of the genetic differences in EAE susceptibility that are expressed by the CNS, we have developed a transplantation model in which brain is heterotopically transplanted to the anterior chamber of the eye. In this protocol, day 13-15 fetal brainstem or spinal cord tissue from EAE-susceptible SJL or (SJL × BALB/c)F1 mice is transplanted to the anterior eye chamber of anesthetized adult animals.[4] The transplant is allowed to mature over the course of the next 6-8 weeks. Following maturation of the transplant, some mice were immunized with 5 mg of mouse spinal cord homogenate in complete Freund's adjuvant. Each immunized mouse received an intravenous injection of pertussis vaccine (2.7×10^{10} organisms) on the day of immunization and 48 hr later. This immunization protocol produces clinical and pathological signs of acute EAE in 80-90% of the mice so immunized. Control mice were neither immunized nor injected with pertussis.

In the transplant, the normal architecture of the CNS neurons, astrocytes, oligodendrocytes, and neuropil is formed (FIG. 1A), and normal-appearing myelin sheaths are observed surrounding nerve fibers (FIG. 1B). Clinical signs of EAE occurred 2 weeks after immunization for EAE in animals with transplants, following

[a] This work was supported by Grant RG-1801-A from the National Multiple Sclerosis Society; by Biomedical Research Support Grant S07-RR05414 (to Jefferson Medical College) and Teacher Investigator Development Awards NS-00271 and NS-00961 from the National Institutes of Health; and by the Pfizer Foundation.

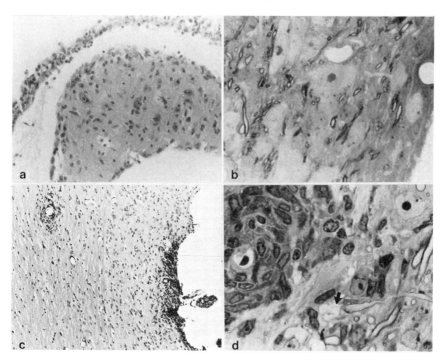

FIGURE 1. (A) A photomicrograph of a paraffin section through a mature brain transplant into the anterior eye chamber. A portion of the iris can be seen beneath the transplant. The transplant contains intact neural and glial cells. Hematoxylin and eosin; original magnification: 280×. (B) A photomicrograph of a plastic section through a mature brain transplant into the anterior eye chamber. Intact neurons and normally myelinated axons are visualized. Toluidine blue; oil immersion; original magnification: 1500×. (C) A photomicrograph of a paraffin section through the spinal cord of a mouse 2 weeks after immunization for EAE. Perivascular and subpial cuffs of inflammatory cells that invade the surrounding tissue are visualized. This mouse was a recipient of a brain transplant to the anterior chamber of the eye. This photomicrograph demonstrates the typical histopathological features of acute EAE in the mouse, indicating that the presence of the transplant did not interfere with the development of EAE. Hematoxylin and eosin; original magnification: 180×. (D) A photomicrograph of a plastic-embedded section through a brain transplant to the anterior eye chamber 2 weeks after immunization for acute EAE. There is an accumulation of perivascular inflammatory cells into the transplant, with cystic degeneration of myelin becoming apparent at this time (arrow). Toluidine blue; oil immersion; original magnification: 1500×. (Figure reduced to 41% of original size.)

an identical time course of disease in animals without transplants. The neuropathological lesions of EAE, characterized by subpial, perivascular, and infiltrating mononuclear cells, are demonstrated in FIGURE 1C. This figure shows the spinal cord of a transplant recipient immunized for EAE. Similar perivascular and infiltrating mononuclear cells are demonstrated in a transplant into the anterior eye chamber of the same animal (FIG. 1D). Tissues of the eye were unaffected by this inflammatory process. Thus, there is no limitation to the onset of either the clinical or pathological signs of EAE in the native CNS or the brain transplant when susceptible mice contain a brain transplant in the anterior eye chamber. There is no evidence of suppression of these specific immune responses as has been reported in other experimental systems when the antigens were placed into the anterior eye chamber.[5]

The survival of the transplant, and accessibility to immune effector cells is dependent upon its vascularity. Blood vessels in the native CNS effectively exclude marker molecules, such as horseradish peroxidase (HRP), when injected intravenously (FIG. 2A). In the transplant, however, there is free communication of HRP into the extra-

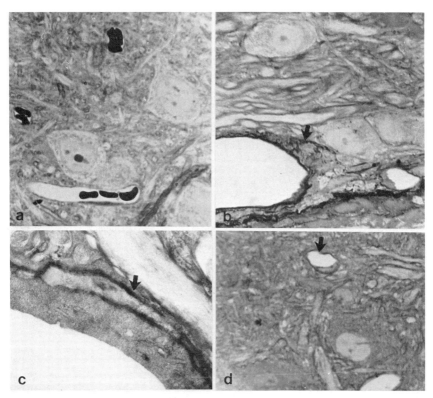

FIGURE 2. (A) A photomicrograph of mouse spinal cord, showing anterior horn neurons, from a mouse that contained a brain transplant into the anterior eye chamber, but was not immunized for EAE. This mouse received 10 mg of HRP intravenously 1 hr before sacrifice and perfusion. HRP reaction product was developed in the tissues with exposure to diaminobenzidine and hydrogen peroxide. This picture demonstrates that HRP is excluded from the CNS, but indicates endogenous peroxidase activity in red blood cells. Toluidine blue; oil immersion; original magnification: 1500×. (B) A photomicrograph through the brain transplant of the mouse in A, perfused with HRP before sacrifice. HRP reaction product is demonstrated in the intercellular space of the iris-transplant border (arrow), and in the surrounding neuropil, indicating that HRP is not excluded from the brain transplant of this nonimmunized animal. Toluidine blue; oil immersion; original magnification: 1500×. (C) An electron micrograph showing HRP reaction product in the perivascular space (arrow) of the brain transplant neuropil shown in B. Original magnification: 28 000× (D) A photomicrograph showing HRP reaction product surrounding blood vessels (arrow) from deep within the transplant, suggesting that these vessels are not as effective at excluding HRP as the vessels of the native spinal cord shown in A. Toluidine blue; oil immersion; original magnification: 1500×. (Figure reduced to 52% of original size.)

cellular space at the iris-transplant interface (FIGS. 2B & 2C). HRP also leaks through the vessel wall deeper within the transplant, albeit to a much lesser degree than at the iris-transplant border (FIG. 2D).

Studies of EAE induction and blood-brain barrier integrity in reciprocal transplants of brain tissue from histocompatible EAE-resistant and EAE-susceptible mice will allow determination of which brain cells, and ultimately which molecules, mediate genetic differences in susceptibility to EAE.

REFERENCES

1. PATERSON, P. Y. 1976. Experimental autoimmune (allergic) encephalomyelitis: Induction, pathogenesis and suppression. *In* Textbook of Immunopathology. P. A. Miescher & H. J. Muller-Eberhard, Eds.: 179-213. Grune & Stratton, New York, NY.
2. KNOBLER, R. L., D. S. LINTHICUM & M. COHN. 1985. Host genetic regulation of acute MHV-4 viral encephalomyelitis and acute experimental autoimmune encephalomyelitis in (BALB/cKe × SJL/J) recombinant inbred mice. J. Neuroimmunol. **8:** 15-28.
3. KORNGOLD, R., A. FELDMAN, L. RORKE, F. LUBLIN & P. DOHERTY. 1986. Acute experimental allergic encephalomyelitis in radiation bone marrow chimeras between high and low susceptible strains of mice. Immunogenetics **24:** 309-315.
4. OLSON, L., A. SEIGER & I. STROMBERG. 1983. Intraocular transplantation in rodents: A detailed account of the procedure and examples of its use in neurobiology with special reference to brain tissue grafting. Adv. Cell. Neurobiol. **4:** 407-442.
5. WETZIG, R. P., C. S. FOSTER & M. I. GREENE. 1982. Ocular immune responses: Priming of A/J mice in the anterior chamber with azobenzenearsonate-derivatized cells induces second-order-like suppressor T-cells. J. Immunol. **128:** 1753-1757.

Embryonic Cortical Transplants Survive in Middle Cerebral Artery Territory after Permanent Arterial Occlusion in Adult Rats

MOSHE HADANI,[a] THOMAS FREEMAN,[a,b] JOHN
PEARSON,[c] WISE YOUNG,[a] AND EUGENE FLAMM[a]

[a]Department of Neurosurgery
and
[c]Department of Pathology
New York University Medical Center
New York, New York 10016

INTRODUCTION

In rats, unilateral occlusion of the middle cerebral artery (MCAO) causes a reproducible focal ischemic lesion in the neocortex and the lateral part of the basal ganglia. In the present study, we used the rat MCAO model to study the survival of embryonic cells in chronically ischemic brain regions. The rationale behind this experiment is based on previous studies showing that embryonic grafts play a role in neuronal regeneration[1] and can restore function in ablated frontal cortex in rats.[2]

METHODS

The middle cerebral artery was microsurgically occluded in adult male outbred Sprague-Dawley rats (300 g) through a subtemporal craniotomy.[3] The proximal trunk was coagulated and divided distal to the lateral striate branch. Fetal cortical cells were harvested from the anterolateral aspect of the telencephalic vesicle of outbred Sprague-Dawley rat embryos at E16 and E17. The developing basal ganglia were not included in the graft. Tissues from 12 to 14 fetuses were collected in glucose-phosphate-buffered saline and were mechanically dissociated in a suspension. Debris was removed by centrifugation. The suspension was diluted to 40 000 cells/μl. The trypan blue exclusion test was used to assure that donor tissue showed at least 80% viability when transplanted. Host animals were divided into three groups: M24: 4 rats, grafted 24 hr after MCAO; M7: 5 rats, grafted 7 days after MCAO; N: 2 normal rats without MCAO that received graft.

[b]To whom correspondence should be addressed.

711

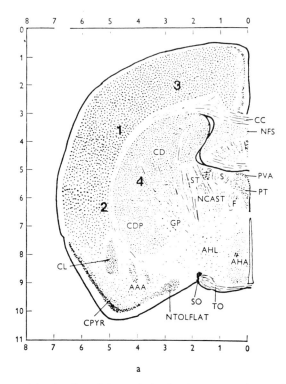

a

FIGURE 1. A coronal hemisection of the rat brain showing stereotactic coordinates of trans-plants (the caudal-rostral zero point is at the bregma; the tooth bar is 5.0 mm above the interaural line). Area 1: Cortex at the center of ischemia (A: 2.2 mm rostral to bregma; L: 4.7 mm lateral to midline; V: 2.0 mm ventral to dura). Area 2: More ventral cortex at the center of ischemia (A: 2.2; L: 4.7; V: 6.0). Area 3: Cortex at the periphery of the ischemic lesion (A: 2.2; L: 2.5; V: 2.0). Area 4: Caudate nucleus at the periphery of ischemia (A: 2.2; L: 2.5; V: 6.0). Each site received a 2.5-μl injection of the suspension (100 000 cells).

RESULTS

Nine out of 11 rats lived until sacrificed at 5 weeks after transplantation. Two of the four rats in group M24 died within a week after the procedure. Thus the mortality in this group was 50%, and the overall mortality was 15%. Viable cortical grafts were found in the two rats in group M24 that survived, and in four out of five rats in group M7. Thus 86% of the lesioned hosts that survived had viable grafts. Trans-plants survived in the periphery of the ischemic zone (areas 3 and 4) (FIGS. 1 & 2). No graft survived at the center of the infarct (areas 1 and 2) which was transformed into a fluid-filled cyst. Such cysts were also seen in animals that had received lesions but did not receive transplants. In two hosts that received transplants 7 days after MCAO, however, grafts survived at the edge of the cyst (area 2). Grafts survived in all four sites when transplanted into two control nonlesioned rats.

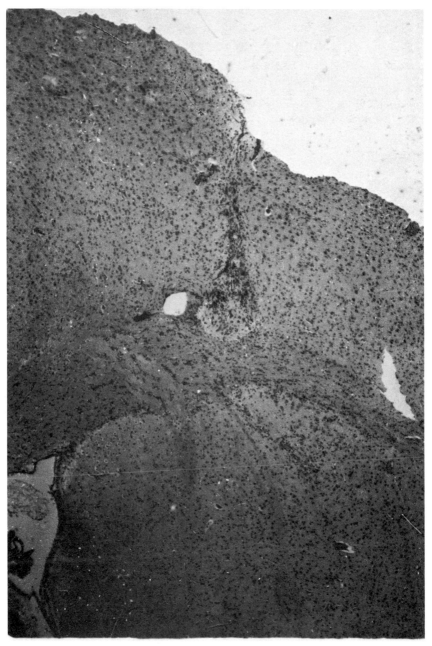

FIGURE 2. The graft at the cortex (area 3) composed of a highly cellular tissue, rich in large neurons, which lack the columnar arrangement of the preexisting cortex. Note the ischemic changes of the surrounding cortex: loss of neurons, large degenerated neurons, and glial proliferation. Original magnification: ×160; enlarged to 130% of original size.

CONCLUSIONS

A new model of neuronal grafting in ischemic brain is presented. Embryonic cortical cells of E16 and E17 in dissociated suspension survived and developed in the periphery of a chronically ischemic region. Embryonic grafts did not survive at the center of the infarct, but there was some evidence for occasional graft survival at the margin of the necrotic cyst. Cells transplanted as early as 24 hr after MCAO survived in the ischemic region despite the presence of edema and despite ionic and metabolic imbalance.

REFERENCES

1. HADANI, M. & A. HAREL. 1984. Proc. Natl. Acad. Sci. USA **84:** 7965-7969.
2. LABBE, R., A. FIRL, E. J. MUFSON & D. G. STEIN. 1983. Science **221:** 470-472.
3. TAMURA, A. & D. I. GRAHAM. 1981. J. Cereb. Blood Flow Metab. **1:** 61-69.

Transplantation of PC12 Pheochromocytoma and B-16/C Melanoma Cells to the Rat Brain

RONALD W. HARGRAVES,[a] HERBERT M. GELLER,[b]
JEFFREY LASKIN,[b] URMI PATEL-VAIDYA,[c]
ANTHONY M. ADINOLFI,[c] AND WILLIAM J. FREED[c]

[a]Department of Neurosurgery
Naval Hospital
Bethesda, Maryland

[b]Department of Pharmacology
UMDNJ-Rutgers Medical School
Piscataway, New Jersey

[c]Preclinical Neurosciences Section
Neuropsychiatry Branch
National Institute of Mental Health
Saint Elizabeth's Hospital
Washington, DC

INTRODUCTION

The purpose of the present experiment was to examine the properties of cultured PC12 pheochromocytoma cells and B-16/C3 melanoma cells after transplantation into the rat brain.

METHODS

Host rats received unilateral lesions of the substantia nigra by stereotaxic administration of 6-hydroxydopamine. Cultured PC12 cells and B-16/C3 melanoma cells were transplanted into the striatum by slow infusion through a 22-gauge cannula. Recipients were sacrificed after 1 day to 5 months and processed for glyoxylic acid-induced fluorescence histochemistry and immunocytochemical staining. Both fluorescence and staining—the latter being carried out with an antibody to a surface antigen of PC12 cells (C-10-2 antibody)—were used to detect tyrosine hydroxylase.

TABLE 1. PC12 Cells

Time after Transplantation	Number of Cells	Description
1-7 days	800-3000	Some cells with processes
2-3 weeks	87-60 000	Apparent continued cell division *or* loss of some cells
7.5-20 weeks	0-500	Small numbers of surviving cells in some animals; most surviving cells had processes
		Very large hemosiderin deposits in some of the animals with no surviving cells, a possible residue of earlier tumor growth

RESULTS

PC12 cells survived and persisted relatively unchanged for about 1 week. Subsequently, there was a slow, gradual decrease in the number of surviving cells. In some rats, the grafted cells apparently increased in number, ultimately leading to the rejection of the graft. There was no evidence of continued unrestricted tumor growth. Between 1 and 7 days after implantation, most of the implanted cells were teardrop shaped, some bearing small processes. After 2 to 3 weeks, the number of surviving cells per animal was extremely variable and the percentage of cells bearing processes had decreased (TABLE 1). Within 4 to 5 months after transplantation, however, most of the surviving cells had processes. The number of cells that stained for C-10-2 antibody usually exceeded the number that reacted with tyrosine hydroxylase antibody.

B-16/C3 cells survived implantation and contained catecholamines immediately after transplantation. One week after implantation, the cells were more rounded with fewer irregularly shaped cells and with a notable decrease in the amount of processes as compared to 1 day after implantation. Within 2 to 3 weeks, the number of catecholamine-containing cells was markedly decreased, and a large increase in the number of pigmented cells was apparent (TABLE 2). Notably, catecholamine-containing cells did not contain pigment, and pigmented cells did not contain catecholamines. Within 6 weeks after transplantation, all cells had become densely pigmented and round in shape. Attempts to retrieve melanoma cells from the grafts and reinitiate growth in tissue culture were unsuccessful.

TABLE 2. B-16/C3 Cells

Time after Transplantation	Number of Cells	Description[a]
1 day	200-3000	All contain C
1 week	2000-3600	All contain C
2-3 weeks	900-20 000	Most contain M granules, some cells contain C
6-14 weeks	5000-60 000	All contain dense M; very few or no cells with C

[a] C: catecholamines; M: melanin.

CONCLUSIONS

The main findings were that PC12 cells can survive transplantation and display a differentiated morphology, including process formation and catecholamine synthesis, for extended periods after implantation. The number of surviving PC12 cells in most cases, however, does decrease with time after implantation.

B-16/C3 cells appeared to undergo several stages of differentiation, ultimately leading to the formation of a consolidated mass of rounded cells densely filled with melanin. These cells did not continue to produce catecholamines beyond 3 weeks after implantation into the brain.

REFERENCES

1. LASKIN, J. D., L. PICCININI, D. L. ENGLEHARDT & I. B. WEINSTEIN. 1982. Control of melanin synthesis and secretion by B-16/C3 melanoma cells J. Cell. Physiol. **113:** 481-486.
2. HU, F. & P. B. LESNEY. 1964. The isolation and cytology of two pigment cell strains from B-16 mouse melanomas. Cancer Res. **24:** 1634-1643.
3. FUJII, D. K., S. L. MASSOYLIA, N. SAVION & D. GOSPORADOWICZ. 1982. Neurite outgrowth and protein synthesis by PC12 cells as a function of substriatum and nerve growth factor. J. Neurosci. **2:** 1157-1175.
4. GREENE, L. A. & G. REIN. 1977. Release, storage, and uptake of catecholamines by a clonal cell line of nerve growth factor (NGF)-responsive pheochromocytoma cells. Brain Res. **129:** 2424-2428.

Evolutionary Learning in Simulated Neural Networks[a]

HAROLD M. HASTINGS[b] AND STEFAN WANER

Department of Mathematics
Hofstra University
Hempstead, New York 11550

Biological systems routinely solve problems involving pattern recognition and feature extraction. Such problems do not appear to admit similarly routine algorithmic solutions; the power of biological systems in this regard apparently arises from nonalgorithmic dynamics.

We developed a set of principles that yield such behavior and implemented these principles via a network of stochastic formal neurons.[1] Previously, J. J. Hopfield studied the statistical mechanics of large formal networks, and in particular the problem of information storage.[2] S. Geman and D. Geman introduced the use of annealing machines to solve problems of image enhancement and pattern recognition.[3] These ideas were further developed and formalized by G. F. Hinton, T. J. Sejnowski, and D. H. Ackley under a theory of "Boltzmann" machines.[4] An annealing system consists of a state space S, a potential energy function V on S, and stochastic noise parametrized by a temperature T, which decreased with time.

Regions of stability in state space correspond to "potential wells," or local energy minima. Further, the tendency of the system to gravitate toward such equilibria is influenced by their relative stability and energy—deeper and broader wells are broader attractors. The system is able to penetrate potential barriers in the course of its evolution because of thermal noise, which gradually decreases as the system evolves toward deeper attractors.

In learning systems the potential function V is modified through feedback and interaction with the environment. An evolutionary learning system is a system in which the states are modes of information processing and in which state transitions depend upon a combination of environmental inputs and ergodic searching. Learning corresponds to changes in the probability distribution underlying the ergodic component of dynamics. This may be formalized in the computer algorithm of simulated annealing. Biological systems can apparently perform physical, nonsimulated annealing very efficiently.[5]

Furthermore, these evolutionary learning dynamics have been realized in a simulated neural net in which the formal neurons are threshold devices and ergodicity is provided by making conduction across synapses stochastic.

We demonstrated path learning and associative learning in stochastic neural networks implemented on a VAX 11/780 and on NASA's Massively Parallel Processor.

---

[a]The computer time used in this study was partially provided by NASA's Massively Parallel Processor Working Group.

[b]To whom correspondence and reprint requests should be addressed.

We extended the theoretical basis to include the learning of arbitrary learning systems via annealing through modes of information processing.[6] These latter results have, as a consequence, the evolutionary learning of knowledge bases and reasoning methods from case studies or, more simply, the evolutionary learning of expert systems.

REFERENCES

1. HASTINGS, H. M. & S. WANER. 1985. Principles of evolutionary learning. BioSystems **18**: 105-109.
2. HOPFIELD, J. J. 1982. Neural networks and physical systems with emergent collective properties. Proc. Natl. Acad. Sci. USA **79**: 2554-2558.
3. GEMAN, S. & D. GEMAN. 1984. Stochastic relaxation, Gibbs distributions, and the Bayesian restoration of images. IEEE Trans. Pattern Anal. Mach. Intell. **6**: 721-741.
4. HINTON, G. F., T. J. SEJNOWSKI & D. H. ACKLEY. 1985. Boltzmann machines: Constraint satisfaction networks that learn. Congnit. Sci. **9**: 147-164.
5. HASTINGS, H. M. & S. WANER. 1984. Low dissipation computing in biological systems. BioSystems **17**: 241-244.
6. WANER, S. & H. M. HASTINGS. 1987. Evolutionary learning of complex modes of information processing. *In* Advances in Cognitive Science. M. Kochem & H. M. Hastings, Eds. AAAS Selected Symposia Series. Westview Press. Boulder, CO. In press.

Age-related Changes in Neuroplasticity and the Progression of Neurodegenerative Diseases

BARRY HORWITZ

Laboratory of Neurosciences
National Institute on Aging
National Institutes of Health
Bethesda, Maryland 20892

In Alzheimer's disease (AD), it has been proposed that axons from cholinergic neurons projecting to cortex are involved in the formation of some neuritic plaques,[1] and it has been found that there is extensive cell loss in the cholinergic basal forebrain,[2] which provides the main cholinergic input to limbic and neocortical neurons. Mesulam *et al.*[3] found in monkey that the cholinergic cells in the basal forebrain (henceforth designated CH) could be divided into six subpopulations, which project to different cortical areas (TABLE 1). Arendt *et al.*[4] determined the percentage cell loss in each CH subregion in 10 AD brain hemispheres, and found a strong nonlinear relation to the density of neuritic plaques in the corresponding cortical target area. Thus, as neurons in the cholinergic forebrain die in AD, the rate of plaque formation in cortical areas increases.

The following neurobiological hypothesis is proposed to account for the relation, described above, found by Arendt *et al.*[4] When cells in CH die, their cortical target sites can be reoccupied by axonal sprouting, some of which derives from other neurons in CH. We further assume that when a CH cell degenerates because of AD, each major axon collateral gives rise to a neuritic plaque. To simplify the equations that are obtained from this hypothesis, it also is assumed that a constant fraction (f) of newly available synaptic sites are reinnervated by CH neuronal projections. The following equation results:

$$d = d_0 + D_0[1 - (1 - p)^{(1-f)}]/(1-f)$$

where d is the density of neuritic plaques in a cortical target area, d_0 is the density of neuritic plaques in the target area due to degeneration of non-CH neurons, D_0 is the initial density of CH axon collaterals in the target area, and p is the fractional cell loss in the specific CH subpopulation that projects to the cortical target area. Best-fit parameters were obtained by fitting this equation to the data of Arendt *et al.*[4] The results are given in TABLE 1 and illustrated for one of the CH subpopulation-cortical target pairs in FIGURE 1.

Because there is an age-related decline in neuronal plasticity,[5] presenile AD patients initially would have greater ability to reoccupy denervated synaptic target sites than would senile AD patients. Thus, presenile patients will have larger axonal arbors than senile patients. The probability of a neuron developing the pathology of AD may increase as the metabolism of the neuron increases, which it will do if it has to support a larger axonal arbor. Hence, greater neural plasticity in presenile AD may lead to more rapid decline, and more severe pathology. Thus, the greater clinical and neuropathological severity in the presenile form of AD may represent primarily a difference in the age-dependent nature of neural plasticity.

This hypothesis should be applicable to other neurodegenerative diseases. For example, older age-of-onset patients with Huntington's disease show less pathology than do younger patients.[6]

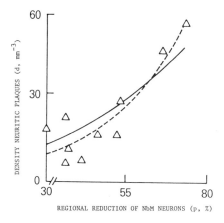

FIGURE 1. Graph of percentage cell loss in the Ch 4am subpopulation of the cholinergic basal forebrain versus density of cortical plaques (mm^{-3}) in parietal lobe. The triangles correspond to the data of Arendt et al.[4] The solid line corresponds to the equation, with the best-fit parameters of TABLE 1. The dotted line corresponds to a fitting of the data with an exponential function [$d = a \exp(bp)$], as was done by Arendt et al.[4]

REGIONAL REDUCTION OF NbM NEURONS (p, %)

TABLE 1. Best-fit Parameters[a]

Subpopulation	Cortical Area[b]	d_o	D_o	f	R^2
Ch 1/2	Hip	0	56	1.0	.61
Ch 4am	Par	0	37	1.0	.76
Ch 4a1	Frb	0	64	0.2	.52
Ch 4i	Frd	0	60	1.0	.65
Ch 4p	Tem	0	34	1.0	.93

[a] These parameters were obtained by fitting the equation to the data from Arendt et al.[4] The parameters d_o, D_o, and f are defined in the text; R^2, the fraction of the sum of squares accounted for by the fit, is a measure of the goodness of the fit.

[b] Hip: hippocampus; Par: parietal lobe; Frb: frontobasal cortex; Frd: frontodorsal cortex; Tem: temporal lobe.

REFERENCES

1. STRUBLE, R. G., L. C. CORK, P. J. WHITEHOUSE & D. L. PRICE. 1982. Science **216:** 413-415.
2. WHITEHOUSE, P. J., D. L. PRICE, R. G. STRUBLE, A. W. CLARK, J. T. COYLE & M. R. DELONG. 1982. Science **215:** 1237-1239.
3. MESULAM, M. M., E. J. MUFSON, A. I. LEVEY & B. H. WAINER. 1983. J. Comp. Neurol. **214:** 170-197.
4. ARENDT, T., V. BIGL, A. TENNSTEDT & A. ARENDT. 1985. Neuroscience **14:** 1-14.
5. COTMAN, C. W. & S. W. SCHEFF. 1979. Mech. Ageing Dev. **9:** 103-117.
6. MYERS, R. H., D. S. SAX, M. SCHOENFELD, E. D. BIRD, P. A. WOLF, J. P. VONSATTEL, R. F. WHITE & J. B. MARTIN. 1985. J. Neurol. Neurosurg. Psychiatry **48:** 530-534.

The Astrocyte and the Failure of CNS Neural Regeneration

A Study of Inoculated Astrocytes in a PNS Regenerating Model System[a]

N. KALDERON

Rockefeller University
New York, New York 10021

Repair of injured neurons is achieved in the peripheral nervous system (PNS) but is abortive in the central nervous system (CNS). The glial cellular component seems to play a major role in the regeneration process. In response to injury, Schwann cells proliferate: these cells seem to support neural regeneration in the periphery as well as in the CNS when implanted there. In CNS injury, however, the astrocytes proliferate and form a scar tissue—glial scar—that seems to be the major impediment for CNS neural regeneration.[1] The role of extracellular proteolysis as a modulator of the cytoarchitecture of the developing and regenerating nervous system is being studied, specifically, of the serum proteolytic system, the plasmin-generating system. The components of this system are plasminogen and plasminogen activator (PA), and the product of these components is the protease plasmin. It has been established by studies performed in this laboratory that the plasmin-generating system is expressed as well as modulated at certain developmental stages by the differentiating nervous system,[2,3] and that this system is predominantly elaborated by the glial component of the PNS[4] and CNS.[5]

Results so far suggest that the Schwann cell[4] (predominantly in the proliferating cell populations) and the immature astrocytes[5] are the "suppliers" of extracellular proteolysis in the developing nervous tissues. Proteolytic activity was detected in regenerating injured sciatic nerve but not in the injured optic nerve.[6] It is suggested that the capacity of a glial cell to express PA activity is an essential component in its ability to support a repair in injured nervous tissue. To test this hypothesis, the effect of the astrocyte, at different cell maturation stages, on neural regeneration is being studied by implanting various rat astrocytic populations in a PNS model system (developed by Lundborg *et al.*[7]), that is, in a silicone chamber between the regenerating rat sciatic nerve stumps (FIG. 1A).

Immature glial cell populations,[8] astrocytes and oligodendrocytes at 13 days (FIG. 1B), astrocytes at 15 days (FIG. 1C), and mature astrocytes at 35 days in culture (FIG. 1D) were implanted, and 45 days later neural regeneration within the chamber was examined (FIGS. 1E-1H). The regeneration process was strongly inhibited by the

[a]This work was supported by a grant from the Spinal Cord Research Foundation. The author is the recipient of a Career Scientist Award from the Irma T. Hirschl Trust.

722

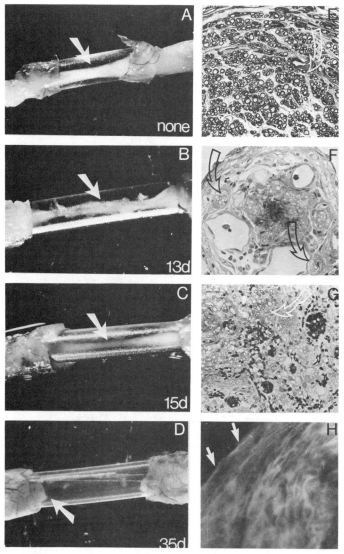

FIGURE 1. The effect of different astrocytic populations on neural regeneration through a silicone chamber (**A-D**) and the corresponding cytological analysis of this process (**E-H**). Neural regeneration through a chamber with a 5-mm gap between the stumps (**A** & **E**) serves as the control experiment. Neural regeneration was obtained in the presence of inoculated glial cells (astrocytes and oligodendrocytes) 13 days *in vitro* (**B** & **F**) and purified astrocytes 15 days *in vitro* (**C** & **G**); these cell populations express high levels of PA activity.[4] Regeneration was strongly inhibited by "mature" astrocytes (maintained 35 days in culture) (**D** & **H**). The regeneration process was examined, at the site indicated by arrows in **A-D**, 44 days (**A**) and 48 days (**B-D**) after surgery. Myelinated fibers (clear arrows) can be seen in thick sections (**E-G**) of the regenerated nerves. Immunocytochemical staining of frozen sections of the nerve stump (**D**) with antiglial fibrillary acidic protein (**H**) reveals layers of astrocytes that encapsulate the stump (arrows). Gap sizes between the stumps: 8 mm (**B** & **C**) and 6 mm (**D**).

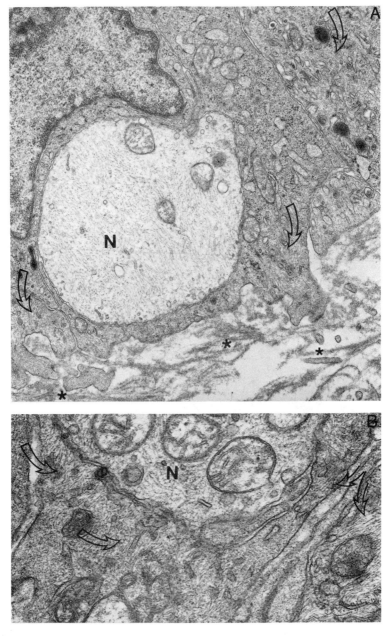

FIGURE 2. Electron micrographs of thin sections cut from the tip of the stump in which neural regeneration was inhibited by the purified "mature" astrocytes (32 days in culture). The astrocytes encapsulated the neurons (N) and formed a "glia limitans" membrane (**A**). Note the collagen fibers (asterisks) (**A**) and the numerous clusters of the intermediate filaments (arrows), which are characteristic of reactive astrocytes. Original magnifications for **A** and **B**: × 13 200 and ×40 000, respectively; figure reduced to 81% of original size.

mature astrocytic population (FIG. 1D), whereas it did take place in the presence of the immature cell populations (FIGS. 1B & 1C). In the cases where regeneration was blocked, the astrocytes formed enveloping layers on the nerve stumps as revealed by immunocytochemistry (FIG. 1H), and these layers resembled the glia limitans membrane as determined by ultrastructural analysis (FIG. 2).

The capacity of the different astrocytic populations to support or to impair regeneration appears to correlate with the activity levels of the extracellular proteolytic tool, PA, in these cell populations.[5] It is hypothesized that the PA-activity-deficient astrocyte that inhibits neural regeneration is probably the "reactive astrocyte" responsible for glial scar formation.

REFERENCES

1. SMITH, G. M., R. H. MILLER & J. SILVER. 1987. Ann. N.Y. Acad. Sci. This volume.
2. KALDERON, N. 1979. Proc. Natl. Acad. Sci. USA 76: 5992-5996.
3. KALDERON, N. & C. A. WILLIAMS. 1986. Dev. Brain Res. 25: 1-9.
4. KALDERON, N. 1984. Proc. Natl. Acad. Sci. USA 81: 7216-7220.
5. KALDERON, N. 1985. Soc. Neurosci. Abstr. 11: 1148.
6. BIGNAMI, A., G. CELLA & N. H. CHI. 1982. Acta Neuropathol. (Berlin) 58: 224-228.
7. LUNDBORG, G., R. H. GELBERMAN, F. M. LONGO, C. H. POWELL & S. VARON. 1982. J. Neuropathol. Exp. Neurol. 41: 412-422.
8. MCCARTHY, K. D. & J. DE VELLIS. 1980. J. Cell Biol. 85: 890-902.

Cerebellar Anlage Transplanted into Mature Cerebellum

K. KAWAMURA

Department of Anatomy
School of Medicine
Okayama University
Okayama 700, Japan

T. NANAMI, Y. KIKUCHI, AND M. SUZUKI

Department of Anatomy
School of Medicine
Iwate Medical University
Morioka 020, Japan

Cerebellar primordia (E14-19) were transplanted into mature cerebella in Fischer 344 rats. After 1-6 months, development of the graft was examined by light and electron microscopy. Experimental procedures were the same as described previously.[1] In some experiments, transplanted cerebellar tissues developed to form a typical trilaminar appearance and foliation. Within the graft, mossy terminals formed synaptic contacts with dendrites of granule cells, and axons of basket cells made synaptic contacts with the somata of Purkinje cells. Many spines of Purkinje dendrites were contacted with parallel fibers, whereas others were surrounded by processes of astroglia. When parts of the brainstem structure were grafted together with the rhombic lip, the development of the white matter and the granular layer of the implanted cerebellum was prominent.

In other experiments, the cerebellar graft appeared to invade the host molecular layer and formed "ectopic" granular and Purkinje cell layers (FIG. 1A). Mossy terminals in the ectopic granular layer were characterized by normal synaptic arrangement of granule cell dendrites and Golgi axons (FIG. 1C). In the newly formed ectopic molecular layer, courses of parallel fibers were multidirectional (FIG. 1B), and many spines of Purkinje cells were enshrouded in glial processes. Some Purkinje cells were scattered in the host molecular layer, whose structure was not disarranged, at the ultrastructural level, by these invading elements. Basket axon terminals formed synaptic contacts with ectopic Purkinje cell somata (FIG. 1D).

Some granule cells implanted in the cortical surface of the cerebellum migrated down the host molecular layer along the process of radial glia (FIG. 2A), which resembles the pattern of migrating external granule cells observed during the course of normal development.[2] It was also observed that migrating granule cells were lined along neuroglial processes that ensheathed the capillary wall (FIG. 2B).

Based upon the present results, it can be said that the histological organization of the cerebellar cortex is preserved even in the absence of afferent fibers, and that granule

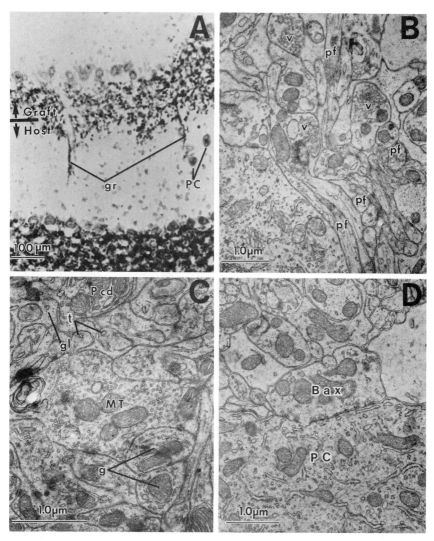

FIGURE 1. (**A**) An embryonic (E17) cerebellar graft survived in the adult cerebellum 6 months after the transplantation (PC: Purkinje cell; gr: granule cell). (**B**) In the ectopic molecular layer, courses of parallel fibers (pf) are multidirectional. Some of them are cut longitudinally, whereas others are cut transversely. Varicosities (v) are also evident. (**C**) In the ectopic granular layer, a mossy terminal (MT) forms synaptic contact with granule cell dendrites (g), and thorns (t) of Purkinje cell dendrite (Pcd) are often seen to be engulfed by astroglia (gl). (**D**) An ectopic Purkinje cell (PC) in the host molecular layer receives a basket cell axon (Bax) on the soma.

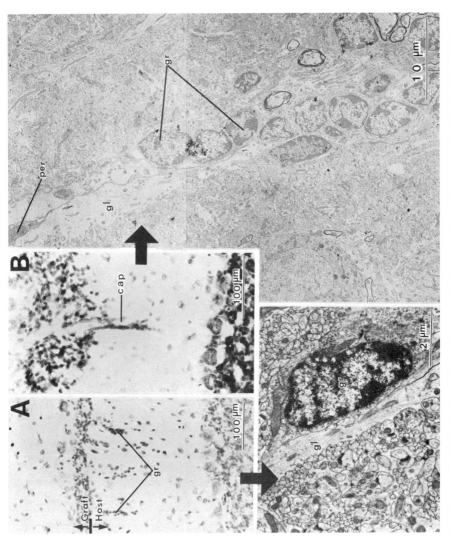

FIGURE 2. (**A**) Ectopic granule cells (gr) migrate down the host molecular layer along the process of radial glia (gl). (**B**) Elongated glial processes (gl) that cover the capillary wall (cap) are probably related to the migration of developing granule cells (gr) (per: capillary pericyte).

cells and Purkinje cells of immature type can migrate down the molecular layer along neuroglial processes of mature brain.

REFERENCES

1. KAWAMURA, K., M. SUZUKI, K. TANIGUCHI & S. NINOMIYA. 1984. Neural transplantation in cerebellum. Seitai No Kagaku **35:** 338-347.
2. RAKIC, P. 1971. Neuron-glia relationship during granule cell migration in developing cerebellar cortex: A Golgi and electron microscopic study in the macacus rhesus. J. Comp. Neurol. **141:** 283-312.

Injury of Catecholaminergic Neurons after Acute Exposure to MPTP

A TH Immunocytochemical Study in Monkey

CHERYL A. KITT,[a] LINDA C. CORK,[a] EDUARDO
EIDELBERG,[b] TONG H. JOH,[c] AND
DONALD L. PRICE[a]

[a]Neuropathology Laboratory
The Johns Hopkins University School of Medicine
Baltimore, Maryland 21205

[b]Division of Surgery
University of Texas Health Science Center
San Antonio, Texas 78284

[c]Department of Neurology
Cornell University Medical College
New York, New York 10021

Recent studies have shown that acute exposure to 1-methyl-4-phenyl-1,2,3,6-tetrahy-dropyridine (MPTP) produces severe parkinsonian symptoms in both man and monkey.[1-13] Neuropathological examinations of parkinsonian brains in these studies revealed marked cell loss in the substantia nigra pars compacta. The present study employed immunocytochemical methods to assess structural changes in catecholaminergic systems after acute MPTP exposure in nonhuman primates.

Six monkeys received intravenous injections of MPTP and subsequently developed a parkinsonian syndrome. Group 1 monkeys received high doses of MPTP (1 mg/kg MPTP on day 1 and 5 mg/kg on day 2), whereas group 2 monkeys received lower doses of the drug (0.5 mg/kg MPTP for 3-4 consecutive days). At high-dose levels, group 1 monkeys developed rigidity and akinesia and died 10, 15, or 60 hr after the last dose of MPTP. Group 2 monkeys showed bradykinesia, loss of facial expression (threat response), rigidity, and had a low-amplitude resting tremor in arms or legs or both after the third dosage of the drug. Group 2 monkeys were euthanized 1, 6, or 7 days after the last dosage of MPTP. Two drug-free control monkeys were also evaluated.

Using immunocytochemical methods and a polyclonal anti-tyrosine hydroxylase (TH) antibody, we examined the effects of acute exposure to MPTP on immunostaining of catecholaminergic neurons in the substantia nigra (SN), ventral tegmental area, and locus ceruleus. In both high- and low-dose groups, neurons in the SN were affected. In group 1, SN cells were severely damaged. Since all of these animals died, the evolution of pathological changes could not be studied in detail. In group 2, many SN neurons survived. The majority of these cells, however, did not stain for TH-like immunoreactivity. Axonal pathology along the course of the nigrostriatal pathway was conspicuous, and there was a dramatic decrease in TH-like immunostaining within the striatum as compared to controls. In addition, TH-like immunoreactivity was reduced somewhat within neurons located within the ventral tegmental area and locus ceruleus.

Loss of TH-like immunoreactivity in catecholaminergic neurons may represent a retrograde axonal reaction, a potentially reversible response. MPTP may damage axons and terminals, causing a retrograde reaction in neurons, that is, a reduction in TH-like immunoreactivity. If, as our results suggest, some neurons can survive the acute insult, they may be able to reconstitute their axons and eventually manufacture and deliver TH to terminals that can then, in turn, synthesize dopamine.

REFERENCES

1. BURNS, R. S., C. C. CHIUEH, S. P. MARKEY, M. H. EBERT, D. M. JACOBOWITZ & I. J. KOPIN. 1983. A primate model of parkinsonism: Selective destruction of dopaminergic neurons in the pars compacta of the substantia nigra by N-methyl-4-phenyl-1,2,3,6-tetrahydropyridine. Proc. Natl. Acad. Sci. USA **80**: 4546-4550.
2. BURNS, R. S., S. P. MARKEY, J. M. PHILLIPS & C. C. CHIUEH. 1984. The neurotoxicity of 1-methyl-4-phenyl-1,2,3,6-tetrahydropyridine in the monkey and man. Can. J. Neurol. Sci. **11**: 166-168.
3. CHIUEH, C. C., R. S. BURNS, S. P. MARKEY, D. M. JACOBOWITZ & I. J. KOPIN. 1985. Current Concepts III. Primate model of parkinsonism: Selective lesion of nigrostriatal neurons by 1-methyl-4-phenyl-1,2,3,6-tetrahydropyridine produces an extrapyramidal syndrome in rhesus monkeys. Life Sci. **36**: 213-218.
4. DAVIS, G. C., A. C. WILLIAMS, S. P. MARKEY, M. H. EBERT, E. D. CAINE, C. M. REICHERT & I. J. KOPIN. 1979. Chronic parkinsonism secondary to intravenous injection of meperidine analogues. Psychiatry Res. **1**: 249-254.
5. HEIKKILA, R. E., A. HESS & R. C. DUVOISIN. 1984. Dopaminergic neurotoxicity of 1-methyl-4-phenyl-1,2,5,6-tetrahydropyridine in mice. Science **224**: 1451-1453.
6. IRWIN, I. & J. W. LANGSTON. 1985. Current Concepts II. Selective accumulation of MPP+ in the substantia nigra: A key to neurotoxicity? Life Sci. **36**: 207-212.
7. JENNER, P., N. M. J. RUPNIAK, S. ROSE, E. KELLY, G. KILPATRICK, A. LEES & C. D. MARSDEN. 1984. 1-Methyl-4-phenyl-1,2,3,6-tetrahydropyridine-induced parkinsonism in the common marmoset. Neurosci. Lett. **50**: 85-90.
8. KITT, C. A., L. C. CORK, E. EIDELBERG, T. H. JOH & D. L. PRICE. 1986. Injury of nigral neurons exposed to 1-methyl-4-phenyl-1,2,3,6-tetrahydropyridine: A tyrosine hydroxylase immunocytochemical study in monkey. Neuroscience **17**: 1089-1103.
9. LANGSTON, J. W. 1985. Current Concepts I. MPTP neurotoxicity: An overview and characterization of phases of toxicity. Life Sci. **36**: 201-206.
10. LANGSTON, J. W., P. BALLARD, J. W. TETRUD & I. IRWIN. 1983. Chronic parkinsonism in humans due to a product of meperidine analogue synthesis. Science **219**: 979-980.
11. LANGSTON, J. W., L. S. FORNO, C. S. REBERT & I. IRWIN. 1984. Selective nigral toxicity after systemic administration of 1-methyl-4-phenyl-1,2,5,6-tetrahydropyridine (MPTP) in the squirrel monkey. Brain Res. **292**: 390-394.
12. LANGSTON, J. W., I. IRWIN & E. B. LANGSTON. 1984. A comparison of the acute and chronic effects of 1-methyl-4-phenyl-1,2,5,6-tetrahydropyridine (MPTP)-induced parkinsonism in humans and the squirrel monkey. Neurology **34**(Suppl. 1): 268.
13. MARKEY, S. P., J. N. JOHANNESSEN, C. C. CHIUEH, R. S. BURNS & M. A. HERKENHAM. 1984. Intraneuronal generation of a pyridinium metabolite may cause drug-induced parkinsonism. Nature **311**: 464-467.

Transplants of Normal Fetal Cerebral Cortical Tissue into Congenitally Malformed Brains of Infant Rats

M. H. LEE, A. RABE, J. R. CURRIE, J. SHEK,
AND H. M. WISNIEWSKI

*New York State Office of Mental Retardation
and Developmental Disabilities
Institute for Basic Research in Developmental Disabilities
New York, New York 10314*

Transplantation of neural tissue may offer a possibility to correct certain congenital brain abnormalities and their functional consequences. This communication summarizes our initial effort to produce large viable solid transplants in infant rats with transplacentally induced micrencephaly. A single intraperitoneal injection of 30 mg/kg of methylazoxymethanol acetate into a pregnant rat on gestation day 15 produces severe micrencephaly in the offspring. The posterior cerebral cortex is drastically reduced, leaving a large intracranial space over the midbrain tectum. Layers II to IV of the posterior cortex are eliminated and the laminar appearance obliterated. The corpus callosum is also severely hypoplastic, and the lateral ventricles are enlarged.[1,2] These structural abnormalities are accompanied by increased concentrations of norepinephrine and acetylcholine in the brain,[3] as well as by cognitive and other behavioral deficits.[4–6]

Using the procedure developed by Das *et al.,*[7] tissue from normal fetal (E18) cerebral cortex was placed into the posterior cerebrum of over 60 infant (P10-12) micrencephalic rats of the Long-Evans strain. Almost one whole hemisphere of the fetal cortex was used for one transplant site. Single transplants were placed unilaterally either in the left or right posterior aspect of the hemisphere, or under the dura along the midline at the posterodorsal junction of the two hemispheres. Some brains received bilateral transplants. The host cortex was slightly damaged in the case of the unilateral and bilateral cortical placements, but the midline insertion produced no gross damage to the host cortex. The transplants were allowed to grow for 6-10 weeks before the host animals were sacrificed. A sample of 20 brains with transplants have been sectioned and stained for histological analysis.

All host animals survived, most with solid transplants larger than 100 mm³ that always occupied the space above the colliculi between the cerebrum and cerebellum (FIG. 1). The size and external appearance of the transplants varied considerably, in spite of an effort to place the same amount of tissue in specific loci. Single transplants increased the total brain weight by up to 15% and bilateral transplants up to 25%, as compared to ungrafted litter mates.

Light microscopic examination of serial sections of two brains and sample sections

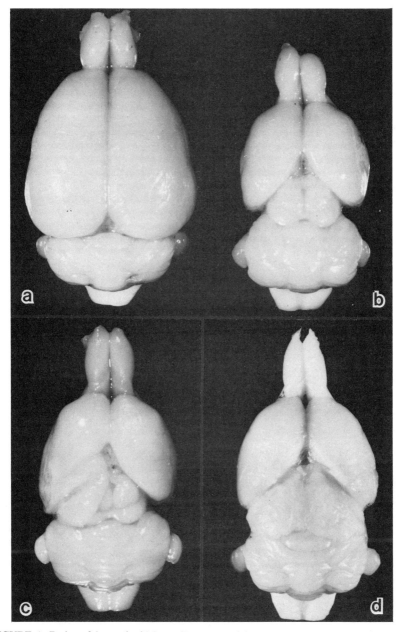

FIGURE 1. Brains of 2-month-old Long-Evans rats: (**a**) Normal; (**b**) Micrencephalic. Note how the drastic reduction of the posterior aspect of the cerebral hemispheres exposes the midbrain tectum and forms a large open space between the cerebrum and cerebellum. (**c**) Unilateral transplant placed in the left hemisphere; the groove on the transplant was formed by the transverse sinus. (**d**) Bilateral transplants, placed one in each hemisphere.

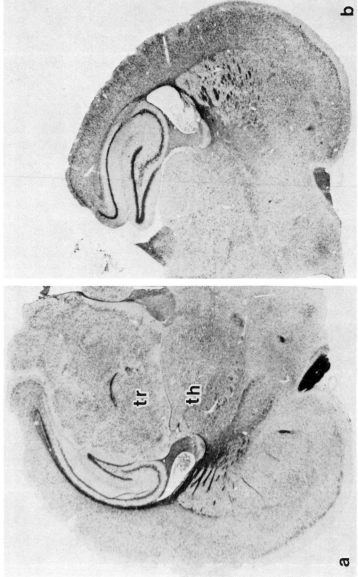

FIGURE 2. Half of a coronal section of a single midline graft (**a**) juxtaposed to a comparable coronal section from a control micrencephalic brain (**b**), Kluver-Barrera stain. A large transplant (tr) sits on the dorsal aspect of the host thalamus (th) and is also apposed to the hippocampus and cerebral cortex. The transplant was bilaterally symmetrical. Note the dense population of cells and the presence of fiber bundles in the transplant, and note how the graft has displaced the dorsal hippocampus and the adjoining cortex from a dorsal to a much more lateral position, whereas the diencephalon has remained unaffected.

of 18 brains showed that the transplants consisted of a dense population of large normal-appearing neurons, myelinated fiber bundles, glia cells, and neuropil. They were well vascularized. There was no readily discernible cerebral cortical laminar organization (FIG. 2); however, several transplants, which apparently also contained fetal hippocampal tissue, showed the typical hippocampal cytoarchitecture.

In most transplants, at least a half of the transplant surface was in apposition to the host brain. The transplants interfaced with the host cerebral cortex and sometimes with the host hippocampus. There were also interfaces between the transplant and the colliculi, as well as the posterior thalamus. Although a characterization and quantification of the interfaces between transplant and host still remains to be made, our findings are consistent with the earlier results from another laboratory showing that small cortical grafts are integrated into the micrencephalic host brain.[8]

In conclusion, our data demonstrate that the brain of the infant micrencephalic rat readily accepts normal fetal brain tissue and promotes good transplant growth. The potential of the transplants for morphological, neurochemical, and functional restitution of the micrencephalic brain, and the conditions under which this may occur, are still to be determined.

REFERENCES

1. DAMBSKA, M., R. HADDAD, P. B. KOZLOWSKI, M. H. LEE & J. SHEK. 1982. Telencephalic cytoarchitectonics in the brains of rats with graded degrees of micrencephaly. Acta Neuropathol. (Berlin) **58:** 203-209.
2. YURKEWICZ, L., K. L. VALENTINO, M. K. FLOETER, J. W. FLESHMAN, JR. & E. G. JONES. 1984. Effects of cytotoxic deletions of somatic sensory cortex in fetal rats. Somatosensory Res. **1:** 303-327.
3. JOHNSTON, M. V. & J. T. COYLE. 1980. Ontogeny of neurochemical markers for noradrenergic, GABA-ergic, and cholinergic neurons in neocortex lesioned with methylazoxymethanol acetate. J. Neurochem. **34:** 1429-1441.
4. RABE, A. & R. K. HADDAD. 1972. Methylazoxymethanol-induced micrencephaly in rats: Behavioral studies. Fed. Proc. **31:** 1536-1539.
5. VORHEES, C. V., K. FERNANDEZ, R. M. DUMAS & R. K. HADDAD. 1984. Pervasive hyperactivity and long-term learning impairments in rats with induced micrencephaly from prenatal exposure to methylazoxymethanol. Dev. Brain Res. **15:** 1-10.
6. PLONSKY, M., E. P. RILEY, M. H. LEE & R. K. HADDAD. 1985. The effects of prenatal methylazoxymethanol acetate (MAM) on holeboard exploration and shuttle avoidance performance in rats. Neurobehav. Toxicol. Teratol. **7:** 221-226.
7. DAS, G. D., B. H. HALLAS & K. G. DAS. 1979. Transplantation of neural tissues in the brains of laboratory mammals: Technical details and comments. Experientia **35:** 143-145.
8. FLOETER, M. K. & E. J. JONES. 1984. Connections made by transplants to the cerebral cortex of rat brains damaged *in utero*. J. Neurosci. **4:** 141-150.

Survival and Integration of Transplanted Hypothalamic Cells in the Rat CNS after Sorting by Flow Cytometry[a]

JUAN J. LOPEZ-LOZANO, DON M. GASH, JAMES F.
LEARY, AND MARY F. D. NOTTER

Department of Neurobiology and Anatomy
University of Rochester School of Medicine
Rochester, New York 14642

Our research group is developing procedures to isolate discrete populations of embryonic or neonatal central neurons for transplantation into the central nervous system (CNS). To this end, flow cytometry has been found to be an appropriate tool for the study of large numbers of cells, and especially for dissociation and separation among heterogeneous cell populations.[1] This report examines the influence of flow cytometry and cell sorting techniques on a population of sorted anterior hypothalamic (AH) cells by studying the anatomicohistological characteristics of sorted AH cells implanted in the CNS.

Pregnant female Long-Evans rats were injected with 1 μCi/g body weight of [^{3}H]thymidine 12-14 days after coitus. Seventeen days after coitus, rats were decapitated and the anterior hypothalamus, free of meninges, was quickly dissected out, minced, and placed in a cold Ca^{2+}- and Mg^{2+}-free buffer. Tissue was dispersed by a trypsin-DNase procedure that provided a viability of better than 90% and produced a minimum of debris.[2] Then, a single suspension of cells (1×10^6 cells/mm^3) flowing at a rate of 1000 cells/sec was analyzed in an EPIC V (Coulter Electronics) multiparameter flow cytometry system. Cells were exposed to an argon ion laser and were sorted on the basis of the combination of light scatter and light scatter pulse width (time of flight)[3] according to specific, previously determined windows. In order to label the suspension of cells to be transplanted, the recovered sorted AH cells were incubated in 0.03% Fast Blue (J. J. Lopez-Lozano, unpublished data). After the excess dye was carefully washed away, cells were implanted into the posterior hypothalamus, lateral to the third ventricle and in the vicinity of the median eminence, of previously neurohypophysectomized adult (200 g) Long-Evans rats. At time periods of 1 day, 3 days, 7 days, 14 days, and 28 days, animals were intracardially perfused with 4% paraformaldehyde. The study of the structural organization of the implanted sorted cells was made by means of fluorescence microscopy and immunocytochemistry of neurophysin. The suspension of sorted cells became structurally well integrated with

[a]This work was supported by Grants NS 19711 (to M. F. D. Notter) and NS 15109 (to D. M. Gash) from the U.S. Public Health Service. J. J. Lopez-Lozano is a Fulbright-MEC and FISS fellow (86/680).

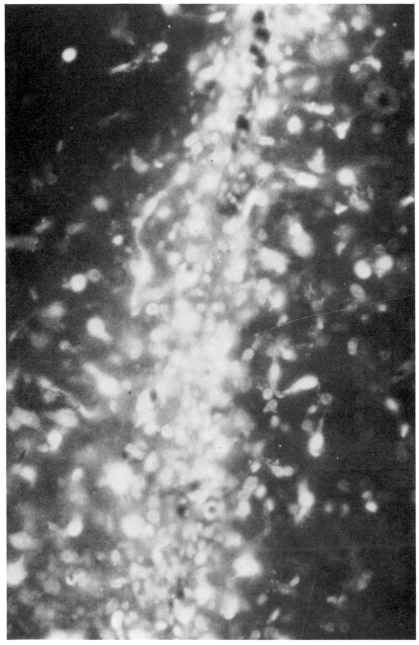

FIGURE 1. This low-power fluorescence photomicrograph depicts the labeled Fast Blue anterior hypothalamic cells a few days after being transplanted in the posterior hypothalamus of previously neurohypophysectomized rats. Cells had become elongated, some wearing an extensive fiber outgrowth.

the host parenchyma. The implanted cells looked morphologically healthy and showed the presence of new blood vessels. In the first few days, red blood cells and inflammatory cells were observed in the needle tract. No signs of gliosis were observed. A typical example of the fluorescent, implanted cells is shown in FIGURE 1 where a few elongated cells can be seen, some wearing an extensive fiber outgrowth.

Neurophysin-containing neurons were present in the grafts. The number of neurons that could be identified in coronal sections varied, and the neurons themselves were predominantly located in the region of the ventromedial hypothalamic nucleus, arcuatus nucleus, and fimbria. FIGURE 2 shows an example of immunocytochemistry

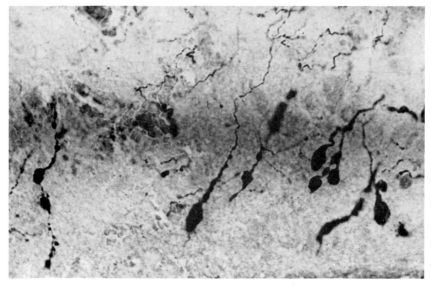

FIGURE 2. This photomicrograph illustrates the grafted suspension of the cells stained for vasopressin-associated neurophysin. Note the densely stained vasopressin neurons in the needle tract (posterior hypothalamus) and the extensive fiber outgrowth. Also, note the presence of beaded axons.

staining where elongated neurophysin-containing cells placed in the needle tract (that is, in the ventromedial hypothalamic area) show fiber outgrowth.

This report demonstrates the ability of the aforementioned sorted cells to survive, migrate, and become differentiated and structurally integrated into the host tissue. Neurons did not appear to be affected by the flow cytometry and cell sorting techniques and retained differentiated properties. The results of this study raise the possibility that flow cytometry can be used to sort specific populations of cells to provide a source of donor tissue for transplantation.

REFERENCES

1. MELAMED, M. R., P. F. MULLANEY & M. L. MENDELSHON, EDS. 1979. Flow cytometry and cell sorting. John Wiley & Sons. New York, NY.
2. NOTTER, M. F. D., D. M. GASH, C. D. SLADEK & S. L. SHAROUN. 1984. Vasopressin in reaggregated cell cultures of the developing hypothalamus Brain Res. Bull. **12:** 307-313.
3. LEARY, J. F., P. TODD, J. C. G. WOOD & J. H. JETT. 1979. Flow cytometric light scatter and fluorescence pulse width and pulse rise time sizing of mammalian cells. J. Histochem. Cytochem. **27:** 315-320.

Cerebellar Transplants into Mutant Mice with Purkinje and Granule Cell Degeneration[a]

WALTER C. LOW,[b,d] LAZAROS C. TRIARHOU,[c,d] AND
BERNARDINO GHETTI[c,d]

[b]*Department of Physiology and Biophysics*
[c]*Department of Pathology, Division of Neuropathology*
[d]*Program in Medical Neurobiology*
Indiana University School of Medicine
Indianapolis, Indiana 46223

INTRODUCTION

Among cerebellar mutant mice, the "Purkinje cell degeneration" (*pcd*) is characterized by the selective loss of Purkinje cells,[1,2] and the weaver (*wv*) is characterized by the loss of granule cells.[3,4] The degeneration of Purkinje cells in *pcd* mutants takes place between the 17th and 45th postnatal days. In *wv* mutants, the degeneration of granule cells occurs within the first 2 postnatal weeks. The loss of these neuronal populations results in a marked atrophy of the mutant cerebella and an alteration in cerebellar connectivity. Behaviorally, the *pcd* is characterized by a moderate ataxia of gait, and the *wv* by ataxia, hypotonia, and tremor.

The recent developments in neural transplantation[5-8] suggest that grafting of normal cerebellar tissue can be applied to these mutants in an attempt to correct motor abnormalities, provided that the transplanted cellular elements are capable of 1) surviving and growing in the mutant host environment, 2) forming appropriate synapses within the graft, and 3) establishing functional synaptic interconnections with the host cerebellum. In the present study, we addressed the first two issues by grafting normal embryonic cerebellum into the cerebellomedullary cistern of adult *pcd* and *wv* recipients.

MATERIALS AND METHODS

Fifteen adult *pcd* mutants (C57BL/6J strain) and 12 *wv* mutants (hybrid B6CBA-A^{w-J}/A strain) were used as recipients. Donor tissue was obtained from normal fetal

[a]This research was supported in part by Grants R01-NS14426, S07-RR5371, and R03-AG5575 from the U.S. Public Health Service and by Grant 85-174 from Eli Lilly and Co.

740

mice of the respective strains at 15 days of gestation and placed into the cavity between the uvula vermis and the dorsal surface of the brainstem. At postoperative times ranging from 27 to 39 days, recipient mice were heparinized, anesthetized with pentobarbital sodium (50 mg/kg, i.p.), and perfused transcardially with aldehydes. Brains were dissected out, postfixed, dehydrated, and embedded in paraffin or Epon. Ten-micrometer-thick paraffin sections and 1-μm-thick plastic sections were examined by light microscopy. Ultrathin Epon sections from two grafts implanted into *pcd* mutant hosts were also examined by electron microscopy.

RESULTS

The grafted cerebella in both mutants were found adhering to the dorsal surface of the brainstem, beneath the uvula vermis of the host cerebellum, which was markedly atrophic. The cerebellar cortex of the *pcd* recipients was devoid of Purkinje cells (FIG. 1A); that of the *wv* was granuloprival (FIG. 1B). In both mutants, the grafts displayed a layered cellular organization reminiscent of the normal cerebellar cortex (FIGS. 1C & 1D). Molecular, Purkinje, and granule cell layers were identified; both Purkinje and granule cell perikarya were found in grafts placed into each mutant (FIGS. 1E & 1F).

In the molecular layer of cerebella transplanted into *pcd* mutant hosts, small axons the caliber of parallel fibers were observed, but were not oriented in a parallel fashion; the majority of their axon terminals were presynaptic to small profiles that were identified as dendritic spines. These axospinous synapses were numerous; in contrast, only a few axodendritic synapses were found. The overall picture was characterized by a relative paucity of dendrites, and of parallel fiber-like axons.

In the Purkinje cell layer, the cytology of grafted Purkinje cell perikarya appeared identical to that of the mature mouse Purkinje cells with the exception of the occasional presence of stubby somatic thorns. Rough endoplasmic reticulum was well developed with abundant cisterns; the polyribosomal accumulations that characteristically persist in the Purkinje cells of *pcd* mutants beyond the 15th postnatal day[2] were not observed in transplanted Purkinje cells. Hypolemmal cisternae were seen in association with mitochondria (FIG. 2A). Axosomatic synapses were found on Purkinje cells (FIGS. 2A & 2B); some of the presynaptic endings contained neurofilaments and were thought to be basket axon terminals.

In the granule cell layer, Purkinje cell axons were often identifiable by the presence of lamellar structures consisting of orderly arranged tubular elements (FIG. 2C). Within the neuropil of the granule cell layer, glomerular arrangements were seen, composed of mossy fiber-like terminals and small postsynaptic dendritic profiles (FIG. 2D).

In some of the preparations, clusters of large neurons were located at a distance from the granule cell layer, interspersed among myelinated axons. Based on their topography, their size, the relative paucity of cisterns in stacks of rough endoplasmic reticulum, and the lack of hypolemmal cisternae associated with mitochondria, these cells were tentatively identified as deep nuclear neurons. Synapses upon these neurons were seen on the initial segment of dendrites (FIG. 2E) and on somata (FIG. 2F).

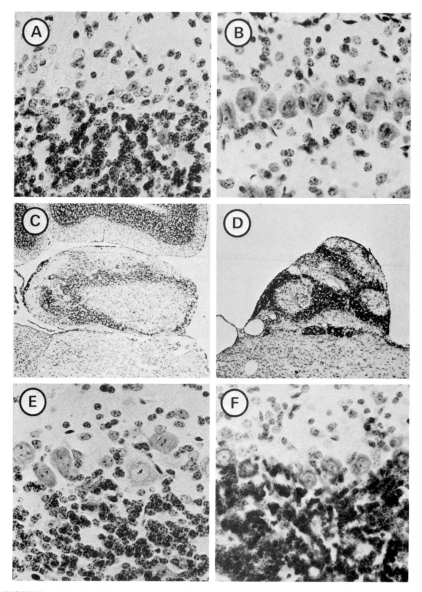

FIGURE 1. (A) Cerebellar cortex of a *pcd* mutant host at postnatal day 122. Note the presence of granule cells and lack of Purkinje cells (×400). (B) Cerebellar cortex of a *wv* mutant host at postnatal day 89. Note the presence of Purkinje cells and lack of granule cells (×400). (C) Cerebellar graft in a *pcd* recipient 39 days after transplantation (×40). (D) Cerebellar graft in a *wv* recipient 27 days after transplantation (×50). (E) High-power view of cerebellar transplant in a *pcd* recipient. The transplant contains both Purkinje and granule cells (×400). (F) High-power view of cerebellar transplant in a *wv* recipient with both Purkinje and granule cells (×400). Paraffin sections; gallocyanin Nissl stain. Original magnifications shown in parentheses; figure reduced to 90% of original size.

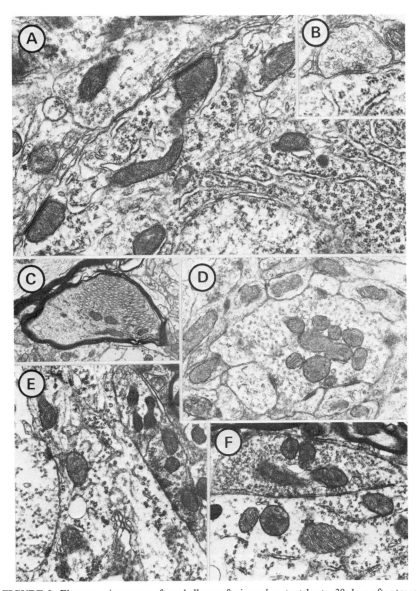

FIGURE 2. Electron microscopy of cerebellar grafts in *pcd* mutant hosts, 39 days after transplantation. (**A**) Axon terminal containing neurofilaments impinging on a Purkinje cell soma. Note the typical association of hypolemmal cisternae with mitochondria ($\times 20\ 750$). (**B**) Axosomatic synapse on Purkinje cell ($\times 31\ 800$). (**C**) Myelinated Purkinje axon containing the characteristic lamellar structures ($\times 8000$). (**D**) Mossy fiber rosette in the granule cell layer ($\times 16\ 600$). (**E**) Axodendritic synapses on deep nuclear neuron ($\times 14\ 110$). (**F**) Axosomatic synapse on deep nuclear neuron ($\times 15\ 810$). Ultrathin sections stained with uranyl acetate and lead citrate. Original magnifications shown in parentheses; figure reduced to 90% of original size.

DISCUSSION

Cerebellar anlagen grafted into adult *pcd* and *wv* mutant hosts are capable of growing and forming organized layers of Purkinje and granule cells. These findings suggest that the adult mutant host environment may not affect the survival of genetically normal Purkinje and granule cells.

Within the grafted tissue, synaptic connections are formed. In the molecular layer, the axospinous connections observed are most likely synapses between granule cell axons and Purkinje cells. These synapses bear a morphologic resemblance to parallel fiber ending-Purkinje spine contacts normally seen in the cerebellum; however, it is apparent that the quantity of such synapses may be deficient. Other types of synapses found in the grafts are those formed by basket-like axon terminals upon Purkinje cell somata. The occurrence of these synapses suggests that qualitatively appropriate connections can be established among grafted cerebellar neurons even in genetically abnormal environments.

REFERENCES

1. MULLEN, R. J., E. M. EICHER & R. L. SIDMAN. 1976. Purkinje cell degeneration, a new neurological mutation in the mouse. Proc. Natl. Acad. Sci. USA **73:** 208-212.
2. LANDIS, S. C. & R. J. MULLEN. 1978. The development and degeneration of Purkinje cells in *pcd* mutant mice. J. Comp. Neurol. **177:** 125-144.
3. SIDMAN, R. L. 1968. Development of interneuronal connections in brains of mutant mice. *In* Physiological and Biochemical Aspects of Nervous Integration. F. D. Carlson, Ed.: 163-193. Prentice-Hall. Englewood Cliffs, NJ.
4. RAKIC, P. & R. L. SIDMAN. 1973. Sequence of developmental abnormalities leading to granule cell deficit in cerebellar cortex of weaver mutant mice. J. Comp. Neurol. **152:** 103-132.
5. DAS, G. D. & J. ALTMAN. 1972. Studies on the transplantation of developing neural tissue in the mammalian brain. I. Transplantation of cerebellar slabs into the cerebellum of neonate rats. Brain Res. **38:** 233-249.
6. WELLS, J. & J. P. MCALLISTER. 1982. The development of cerebellar primordia transplanted to the neocortex of the rat. Dev. Brain Res. **4:** 167-179.
7. ALVARADO-MALLART, R. M. & C. SOTELO. 1982. Differentiation of cerebellar anlage heterotopically transplanted to adult rat brain: A light and electron microscopic study. J. Comp. Neurol. **212:** 247-267.
8. KROMER, L. F., A. BJÖRKLUND & U. STENEVI. 1983. Intracephalic embryonic neural implants in the adult rat brain. I. Growth and mature organization of brainstem, cerebellar, and hippocampal implants. J. Comp. Neurol. **218:** 433-459.

Tritiated Thymidine Identification of Embryonic Neostriatal Transplants

JAMES P. McALLISTER II

Departments of Anatomy and Neurosurgery
Temple University School of Medicine
Philadelphia, Pennsylvania 19140

Previous identification of embryonic neostriatal tissue transplanted into either intact neostriata or neostriata in which lesions had been created has been based purely on cytoarchitectural criteria.[1-4] These striatal implants are usually differentiated from the host neostriatum by their paucity of myelinated fiber bundles and by having a denser population of cells. The host-transplant interface is characterized by gliosis and the close packing of myelinated corticofugal fibers. The possibility remains that the neurons constituting the apparent implant could have arisen from the adjacent host. Host neurons could have migrated into the transplant site or been displaced by cells of the implant. To unequivocally determine the origin of the transplanted neurons, donor tissue was tagged with [^{3}H]thymidine and the transplant and host neostriatum examined for labeled cells.

Pregnant rats received two intraperitoneal injections of [^{3}H]thymidine (specific activity: 6.7 Ci/mM; dose: 5 μCi/g body wt.) on days 12 and 13 of gestation (E12 and E13), day 0 being the day of sperm positivity. On E14 striatal ridges were dissected from the embryos, dissociated in 0.1% trypsin, and transplanted into the intact neostriatum of adult hosts. Hosts were sacrificed 78-79 days after transplantation; their brains were embedded in paraffin, sectioned at a thickness of 15 μm, and processed by routine autoradiographic methods.

Transplants up to 2 mm in diameter were located in the middle of the host neostriatum and within the overlying cerebral cortex along the needle track (FIGS. 1A & 1B). These transplants were usually separated from the adjacent host tissue by a region of intense gliosis. Intensely, moderately, and lightly labeled neurons were found in all parts of the transplants (FIGS. 1C & 1D). These cells were similar to host neostriatal neurons by being round or polygonal in shape, 12-15 μm in diameter, and containing a thin rim of cytoplasm. Larger neurons were occasionally found within the implants. Approximately 40-50% of all neurons within the transplant contained some label.

Occasionally, labeled neurons were located within the surrounding gliotic region, but never more than 100 μm into the adjacent host neostriatum or cerebral cortex (FIG. 2A). In one case, labeled neurons were intermingled with glial cells and unlabeled neurons in a transition region between an obvious transplant and the host external capsule (FIG. 2B). Although this region was near the needle track, the absence of a clear glial boundary between the implant and host gave the impression that the labeled neurons were integrated somewhat into the host neostriatum. Labeled glial cells were seldom found within the transplant and the host brain. In the glial scar, however, label was present in cellular fragments and within glial cells. Since donor tissue was obtained before the onset of gliogenesis, glial labeling may represent debris from transplanted cells that had died.

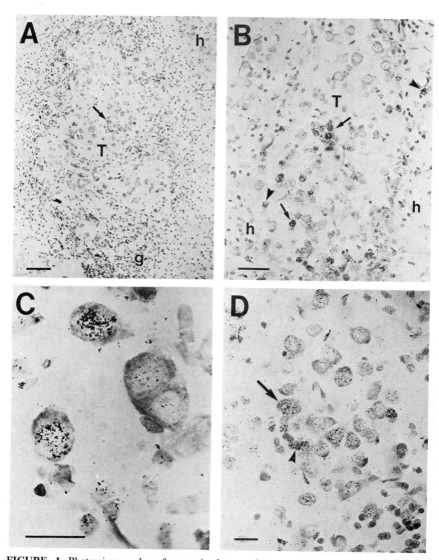

FIGURE 1. Photomicrographs of neostriatal transplants containing cells labeled with [³H]thymidine. (**A**) Low magnification of transplant (T) separated from the host neostriatum (h) by a region of gliosis (g). The arrow locates the intensely labeled neuron shown in **D**. (**B**) A transplant (T) located within the host neocortex (h) containing intensely labeled neurons (arrows). Some labeled neurons (arrowheads) seem to be integrated with the adjacent host tissue. (**C & D**) Intensely, moderately, and lightly labeled neurons in a transplant located within the host neostriatum. In **D**, notice the intensely labeled neuron (arrow) shown in **A** and the labeled glial cells (arrowhead). Scale bars: 100 μm in **A**; 50 μ in **B**; and 25 μm in **C** and **D**. Cresyl violet stain.

These results demonstrate that at least part, if not all, of the neurons constituting neostriatal implants are derived from embryonic donors. We have previously shown that these cells differentiate into neurons whose dendritic morphology is similar to that of the spiny and aspiny neurons that populate the normal neostriatum.[4] Furthermore, cells within striatal transplants contain glutamic acid decarboxylase and substance P[2] as well as acetylcholinesterase.[5] In transplants placed into intact neostriata, the donor neurons are confined to the implant and do not migrate any appreciable distance into the adjacent host tissue. Presumably, this phenomenon holds for striatal transplants that exhibit similar cytoarchitectural features as shown here but are located in lesion sites within the host neostriatum.

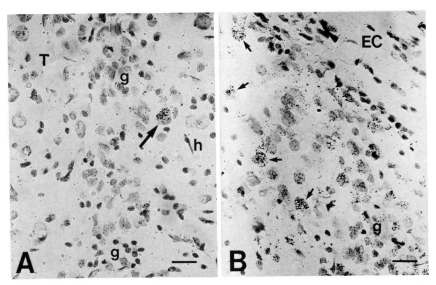

FIGURE 2. Photomicrographs of the host-transplant interface. (A) A neostriatal transplant (T) is separated from the host neocortex (h) by a region of sparse gliosis (g). A labeled neuron (arrow) is situated about 50 μm from the transplant. (B) Labeled neurons (arrows) ventral to the external capsule (EC) that appear intermingled with glial cells (g) and other neurons of the host neostriatum. Scale bar: 25 μm. Cresyl violet stain.

REFERENCES

1. DECKEL, A. W., R. G. ROBINSON, J. T. COYLE & P. R. SANBERG. 1983. Reversal of long-term locomotor abnormalities in the kainic acid model of Huntington's disease by day 18 fetal striatal implants. Eur. J. Pharmacol. **93**: 287-288.
2. ISACSON, O., P. BRUNDIN, D. DAWBARN, P. A. T. KELLY, F. H. GAGE, P. C. EMSON & A. BJÖRKLUND. 1985. Striatal grafts in the ibotenic acid-lesioned striatum. *In* Neural Grafting in the Mammalian CNS. A. Björklund & U. Stenevi, Eds.: 539-549. Elsevier. Amsterdam.
3. ISACSON, O., P. BRUNDIN, F. H. GAGE & A. BJÖRKLUND. 1985. Neural grafting in a rat model of Huntington's disease: Progressive neurochemical changes after neostriatal ibotenate lesions and striatal tissue grafting. Neuroscience **16**: 799-817.

4. McALLISTER, J. P., II, P. D. WALKER, M. C. ZEMANICK, A. W. WEBER, L. I. KAPLAN & M. A. REYNOLDS. 1985. Morphology of embryonic neostriatal cell suspensions transplanted into adult neostriata. Dev. Brain Res. **23:** 282-286.
5. McALLISTER, J. P., II, P. D. WALKER & G. I. CHOVANES. 1987. Transplants of neostriatal primordia contain acetylcholinesterase-positive neurons. Ann. N.Y. Acad. Sci. This volume.

Transplants of Neostriatal Primordia Contain Acetylcholinesterase-positive Neurons

JAMES P. McALLISTER II, PAUL D. WALKER, AND
GEORGE I. CHOVANES

Departments of Anatomy and Neurosurgery
Temple University School of Medicine
Philadelphia, Pennsylvania 19140

The normal neostriatum is characterized by a dense neuropil that is highly reactive for acetylcholinesterase (AChE). Grafts of embryonic neostriatal tissue also contain patches of AChE-positive neuropil,[1] but it is not known if neurons of the transplant contribute to this plexus. Our previous Golgi studies[2] have demonstrated that embryonic neostriatal neuroblasts transplanted into neostriatum of adult hosts in which lesions had been created will differentiate into many of the normal types of neostriatal neurons. These include the large and medium-sized aspiny neurons that normally contain AChE. The current study was designed to determine whether AChE-positive neurons are present within the transplants.

Adult host rats received intrastriatal injections of embryonic (E14) neostriatal cell suspensions 5 days after unilateral kainic acid lesions of the implant site. Two months later, 7 of 10 hosts were given injections of the AChE inhibitor diiosopropyl fluorophosphate (DFP, 2.0 mg/kg) and sacrificed 7 hr later. Frozen sections through the neostriatum were processed to demonstrate intraneuronal AChE according to the methods of Satoh *et al.*[3]

All recipients contained large transplants that occupied most of the lesion site (FIG. 1). These grafts were surrounded medially, ventrally, and laterally by regions of intact host neostriatum, and extended dorsally into the cerebral cortex. The caudal pole of these transplants was usually located within the rostral globus pallidus. In DFP-treated animals, two types of AChE-positive neurons were found throughout the transplants. The most reactive neurons had medium-sized round or polygonal somata with long, sparsely branched dendrites (FIG. 2C). These neurons were identical in morphology and staining characteristics to those that occupy the contralateral neostriatum (FIG. 2A) and that Bolam *et al.*[4] classify as type I in the normal neostriatum. Less reactive neurons usually had smaller round or polygonal somata, with dendrites that were not stained for any appreciable distance (FIG. 2D). These neurons were similar to the neostriatal cells that Bolam *et al.*[4] classify as type II, as well as to those cells that abundantly populate the normal globus pallidus.

Type I and II neurons were located conspicuously in segregated clusters (FIG. 2B). Type I neurons appeared less frequently than observed in the contralateral neostriatum, and were usually found in groups of three to five. Compared to the contralateral neostriatum, type II neurons were much more numerous, and clusters of these cells seldom contained any type I neurons. The neuropil staining in the region of type I clusters was faint, but slightly more intense than that observed in the area of type II neurons. In sections counterstained with cresyl violet, it was estimated that type II AChE-positive neurons constituted about 50% of the total population.

In non-DFP-treated animals, all transplants contained islands or swirls of intensely reactive neuropil separated by regions of lightly staining neuropil (FIG. 1A). In caudal portions of some transplants, which were usually embedded in the host globus pallidus, the intensely reactive neuropil was located only in the periphery of the graft. In these sections, bundles of AChE-positive fibers could be seen connecting the transplant and the adjacent neostriatum of the host.

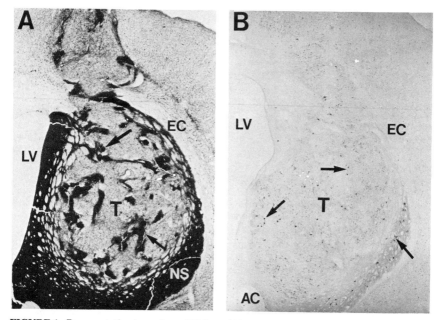

FIGURE 1. Representative transplants (T) from (**A**) non-DFP- and (**B**) DFP-treated animals. (**A**) Intensely reactive AChE neuropil can be seen throughout the host neostriatum (NS) and in patches (arrows) within the transplant. Areas of less reactivity within the transplant are seen surrounding dark AChE neuropil. (**B**) Note the intensely reactive AChE neurons (arrows) in the transplant and host neostriatum. AC: anterior commissure; EC: external capsule; LV: lateral ventricle.

These results demonstrate that AChE-positive neurons populate neostriatal transplants. Type I neurons appear in reduced numbers whereas type II neurons are much more numerous relative to controls. This disparity in numbers, combined with the clear segregation of these two cell types, may indicate that the cell suspensions contain a mixture of both neostriatal and globus pallidus anlagen. Conversely, the increased frequency of type II neurons may be due to synthesis of AChE by striatal neurons that normally do not produce high levels of this enzyme. Nevertheless, the presence of AChE-positive neurons suggests that cells of the transplant may be the source of the AChE neuropil in the graft, and may contribute to the intrinsic circuitry of the transplant.

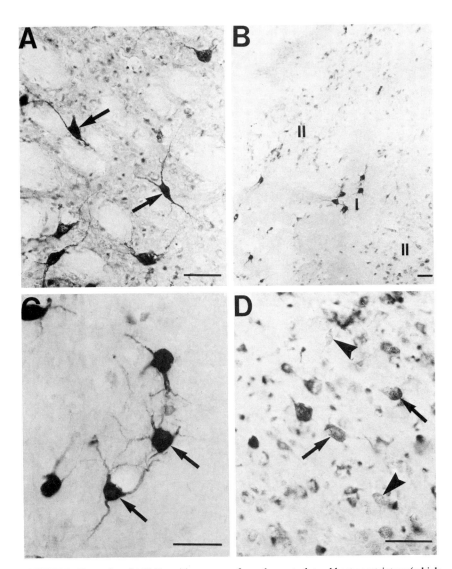

FIGURE 2. Examples of AChE-positive neurons from the contralateral host neostriatum (which had not received lesions) and transplanted neostriatum. (**A**) Large neurons (arrows) intensely reactive for AChE are characteristic of type I cells according to Bolam *et al.*[4] Cresyl violet counterstain. (**B**) Segregated clusters of type I- and type II-like neurons are seen within neostriatal transplants. Note the darker neuropil staining surrounding type I cells compared to the lighter neuropil in type II clusters. (**C**) Type I-like AChE neurons (arrows) within the transplant. (**D**) small (arrowheads) and medium (arrows) lightly reactive AChE neurons within type II clusters in the transplant. Scale bar: 50 μm.

REFERENCES

1. ISACSON, O., P. BRUNDIN, F. H. GAGE & A. BJÖRKLUND. 1985. Neural grafting in a rat model of Huntington's disease: Progressive neurochemical changes after neostriatal ibotenate lesions and striatal tissue grafting. Neuroscience 16(4): 799-817.
2. MCALLISTER, J. P., II, P. D. WALKER, M. C. ZEMANICK, A. B. WEBER, L. I. KAPLAN & M. A. REYNOLDS. 1985. Morphology of embryonic neostriatal cell suspensions transplanted into adult neostriata. Dev. Brain Res. 23: 282-286.
3. SATOH, K., D. M. ARMSTRONG & H. C. FIBIGER. 1983. A comparison of the distribution of central cholinergic neurons as demonstrated by acetylcholinesterase pharmohistochemistry and choline acetyltransferase immunohistochemistry. Brain Res. Bull. 11: 693-720.
4. BOLAM, J. P., C. A. INGHAM & A. D. SMITH. 1984. The section-Golgi-impregnation procedure. III. Combination of Golgi impregnation with enzyme histochemistry and electron microscopy to characterize acetylcholinesterase-containing neurons in the rat neostriatum. Neuroscience 12(3): 687-709.

Why Don't Axons Regenerate in the Adult Mammalian Visual System?[a]

STEVEN C. McLOON,[b,c] LINDA K. McLOON,[d] AND
DANIEL M. WOLNER[c]

[c]Department of Cell Biology and Neuroanatomy
and
[d]Department of Ophthalmology
University of Minnesota
Minneapolis, Minnesota 55455

Retinal axons fail to regenerate successfully after injury to the mature mammalian visual system. The basis for this lack of axonal regeneration is unknown, but two possibilities are most likely. First, mature retinal ganglion cells could intrinsically lack the ability to regrow an axon, or, second, factors in the environment of the mature visual system may not be conducive to axonal growth. Several studies suggest that the latter is true. We have transplanted embryonic day 14 retinas adjacent to the superior colliculus of newborn or adult host rats. One to 3 months later, axonal tract tracing techniques were used to identify the transplant projections in the host brain. Axons from transplants to newborn hosts entered the host superior colliculus, projected rostrally along the optic tract, and innervated most of the primary visual nuclei.[1] Axons from transplants to adult hosts entered the host colliculus but never coursed over 200 μm into the host brain.[2] The recent finding that mature retinal ganglion cells will grow axons into peripheral nervous system grafts[3–6] shows that they have the intrinsic ability to grow an axon. This result coupled with the finding that young actively growing retinal axons fail to penetrate significantly into the mature brain suggests that factors in the environment are responsible for the lack of retinal axon regeneration.

Environmental factors that prevent retinal axon growth could be of two types. First, something in the environment of the mature visual system could actively inhibit retinal axon growth. This inhibitory factor could be in the form of a barrier such as gliosis (the hypertrophy or proliferation or both of astrocytes) or a glial scar (one or more layers of astrocytic processes covered by a basal lamina) that might result from the injury. We examined the interface between transplants of embryonic visual system tissue placed in the mature host superior colliculus for the presence of a glial barrier to axonal growth.[7] Ultrastructurally the interface, in some places, can be identified by parallel processes of reactive astrocytes. This glial interface was discontinuous, and axons crossed the interface through the discontinuities. In other regions, there were

[a]This work was supported by Grants EY05371, EY05372, and EY05432 from the National Institutes of Health and by a grant from Research to Prevent Blindness to the Department of Ophthalmology.

[b]Address for correspondence: Department of Cell Biology and Neuroanatomy, University of Minnesota, 4-135 Jackson Hall, 321 Church Street S.E., Minneapolis, Minnesota 55455.

no glial processes marking the boundary between the transplant and host brain. This interface was also studied for the presence of glial fibrillary acidic protein (GFAP)-positive astrocytes and a laminin-positive basal lamina using immunohistochemistry at the light microscopic level. Very little GFAP immunoreactivity was present until about 7 days after transplantation. From other studies we know that axon outgrowth begins by 2 days after transplantation.[8] In all cases GFAP immunoreactivity was significantly reduced in the host brain adjacent to a fetal transplant (FIG. 1A) compared to sham-operated controls (FIG. 1B). This suggests that transplants of fetal central nervous system tissue may actually reduce the glial response to injury in the mature brain. At no time was a laminin-positive basal lamina interposed between the transplant and host brain. There was no indication that gliosis or glial scar formation could be a significant factor in the inhibition of the growth of axons from transplants into the adult brain.

It could also be that a particular cell type that inhibits axonal growth is normally present in the mature visual system. The two main cell types present in the mature optic nerve and optic tract are astrocytes and oligodendrocytes. Astrocytes are present in the developing pathway when optic axons are growing, so it is unlikely that they inhibit axon growth. Oligodendrocytes, however, do not appear until relatively late in development. Also, mature retinal axons will regenerate in the optic fiber layer of the retina, which contains astrocytes, but they stop at the optic nerve head, which contains oligodendrocytes.[9,10] Thus, oligodendrocytes or their myelin may inhibit retinal axon growth. The ability of retinal axons to regenerate in the absence of oligodendrocytes was tested in Shiverer mice (Wolner and McLoon, unpublished results). Approximately 95% of the oligodendrocytes and their accompanying myelin fails to develop in Shiverer mice. The optic nerve at the midpoint between the retina and chiasm was crushed in these animals. Between 1 week and 2 months later, an axon tracer substance was injected into the eyes associated with the injury. These animals were processed to show the projection of the retinal axons in the optic nerve and brain. There was no indication of axon growth in these animals at short or long

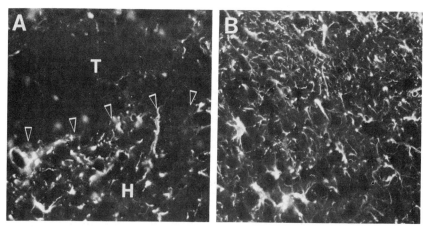

FIGURE 1. Fluorescence photomicrographs of GFAP immunoreactivity. (**A**) The interface (arrowheads) between a transplant (T) and the host superior colliculus (H). (**B**) The superior colliculus of a sham-operated control animal. The GFAP reactivity is reduced in animals with transplants.

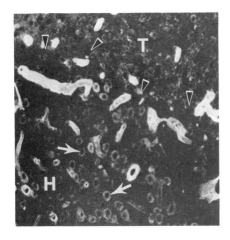

FIGURE 2. Fluorescence photomicrograph of laminin immunoreactivity at the interface (arrowheads) between a transplant (T) and host superior colliculus (H). Laminin-positive cells (arrows) are present in the host brain around the area of injury induced during the transplantation procedure.

survival times after injury. These results do not support the idea that oligodendrocytes inhibit axon growth in the mature visual system.

The second type of environmental factor that might prevent retinal axon regeneration is that some substance required for axon growth, which may be present during development, is lacking from the environment of the mature visual system. Such a substance could be a cell survival factor (analogous to nerve growth factor) or a substrate factor required for adhesion of growing axons. A growing axon requires a substrate to which it can adhere in order to extend.[11] Retinal ganglion cells survive a considerable time after their axons are severed, as demonstrated by the study with the Shiverer mice described above. This suggests that substrate factors may be more important than survival factors in the problem of axon regeneration. We have been screening for molecules that are present in the developing visual pathway, are absent in the mature system, and can support retinal axon growth in culture. Laminin is transiently present on cells within the rat optic nerve during the time retinal axons are growing.[12] In the adult optic nerve, laminin immunoreactivity is confined to the basal lamina surrounding blood vessels and the outside of the nerve. Laminin has also been shown to support retinal axon growth in culture, an activity that is blocked by antibodies to laminin.[13–15] Other results are also consistent with laminin having an essential role in retinal axon growth. The procedure of transplanting retina to adult hosts results in induction of laminin immunoreactivity in the host superior colliculus, and its distribution correlates with the pattern of axon growth from these transplants (FIG. 2).[7] Laminin has also been shown to be present in the optic nerve of goldfish during retinal axon regeneration.[16] These results give intriguing support to the notion that the inability of retinal axons to grow in the mature visual system may be due to the lack of an appropriate substrate molecule, possibly laminin.

REFERENCES

1. McLOON, S. C. & R. D. LUND. 1980. Specific projections of retina transplanted to rat brain. Exp. Brain Res. **40:** 273-282.
2. McLOON, S. C. & R. D. LUND. 1983. Development of fetal retina, tectum and cortex transplanted to the superior colliculus of adult rats. J. Comp. Neurol. **217:** 376-389.

3. So, K.-F. & A. J. AGUAYO. 1985. Lengthy regrowth of cut axons from ganglion cells after peripheral nerve transplantation into the retina of adult rats. Brain Res. **328:** 349-354.
4. STEVENSON, J. A. 1985. Growth of optic tract axons in nerve grafts in hamsters. Exp. Neurol. **87:** 446-457.
5. BERRY, M., L. REES & J. SIEVERS. 1986. Unequivocal regeneration of rat optic nerve axons into sciatic nerve isografts. *In* Neural Transplantation and Regeneration. G. D. Das & R. B. Wallace, Eds.: 63-79. Springer-Verlag. New York, NY.
6. POLITIS, M. J. & P. S. SPENCER. 1986. Regeneration of rat optic axons into peripheral nerve grafts. Exp. Neurol. **91:** 52-59.
7. MCLOON, L. K. & S. C. MCLOON. 1986. Alteration of reactive gliosis by transplants of embryonic tectum or cortex to the mature brain of rats. Submitted for publication.
8. MCLOON, L. K. & S. C. MCLOON. 1984. Early development of projections from embryonic retina transplanted into the host brain of rats. Soc. Neurosci. Abstr. **10:** 373.
9. GOLDBERG, S. & B. FRANK. 1980. Will central nervous system axons in the adult mammal regenerate after bypassing a lesion? A study in the mouse and chick visual systems. Exp. Neurol. **70:** 675-689.
10. MCCONNELL, P. & M. BERRY. 1982. Regeneration of ganglion cell axons in the adult mouse brain. Brain Res. **241:** 362-365.
11. LETOURNEAU, P. C. 1975. Cell-to-substratum adhesion and guidance of axonal elongation. Dev. Biol. **44:** 92-101.
12. MCLOON, S. C., L. K. MCLOON, L. T. FURCHT & S. L. PALM. 1986. Laminin is transiently expressed along the pathway of growing optic axons in the developing rat. Soc. Neurosci. Abstr. **12:** 1211.
13. MANTHORPE, M., E. ENGVALL, E. RUOSLAHTI, F. M. LONGO, G. E. DAVIS & S. VARON. 1983. Laminin promotes neuritic regeneration from cultured peripheral and central neurons. J. Cell Biol. **97:** 1882-1890.
14. ROGERS, S. L., P. C. LETOURNEAU, S. L. PALM, J. MCCARTHY & L. T. FURCHT. 1983. Neurite extension by peripheral and central nervous system neurons in response to substratum-bound fibronectin and laminin. Dev. Biol. **98:** 212-220.
15. SMALHEISER, N. R., S. M. CRAIN & L. M. REID. 1984. Laminin as a substrate for retinal axons *in vitro.* Dev. Brain Res. **12:** 136-140.
16. HOPKINS, J. M., T. S. FORD-HOLVINSKI, J. P. MCCOY & B. W. AGRANOFF. 1985. Laminin and optic nerve regeneration in the goldfish. J. Neurosci. **5:** 3030-3038.

Fetal Noradrenergic Cell Suspensions Transplanted into Amine-depleted Nuclei of Adult Rats

Restoring the Drinking Response to Angiotensin II

A. McRAE-DEGUEURCE

*Institut National de la Santé
et de la Recherche Médicale Unité 259
Bordeaux, France*

J. T. CUNNINGHAM, S. BELLIN,
S. LANDAS, L. WILKIN, AND A. K. JOHNSON[a]

*Departments of Psychology and Pharmacology
and the Cardiovascular Center
University of Iowa
Iowa City, Iowa 52242*

It is now well established that transplanted neuronal tissue survives, differentiates, and forms connections in the mammalian central nervous system (CNS). Few models, however, demonstrate the functional significance of the transplants in the host. In our laboratory, we have recently focused on developing a transplant preparation specifically targeted to a CNS region known to contain neural systems involved in the maintenance of body fluid balance and cardiovascular homeostasis.

The periventricular tissues of the anteroventral portion of the third ventricle (AV3V) are critically involved in the control of body fluid homeostasis, electrolyte balance, and arterial blood pressure.[1] Specific disruption of the catecholamine innervation in the organum vasculosum of the lamina terminalis (OVLT) and the ventral median preoptic nuclei (VMPN), which are contained within the AV3V region, attenuates drinking and pressor responses elicited by angiotensin II.[2] These findings suggest that the noradrenergic innervation of the AV3V region may play a critical role in modulating these responses. We investigated if dissociated fetal noradrenergic cell suspensions transplanted into these amine-depleted nuclei would reestablish noradrenergic input into these nuclei and restore drinking responses to systemically and centrally administered angiotensin II.

Initially, animals were prescreened for water consumption of 2.5 ml or more in 2 hr after the administration of angiotensin II (1.5 mg/kg). Two weeks after vehicle or 6-hydroxydopamine (6-OHDA) injections into the OVLT/VMPN, a second drink-

[a] To whom correspondence and reprint requests should be addressed.

ing test was conducted, and the following results for water consumption were obtained: vehicle controls: 5.3 ± .6 ml (N = 5); 6-OHDA-treated rats: 0.71 ± .6 ml (N = 23). The 23 6-OHDA-treated animals were divided into three groups: locus ceruleus (LC)-transplanted rats: 12 rats that received dissociated cell suspensions that were prepared from the LC of 17-day-old fetuses and injected into the OVLT/VMPN; cortical-transplanted rats: 5 rats that received dissociated cortical tissue prepared from 17-day-old fetuses; treatment controls: the remaining 6 rats. Two months later, seven of the LC-transplanted rats drank significantly more than both the treatment controls and the cortical-transplanted rats, as depicted in FIGURE 1A [F(6,19) = 35.6, p <

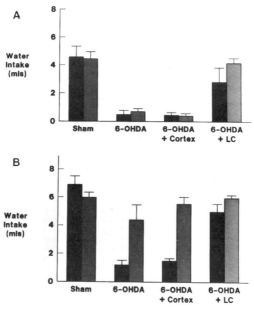

FIGURE 1. (A) Water intake during 2-hr-long drinking tests. The response to subcutaneously injected angiotensin II (1.5 mg/kg) was evaluated for each of the following groups: vehicle controls, treatment controls, cortical-transplanted rats, and LC-transplanted rats. Dark bars: water intake 1 month after transplantation; light bars: water intake by the same animals 2 months after transplantation. (B) Water intake during 30-min-long drinking tests. Dark bars: water intake after intraventricular injection of angiotensin II (100 ng in 2 μl of saline); light bars: water intake after intraventricular injection of carbachol (250 ng in 2 μl of saline). These drinking tests were conducted on the same animals described in A, 3 months after transplantation.

.01; Newman-Keuls, p < .05]. After these tests, the rats were implanted with cannulae in the lateral ventricle. All four groups of rats received central injections of carbachol (250 ng in 2 μl of saline) and angiotensin II (100 ng in 2 μl of saline). At least 24 hr intervened between these two tests. None of the groups showed a drinking response to carbachol that differed significantly from the responses shown by the other groups. After angiotensin II was centrally administered, however, the vehicle controls and the LC-transplanted rats drank significantly more than either treatment controls or cortical-transplanted rats, as depicted in FIGURE 1B [F(3,16) = 10.6, p < .01; Newman-Keuls, p < .05].

Histofluorescence examination of the brains of those animals that received transplants and subsequently responded to angiotensin II (that is, the LC-transplanted rats) indicated the presence of clusters of catecholamine-fluorescent cells in the previously denervated OVLT/VMPN region. The nonresponding cortical-transplanted rats and the treatment controls evidenced large reductions in catecholamine fluorescence within this brain region.

From these observations we have drawn the following conclusions: 1) transplanted fetal cells from the LC survive in previously denervated OVLT/VMPN nuclei; 2) transplanted LC cells can reverse drinking deficits to both systemically and centrally administered angiotensin II; and 3) the noradrenergic innervation in this brain region plays a significant role in mediating the drinking response elicited by angiotensin II but not that elicited by carbachol.

This functional transplant model has significance for understanding the neural control of behavior (that is, thirst and drinking behavior), pituitary control (vasopressin secretion), and cardiovascular pathology (hypertension).

REFERENCES

1. JOHNSON, A. K. 1982. Neurobiology of the periventricular tissue surrounding the anteroventral third ventricle (AV3V) and its role in behavior, fluid balance and cardiovascular control. *In* Circulation, Neurobiology and Behavior, O. A. Smith, R. A. Galosy & S. M. Weiss, Eds. Vol. **15:** 277-295. Elsevier. New York, NY.
2. BELLIN, S., S. LANDAS, R. BHATNAGAR & A. K. JOHNSON. 1984. The role of catecholamines in discrete AV3V nuclei: Alterations in drinking and pressor responses to angiotensin following 6-hydroxydopamine. Fed. Proc. **43:** 1070.

The Role of Target-Graft Interactions in the Functional Development of Transplanted Vasopressin Neurons

FREDERICK F. MARCIANO,[a] STANLEY J.
WIEGAND, AND DON M. GASH

*Department of Neurobiology and Anatomy
University of Rochester School of Medicine
Rochester, New York 14642*

Our research group has demonstrated that the diabetes insipidus associated with surgical disruption of the supraoptico-hypophysial tract via neurohypophysectomy can be ameliorated with third ventricular grafts of fetal anterior hypothalamic tissue.[1] Interestingly, grafts were ineffective in alleviating the fluid and electrolyte imbalances of hosts that had received anterior hypothalamic deafferentations, a surgical lesion that denervates the median eminence-neurohypophysial region of vasopressinergic inputs. After neurohypophysectomy there is a proliferation of fenestrated capillaries in the median eminence[2,3] that could be of vital importance in producing the functional response seen after tissue grafting. Given the apparent association between functional development and median eminence vasculature, the lack of a physiologically favorable response of hosts with anterior hypothalamic deafferentations may also be attributable to changes in this vascular target. The present study examined the effect of these lesions on the vasculature of the median eminence and investigated the importance of target manipulation in the functional development of transplanted vasopressin-containing neurons.

One to 2 weeks before transplantation, male adult Long-Evans rats (250-275 g) received either a neurohypophysectomy ($N = 15$) or an anterior hypothalamic deafferentation ($N = 14$). Tissue blocks of 17 day fetal anterior hypothalamus were stereotaxically positioned into the third cerebral ventricle of the operated animals. Control animals received either a surgical procedure or a sham graft consisting of sterile culture media. Forty to 50 days after transplantation, the recipients were perfused transcardially with a paraformaldehyde-picric acid fixative followed by a warmed 2% gelatin ink solution for the demonstration of brain microvasculature. After the appropriate postfixation, 50-μ-thick frozen sections were collected and processed immunocytochemically with antisera specific for either arginine vasopressin or vasopressin-associated neurophysin. Reference sections were stained with an antiserum that reacted with both vasopressin and oxytocin neurophysin.

[a] Address for correspondence: Department of Neurobiology and Anatomy, Box 603, 601 Elmwood Avenue, University of Rochester School of Medicine, Rochester, New York 14642.

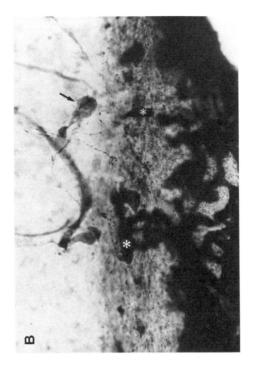

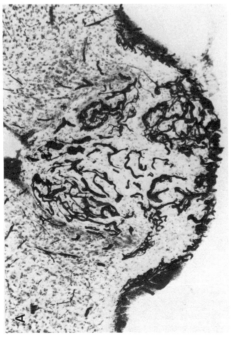

FIGURE 1. (*Continued.*)

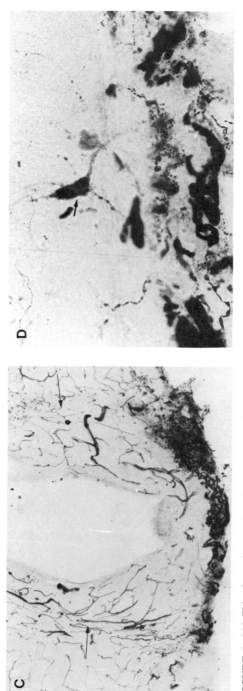

FIGURE 1. (**A**) This photomicrograph depicts the median eminence of a neurohypophysectomized, sham-grafted rat processed for demonstration of brain microvasculature. The median eminence is grossly enlarged because of a proliferation of blood vessels and glial elements (×200). (**B**) This high-power photomicrograph (×400) illustrates the graft-host median eminence interface of an animal that was neurohypophysectomized and received a transplant of 17 day fetal anterior hypothalamus 1 week later. The brain was perfused with a 2% gelatin ink solution to demonstrate the vasculature. This section was processed immunocytochemically with an antiserum that reacts with arginine vasopressin and was counterstained with cresyl violet acetate. The magnocellular neurons (arrow) present are in close association to the underlying gelatin-ink-filled vessels (asterisks) intrinsic to the host median eminence (**C**). This photomicrograph (×100) of a section from the brain of a rat that received an anterior hypothalamic deafferentation and a graft of fetal anterior hypothalamus demonstrates the effect of this lesion on the vasculature and vasopressin-neurophysin immunohistochemistry of the host median eminence. The tract left by the knife used to deafferent the median eminence is present (arrow). The vascularity of the median eminence, in comparison to that of the neurohypophysectomized host, is significantly different. The median eminence is also devoid of the normally robust vasopressin-neurophysin staining. (**D**) This high-power photomicrograph (×400) depicts an immunocytochemically stained, implanted, vasopressin-neurophysin-containing neuron in close association with the gelatin-ink-filled blood vessels in the median eminence of a rat that received an anterior hypothalamic deafferentation 2 weeks before transplantation. This neuron (arrow) can be seen to send processes into the host median eminence. Original magnifications are shown in parentheses; figure reduced to 53% of original size.

Neurohypophysectomized animals presented with a proliferation of vasculature in the median eminence and reorganized stalk as compared to anterior hypothalamic deafferented animals, whose median eminence appeared regressed because of the loss of axonal projections through the zona interna or the collapse of the intrinsic fenestrated capillaries or both. Neurohypophysectomized hosts, whose grafts were in apposition to the median eminence, presented with well-developed vasopressin- and neurophysin-positive magnocellular neurons with extensive axonal arborizations. The implants of animals that had received anterior hypothalamic deafferentations contained immunocytochemically identifiable vasopressin and neurophysin magnocellular and parvicellular neurons. Given the lack of endogenous staining in the host median eminence of deafferented animals, axonal processes from the transplanted neurons could be seen in apposition to the gelatin-ink-filled blood vessels (FIG. 1).

As demonstrated in our previous study, the neurohypophysectomized hosts responded functionally when the grafts were in juxtaposition to the enriched vasculature of the median eminence and contained vasopressin magnocellular neurons. In contrast to this situation, the fluid imbalances of the anterior hypothalamic deafferented animal persisted even though magnocellular neurons reinnervated, to some degree, the host median eminence.

The results of the present study suggest that the availability of an appropriate neurovascular target is a necessary condition for the functional development of transplanted vasopressinergic neurons. Grafts of fetal anterior hypothalamic tissue were unable to reverse the fluid and electrolyte deficits of recipients that had been subjected to anterior hypothalamic knife lesions, which caused a regression of target vasculature, even though the host median eminence was reinnervated, albeit sparsely, by the implanted vasopressin neurons. In contrast, hosts whose hypothalamic neurosecretory system was damaged via neurohypophysectomy, which resulted in a proliferation of vessels in the median eminence, responded functionally after implantation of fetal hypothalamic tissue that was structurally integrated with this enriched vascular target. Another interesting and contrasting condition between the two surgical manipulations that could also influence the function of the graft is the fact that following neurohypophysectomy alone there is a considerable degree of recovery[4] by the host hypothalamic neurosecretory system that is not seen after anterior hypothalamic deafferentation. The same stimulus that is guiding the regeneration of the damaged host magnocellular neurons in the case of neurohypophysectomy could also influence the development and function of the implanted magnocellular vasopressinergic neurons. This same trophic influence may not be present in the anterior hypothalamic deafferentation situation given the lack of host system recovery after the lesion.

REFERENCES

1. MARCIANO, F. F. & D. M. GASH. 1986. Brain Res. **370**(2): 338-342.
2. RAISMAN, G. 1973. Brain Res. **55**: 245-261.
3. RAISMAN, G. 1973. J. Comp. Neurol. **147**: 181-208.
4. MOLL, J. & D. DEWIED. 1962. Gen. Comp. Endocrinol. **2**: 215-228.

Receptors for Bombesin-like Peptides Are Present on Fetal Transplants[a]

TERRY W. MOODY,[b] REINA GETZ,[b] JAMES R. CONNER,[c,e] AND JERALD J. BERNSTEIN[c–e]

Departments of [b]Biochemistry, [c]Physiology, and [d]Neurosurgery
George Washington University School of Medicine
Washington, DC 20037
and
[e]Laboratory of Central Nervous System Injury and Regeneration
Veterans Administration Medical Center
Washington, DC 20422

Transplantation of fetal central nervous system (CNS) tissue into the nervous system of adult animals can be utilized as a mechanism to study the development of the nervous system both morphologically and chemically.[1] This research tool can be utilized to study phenotypic expression of peptides, receptors, and cellular organization of transplants of various fetal CNS tissues in ectopic locations. The following experiments study the development of receptors on 14 day gestation cerebral cortex homografts transplanted into the spinal cord of adult rats.

After 12 Sprague-Dawley male rats (~ 350 g) underwent deep pentabarbitol anesthesia, the spinal cord (under the sixth thoracic vertebra) was exposed within the dura incised from each rat. The transplants these rats were to receive were 1.0 mm³ homografts of 14 day gestation cerebral cortex from timed pregnant dams. The transplants were aspirated into a 30-gauge needle, which was mounted on a 50-μl Hamilton syringe. Transplants were pressure injected between the dorsal horn and the dorsal column of the host. The animals were closed and injected with Longicil.

Animals were utilized 14 and 30 days after surgery. Neuropeptides were characterized using immunocytochemical techniques. Animals were perfused with 4% paraformaldehyde through the ascending aorta. The tissue was removed immediately and sectioned on a Vibratome at 50 μm. Sections were pretreated in NaIO$_4$, NaBH$_4$, dimethyl sulfoxide, and 1:30 goat serum. The primary antibodies were bombesin (1:1000), vasoactive intestinal polypeptide (VIP) (1:1000), and substance P (1:1000). The tissue was incubated at 4° C in the primary antibody overnight and developed the following day using the peroxidase-antiperoxidase method.

Neuropeptide receptors were characterized using *in vitro* autoradiographic techniques. Fresh frozen rat spinal cord was sectioned using an IEC minotome. Twelve-micrometer-thick sections were thaw mounted onto coverslips and air dried. The sections were incubated in a Krebs-Ringer buffer that contained 100 μg/ml bacitracin

[a]This work was supported by Grant BNS 8500552 (to T. W. Moody) from the National Science Foundation. J. J. Bernstein was supported by the Veterans Administration.

and 0.25% bovine serum albumin plus radiolabeled peptide. Bound peptide was separated from free peptide by two consecutive washes in buffer. ^{125}I-VIP was employed as a probe for VIP receptors; ^{125}I-physalemin, as a probe for substance P receptors; and (^{125}I-Tyr 4)bombesin as a probe for bombesin receptors.

The times at which VIP- and somatostatin-positive neuron cell bodies appeared in the cortical transplants were similar to times at which these cell bodies appeared in the cortical controls.[2,3] The peptide was first seen 8 days after birth in controls and between 14 and 30 days after birth in the transplanted cortex. No bombesin-positive nerve cell bodies were observed at either time period.[4] Substance P nerve fibers do enter transplants from the host spinal cord,[5] but no substance P nerve cell bodies were observed in the transplants.

Receptors for VIP were present in low density in the fetal transplant tissue. In contrast, VIP receptors are normally present in moderate density in the adult rat cerebral cortex, especially in lamina I.[6] TABLE 1 shows that substance P receptors were not present in the fetal tissue, although they were present in moderate densities in their normal position in the dorsal horn of the host spinal cord.[7] Receptors for bombesin-like peptides were also present in high densities in the fetal transplant tissue.[8] These receptors appeared to develop on the transplant as they were not abundant 2

TABLE 1. Distribution of Neuropeptides and Receptors in Neocortex Fetal Transplants

Marker	Relative Density[a]
VIP	+ +
VIP receptors	+
Substance P	+
Substance P receptors	−
Bombesin	−
Bombesin receptors	+ + +

[a] The relative density of the peptides and receptors 30 days after transplantation is indicated: + + +: high density; + +: moderate density; +: low density; −: absent.

weeks after the transplant was injected into the spinal cord, were present in moderate density after 3 weeks, and were present in high density after 4 weeks.

In summary, fetal transplants into the spinal cord contain VIP receptors but not substance P receptors. Because VIP functions as a vasodilator of cerebral arteries,[9] these VIP receptors may be activated by endogenous VIP present in the transplant and stimulate blood flow to the transplant. Also, the fetal transplant contains high densities of bombesin receptors but not bombesin-like peptide content. These receptors may be activated, however, by the bombesin-like peptides that are present in high densities in the dorsal horn of the host spinal cord. Because bombesin functions as a growth factor for normal and malignant cells,[10] the bombesin receptors may facilitate growth or differentiation or both of the transplant.

REFERENCES

1. BJÖRKLUND, A. & U. STENEVI, EDS. 1985. Neural Grafting in the Mammalian CNS. Elsevier. Amsterdam.
2. CONNOR, J. R. & J. J. BERNSTEIN. 1986. Brain Res. 367: 214-221.

3. BERNSTEIN, J. J. & J. R. CONNOR. 1986. Brain Res. **374:** 147-152.
4. MCDONALD, J. K., J. G. PARNAVELAS, A. N. KARAMANLIDIS & N. J. BRECHA. 1982. Neurocytology **11:** 825-837.
5. CONNOR, J. R. & J. J. BERNSTEIN. 1987. *In* Neural Regeneration. F. Seil, E. H. Herbert & B. Carlson, Eds.: 359-371. Elsevier. Amsterdam.
6. MCGRANE, M. & T. MOODY. 1986. Peptides. **7:** 283-288.
7. WOLF, S., T. MOODY, R. QUIRION & T. O'DONOHUE. 1985. Brain Res. **332:** 299-307.
8. ZARBIN, M., M. KUHAR, S. WOLF & T. MOODY. 1985. J. Neurosci. **5:** 429-437.
9. LARSSON, L. I., L. EDVINSSON, J. FAHRENKRUG, R. HAKANSON, C. OWMAN, O. SCHAFFALITZKY DE MUCKKADELL & F. SUNDLER. 1976. Brain Res. **113:** 400-409.
10. CUTTITTA, F., D. CARNEY, J. MULSHINE, T. MOODY, J. FEDORKO, A. FISCHLER & J. MINNA. 1985. Nature **316:** 823-826.

Differentiated Neuronal Cell Lines as Donor Tissue for Transplantation into the CNS[a]

MARY F. D. NOTTER,[b] JEFFREY H. KORDOWER,
AND DON M. GASH

Department of Neurobiology and Anatomy
University of Rochester School of Medicine and Dentistry
Rochester, New York 14642

We are investigating the use of specific neural cell lines for transplantation into the damaged central nervous system (CNS). Treatment of neuronal cell lines *in vitro* with various growth modulators and antimitotic drugs has been shown to render cells amitotic and to induce the normal neuronal phenotype.[1-3] In this study, several mouse and human neuroblastomas and a rat pheochromocytoma were treated with either 0.5 μg/ml mitomycin C (mito) and 10^{-5} M bromodeoxyuridine (Brdu) or 10 μg/ml prostaglandin E_1 and 500 μg/ml dibutyryl cyclic adenosine monophosphate for examination of their neuronal properties before implantation into the lesioned CNS. The pheochromocytoma cells (PC12 cells) were first treated with 100 ng/ml nerve growth factor (NGF) to induce neuritic sprouting. Maximum neurite outgrowth occurred over 4 days, after which time PC12 cells were exposed to mito-Brdu for an additional 3 days. FIGURE 1a shows the normal appearance of mitotic PC12 cells. Cells are round with only a few anchoring extensions arising from some cells. When PC12 cells are treated as described, neuritic extensions can be quite long and branched. Significantly, removal of all drugs and NGF from the culture does not induce a reversion to the undifferentiated, mitotic state (FIG. 1b), and differentiated cells can be maintained *in vitro* for at least 1 month after drug removal. These cells show typical tyrosine hydroxylase immunocytochemical staining (FIG. 1c) and produce 4.3 μg dopamine/mg protein as measured by high-performance liquid chromatography.

N_2AB-1 cells, a mouse neuroblastoma subclone of Neuro 2a, is an adrenergic line that extends bipolar, unbranched neurites for more than 50 μm when treated with either drug combination for 4 days. These cells become arrested in G_0G_1 of the cell cycle as measured by flow cytometry of propidium iodide-stained DNA[4] and show a significant change in cell surface glycoproteins. Living, control N_2AB-1 cells bound fluorescein-labeled wheat germ agglutinin (FL-WGA) in a discontinuous pattern around the cell body (FIG. 2a) whereas differentiated cells showed an intense green fluorescence outlining both neurites and cell body completely (FIG. 2b). Differentiated

[a] This work was supported by Grants NS19711 (to M. F. D. Notter) and NS15109 (to D. M. Gash) from the U.S. Public Health Service. J. H. Kordower received a fellowship from the John Douglas French Foundation for Alzheimer's disease research.

[b] Address for correspondence: Department of Neurobiology and Anatomy, University of Rochester School of Medicine and Dentistry, 601 Elmwood Avenue, Rochester, New York 14642.

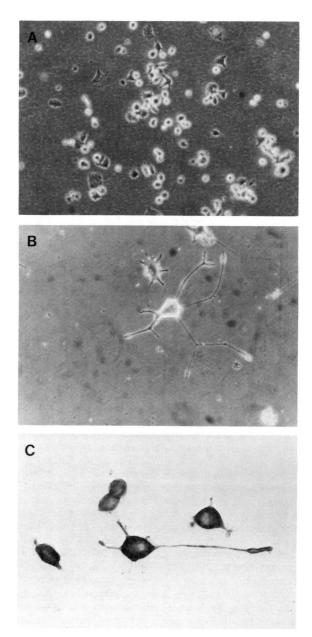

FIGURE 1. (**A**) Control PC12 cells growing *in vitro*. Cells are round and clustered. (**B**) PC12 cells that were in growth medium for 1 month after drug and NGF removal. Cells were first treated with NGF for 4 days and subsequently with mito-Brdu for an additional 3 days. (**C**) PC12 cells stained for tyrosine hydroxylase by immunocytochemistry. Cells were differentiated as described in **B**. Original magnifications: ×320; figure enlarged to 105% of original size.

N$_2$AB-1 cells bound more FL-WGA than mitotic cells as revealed by quantitative fluorescence measurements, indicating that there is more N-acetylglucosamine on the surface of these cells compared to mitotic cells. N$_2$AB-1 cells have also recently been shown to have more specific surface gangliosides after differentiation.[4] When taken together, these ganglioside and glycoprotein alterations indicate that differentiation induced a pattern of cell surface changes similar to that found in developing brain *in vivo.* [5,6]

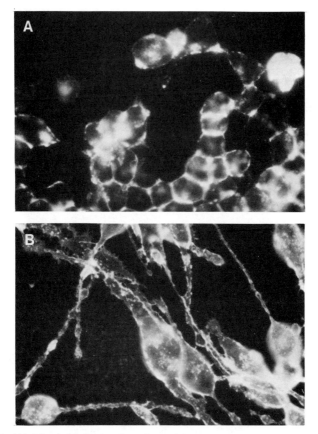

FIGURE 2. (A) Mitotic N$_2$AB-1 cells stained with 50 μg/ml FL-WGA. These living cells show discontinuous fluorescent staining around the cell body. (B) Differentiated N$_2$AB-1 cells show FL-WGA binding along all neurites and the cell body. Original magnifications: $\times$800; figure enlarged to 105% of original size.

Human IMR-32 cells have been examined for optimal differentiation both *in vitro* and *in vivo.* When replated after subculture, drug-treated IMR-32 cells reattach, extend neurites, and remain amitotic. Most importantly, when given the ultimate test of differentiation, drug-treated human IMR-32 cells survive in rat hippocampus in which lesions have been created without reversion to the neoplastic state.[7]

Therefore, these findings suggest that manipulation of neuroblastoma cells *in vitro* can provide us with nondividing cells that have a more appropriate neuronal cell surface which may potentiate recognition and integration of these transplanted cells by the host brain.

REFERENCES

1. PRASAD, K. N. & A. W. HSIE. 1971. Morphological differentiation of mouse neuroblastoma cells induced *in vitro* by dbcAMP. Nature (London) **233**: 141-142.
2. BOTTENSTEIN, J. E. 1981. Differentiated properties of neuronal cell lines. *In* Functionally Differentiated Cell Lines. G. H. Sato, Ed.: 155-184. Alan R. Liss. New York, NY.
3. PRASAD, K. N. & S. KUMAR. 1975. Role of cyclic AMP in differentiation of human neuroblastoma cells in culture. Cancer **36**: 1338-1343.
4. NOTTER, M. F. D. & J. F. LEARY. 1986. Tetanus toxin binding to neuroblastoma cells differentiated by antimitotic agents. Dev. Brain Res. **26**: 59-68.
5. DE SILVA, N. S., J. W. GURD & L. SCHWARTZ. 1979. Developmental alterations of rat brain synaptic membranes: Reaction of glycoproteins with plant lectins. Brain Res. **165**: 283-293.
6. YAVIN, E. & Z. YAVIN. 1979. Ganglioside profiles during neural tissue development. Dev. Neurosci. **2**: 25-37.
7. KORDOWER, J. H., M. F. D. NOTTER, H. H. YEH & D. M. GASH. 1987. An *in vivo* and *in vitro* assessment of differentiated neuroblastoma cells as a source of donor tissue for transplantation. Ann. N.Y. Acad. Sci. This volume.

Human Fetal Adrenal Medulla for Transplantation in Parkinsonian Patients

GIANNI PEZZOLI,[a] VINCENZO SILANI,[a] ENRICO
MOTTI,[b] CLAUDIO FERRANTE,[a] ANTONIO
PIZZUTI,[a] ANDREA FALINI,[a] ANNA ZECCHINELLI,[a]
FRANCO MAROSSERO,[b] AND GUGLIELMO
SCARLATO[a]

[a]Institute of Neurology
and
[b]Institute of Neurosurgery
University of Milan Medical School
Milan 20122, Italy

Adrenal chromaffin tissue, when transplanted into the lateral ventricle or into the striatum of rat, can reduce apomorphine-induced rotational behavior after substantia nigra lesion.[1] This rotational behavior of rats with lesions is a widely recognized experimental model of hemiparkinsonism,[2] and grafted adrenal chromaffin cells are able to reduce the neurological deficit strictly depending on the immaturity of the tissue donor.[3] The age of the cells, a possible limitation to successful transplantation in man, led us to evaluate human fetal adrenal medullary chromaffin cells as a dopaminergic grafting donor in parkinsonian patients. Chromaffin cells were exposed *in vitro* to the striatal human target.

Human fetal adrenal cells were dissociated with collagenase (4 mg/ml) and DNase (0.1 mg/ml) in Medium 199. Partial purification of the medullary cells was obtained by the Percoll gradient method. The enzymatic digestion of fetal adrenal glands and subsequent mechanical dissociation were unable to reduce the medullary cell clusters to single cells. This characteristic of the human medullary tissue allowed cell clusters to be purified simply by filtration on nylon mesh. The use of this reliable method of purification greatly reduced preparation time compared to the Percoll gradient technique. Caudate nucleus explants from biopsies, obtained during neurosurgical thalamotomy carried out in parkinsonian patients (after informed consent), were cultured as previously described.[4] Isolated human adrenal medullary cells were added to caudate explants at day 10 *in vitro* to characterize reciprocal interactions. Adrenal clusters developed long, branching, neurite-like processes and a phase-dark agranular cytoplasm with positive fluorescence to glyoxylic acid conjugation.

The relative levels (on a scale of 100) of three catecholamines in human fetal adrenal glands were determined: the dopamine:norepinephrine:epinephrine ratio was 1.9:82.7:15.4. The high standard deviations of the values may be due to the different gestational ages (between 13-18 weeks). Fetal dopamine was about 2% of the total catecholamine content with a prevalence of norepinephrine (80%); however, epi-

TABLE 1. Catecholamine Content

	Adult Rat Adrenal Glands		Human Fetal Adrenal Glands	
	Content (ng/mg)	Relative Level	Content (ng/mg)	Relative Level
Dopamine	161.30 ± 5.50	2.58	7.50 ± 3.63	1.94
Norepinephrine	1693.80 ± 27.15	27.15	319.28 ± 257.61	82.66
Epinephrine	4381.40 ± 455.80	70.25	59.44 ± 42.04	15.39

NOTE: Catecholamine content is expressed in ng of protein per mg of adrenal gland tissue (mean ± SD). The relative levels are scaled to 100.

nephrine predominates in the adult gland (90%), as the data in the literature show (TABLE 1).

Tissue culture studies have demonstrated the relative ease with which small fragments of human parkinsonian caudate nucleus can be grown *in vitro* and survive as explants for at least 30 days. Around the explants, glial and neuronal cells were observed with long, branching processes. When purified fetal adrenal medullary cells were added to caudate explants, medullary chromaffin cells differentiated with extensive neurite-like formations after 48 hr (FIG. 1). These cells, whether in the soma or along the cellular processes, were positive for catecholamine fluorescence induced by glyoxylic acid conjugation.

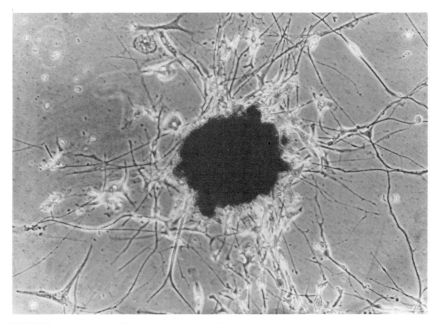

FIGURE 1. Human parkinsonian caudate nucleus co-cultured at day 10 *in vitro* with human fetal adrenal medullary cells. Chromaffin cells, with positive catecholamine fluorescence, after exposure to the human target for 48 hr, differentiated with extensive neurite-like formations compared to controls. Original magnification: ×100; reduced to 77% of original size.

The *in vitro* model of co-culturation with caudate explants has shown that medullary cells are responsive to target signals and extend neurite-like processes within 48 hr.

The neuronal-like behavior of the medullary cells exposed to the target signals suggested there should be further investigation on the synaptic-related events underlying the interaction between donor and host tissues. In particular, we are interested in demonstrating specific synaptic connections and the presence of dopamine receptors on the chromaffin cells after caudate exposure.

REFERENCES

1. FREED, W. J., J. M. MORIHISA, H. E. SPOOR, B. J. HOFFER, L. OLSON, A. SEIGER & R. J. WYATT. 1981. Nature 292: 351-352.
2. UNGERSTEDT, U. 1976. Pharmacol. Ther. B 2: 37-40.
3. FREED, W. J. 1983. Biol. Psychiatry 18: 1205-1267.
4. SILANI, V., G. PEZZOLI, A. FALINI, E. MOTTI, A. PIZZUTI, C. FERRANTE, A. ZECCHINELLI, F. MAROSSERO & G. SCARLATO. J. Neurol. 1986. Submitted for publication.

Fetal Dopamine Neurons Implanted Unilaterally into the Nucleus Accumbens Drive Amphetamine-induced Locomotion and Circling

E. POULSEN, P. BRUNDIN, R. E. STRECKER,
AND A. BJÖRKLUND

Department of Histology
University of Lund
S-223 62 Lund, Sweden

The nucleus accumbens septi (NAS) receives a major innervation from A10 ventral tegmental neurons of the mesolimbic dopaminergic system and is considered to act as an interface between limbic and striatal sensorimotor structures. The NAS has been proposed to act as an "amplifier" in locomotor behaviors because dopamine (DA) injections into the NAS induce locomotion, and because local 6-hydroxydopamine (6-OHDA) lesions of the NAS can block the increases in locomotor or rotational behavior caused by peripheral amphetamine injection. Unilateral lesions of the ascending mesostriatal DA pathway (indicated here as MS lesion) produce rotational asymmetry characterized by ipsilateral rotation (toward side with the lesion) that can be increased by giving amphetamine. Moore and Kelly[1,2] have suggested that in this MS lesion rotational paradigm, depletion of DA in the caudate-putamen is responsible for the postural asymmetry and direction of rotation, whereas levels of DA in the NAS determine the magnitude or speed of rotation. In addition, Moore and Kelly[1,2] proposed that the NAS complex acts only as an "amplifier" in turning behavior, such that an asymmetry of the NAS system alone will not cause turning.

Previous studies have shown that intracerebral DA neuron grafts can survive and compensate for behavioral deficits resulting from prior damage to the host intrinsic DA systems.[3,4] The rotational behavior, seen in rats with unilateral destruction of mesostriatal DA pathway (after administration of amphetamine and apomorphine), can be ameliorated or reversed by transplants of fetal DA neurons to the caudate-putamen.[3,4] Nadaud et al.[5] transplanted DA neurons to a previously 6-OHDA-denervated NAS and observed total restoration of amphetamine-induced locomotor behavior, which, before transplantation, had been abolished by the initial lesion. The purpose of the present study was to investigate the role of the NAS as a modulator of the amplitude of rotational behavior and locomotor activity by implanting fetal DA-rich mesencephalic cells unilaterally into the NAS of rats.

First, all the rats received unilateral 6-OHDA lesions (8 μg in 4 μl) of the ascending mesostriatal DA pathway (MS lesion); these lesions produced ipsilateral rotational asymmetry. Rotation was monitored over 90 min in automated rotometer bowls after an injection of amphetamine (5 mg/kg, i.p.). Only rats performing a mean of > 7 full turns/min were included in the study. Rats were also tested over 60 min for amphetamine-induced locomotor activity (1.5 mg/kg, i.p.) in automated activity boxes, after 60 min habituation. In the second step, all the rats received a local bilateral 6-OHDA lesion of the NAS (8 μl in 3 μl), which, as expected, caused a significant attenuation of the amphetamine-induced locomotor and circling behavior. Finally, a subgroup of the rats received fetal ventral mesencephalic DA grafts, according to the suspension technique,[3] in the NAS, ipsilateral to the original MS lesion. Our hypotheses were as follows: If the NAS acts only as an amplifier in locomotor behavior and does not play a directional role, then DA grafts into the NAS should actually produce an *increase* in ipsilateral rotation (opposite to the direction of rotation produced when a graft is placed in the ipsilateral caudate). Similarly, in open-field locomotion, this graft was predicted to normalize the level of amphetamine-induced locomotor activity, which had been suppressed by the previous MS and NAS lesions. Both of these hypotheses were confirmed by our results.

Six weeks after transplantation, the rats with DA-rich neural grafts showed complete restoration of amphetamine-induced locomotor activity (FIG. 1); furthermore,

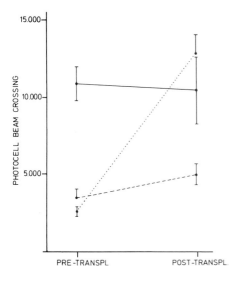

FIGURE 1. Amphetamine-induced locomotor activity measured for "normal rats" (solid line), "MS + NAS-lesioned rats" (dashed line), and "MS + NAS-lesioned + unilateral NAS-transplanted rats" (dotted line) at timepoints corresponding to before and after grafting. Unilateral NAS transplants restored locomotor activity to normal levels (two-way ANOVA, group $\times$ time F(2,18) = 19.5, p < .01).

rotation levels were restored to those seen before the NAS lesion. A change in maximum rotation speed (Δ-peak rotation value: measured as highest rotation score/min when transplanted, or as control, minus highest rotation score with only mesostriatal and NAS lesions) was significantly greater in the transplanted rats (FIG. 2). At subsequent fluorescence histochemical analysis, all the grafted animals had surviving transplants in the NAS area, containing between 64 and 703 DA neurons.

In summary, the results suggest that reinstatement of DA innervation in only one NAS is sufficient to drive amphetamine-induced locomotion in rats. The results also extend previous findings demonstrating a regional functional specificity of the striatal complex in circling behavior, and support an amplification role of the NAS in locomotion. Moreover, the results highlight the previous suggestion that intraparenchymal DA grafts exert their functional effects only within the restricted zone that they actually reinnervate, rather than by a diffuse release of DA over a larger area.

FIGURE 2. Change in peak rotation for individual rats (dots) is plotted showing that after transplantation the graft group had a significantly greater change in peak rotation than the lesion group ($p < .01$, Mann-Whitney U-test, the rat represented by the open dot was excluded from the analysis as it was found to be over five standard deviations from the mean). Change in peak rotation was calculated for each rat as follows: the maximum rotation speed during the 90-min session (turns/min) after transplantation, minus the maximum rotation speed before transplantation (values below zero indicate a decrease in peak rotation rate). The arrow points to the rat with the smallest graft (64 DA neurons compared to group mean of 405).

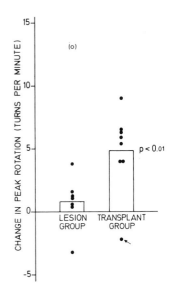

REFERENCES

1. KELLY, P. H. 1975. Unilateral 6-hydroxydopamine lesions of nigrostriatal or mesolimbic dopamine-containing terminals and the drug-induced rotation of rats. Brain Res. **100:** 163-169.

2. MOORE, K. E. & P. H. KELLY. 1978. Biochemical pharmacology of mesolimbic and mesocortical dopaminergic neurons. *In* Psychopharmacology: A Generation of Progress. M. A. Lipton, A. DiMascio & K. F. Killam, Eds.: 221-234. Raven Press. New York, NY.

3. BJÖRKLUND, A., R. H. SCHMIDT & U. STENEVI. 1980. Functional reinnervation of the neostriatum by use of intraparenchymal grafting of dissociated cell suspensions from the substantia nigra. Cell Tissue Res. **212:** 39-45.

4. DUNNETT, S. B., A. BJÖRKLUND, F. H. GAGE & U. STENEVI. 1985. Transplantation of mesencephalic dopamine neurons to the striatum of adult rats *In* Neural Grafting in the Mammalian CNS. A. Björklund & U. Stenevi, Eds.: 451-469. Elsevier. Amsterdam.

5. NADAUD, D., J. P. HERMAN, H. SIMON & M. LE MOAL. 1984. Functional recovery following transplantation of ventral mesencephalic cells in rats subjected to 6-OHDA lesions of the mesolimbic dopaminergic neurons. Brain Res. **304:** 137-141.

Modulation of Systemic Antibody Response and Tolerance by Brain Injury[a]

T. QUÍRICO-SANTOS

Departmento de Patologia
Hospital Universitário Antonio Pedro, UFF
Rio de Janeiro, Brazil

H. VALDIMARSSON

Department of Immunology
National University Hospital
Reykjavík, Iceland

Injections of thymus-dependent antigens into the subarachnoid space (SAS) of mice give rise to higher systemic antibody responses than do injections into other sites commonly used for immunization.[1] Moreover, suppressor-dependent low-zone tolerance is abrogated when antigens are injected into the SAS.[2] Control experiments suggested that the increased antibody responses observed after SAS antigen injections might, in part, be due to the release from brain tissues of substances with adjuvant activity. It was therefore decided to study the effects of brain injury and brain extracts on systemic antibody production and low-zone tolerance. We now report that low-zone tolerance can be broken in animals that suffer brain injury at the time of the antigenic challenge.

Mice immunized by injections of sheep red blood cells into the SAS showed greater antibody production than did mice immunized by intraperitoneal injections. Similar increases were observed in mice immunized by intraperitoneal injections of sheep red blood cells mixed with brain extracts. Extracts from brain-damaged mice had a greater effect than did extracts from normal brains. Serum or cerebrospinal fluid (CSF) collected from brain-damaged mice also significantly ($p < .02$) increased the numbers of spleen PFC compared with serum or CSF obtained from animals that had not received brain injury (data not shown).

Irradiation of the brain caused a marked increase in systemic antibody production in mice that received intraperitoneal injections but not in mice that received injections into the SAS. Irradiation of the trunk alone, which was accomplished by shielding the animal's head, did not give rise to enhanced antibody responses whether the animal received an intraperitoneal injection or received an injection into the SAS (TABLE 1). It should be noted that animals that received an injection into the SAS and that

[a]This work was supported by Grant 1627/79 from the Brazilian Government CAPES and by Grant 400253-83 from the CNPQ.

TABLE 1. Effects of Brain Extracts on Systemic Antibody Production

Route of Immunization	Brain Extracts	$PFC/2 \times 10^7$ SRBC				Antibody Titers	Significance
		Direct	Significance	Indirect	Significance		
SAS	None	2.80 ± 0.06		3.07 ± 0.08		7.54 ± 0.04	$p < .001$
IP	None	2.00 ± 0.10		2.19 ± 0.08		5.16 ± 0.14	
IP	Normal brain	2.22 ± 0.06	$p < .05$	2.48 ± 0.07	$p < .02$	6.45 ± 0.14	$p < .001$
IP	Damaged brain	2.37 ± 0.10	$p < .02$	2.65 ± 0.09	$p < .001$	6.33 ± 0.05	$p < .001$

NOTE: Each of the four groups above included four (CBA × C57BL) F1 adult mice that were primed and challenged by 10-μl injections into the subarachnoid space (SAS) or by 200-μl intraperitoneal (IP) injections. Each injection included 2 × 10⁷ sheep red blood cells (SRBC), which were either alone or mixed with an equal volume of saline brain extracts prepared from normal or brain-damaged mice. A horizontal transcranial brain injury was inflicted with a 27-gauge needle in the right parietal lobe of anesthetized mice 2 days before the latter extract was prepared. The protein content of the extract was adjusted to 1.5 mg/ml. Antibody production was measured 5 days after immunization by microhemagglutination and by direct and indirect spleen plaque assays.[1] Indirect plaques were developed with 1:100 dilutions of a rabbit antimouse immunoglobulin G serum. Each value above was calculated from a mean of values taken from three experiments (direct plaque value: log₂ (mean ± SEM; indirect plaque value: log (mean ± SEM)). The p values refer to intraperitoneally immunized mice that did not receive brain extracts.

received irradiation of the brain showed significantly lower antibody production than did animals in the corresponding control group (TABLE 2).

Low-zone tolerance is known to be mediated by a cyclophosphamide-sensitive suppressor mechanism acting on carrier-specific T-helper cells.[3] Abrogation of low-zone tolerance can be achieved with treatment that selectively impairs suppressor mechanisms or enhances helper cell function.[4,5] Injection of a brain extract or infliction of brain injury by a stab or by irradiation proved as effective as cyclophosphamide in breaking low-zone tolerance (TABLE 3).

We have previously demonstrated that subarachnoid inoculation of thymus-dependent antigens gives rise to more vigorous systemic antibody responses than does immunization in other sites. This does not apply to thymus-independent antigens.[1] Subarachnoid immunization can also abrogate low-zone tolerance mediated by sup-

TABLE 2. Effects of X-irradiation on Systemic Antibody Production

Route of Immunization	X-irradiation	PFC/Spleen			
		Direct	Significance	Indirect	Significance
SAS	None	4.40 ± 0.06		4.92 ± 0.11	
	Trunk only (200 R)	3.86 ± 0.02	$p < .02$	4.51 ± 0.12	$p < .01$
	Head only (200 R)	3.91 ± 0.17	$p < .05$	4.22 ± 0.21	$p < .02$
	Head only (2000 R)	4.10 ± 0.10	$p < .05$	4.28 ± 0.07	$p < .001$
IP	None	3.32 ± 0.04		3.44 ± 0.16	
	Trunk only (200 R)	3.54 ± 0.30	NS	4.01 ± 0.20	NS
	Head only (200 R)	4.39 ± 0.04	$p < .001$	4.69 ± 0.05	$p < .001$
	Head only (2000 R)	4.26 ± 0.17	$p < .001$	4.97 ± 0.11	$p < .001$

NOTE: Each of the groups above included four to six adult (CBA × C57BL) F1 mice that were primed and challenged by 10-μl injections into the subarachnoid space (SAS) or by 200-μl intraperitoneal (IP) injections. Each injection included 2×10^7 sheep red blood cells. The numbers of spleen PFC were determined 5 days after challenge. All mice were anesthetized with sagittal intraperitoneal injections of 10 mg/kg, and the X-irradiation was conducted with a Stabiliplan machine operated at 240 kV constant potential and with 10 mm aluminum filters. The irradiation field was uniform within 3% over 15 cm. A lead box with sides 2-mm thick was used to shield the trunk or the head of each mouse. Irradiation (200 or 2000 R) was performed 24 hr before the antigen challenge. Each value above was calculated from a mean of values taken from three experiments (log (mean ± SEM)). The p values refer to the control groups, which did not receive irradiation.

pressor mechanisms.[2] The experiments presented here show that brain injury is associated with enhanced systemic antibody responses to intraperitoneally inoculated thymus-dependent antigen. Furthermore, animals that are tolerant to haptenated bovine serum albumin respond by vigorous systemic antibody production when the intraperitoneal immunization coincides with brain injury inflicted by a stab or by irradiation.

It should be noted that irradiation of the head alone, or of the body with the head shielded, although markedly increasing the numbers of PFC in intraperitoneally immunized mice, had an opposite effect in animals immunized by injections into the SAS (TABLE 2). This paradoxical effect indicates that the mechanism responsible for the systemic hyperactivity associated with subarachnoid inoculations is sensitive to X-rays and is operating both within and outside the central nervous system.

Hyperreactivity is also observed when antigens are mixed with saline extracts of brain tissues. Brain homogenates have been shown to contain mitogenic activity,[6] and an interleukin-1-like substance has been detected in culture supernatants from astrocytes.[7] It is therefore postulated that the hyperimmune phenomena associated with injections of antigens into the SAS are at least in part due to adjuvant activity released from injured brain tissue. This might in turn give rise to vigorous induction of systemic T-helper cell activity relative to that of the suppressor mechanism. It is conceivable that brain injury might sometimes initiate or contribute to autoimmune responses against self-antigens that are tolerated with suppressor-dependent mechanisms.

TABLE 3. Effect of Brain Injury or Brain Extract on Systemic Low-zone Tolerance

Groups	BSA Reactivity	Treatment	Indirect (TNP-PCF/10^7)	Significance
1	Primed	Cyclophosphamide	3.31 ± 0.10	
2	Tolerant	None	2.07 ± 0.13	$p < .001$
3	Tolerant	Cyclophosphamide	3.12 ± 0.15	$p < .001$
4	Tolerant	Transcranial stab	2.68 ± 0.16	$p < .02$
5	Tolerant	Head irradiation (400 R)	3.10 ± 0.10	$p < .001$
6	Tolerant	Brain extract	3.25 ± 0.14	$p < .001$

NOTE: Each of the groups above included five mice. Low-zone tolerance was induced in each mouse by a pretreatment in which 2.5 mg of hydrocortisone acetate was injected intraperitoneally. This injection was followed by daily intraperitoneal injections of 10 μg of deaggregated bovine serum albumin (BSA).[3] These injections continued up to day 8. On day 8, groups 1 and 3 received 10 mg of cyclophosphamide (intraperitoneally), and groups 4 and 5 received brain injury (by a stab or by irradiation). The controls (group 1) received 2.5 mg of hydrocortisone acetate on day 0 and 100 μg of BSA on day 1, followed by saline on days 2 through 7. On day 10, all groups were challenged with an intraperitoneal injection of 1 mg of TNP-BSA. The mice in group 6 were immunized with TNP-BSA mixed with brain extracts. Anti-TNP spleen PFC responses were determined in all groups 6 days after the TNP-BSA challenge. All p values refer to group 2.

REFERENCES

1. QUÍRICO-SANTOS, T. & H. VALDIMARSSON. 1982. J. Neuroimmunol. 2: 215-222.
2. QUÍRICO-SANTOS, T. & H. VALDIMARSSON. 1984. Cell. Immunol. 83: 442-446.
3. BRÜNER, K. & E. KÖLSCH. 1981. Cell. Immunol. 62: 436-447.
4. WEIGLE, W. D. 1973. Adv. Immunol. 16: 61-122.
5. SCIBIENSKI, R. J. 1981. Cell. Immunol. 58: 293-301.
6. MIRSKY, R. 1980. Trends Neurosci. 3(8): 190-192.
7. FONTANA, A., H. HENGARTNER, N. TRIBOLET & E. WEBER. 1984. J. Immunol. 132(4): 1837-1844.

Multiple Transplants of Fetal Striatal Tissue in the Kainic Acid Model of Huntington's Disease

Behavioral Recovery May Not Be Related to Acetylcholinesterase[a]

PAUL R. SANBERG,[b] MARK A. HENAULT,
STARR H. HAGENMEYER-HOUSER,
MAGDA GIORDANO,
AND KRISTANNE H. RUSSELL

Behavioral Neuroscience Laboratory
Department of Psychology
Ohio University
Athens, Ohio 45701

Earlier research has demonstrated that rats which received injections of kainic acid (KA) into the striatum displayed many of the anatomical, biochemical, and behavioral abnormalities seen in patients with Huntington's disease (HD).[1,2] Subsequently, it was found that fetal transplants could reverse some of the behavioral deficits caused by KA-induced[3,4] or ibotenic acid-induced[5] lesions of striatal neurons. Deckel *et al.*[3] indicated that fetal transplants in female rats with KA lesions could actually partially reverse some of the profound locomotor hyperactivity. They also demonstrated that the amount of recovery of function was correlated with the number of transplanted neurons surviving in the striatum.[3] In that study, only a small amount of fetal tissue was injected into one area of the striatum in female rats. The present study observed the effects of larger transplants in male rats on spontaneous and drug-induced locomotor deficits and acetylcholinesterase (AChE) staining.

Four weeks after the KA lesion (2 nmole/0.8 μl saline/side), all experimental rats received four 1-μl injections of fetal day 17 striatal ridge tissue along the ventral-dorsal plane into each striatum. Appropriate sham animals were used for the lesion and transplant control conditions. Three, 6, and 9 weeks after transplantation, the rats were tested in Digiscan monitors (Omnitech Electronics) for their locomotor behavior during the nighttime at peak activity periods, under spontaneous and am-

[a] This work was supported by the Hereditary Disease Foundation, the Huntington's Disease Society of America, Grant MH40127 from the National Institutes of Health, the Pratt Family and Friends, and Omnitech Electronics, Inc.

[b] Present address: Laboratory of Behavioral Neuroscience, Department of Psychiatry, University of Cincinnati College of Medicine, Cincinnati, Ohio 45267-0559.

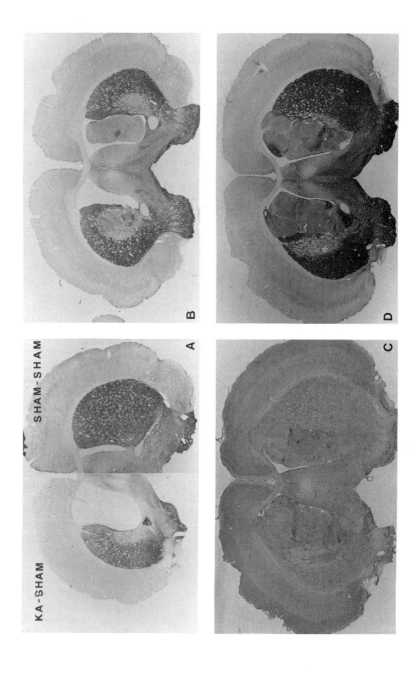

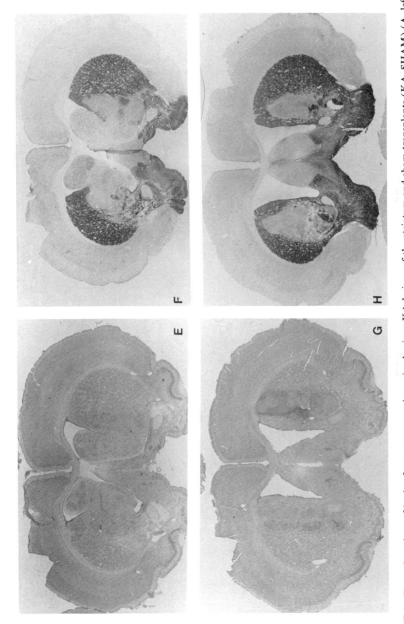

FIGURE 1. Coronal sections of brains from representative animals given KA lesions of the striatum and sham transplants (KA-SHAM) (A, left side) or KA lesions followed by day 17 fetal striatal transplants (B-H). SHAM-SHAM represents a control animal (A, right side). Sections **A**, **B**, **D**, **F**, and **H** are stained for AChE. Sections **C**, **E**, and **G** are cresyl violet-stained sections of the same brains as sections **D**, **F**, and **H**, respectively.

TABLE 1. Effect of Day 17 Fetal Striatal Transplants on Various Aspects of Locomotion in Rats with KA-induced Striatal Lesions

Locomotor Variables	Spontaneous Activity			Amphetamine Activity		
	Sham-Sham	KA-Sham	KA-Transplant	Sham-Sham	KA-Sham	KA-Transplant
HA	4411.5 ± 408.7	11 093 ± 874.7	4828.3 ± 568.0[a]	16 200 ± 2223	35 840 ± 3268	14 850 ± 3691[a]
VA	138.1 ± 18.8	279.3 ± 50.7	209.8 ± 30.3	381.9 ± 98.7	853.7 ± 227.3	275.7 ± 123.6[a]
TD	1200.0 ± 129.2	3486 ± 330	1387.0 ± 256.9[a]	5279.0 ± 820.8	12 170 ± 1227	4671 ± 1940[a]
MT	55.4 ± 45.9	1240.5 ± 90.3	632.7 ± 113.4[a]	1853.0 ± 174.4	2702.0 ± 23.9	1686 ± 506
AS	2.11 ± 0.06	2.84 ± 0.28	2.12 ± 0.11	2.70 ± .23	4.5 ± 0.4	2.60 ± .39[a]
RT	3051 ± 45	2369.0 ± 89.6	2974.4 ± 112.7[a]	1760.0 ± 174.7	906.7 ± 24.5	1925.0 ± 505.6
NM	347.8 ± 22.6	478.2 ± 39.0	363.7 ± 43.5	696.6 ± 40.1	488.7 ± 33.8	584.3 ± 37.5
AD	3.4 ± 0.22	7.67 ± 1.28	3.74 ± 0.48[a]	8.0 ± 1.8	25.4 ± 4.0	7.7 ± 2.9
VT	99.6 ± 15.4	110.8 ± 9.1	106.4 ± 18.9	124.5 ± 37.4	324.0 ± 72.1	84.0 ± 39.4[a]
VM	25.1 ± 3.8	47.30 ± 5.74	29.4 ± 3.9	74.1 ± 17.6	220.0 ± 19.0	40.3 ± 14.8[a]
ST	278.1 ± 19.6	502.8 ± 62.4	219.0 ± 43.3[a]	462.9 ± 53.3	549.7 ± 41.9	509.0 ± 42.2
NS	221.9 ± 16.7	367.8 ± 36.1	193.4 ± 25.9[a]	413.9 ± 17.9	510.3 ± 15.7	419.7 ± 49.1
CR	49.2 ± 5.3	135.00 ± 8.05	55.0 ± 11.9[a]	212.0 ± 29.0	382.0 ± 18.2	159.7 ± 76.9[a]
AR	50.6 ± 5.4	117.0 ± 8.0	50.0 ± 10.4[a]	216.0 ± 29.2	399.7 ± 16.5	161.0 ± 70.3[a]

NOTE: Each value is a mean ± SEM. Values obtained 9 weeks after transplantation are shown for 16 control transplant (sham-sham) rats, 6 KA lesion control transplant (KA-sham) rats, and 7 KA lesion fetal striatal transplant (KA-transplant) rats. Spontaneous activity represents activity testing without drug from 10:00 P.M. to 11:00 P.M. Amphetamine activity represents activity testing from 11:00 P.M. to 12:00 P.M. under 1 mg/kg d-amphetamine sulfate. HA: horizontal activity; VA: vertical activity; TD: total distance traveled (inches); MT: movement time (sec); AS: average speed (inches/sec); RT: rest time (sec); NM: number of movements; AD: average distance; VT: vertical time (sec); VM: vertical movements; ST: stereotypy time (sec); NS: number of stereotypy movements; CR: clockwise revolutions; AR: counterclockwise revolutions. See reference 8 for further details.
[a] Significantly different from KA-sham ($p < .05$).

phetamine-induced conditions. At the conclusion of the experiment, the rat brains were histologically analyzed by staining alternate coronal section with cresyl violet and AChE techniques, respectively.[5]

The hyperactivity exhibited on many aspects of ambulatory, stereotypical, and rotational behaviors by the striatal transplant group before transplantation decreased gradually after transplantation in seven animals until they reached control levels 9 weeks later (TABLE 1). Furthermore, when tested with amphetamine (1.0 mg/kg), the exaggerated locomotor response exhibited by the sham transplant KA lesion group was not present in the striatal transplant group 9 weeks after transplantation (TABLE 1). Upon histological examination, the striatal transplants in recovered animals had reconstructed much of the gross morphology of the striatum in which lesions had been created. No longer was ventricular expansion present, either. However, AChE was much less apparent within the transplanted tissue than in the host brain (FIG. 1). Although AChE did not correlate with behavioral recovery, it appeared that the location and integration of the transplant within the brain were critical factors. Behavioral recovery was diminished if 1) the transplant did not integrate within the area of the striatum in which a lesion had been created (that is, remained primarily in the ventricles) or 2) the transplant encroached on normal extrastriatal tissue.

The histological results indicated that although cell bodies were distributed abundantly throughout the nontrypsinized transplanted material, few stained for AChE. Lehmann and Fibiger[7] reported that only large aspiny neurons contained within the normal striatum stain intensely for AChE. Therefore, the presence of these cells may not be a necessary or sufficient condition for the mediation of transplant-induced recovery of function.

REFERENCES

1. SANBERG, P. R. & J. T. COYLE. 1984. CRC Crit. Rev. Clin. Neurobiol. **1:** 1-44.
2. SANBERG, P. R. & G. A. JOHNSTON. 1981. Med. J. Aust. **2:** 460-466.
3. DECKEL, A. W., R. G. ROBINSON, J. T. COYLE & P. R. SANBERG. 1983. Eur. J. Pharmacol. **93:** 287-288.
4. DECKEL, A. W., T. H. MORAN, J. T. COYLE, P. R. SANBERG & R. G. ROBINSON. 1986. Brain Res. **365:** 249-258.
5. ISACSON, O., P. BRUNDIN, P. A. T. KELLY, F. H. GAGE & A. BJÖRKLUND. 1984. Nature **311:** 458-460.
6. PAXINOS, G. & C. WATSON. 1984. The Rat Brain in Stereotaxic Coordinates. Academic Press. Sydney.
7. LEHMANN, J. & H. C. FIBIGER. 1979. Life Sci. **25:** 1939-1947.
8. SANBERG, P. R., S. H. HAGENMEYER & M. A. HENAULT. 1985. Neurobehav. Toxicol. Teratol. **7:** 87-94.

Neonatally Transplanted Brain Tissue Protects the Adult Rat from a Lesion-induced Syndrome of Adipsia, Aphagia, and Akinesia

SAUL S. SCHWARZ

Department of Neurosurgery
Naval Hospital
Bethesda, Maryland 20814

WILLIAM J. FREED

Preclinical Neurosciences Section
Neuropsychiatry Branch
National Institute of Mental Health
Saint Elizabeth's Hospital
Washington, DC 20032

In previous transplantation experiments, animals have been grafted after lesion-induced behavioral abnormalities have first been established, so that the extent of denervation can be first measured and the restorative properties of the transplant then derived.[1-2] In the present study, transplantation was performed in intact neonatal rats to allow incorporation of the grafted fetal substantia nigra (SN) into the immature host brain.[3] After maturation, bilateral nigrostriatal lesions were made to uncover the functional contribution of the transplant tissue. This design also provided an opportunity to study the interaction between embryonic donor tissue and neonatal recipient brain when allowed to mature together.

Twenty litters of 1-day-old Sprague-Dawley rat pups received bilateral intraventricular grafts of embryonic SN or sciatic nerve (controls). After 3-4 months, adult male and female rates (300-550 g) that were to receive bilateral lesions of the SN were selected randomly. Lesions were made by stereotactic infusion of 6-hydroxydopamine, a selective catecholamine neurotoxin. In a short-term group, each animal's weight was measured daily, as was its food and water consumption, for 7 days after the operation, and behavioral deficits were noted. Six days after the operation, each animal's spontaneous locomotor activity was measured over 60 min by infrared-activated photocells; animals were sacrificed 7 days after the operation for histochemical analysis. A long-term group was monitored daily or weight change, food and water consumption, and behavioral deficits over a 30-day period, and, at the end of this trial, data were included from all animals tested. Only survivors were sacrificed for fluorescence histochemistry.

Within the short-term group ($N = 32$), 11 SN-transplanted animals and 7 controls were completely aphagic and adipsic for a 7-day period of observation, whereas 14 other SN-transplanted animals (56%) and no controls resumed feeding and drinking ($p < .01$, Fisher's exact test). Mean total food and water intake for SN-transplanted animals was 38.7 ± 10.4 g and 73.8 ± 15.7 ml compared with 1.1 ± 0.5 g and 7.9 ± 2.9 ml for controls ($p < .02$, two-tailed Mann-Whitney U test). Spontaneous locomotor activity in SN-transplanted animals was 3.7 times that of controls ($p < .05$, two-tailed Mann-Whitney U test). Control animals and unrecovered SN-transplanted animals were rigid within 2 days after the lesion, with progressive dorsal spinal curvature, splayed limbs, profound somatosensory inattention, and minimal spontaneous movement. Within the long-term group, 6 of 14 SN-transplanted animals (43%) and 1 of 11 control animals (9%) survived the 30-day trial ($p < .073$, Fisher's exact test). Only 1 of 14 SN-transplanted animals (7%) as compared to 7 of 11 control animals (64%) were completely aphagic during this trial ($p < .005$, Fisher's exact test), and only 1 of 14 SN-transplanted animals (7%) as compared to 9 of 11 control animals (82%) were completed adipsic during this trial ($p < .0001$, Fisher's exact test). Mean 30-day total water and food intake for SN-transplanted animals was 409 ± 123 ml and 259 ± 82.6 g compared to 65.7 ± 53.7 ml and 63.6 ± 61.0 g for control animals ($p < .05$ and $p < .01$, respectively, two-tailed Mann-Whitney U tests).

In both the short-term and long-term groups, recovered SN-transplanted animals had bilateral intraventricular grafts with fiber ingrowth into host striatum and septal nuclei, and varying amounts of catecholamines by fluorescence histochemistry. All unrecovered animals demonstrated extensive striatal dopaminergic depletion, whereas striatal fluorescence was present unilaterally or bilaterally in recovered animals, predominantly in the region surrounding the graft (medial striatum and septal nucleus).

These experiments demonstrate that fetal SN can become well integrated in the host brain when transplanted during the neonatal period, and provide an alternate pathway that permits escape from subsequent nigrostriatal lesions. Further neonatal transplantation experiments may reveal a competitive effect of grafted SN on host SN during this crucial period of nigrostriatal synaptogenesis, and thus offer another means of studying progressive and regressive events in the developing nervous system.

REFERENCES

1. PERLOW, M. J., W. J. FREED, B. J. HOFFER, A. SEIGER, L. OLSON & R. J. WYATT. 1979. Science **204:** 643-647.
2. FREED, W. J., M. J. PERLOW, F. KAROUM, A. SEIGER, L. OLSON, B. J. HOFFER & R. J. WYATT. 1980. Ann. Neurol. **8:** 510-519.
3. SCHWARZ, S. S. & W. J. FREED. 1987. Exp. Brain Res. **65:** 449-454.

Catecholamine Fibers Form Synaptic Contacts with Hypothalamic Neurons Transplanted Adjacent to the Medial Forebrain Bundle in Rats

W. F. SILVERMAN, P. F. ARAVICH, T. J. COLLIER,
J. A. OLSCHOWKA, AND J. R. SLADEK, JR.

Department of Neurobiology and Anatomy
University of Rochester School of Medicine and Dentistry
Rochester, New York 14642

The establishment of connectivity between a host brain and a neural graft may be critical to the integration and ultimately the function of the transplanted tissue. It has been well established that neural grafts both receive afferent input from and project efferent fibers to the host.[1-3] Few studies,[4,5] however, have examined the issue of connectivity at the ultrastructural level to determine whether transplanted neurons, in fact, receive a relevant synaptic input from host fibers. We have addressed this problem using ultrastructural immunocytochemistry for tyrosine hydroxylase (TH) applied to fetal rat hypothalamic grafts that were transplanted adjacent to the medial forebrain bundle (MFB) of adult hosts. The grafted tissue, which contained the supraoptic and paraventricular nuclei as well as other portions of the medial basal hypothalamus, is normally richly innervated by noradrenergic fibers from the MFB.

Hypothalamic tissue was dissected from fetal Long-Evans rats (day 17 gestation), and implanted stereotaxically into the brains of young adult hosts according to the previously described protocol used in our laboratory.[6] Following 6-, 12-, and 20-week survival periods, the host animals were anesthetized with sodium phenobarbitol and perfused with 5% acrolein, 4% paraformaldehyde. Sample vibratome sections (50 μm thick) were stained for Nissl substance to locate the grafted tissue. Remaining sections were then processed for preembedded immunocytochemistry and electron microscopy. In addition to those sections stained for TH, some sections were stained for vasopressin-associated neurophysin (NPII) to assess the viability of transplanted vasopressin neurons.

Consonant with previous reports,[3] most of the grafts appeared healthy and increasingly well integrated with the host brain the longer the survival time. Transplants exhibited striking growth in the host environment, and, within 20 weeks, were several times the size of the original implants. At the light level, NPII-positive neurons and fibers were observed in the grafts as were TH-positive fibers. A dense plexus of TH fibers resembling that found in the supraoptic or paraventricular nuclei was observed in a circumscribed region of one 20-week graft (FIG. 1A). Cell bodies staining for TH, however, were rarely found in the transplants. Ultrastructurally, immunochem-

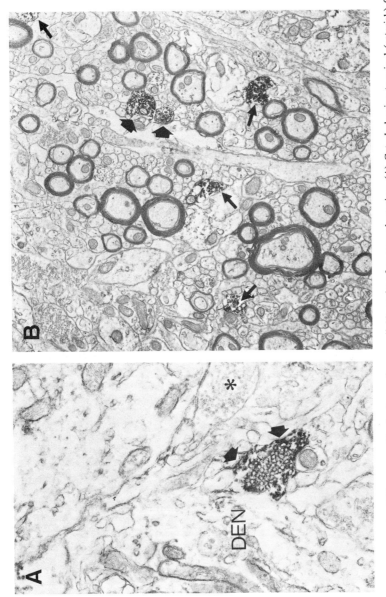

FIGURE 1. Immunoreactive TH axon profiles in the graft neuropil 12 weeks after transplantation. (**A**) Catecholamine terminal (asterisk) forming a synaptic contact (arrows) with a proximal dendrite (DEN) of a large neuron in the graft. Synaptic vesicles are clearly visible in the labeled terminal. (**B**) A number of labeled fibers are evident (arrows); some (wide arrows) appear to form synaptic contact with a segment of transversally sectioned dendrite. Original magnifications for **A** and **B**: ×28 000 and ×12 500, respectively; figure reduced to 63% of original size.

ically stained terminals were readily distinguished from nonlabeled fibers by their peroxidase reaction product (FIGS. 1 & 2). Six-week subjects exhibited a sparse distribution of labeled terminals in the grafts, and only an occasional contact with a neuron or dendrite. In contrast, 12- and 20-week transplants contained a wealth of TH-positive terminals, many of which appeared to make synaptic contact with dendrites and cell bodies in the graft.

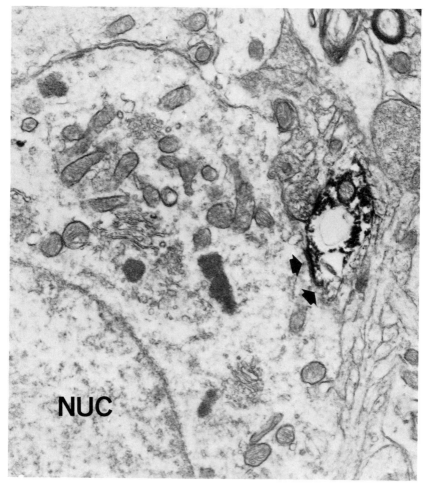

FIGURE 2. Catecholamine terminal contacting a large magnocellular-like neuron in a 20-week transplant. Arrows indicate likely areas of synaptic contact. NUC: nucleus. Original magnification: ×22 000; reduced to 64% of original size.

This investigation suggests that host catecholamine fibers form synaptic contacts with transplanted hypothalamic neurons in the rat. It is likely that these fibers originate in ascending noradrenergic fiber systems, which were in close proximity to the transplanted tissue. The possibility that the fibers arise from catecholamine neurons intrinsic to the grafts is remote because the number of such cells was quite small compared to the number of catecholamine fibers observed. Having established that catecholamine terminals synapse within the transplant, subsequent studies will examine the specificity of the innervation in relation to the afferent terminal and its transplanted target cell. Of particular interest is the degree to which vasopressin neurosecretory neurons, which normally receive a profuse noradrenergic innervation via the MFB, are reinnervated when transplanted. Pre- and postembedding immunolabeling for vasopressin and dopamine β-hydroxylase, an enzyme marker for norepinephrine, is currently underway in our laboratory on the sections previously stained for TH to address these questions.

REFERENCES

1. LUND, R. D. & S. D. HAUSCHKA. 1976. Science **193:** 582-584.
2. JAEGER, C. B. & R. D. LUND. 1980. J. Comp. Neurol. **194:** 571-597.
3. OBLINGER, M. M. & G. D. DAS. 1982. Brain Res. **249:** 31-49.
4. HARVEY, A. R., G. T. GOLDEN & R. D. LUND. 1982. Exp. Brain Res. **47:** 437-445.
5. NISHINO, H., O. TEKATOSHI, J. TAKAHASHI, M. KIMURA, S. HOSAKA, H. YAMASAKI, H. HATANAKA & M. TOHYAMA. 1986. Neurosci. Lett. **64:** 13-16.
6. GASH, D. M. & J. R. SLADEK, JR. 1980. Peptides **1:** 11-14.

The Potential for Causing Slow, Progressive Diseases in Experiments Involving Cell and Tissue Transplants in Brain

ROULETTE W. SMITH

Institute for Postgraduate Interdisciplinary Studies
Palo Alto, California 94306-0846

The prospect of transplanting cells and tissue in brain reveals exciting new approaches for treating certain diseases of brain. Nevertheless, these procedures may place donors and recipients of transplants at risk for slow, progressive diseases. This report presents novel perspectives on transmissible diseases of brain with long incubation periods. These perspectives underscore the need for extraordinary vigilance, skillful surgical technique, and rigorous experimental controls.

Perhaps the best known and least desirable risks for transmissible diseases arising from neurosurgery are risks of Creutzfeldt-Jakob disease (CJD) and other transmissible dementias. Putative agents causing many of these diseases are known to be extraordinarily resistent to degradation. Those agents also elude immune detection by unknown mechanisms, even though the spleen often is laden with infectious particles.[1] Of special significance is the potential risk to neurosurgeons and other care-givers—in addition to the usual risks of these diseases developing in donors and recipients of transplants and in other neurosurgical patients.

Recent recovery from brain of lymphadenopathy viruses (HIV/LAV/HTLV-III)[2] associated with the acquired immune deficiency syndrome (AIDS) poses still further challenges. Because so little is known about the natural repositories of these agents or their mechanisms of action, there also may be significant risks of their transmission when transplanting cells or tissue into brain. Moreover, as these viruses may be transmitted through sexual activity, there may be significant risks to families if transmission of these viruses is associated with tissue used in transplants. Thus, unlike the transmission of CJD, it is conceivable that AIDS may develop secondarily in family members—though with disease developing over very long periods if the profoundness of disease is dose dependent, as is the case in infections by most other "slow viruses."

Perhaps the most unusual risk of slow, progressive diseases developing in donors, recipients, and care-givers (where cells and tissue are transplanted in brain) involves novel mechanisms of autotoxicity and autovirulence.[3] While attempting to disambiguate causation from consequence in AIDS, I discovered[3] that physiochemical properties of unconventional "slow viruses" are remarkably concordant with physiochemical properties of selected small ribonucleoprotein particles (snp-RNPs)—including the putative agent of scrapie (see TABLE 1 in reference 3). Recent demonstration that several small nonprotein-encoding RNAs associated with Epstein-Barr virus (EBV) and several adenoviruses can form complexes mimicking host snpRNPs[4] now raises the extraordinary possibility that classes of autoantigens (that is, autotoxins; see FIG. 1) and particles mimicking autoantigens (that is, autovirions; see FIG. 2) may also cause debilitating transmissible diseases of the central nervous system (CNS). Most important, because there may be multiple copies of those particles in cells and because of their potential toxicity to other cells, release of autotoxins or autovirions (by surgical trauma, viral infection, transplant rejection, drug toxicity, or any other means) could lead to a slow, dose-dependent process of "biological fission" mimicking viral replication. Moreover, those particles have the potential for eluding immune detection and clearance, in part, because of their likeness to "self" and, in part, because of the general absence of immune cells in brain. In short, there are a variety of reasons why autotoxins and autovirions may confuse or defy conventional virological methods (including the Henle-Koch postulates and end-point titration

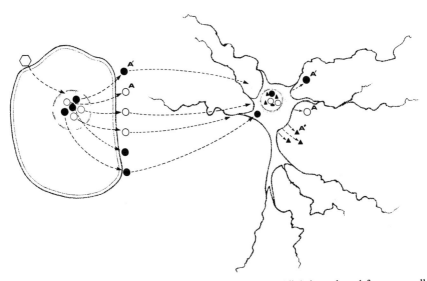

FIGURE 1. Autotoxicity: Diagram of "autotoxins" (A and A') being released from one cell type—by some lytic, genetic, or other neurophysiological event—causing a toxic reaction in some neuron in brain. The diagram shows the uptake and toxicity of A' causing the release of multiple copies of A" (and sometimes A or A').

procedures) while also mimicking autoimmune diseases. A recent report[5] of primary Sjögren's syndrome mimicking multiple sclerosis tends to support this view.
    In an attempt to assess and anticipate diseases caused by autotoxins and autovirions, I discovered that many of those diseases may represent diseases of RNA processing (FIG. 3). Evidence supporting this claim stems from an analysis of snpRNPs and their putative functions. Small RNAs associated with some snpRNPs (for example, the La particle) appear to play a role in the process of translation. These include tRNA, EBER1 and EBER2 (associated with EBV), and VAI and VAII (associated with some adenoviruses). Translational and posttranslational aberrations (FIG. 4B) could produce subtle structural or functional changes or both leading to altered biological activity (for example, psychoses, neuromuscular diseases, tumors). Small RNAs associated with other snpRNPs (for example, the Sm particle) appear to be

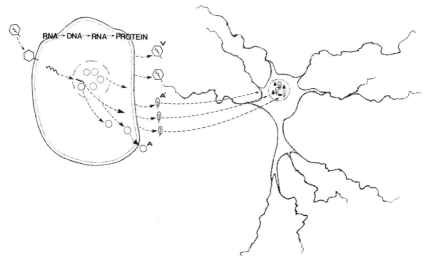

FIGURE 2. Autovirulence: Diagram of viral infection leading to the assembly and release of "autovirions" from one cell type with subsequent uptake in some neuron. Autovirions may be composed of host protein and viral-encoded nucleic acid. V: virus; A: autotoxin; A': autovirion.

associated with splicing of introns from primary RNA transcripts. Aberrations in splicing could produce gross structural aberrations (for example, subacute spongiform change and amyloid fibrils) as depicted in FIGURE 4C.

It should be apparent that retroviruses may be associated with transcriptional aberrations because of the nonspecific integration of their proviral DNA into host DNA. It also should be apparent that the association of La with two small RNAs encoded by EBV presents special challenges because of the ubiquity of EBV and

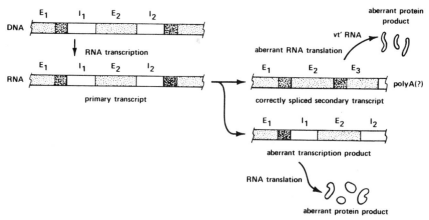

FIGURE 3. Some possible mechanisms of diseases of RNA processing. Note that transcriptional aberrations may cause gross structural change, whereas translational aberrations generally cause subtle structural or functional aberrations or both. E: exons; I: introns; vt' RNA: viral transfer-like RNA (for example, EBER1 and EBER2 encoded by Epstein-Barr virus).

because its cellular repositories remain unknown. Whether this is the basis of EBV, despite its ubiquity, being associated with diverse diseases (infectious mononucleosis, Burkitt's lymphoma, nasopharyngeal carcinoma, Kaposi's sarcoma, CNS lymphomas [especially in AIDS], posttransplant non-Hodgkin's lymphomas, universal reactor syndromes, chronic fatigue syndrome, and perhaps a variety of other unspecified diseases) is now a matter for further investigation. Nevertheless, the important lesson for investigators contemplating transplanting cells and tissue into brain is one of caution, use of surgical techniques that minimize needless surgical trauma, extraordinary vigilance for slow diseases requiring long-term follow-up, and rigorous experimental procedures and controls. The recent discovery[6] of CJD in youngsters receiving growth hormone preparations should provide a sobering example. Although I am not

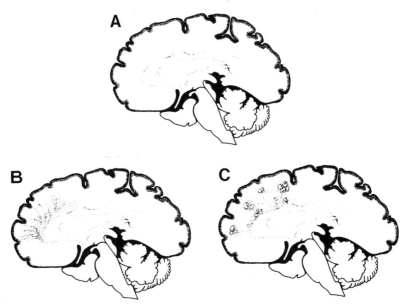

FIGURE 4. Diagram showing the effects of mRNA aberrations on the brain. (**A**) Normal brain. (**B**) Psychophysiological change representing translational aberrations. (**C**) Spongy change representing transcriptional aberrations.

aware of whether its cause and sources have been determined, the mere fact that the growth hormone preparations were made from tissue taken from accident victims[6] serves to underscore possibilities that the infectious particles of CJD, like scrapie, may be spontaneously induced.[3,7] This also could be the basis of unusual proteinaceous particles in scrapie preparations being concordant with host gene products.[3,8]

CONCLUSIONS AND RECOMMENDATIONS

I have attempted to highlight some of the concerns that must be considered if studies of transplants of cells and tissue in brain are to succeed. Even when focusing on transmissible slow, progressive diseases, it is apparent that the spectrum of those diseases could be quite broad. Subtle sequelae may involve diffuse disease processes, slow-onset insidious neuromuscular diseases, dementias and other behavioral changes, immune deficiencies and autoimmune sequelae, and general aberrations of RNA processing causing gross structural lesions or subtle pathophysiological events or both. The challenge does not rest there. Vigilance in slowly developing progressive events may be inherently less reliable in activities involving long periods of time.[9] Equally important, novel biological processes (for example, autotoxicity, autovirulence, and biological fission) and enigmatic brain mechanisms (for example, molecular mechanisms of memory, especially those involving rearrangements in genes[3]) may further complicate matters. These findings argue for 1) the development of techniques for early and rapid detection of changes in brain and behavior associated with slow infections[10]; 2) a need for reliable technologies capable of distinguishing different types of aberrations in RNA processing; 3) having a high index of suspicion for slow infectious diseases and dose-dependent relationships with incubation periods; 4) avoiding needless surgical trauma to minimize risks of transmitting slow diseases to donors, recipients, and care-givers; 5) recognizing that ubiquitous entities may cause diverse and uncommon diseases; 6) recognizing the potential for autoimmune and other sequelae; 7) regulating the rate of the slowness of infections for diagnostic or therapeutic benefits (for example, using thyroxine to shorten incubation periods or using methionazole, HPA 23, and AZT to prolong incubation periods).

REFERENCES

1. OUTRAM, G. W. 1976. *In* Slow Virus Diseases in Animal and Man. R. H. Kimberlin, Ed.: 325-357. Elsevier/North-Holland. New York, NY.
2. LEVY, J. A. *et al.* 1985. Ann. Intern. Med. **103:** 694-699.
3. SMITH, R. W. 1984. Ann. N.Y. Acad. Sci. **437:** 576-607.
4. LERNER, M. R. *et al.* 1981. Proc. Natl. Acad. Sci. USA **78:** 805-809.
5. ALEXANDER, E. L. *et al.* 1986. Ann. Intern. Med. **104:** 323-330.
6. NORMAN, C. 1985. Science **228:** 1176-1177.
7. PATTISON, I. H. 1982. Nature **293:** 200.
8. OESCH, B. *et al.* 1985. Cell **40:** 735-746.
9. WARM, J. S., ED. 1984. Sustained Attention in Human Performance. John Wiley & Sons. New York, N.Y.
10. BROWN, P. *et al.* 1986. New Engl. J . Med. **314:** 547-551.

Successful Grafting of Embryonic Rat Retinal Tissue into the Lesion Site of an Adult Host Retina[a]

JAMES E. TURNER, JERRY R. BLAIR, AND
THOMAS E. CHAPPEL

Department of Anatomy
Bowman Gray School of Medicine
Wake Forest University
Winston-Salem, North Carolina 27103

The grafting of immature neuronal tissue into adult central nervous system in which a lesion has been created may provide a powerful tool for repair and replacement of intrinsic neuronal circuitry initiated by trauma or disease. It has been shown that fetal rat retinal tissue will survive, differentiate, and establish target-specific connections when grafted into the brain of an adult host. We report the successful grafting of fetal and neonatal rat retina into an adult retinal lesion site. A penetrating lesion is made through the sclera, choroid, and retina on the superior surface of the eye of the host (a 225-250 g male Sprague-Dawley rat) and closed with 10 sutures. The lesion site is either allowed to stabilize for 1-8 weeks or immediately receives a retinal graft. Retinas are removed from 14-20-day-old fetuses or 1-10-day-old neonate donors and placed in ice-cold phosphate-buffered saline. Pieces of donor retina are drawn into a 1-µl Hamilton syringe using a 26-gauge needle. The needle is inserted into the lateral edge of the fresh or stabilized lesion and the disrupted retinal tissue injected into the lesion site. Host animals are sacrificed and the eyes processed for light and electron microscopic analysis at 1, 2, and 4 weeks after grafting.

Light microscopic analysis of sections through grafted tissue within the lesion site revealed that the neonatal tissue not only survived at all times examined, but also continued its organotypic development reminiscent of intact littermates. Examination of 4-week-old grafts revealed a clear optic fiber; ganglion cell, inner plexiform, and inner nuclear layers; initiation of outer plexiform layers; and developing receptor neurons. In addition, the plexiform regions of the graft merged with those of the host. Transmission electron microscopic observations of the graft revealed cells in the ganglion cell, inner nuclear, and photoreceptor layers with ultrastructural characteristics very similar to those reported for the *in vivo* and *in vitro* developing rat retina. In addition, our ultrastructural studies revealed the development of normal synaptic relationships within the plexiform layers of the grafts. One of the most curious aspects of this analysis was the absence of a continuous, recognizable optic fiber layer in those areas of the graft facing the vitreous body. Scanning electron microscopy of the graft surface, however, revealed the collection of intermittent fascicles of fibers from the

[a]This work was supported by Grant EY04377 from the National Institutes of Health (to J. E. Turner).

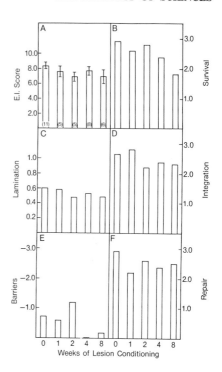

FIGURE 1. A demonstration that successful grafting can occur immediately after lesion or by waiting up to 8 weeks following stabilization of the host retinal lesion site as determined by an EI score. (**A**) Composite EI score showing no significant differences among grafts transplanted from 0-8 weeks following host lesion. (**B-F**) Evaluation of individual components of the EI score. Note that in **E** the trend is toward reduced barriers, which may lead to better host-graft communication, if the transplant is made at later lesion conditioning periods. Each vertical bar represents an SEM, and numbers in parentheses indicate total grafted eyes analyzed.

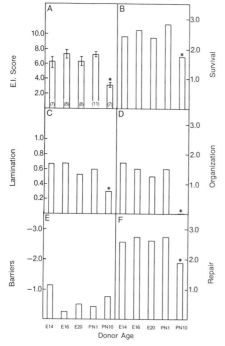

FIGURE 2. A demonstration that retinal transplantation can be initiated over a wide range of donor ages (E14-PN1) as determined by an EI score. (**A**) Composite EI score showing a significant decrease in overall graft success when using PN10 tissue compared to younger transplants. (**B-F**) Evaluation of individual components of the EI score, demonstrating a critical period between PN1 and PN10 when the grafting process begins to dramatically deteriorate. Each vertical bar represents an SEM, and numbers in parentheses indicate total grafted eyes analyzed. Asterisks indicate significant reduction in EI scores ($p < .01$) of PN10 grafts when compared to those of E14 to PN1 time periods.

region of the ganglion cell layer. These fibers were seen to project onto the host vitreal surface and eventually appeared to join with the host optic fiber layer.

The vitreal delivery method initiated through the edge of the closed lesion site or through a second penetrating lesion insures 98% survival of the grafted tissue and a 95% success rate for graft-host integration. Successful grafting can occur immediately after lesion or up to 8 weeks following stabilization of the host retinal lesion site as determined by an evaluation index (EI), which was designed to objectively evaluate grafts at the light level (FIG. 1). In addition, retinal transplantation can also be initiated over a wide range of donor ages (E14 to PN3); however, by PN10 the graft EI score is significantly reduced—by more than 50% (FIG. 2). Also, successful cross-species grafting has been initiated in this model using fetal mouse donor tissue.

These studies show for the first time the feasibility of using a retinal transplantation technique for the possible reconstruction of adult mammalian retina in which a lesion has been created. Also, this model can be used to study numerous retinal developmental phenomena.

Bridging a Transected Rat Optic Nerve with a Semipermeable Guidance Channel

R. F. VALENTINI, P. AEBISCHER, S. R. WINN,
G. PANOL, AND P. M. GALLETTI

Artificial Organ Laboratory
Brown University
Providence, Rhode Island 02912

Entubulation of a central nervous system (CNS) structure with a biocompatible tubular channel can provide axonal guidance and, with proper selection of the material, minimize scar tissue formation. Previous work in our laboratory indicated that a semipermeable acrylic copolymer material (Amicon XM-50 hollow fiber membranes) supported the regeneration of transected peripheral nerves in rodents.[1] Using the adult rat optic nerve as a CNS model, we used the same semipermeable guidance channel to bridge intracranially transected optic nerves. After craniotomy, the sagittal sinus and dura matter were cauterized and cut between the frontal lobes and the olfactory bulb. The optic nerve was visualized after retraction of the frontal lobes and partial aspiration of the olfactory bulb. Upon gentle retraction of the pial plexus of capillaries and the anterior cerebral artery, the optic nerve was irrigated with ice-cold sterile saline and transected with microscissors at its midpoint, between the optic foramen and the optic chiasma. The proximal (retinal) and distal stumps of the nerve were aligned at either end of the semipermeable tube (2-3 mm long, 800 μm ID, 150 μm wall thickness, 50 000 Dalton nominal molecular weight cut-off) and positioned within its lumen by applying suction on the outside of the guidance channel. Animals were sacrificed at 6 weeks and perfused transcardially with a buffered fixative. Cross sections of the nerve and surrounding channel were prepared for light and transmission electron microscopy. Three out of 6 rats showed a cable bridging the gap between the proximal and distal stumps (FIG. 1). The cable diameter tapered gradually as it progressed from the proximal to distal nerve stumps, suggesting that the cellular elements of the cable had migrated primarily from the proximal stump. Cable histology revealed a cellular matrix containing several unmyelinated axons and numerous neuroglial cells and capillaries surrounded by a continuous sheath of circumferentially organized, flattened cells (FIG. 2). The cable was loosely anchored to the inner wall of the guidance channel by a lattice of filamentous cells that budded off the perimeter of the cable and contacted the channel wall at focal points. With the exception of this network of attachment cells, the space between the cable and the internal wall of the channel was devoid of cellular or fibrotic tissue, whereas the outer surface of the channel was covered with fibrous connective tissue. The lumens of the channels without cables contained only an acellular matrix.

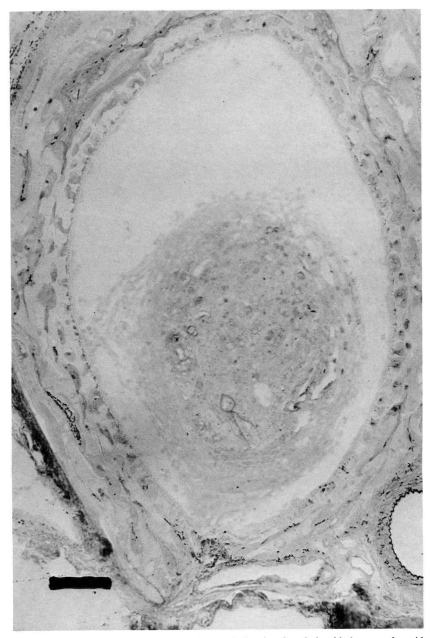

FIGURE 1. Toluidine blue-stained light micrograph showing the relationship between the guidance channel and regenerated cable in cross section. Size bar: 100 μ.

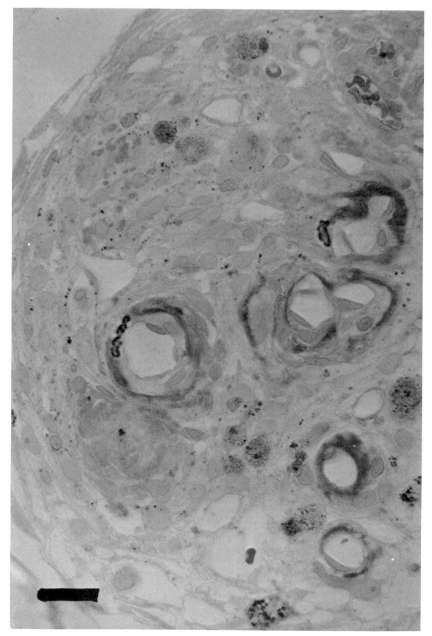

FIGURE 2. Toluidine blue-stained light micrograph of the regenerated cable showing the numerous capillaries and neuroglial cells present. Size bar: 20 μ.

CONCLUSIONS

1) Entubulation of a transected optic nerve with an appropriate biomaterial favors the formation of a cable bridging the nerve stumps; 2) This cable is well vascularized and contains numerous neuroglial cells; 3) The cable is loosely anchored to the inner wall of the guidance channel; 4) The entubulating material does not elicit the luminal invasion of scar-forming tissue, which could create a barrier to impede axonal elongation; 5) The use of a semipermeable channel may favor the retention of endogenous growth-promoting factors within its lumen while allowing metabolic exchange across its wall; 6) Inclusion of various exogenous protein or tissue substrates or both within the lumen of the guidance channel will enable us to evaluate their influence on CNS regeneration.

REFERENCES

1. AEBISCHER, P., R. F. VALENTINI, S. R. WINN, S. K. KUNZ, H. S. SASKEN & P. M. GALLETTI. 1986. Regeneration of transected sciatic nerves through semipermeable nerve guidance channels: Effect of extracellular matrix protein additives. Trans. Am. Soc. Artif. Intern. Organs **32:** 474-477.

Migration and Differentiation of Xenogenic and Homogenic Brain Cells Transplanted into the Adult Rat Hippocampus[a]

JOSEPH WELLS, BRAD P. VIETJE, AND
DAVID G. WELLS

University of Vermont
Burlington, Vermont 05405

Brain cells from the septal-basal forebrain region of embryonic mice and rats were prepared as cell suspensions and labeled by horseradish peroxidase (HRP). The labeled cell suspensions were injected into the hippocampal formation of adult rats that were partially denervated by fornix lesions, and cross-species transplants were compared to transplants between the same species. One to 2 weeks after the transplants were injected, the rat hosts were perfused and the brain processed histochemically to show HRP.

In the transplants between different species, four significant observations were made. First, the mouse cells, labeled by HRP, migrated away from the injection site (FIG. 1). The route of the migration was frequently along the dentate granule cell layer and occurred over considerable distances—up to 1.5 mm. Second, the injection site rarely contained labeled cells that looked like viable neurons. The injection site itself contained cells, but the only HRP reaction product was seen as debris or as particulate matter in phagocytic cells. Third, two types of neurons survived the xenogenic transplants—pyramidal neurons and multipolar neurons. Fourth, some pyramidal neurons had highly differentiated dendritic arbors whereas others had only rudimentary branches. The thick apical dendrites of the pyramidal neurons were preferentially oriented toward the molecular layer of the dentate gyrus, much like the dendrites of the host granule cells. Thus, the cues for migration and orientation must still be present in the adult rat dentate gyrus and available to cells from a different species. The multipolar neurons showed no preferred orientation of their dendrites.

In contrast to the xenogenic transplants, when the transplants were made between animals of the same species, many more labeled cells survived. The labeled cells were largely within the injection site with just a few cells having migrated out of the transplant site (FIG. 2). Those labeled cells that did leave the injection site were still close to the injection site between 1 and 2 weeks after transplantation. The most commonly labeled cell type seen in the homogenic transplants was a fusiform neuron with long dendrites that had few branches. This cell type was not seen in the xenogenic transplants. The homogenic transplants had begun to organize themselves within the injection site itself. Some labeled cells appeared to have started to form a row. The

[a]This work was supported by Grant 23266 from the U.S. Public Health Service.

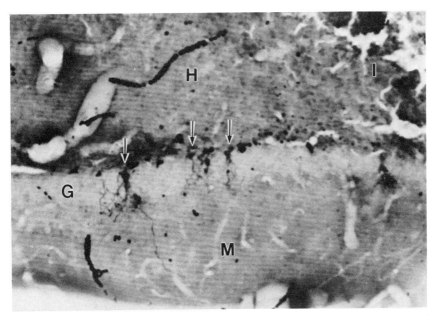

FIGURE 1. A xenogenic transplant showing that HRP-labeled cells (arrows) have migrated away from the injection site (I) along the host granule cell layer (G). Labeled pyramidal cells are oriented toward the molecular layer (M) of the host. In both FIGURE 1 and FIGURE 2, diaminobenzidine was used to show presence of HRP. No counterstain. H: hilus.

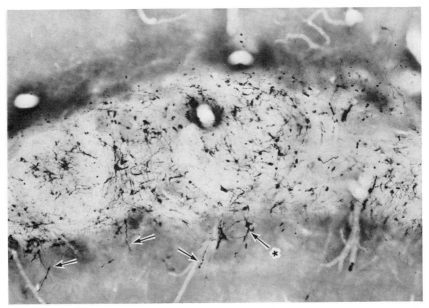

FIGURE 2. A homogenic transplant showing HRP-labeled cells. Fibers (arrows) leave the injection site (pale region) to enter the host tissue. In homogenic transplants, most of the labeled neurons stayed within the injection site. A few labeled neurons (asterisk) migrated a short distance from the injection site.

transplants between different species showed little of this internal organization within the injection site. In the transplants within the same species, many fibers could be seen that had grown out into the host hippocampal formation.

Even with the remarkable differences in the characteristics of the transplants, transplantation of cell suspensions between different species has been shown to be about as effective in restoring function as transplants within the same species.

Intraventricular Transplants of Anterior Hypothalamus

Neurochemical and Connectional Specificity in Morphologically Distinct Subtypes of Neurophysin-containing Neurons[a]

STANLEY J. WIEGAND[b] AND DON M. GASH

Department of Neurobiology and Anatomy
University of Rochester Medical Center
Rochester, New York 14642

In previous experiments, when normal fetal anterior hypothalami were transplanted to the third ventricle-median eminence of adult rats with congenital or experimentally induced diabetes insipidus (DI), an amelioration of the DI symptoms observed in some host animals was correlated with the presence of large neurons containing the antidiuretic hormone, vasopressin (VP), or its associated neurophysin, within the graft.[1] As in the native hypothalamus, however, neurophysin-immunoreactive (NPir) neurons identified within the transplants were not a homogeneous population, but expressed a variety of morphological phenotypes. In our current studies, we have begun to characterize NPir neurons contained in anterior hypothalamic grafts based on the morphology, organization, connectivity, and peptide content of the neurons in order to determine their homology with the known NPir anterior hypothalamic cell groups.

Anterior hypothalami obtained from normal Long-Evans rat fetuses on embryonic day 16 or 17 were transplanted to the lateral, third, or fourth ventricles of adult, VP-deficient Brattleboro rats. Host animals were sacrificed 4-6 weeks after transplantation, and brain sections were processed for the immunohistochemical localization of NP-containing cells. Alternate series of sections were processed for localization of VP, oxytocin (OT), vasoactive intestinal polypeptide (VIP), and corticotropin-releasing factor (CRF) neurons. Fetal hypothalami readily survived transplantation at each site studied and contained numerous NPir neurons (TABLE 1).

The NPir populations of the grafts are heterogeneous, containing both magnocellular and parvicellular subtypes (FIG. 1). Magnocellular NPir neurons, similar in size (20-35 μm) and shape to the magnocellular neurosecretory neurons of the supraoptic and paraventricular nuclei, are observed least frequently. Like endogenous magnocellular neurons,[2] magnocellular NPir neurons within the transplants express

[a] This work was supported by Grant NS 19900 from the National Institutes of Health.

[b] Address for correspondence: Department of Neurobiology and Anatomy, Box 603, University of Rochester School of Medicine, 601 Elmwood Avenue, Rochester, New York 14642.

either OT or VP, and appear to project preferentially to fenestrated capillary plexuses in the host brain, especially the neurohypophysis. Parvicellular NPir neurons are predominant in nearly all grafts, and can be divided into three distinct subtypes. The most frequently encountered parvicellular subtype (type I) consists of VPir neurons exclusively. These neurons exhibit many of the characteristics of the VPir neurons of the endogenous suprachiasmatic nucleus (SCN).[3] These cells are generally organized into well-defined clusters and associated with VIPir neurons of a similar small size (9-13 μm). VPir fibers of very fine caliber ramify extensively around the cell bodies of origin and in their immediate vicinity, and project, almost exclusively, to periventricular areas of the host diencephalon that are normally innervated by the VP-containing neurons of the SCN. A second subtype (type II) of parvicellular NPir

TABLE 1. Characteristics of NPir Cell Types in Intraventricular Anterior Hypothalamic Transplants

NP Cell Subtype	Grafts with Subtype (%)	Peptide Content	Efferent Connections	In Situ Homologue
Magnocellular	33	VP, OT	Neural vasculature (host median eminence)	Magnocellular neuro-secretory system
Parvicellular				
Type I	95	VP	Periventricular diencephalon	Suprachiasmatic nucleus
Type II	67	VP	Neural vasculature (usually intrinsic to the graft)	Paraventricular nucleus (medial parvicellular)
Type III	38	OT (VP)	Not known	Paraventricular nucleus (lateral parvicellular)

NOTE: This table summarizes some of the principal features of morphologically distinct subtypes of NP-containing neurons identified in intraventricular grafts of fetal anterior hypothalamus. This body of data is based on a series of 45 transplants, of which 42 survived to the end of the experimental period. The percentage of the surviving grafts containing each specific type of NP-containing neuron is given in the second column from the left. Note the extreme variance among cell types: magnocellular neurons can be identified in only 33% of surviving grafts whereas type I parvicellular neurons are present in 95%. Efferent connections of type III cells could not be identified unequivocally because the host brain exhibits a normal complement of OT-containing neural elements. The proposed in situ homologue for each NP subtype identified in the grafts is given in the far right-hand column.

neuron identified frequently within the transplants also expresses VP, but not OT. These cells are slightly larger (12-18 μm) and less densely packed than the type I cells, however, and they project preferentially to blood vessels, usually within the graft itself. Type II parvicellular neurons, or a morphologically similar companion population, also contain CRF, but are not associated with VIPir cells. These same characteristics are exhibited by NPir neurons identifiable within the medial parvicellular component of the paraventricular nucleus (PNV) following adrenalectomy.[4] A third subtype (type III) of parvicellular NPir neuron is present in the grafts. This subtype consists of small to moderately sized fusiform and multipolar cells (10-25 μm). In marked contrast to the other parvicellular NPir cells identified within the grafts, type

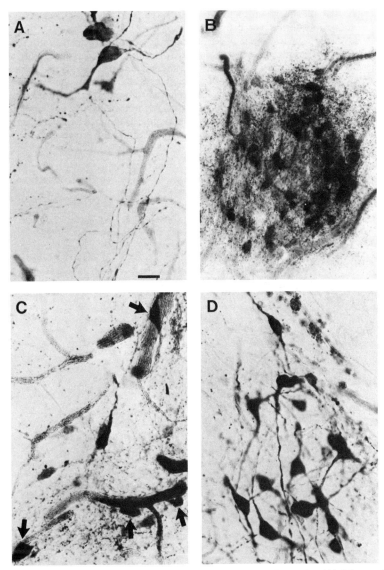

FIGURE 1. The distinct subtypes of NP neurons identified in the grafts. (A) Magnocellular neurons, which are few in number and are most usually found singly or in small groups. (B) In contrast, type I parvicellular neurons are found in distinct aggregations that resemble the endogenous suprachiasmatic nucleus. Note the very fine caliber varicose fibers that ramify extensively among the cell bodies of origin and in their immediate vicinity. (C) Type II cells are somewhat larger and are aggregated into less well defined clusters containing fewer cells. Type II neurons are often found in close apposition to blood vessels (arrows). (D) Collections of type III neurons are morphologically heterogeneous and, unlike types I and II, predominantly oxytocinergic. All sections were 50 μ thick and stained for VP, except the section in D, which was stained for neurophysins. Blood vessels were visualized by perfusing the animals with pigmented inks.

III parvicellular neurons are predominantly oxytocinergic, as are the NPir neurons of the lateral and dorsal parvicellular subnuclei of the PVN.[2]

In summary, the principal NPir populations normally present within the adult anterior hypothalamus have been identified within intraventricular grafts of fetal hypothalamus using morphological, connectional, and neurochemical criteria. The development, within ectopic grafts of anterior hypothalamus, of the normative characteristics of the various classes of NPir neurons suggests that fetal neurons may be phenotypically specified before transplantation, and consequently are restricted as to the nature of the structural and functional relationships they are capable of establishing with the host brain.

REFERENCES

1. GASH, D. M., S. J. WIEGAND, F. F. MARCIANO & J. R. SLADEK, JR. 1984. *In* Fetal Neuroendocrinology. F. Ellendorf, P. Gluckman & N. Parvizi, Eds.: 71-82. Perinatology Press. Ithaca, NY.
2. ARMSTRONG, W. E., S. WARACH, G. I. HATTON & T. H. McNEILL. 1980. Neuroscience **5:** 1931-1958.
3. VAN DEN POL, A. N. & K. L. TSUJIMOTO. 1985. Neuroscience **15:** 1049-1086.
4. SAWCHENKO, P. E., L. W. SWANSON & W. W. VALE. 1984. Proc. Natl. Acad. Sci. USA **81:** 1883-1887.

Index of Contributors

(Italic page numbers refer to comments made in discussion.)